Maternal and Infant Health

Maternal and Infant Health

Editor: Katie Beckett

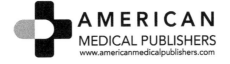

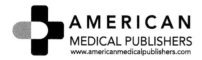

Cataloging-in-Publication Data

Maternal and infant health / edited by Katie Beckett.
   p. cm.
Includes bibliographical references and index.
ISBN 979-8-88740-242-0
1. Pregnancy. 2. Mothers--Health and hygiene. 3. Infants--Care. 4. Infants--Health and hygiene.
5. Maternal and infant welfare. 6. Maternal health services. 7. Infant health services. I. Beckett, Katie.
RG551 .M38 2023
618.2--dc23

© American Medical Publishers, 2023

American Medical Publishers,
41 Flatbush Avenue,
1st Floor, New York,
NY 11217, USA

ISBN 979-8-88740-242-0 (Hardback)

This book contains information obtained from authentic and highly regarded sources. Copyright for all individual chapters remain with the respective authors as indicated. All chapters are published with permission under the Creative Commons Attribution License or equivalent. A wide variety of references are listed. Permission and sources are indicated; for detailed attributions, please refer to the permissions page and list of contributors. Reasonable efforts have been made to publish reliable data and information, but the authors, editors and publisher cannot assume any responsibility for the validity of all materials or the consequences of their use.

Trademark Notice: Registered trademark of products or corporate names are used only for explanation and identification without intent to infringe.

Contents

Preface VII

Chapter 1 **Enhanced dopamine D1 and BDNF signaling in the adult dorsal striatum but not nucleus accumbens of prenatal cocaine treated mice** 1
Thomas F. Tropea, Zeeba D. Kabir, Gagandeep Kaur, Anjali M. Rajadhyaksha and Barry E. Kosofsky

Chapter 2 **Prenatal IV cocaine: Alterations in auditory information processing** 12
Charles F. Mactutus, Steven B. Harrod, Lauren L. Hord, Landhing M. Moran and Rosemarie M. Booze

Chapter 3 **Litter gender composition and sex affect maternal behavior and DNA methylation levels of the *Oprm1* gene in rat offspring** 27
Yanli Hao, Wen Huang, David A. Nielsen and Therese A. Kosten

Chapter 4 **Are behavioral effects of early experience mediated by oxytocin?** 39
Karen L. Bales, Ericka Boone, Pamela Epperson, Gloria Hoffman and C. Sue Carter

Chapter 5 **Technical and conceptual considerations for performing and interpreting functional MRI studies in awake rats** 51
Marcelo Febo

Chapter 6 **Using animal models to disentangle the role of genetic, epigenetic, and environmental influences on behavioral outcomes associated with maternal anxiety and depression** 68
Lisa M. Tarantino, Patrick F. Sullivan and Samantha Meltzer-Brody

Chapter 7 **Impaired neural synchrony in the theta frequency range in adolescents at familial risk for schizophrenia** 78
Franc C. L. Donkers, Shane R. Schwikert, Anna M. Evans, Katherine M. Cleary, Diana O. Perkins and Aysenil Belger

Chapter 8 **Adolescent opiate exposure in the female rat induces subtle alterations in maternal care and transgenerational effects on play behavior** 94
Nicole L. Johnson, Lindsay Carini, Marian E. Schenk, Michelle Stewart and Elizabeth M. Byrnes

Chapter 9 **Mesolimbic dopamine transients in motivated behaviors: Focus on maternal behavior** 104
Donita L. Robinson, Dawnya L. Zitzman and Sarah K. Williams

Chapter 10	**Synergy of image analysis for animal and human neuroimaging supports translational research on drug abuse**..................117 Guido Gerig, Ipek Oguz, Sylvain Gouttard, Joohwi Lee, Hongyu An, Weili Lin, Matthew McMurray, Karen Grewen, Josephine Johns and Martin Andreas Styner	
Chapter 11	**Addiction, adolescence, and innate immune gene induction**..................126 Fulton T. Crews and Ryan Peter Vetreno	
Chapter 12	**Use of high resolution 3D diffusion tensor imaging to study brain white matter development in live neonatal rats**..................137 Yu Cai, Matthew S. McMurray, Ipek Oguz, Hong Yuan, Martin A. Styner, Weili Lin, Josephine M. Johns and Hongyu An	
Chapter 13	**Maternal neural responses to infant cries and faces: Relationships with substance use**..................146 Nicole Landi, Jessica Montoya, Hedy Kober, Helena J.V. Rutherford, W. Einar Mencl, Patrick D. Worhunsky, Marc N. Potenza and Linda C. Mayes	
Chapter 14	**Prenatal stress alters progestogens to mediate susceptibility to sex-typical, stress-sensitive disorders, such as drug abuse**..................158 Cheryl A. Frye, Jason J. Paris, Danielle M. Osborne, Joannalee C. Campbell and Tod E. Kippin	
Chapter 15	**Maternal genetic mutations as gestational and early life influences in producing psychiatric disease-like phenotypes in mice**..................173 Georgia Gleason, Bojana Zupan and Miklos Toth	
Chapter 16	**Epigenetics of early child development**..................183 Chris Murgatroyd and Dietmar Spengler	
Chapter 17	**The emergence of spanking among a representative sample of children under 2 years of age in North Carolina**..................198 Adam J. Zolotor, T. Walker Robinson, Desmond K. Runyan, Ronald G. Barr and Robert A. Murphy	
Chapter 18	**Social behavior of offspring following prenatal cocaine exposure in rodents: A comparison with prenatal alcohol**..................206 Sonya K. Sobrian and R. R. Holson	
Chapter 19	**The impact of childhood maltreatment: A review of neurobiological and genetic factors**..................223 Eamon McCrory, Stephane A. De Brito and Essi Viding	

Permissions

List of Contributors

Index

Preface

This book aims to highlight the current researches and provides a platform to further the scope of innovations in this area. This book is a product of the combined efforts of many researchers and scientists, after going through thorough studies and analysis from different parts of the world. The objective of this book is to provide the readers with the latest information of the field.

Maternal health refers to the well-being of women during pregnancy and after the birth of the child. It also relates to maintaining the health of mothers in the postpartum period. Infant health is an area of study within medicine dealing with the well-being and prevention of diseases in infants. The significant aspect of this field is to reduce maternal morbidity and mortality. Several other health care dimensions such as family planning, preconception, and prenatal and postnatal care are also covered under the domain of maternal and child health. The several factors affecting maternal health include poverty and access to healthcare, pre-existing conditions such as HIV/AIDS and maternal weight. The leading cause of death among women of reproductive age is considered to be complications of pregnancy and childbirth. Maternal bleeding, postpartum infections including maternal sepsis, hypertensive diseases of pregnancy, obstructed labor, and pregnancy with abortive outcome including miscarriage and ectopic pregnancy are some causes that can be attributed to maternal mortality. This book brings forth some of the most innovative concepts and elucidates the unexplored aspects of maternal and infant health. It will help the readers in keeping pace with the rapid developments in this field of study.

I would like to express my sincere thanks to the authors for their dedicated efforts in the completion of this book. I acknowledge the efforts of the publisher for providing constant support. Lastly, I would like to thank my family for their support in all academic endeavors.

Editor

Enhanced dopamine D1 and BDNF signaling in the adult dorsal striatum but not nucleus accumbens of prenatal cocaine treated mice

Thomas F. Tropea[1,2], Zeeba D. Kabir[1,3], Gagandeep Kaur[4], Anjali M. Rajadhyaksha[1,3] and Barry E. Kosofsky[1,3]*

[1] Division of Pediatric Neurology, Department of Pediatrics, Weill Cornell Medical College, New York, NY, USA
[2] College of Osteopathic Medicine, University of New England, Biddeford, ME, USA
[3] Graduate Program in Neurosciences, Weill Cornell Medical College, New York, NY, USA
[4] School of Environmental and Biological Sciences, Rutgers, The State University of New Jersey, New Brunswick, NJ, USA

*Correspondence:
Barry E. Kosofsky, Division of Child Neurology, Weill Cornell Medical College/New York Presbyterian Hospital, 525 East 68th Street, Box 91, New York, NY 10021, USA.
e-mail: bar2009@med.cornell.edu

Previous work from our group and others utilizing animal models have demonstrated long-lasting structural and functional alterations in the meso-cortico-striatal dopamine pathway following prenatal cocaine (PCOC) treatment. We have shown that PCOC treatment results in augmented D1-induced cyclic AMP (cAMP) and cocaine-induced immediate-early gene expression in the striatum of adult mice. In this study we further examined basal as well as cocaine or D1-induced activation of a set of molecules known to be mediators of neuronal plasticity following psychostimulant treatment, with emphasis in the dorsal striatum (Str) and nucleus accumbens (NAc) of adult mice exposed to cocaine *in utero*. Basally, in the Str of PCOC treated mice there were significantly higher levels of (1) CREB and Ser133 P-CREB (2) Thr34 P-DARPP-32 and (3) GluA1 and Ser 845 P-GluA1 when compared to prenatal saline (PSAL) treated mice. In the NAc there were significantly higher basal levels of (1) CREB and Ser133 P-CREB, (2) Thr202/Tyr204 P-ERK2, and (3) Ser845 P-GluA1. Following acute administration of cocaine (15 mg/kg, i.p.) or D1 agonist (SKF 82958; 1 mg/kg, i.p.) there were significantly higher levels of Ser133 P-CREB, Thr34 P-DARPP-32, and Thr202/Tyr204 P-ERK2 in the Str that were evident in all animals tested. However, these cocaine-induced increases in phosphorylation were significantly augmented in PCOC mice compared to PSAL mice. In sharp contrast to the observations in the Str, in the NAc, acute administration of cocaine or D1 agonist significantly increased P-CREB and P-ERK2 in PSAL mice, a response that was not evident in PCOC mice. Examination of Ser 845 P-GluA1 revealed that cocaine or D1 agonist significantly increased levels in PSAL mice, but significantly decreased levels in the PCOC mice in both the Str and NAc. We also examined changes in brain-derived neurotrophic factor (BDNF). Our studies revealed significantly higher levels of the BDNF precursor, pro-BDNF, and one of its receptors, TrkB in the Str of PCOC mice compared to PSAL mice. These results suggest a persistent up regulation of molecules critical to D1 and BDNF signaling in the Str of adult mice exposed to cocaine *in utero*. These molecular adaptations may underlie components of the behavioral deficits evident in exposed animals and a subset of exposed humans, and may represent a therapeutic target for ameliorating aspects of the PCOC-induced phenotype.

Keywords: prenatal cocaine, striatum, nucleus accumbens, D1, TrkB, BDNF, CREB, GluA1

INTRODUCTION

Over the past 25 years since crack cocaine became a drug commonly abused by pregnant women, multiple clinical, and pre-clinical studies have identified alterations in fetal brain development with lasting consequences on brain structure and function resulting from prenatal cocaine (PCOC) exposure (Kosofsky et al., 1994; reviewed in Trask and Kosofsky, 2000; Kosofsky and Hyman, 2001). Identification of a prenatal drug-induced phenotype uniquely attributable to intrauterine cocaine exposure has been elusive. Specifically, only a subset of exposed infants and children demonstrate persistent deficits, and when they do, may manifest ongoing behavioral abnormalities in subtle neurobehavioral domains including deficits in "Affect, Attention, Arousal, and Action" (the 4A's: see Lester, 1998; Bada et al., 2007). Specifically, PCOC exposure has been shown to result in subtle reductions in IQ and cognitive development (Alessandri et al., 1998; Lester et al., 1998), delayed language development (Beeghly et al., 2006), and impairments in tasks requiring sustained attention (Accornero et al., 2007). Such studies support the idea that intrauterine exposure to cocaine most profoundly alters attention, arousal, and reactivity, functions that may negatively impact learning and memory in exposed offspring (Mayes et al., 1998). The implications for public policy are far reaching, as when such deficits are evident in PCOC-exposed individuals they may require longer perinatal hospitalizations and associated increments in healthcare costs (Behnke et al., 1997), as well as increased special education needs and associated expenses (Lester et al., 1998; Levine et al., 2008), making prevention of prenatal exposure to cocaine, and early identification and treatment of resulting adverse outcomes a high priority.

As the primary molecular targets of cocaine action are the uptake pumps for the monoamines dopamine, serotonin, and to a lesser extent norepinephrine (Uhl et al., 2002), neurochemical systems which mediate cocaine-induced behaviors, persistent alterations in aminergic function have been suggested as contributing to the PCOC-induced phenotype (Mayes, 2002). Animal models, including work performed in mice (Wilkins et al., 1998), rats (Spear et al., 2002), rabbits (Harvey, 2004), and non-human primates (Lidow and Song, 2001) have been particularly helpful in identifying the independent contribution of cocaine to such neurobehavioral deficits, as well as in understanding the basic mechanisms underlying such changes (Malanga, 1999). In particular, rodent models have demonstrated persistent alterations in dopaminergic (DA) signaling, primarily via the D1 receptor, in adult animals following PCOC treatment (Friedman and Wang, 1998; Unterwald et al., 2003; Stanwood and Levitt, 2007; Malanga et al., 2008; Tropea et al., 2008a).

The cascade of molecular events initiated in the striatum (Str) and nucleus accumbens (NAc) following acute exposure of adult animals to cocaine has been well characterized (reviewed in McGinty et al., 2008). Specifically, a wealth of experimental data identifies a rapid and robust activation of D1-like cell surface receptors activating intracellular signaling pathways to affect specific patterns of gene expression (Self et al., 1996), and alterations thereof in mice genetically engineered to be deficient in D1 mediated signal transduction in the Str (Drago et al., 1996). High throughput array-based methods have identified sets of genes activated in the Str and NAc following acute cocaine exposure that are distinguishable from those following repeated cocaine exposures (Renthal et al., 2009), emphasizing the persistent molecular adaptations, in part via recurrent D1-mediated neuronal stimulation, in contributing to the "addicted state" (Chao and Nestler, 2004).

One phenomenon that has been extensively investigated in animal models has been the process of sensitization, by which prior psychostimulant exposure augments the subsequent response to a challenge dose of drug (reviewed in Kalivas et al., 1998). Work from our lab and others has identified that signaling via second messenger molecules such as (P-)CREB, (P-)DARPP-32, (P-)ERK, and (P-)GluA1 in the Str and NAc are persistently altered following recurrent psychostimulant exposure, and may underlie aspects of the "sensitized state." These data raise the possibility that following PCOC exposure, such signaling pathways may similarly demonstrate persistent dysregulation, and may render adult animals susceptible to altered behavioral responses to subsequent administration of drugs of abuse (reviewed in Crozatier et al., 2003; Malanga and Kosofsky, 2003).

Consistent with this thinking, we have focused our attention on the effect of PCOC treatment on persistent dysregulation of a set of target genes known to mediate aspects of synaptic plasticity, including growth factors (e.g., brain-derived neurotrophic factor, BDNF), immediate-early genes (e.g., zif-268), and synaptic scaffolding proteins (e.g., homer 1a). Previous work from our group analyzing the Str and NAc has focused on the role of dopamine D1-mediated cyclic AMP (cAMP) regulation, and demonstrated increased cocaine-mediated induction of both zif-268 and homer 1a mRNA in the Str, but not the NAc of adult PCOC treated vs. prenatal saline (PSAL) treated mice (Tropea et al., 2008a). Here we extend that work to identify that an additional set of signaling molecules activated via D1 stimulation including (P-)CREB, (P-)DARPP-32, (P-)ERK, and (P)GluA1 are differentially activated in the Str and NAc of adult PCOC vs. PSAL mice. We found that following acute administration of cocaine (15 mg/kg, i.p.) or D1 agonist (SKF 82958; 1 mg/kg, i.p.) there were significantly higher levels of Ser133 P-CREB, Thr34 P-DARPP-32, and Thr202/Tyr204 P-ERK2 evident in the Str in both prenatal treatment groups. However, this increase was significantly augmented in PCOC vs. PSAL mice. In sharp contrast, neither acute cocaine nor SKF 82958-induced phosphorylation of CREB or ERK2 in the NAc of PCOC mice, but did in the NAc of PSAL mice. Following acute administration of cocaine or D1 agonist there were significantly increased levels of Ser845 P-GluA1 in both the Str and NAc of PSAL mice, in contrast to significantly decreased levels of Ser845 P-GluA1 in both the Str and NAc of PCOC mice. In parallel we have additionally identified that the growth factor pro-BDNF, and TrkB, a BDNF receptor, are upregulated in the Str but not NAc of adult PCOC mice.

Taken together our data identifies region-specific patterns (i.e., Str vs. NAc) in the constitutive expression of a set of proteins and phospho-proteins, as well as their pattern of expression following acute administration of cocaine or the D1 agonist SKF 82958, which distinguish PCOC from PSAL mice. The differential pattern of constitutive as well as inducible proteins and phospho-proteins that we have identified suggest a persistent molecular memory in PCOC mice evidenced as a cocaine-induced augmentation in CREB and ERK phosphorylation in the Str, blunting of CREB and ERK phosphorylation in the NAc, and de-phosphorylation of GluA1 in both the Str and NAc, all via D1 mechanisms. Such data extends the idea that recurrent drug exposure induces abnormal synaptic learning and memory (Berke and Hyman, 2000; Hyman and Malenka, 2001; Hyman, 2005) in a developmental context such that adaptations in Str and NAc neuronal function established in the womb may "feed forward" to induce alterations in dopaminergic neurotransmission and associated behaviors in adulthood.

MATERIALS AND METHODS
PRENATAL COCAINE TREATMENT
Prenatal treatments were performed as previously described (Tropea et al., 2008b). Briefly, timed-pregnant Swiss Webster dams (Taconic Labs, New York) were assigned to one of two treatment groups and received twice-daily subcutaneous (SC) injections (at 7:00 AM and 7:00 PM) from embryonic (E) day E8 to E17, inclusive, of cocaine HCl (Sigma-Aldrich, St. Louis, MO, USA; 20 mg/kg/injection, SC, dissolved in saline) totaling 40 mg/kg per day (offspring referred to as PCOC for prenatal cocaine treated)

or 0.9% saline (offspring referred to as PSAL for prenatal saline treated). All pups were surrogate fostered to control dams (Black Swiss Webster; Taconic Labs), which had delivered within the previous 48 h. Litters were culled to a maximum of 10 pups per dam. Animals were weaned at 28 days in to same sex cages, at which point female animals were euthanized. Only one male animal per litter was used for any of the studies reported, thereby avoiding the problem of litter effects resulting in "oversampling." As a result, the individual animal's data was the unit of statistical measure, and represented the "litter mean" for that data point. All experimental protocols were approved by the Weill Cornell Medical College Institutional Animal Care and Use Committee, and were in accordance with NIH directives for animal studies.

WESTERN BLOT ANALYSES

Western blot analysis was performed as previously described (Tropea et al., 2008b). Briefly, adult (P60) male PSAL and PCOC treated mice were injected with saline, cocaine (15 mg/kg, i.p.), or the D1 agonist SKF 82958 (1 mg/kg, i.p.) followed 15 min later by rapid decapitation, brain dissection and freezing at −40°C in isopentane. All brains were serially cut rostro-caudally in a freezing cryostat to obtain bilateral punches of the dorsal striatum (Str; A/P +1.7 to +1.2; Paxinos and Franklin, 2003), the NAc (A/P stereotactic coordinates +1.7 to +1.2), bilateral 0.5 mm deep tissue punches of somato-sensory cortex (CTX; A/P +1.7 to +1.2 mm), medial prefrontal cortex (mPFC; A/P +1.98 to +1.54 mm), and unilateral ventral tegmental area (VTA; A/P −3.16 to −3.64 mm) punches. All tissue punches were obtained with a 17-gage stainless steel stylet.

For pro- and mature BDNF, TrkB, and p75 Western blot analyses, tissue from the NAc, Str, mPFC, and VTA, of untreated PSAL and PCOC animals was used. Tissue was sonicated in SDS sample buffer (1% SDS in TE pH 7.4) containing protease and phosphatase inhibitors and 25 μg of protein was separated on a 15% gel along with a Kaleidoscope-prestained standard (Bio-Rad, Hercules, CA, USA). For all other protein analyses, protein lysates were isolated on a 12% gel. Blots were incubated in primary antibody [CREB (1:850), Ser133 P-CREB (1:850), DARPP-32 (1:1000), Thr34 P- DARPP 32 (1:500), Thr75 P-DARPP-32 (1:500), Thr202/Tyr204 P-ERK1/2 (1:1000), ERK1/2 (1:1000), Ser 845 P-GluA1 (1:850), GluA1 (1:1000), Cell Signaling, Danvers, MA, USA; BDNF N-20 (1:200), Santa Cruz Biotechnology, Santa Cruz, CA, USA; TrkB (1:500), Upstate Cell Signaling Solutions, Lake Placid, NY, USA; p75 (1:1000), NR2B (1:1000), actin (1:20,000), Chemicon, Temecula, CA, USA] for 12–48 h at 4°C. Secondary antibody incubations were performed at room temperature in blocking buffer for 1 h (horseradish peroxidase-linked IgG conjugated goat anti-rabbit 1:5000 for CREB, P-CREB, DARPP-32, Thr34 P-DARPP-32, BDNF, TrkB, and NR2B and 1:10,000 for p75, or horse anti-mouse 1:30,000 for actin, Vector Laboratories, Burlingame, CA, USA). Membranes were visualized with Western Lightning Chemiluminescence solution (Perkin Elmer Life Science, Boston, MA, USA). Optical density from films was analyzed using NIH Image (NIH, Bethesda, MD, USA). For BDNF, pro-BDNF bands were analyzed at 30 kDa, while mature BDNF bands were analyzed at 14 kDa. To confirm the identity of these bands, striatal cell lysate and recombinant BDNF protein (generously supplied by Dr. Francis Lee, Weill Cornell Medical College, New York, NY, USA) was analyzed as shown in **Figure 3A**.

STATISTICAL ANALYSES

Gestational data were analyzed using t-test, while western blot data were analyzed by one-way ANOVA, and when significant at $p < 0.05$ level, *post hoc* comparisons (Bonferroni–Dunn) between treatment groups was performed.

RESULTS
GESTATIONAL DATA

The average percentage weight gain of dams from E8 to E17 and the number of live pups per litter for each prenatal treatment group were recorded. PCOC dams gained less weight during pregnancy ($p < 0.0001$), and gave birth to less live pups per litter ($p < 0.001$) as compared to PSAL dams (**Table 1**).

ALTERED PROTEIN PHOSPHORYLATION LEVELS IN THE Str OF PCOC MICE

To examine protein phosphorylation levels, adult PSAL and PCOC mice were administered saline (PSAL sal and PCOC sal), cocaine (PSAL coc and PCOC coc) or the dopamine agonist, SKF 82958 (SKF; PSAL skf and PCOC skf). Fifteen minutes later mice were rapidly decapitated and tissue was isolated in a cryostat for Western blot analysis of the Str (**Figure 1**) and NAc (**Figure 2**). To evaluate the effect of PCOC exposure on basal differences in protein levels of CREB/Ser133 P-CREB, DARPP-32/Thr34 and Thr75 P-DARPP-32, ERK2/Thr202/Tyr204 P-ERK, and GluA1/Ser 845 P-GluA1 we compared PCOC sal vs. PSAL sal mice. The effect of PCOC exposure on cocaine and dopamine D1 signaling was evaluated by comparing cocaine- and D1 agonist, SKF 82958-induced changes in phospho-protein levels (P-CREB, Thr34- and Thr75-DARPP-32, P-ERK, and P-GluA1) in PCOC coc vs. PSAL coc, and PCOC skf vs. PSAL skf, respectively.

Striatum

Examination of basal levels of total and phospho-proteins revealed significantly higher levels of CREB and P-CREB in PCOC vs. PSAL mice (**Figures 1A,B**, respectively). Examination of DARPP-32 revealed no effect of PCOC on basal DARPP-32 levels (**Figure 1E**). However, there were significantly higher basal levels of Thr34 P-DARPP-32 in PCOC mice compared to PSAL mice

Table 1 | Effect of prenatal cocaine treatment on dam weight gain and offspring number.

Prenatal Treatment	Average percentage weight gain of dam	Average number of live pups per litter
PSAL	79.7 ± 2.46	13.8 ± 0.48
PCOC	61.6 ± 2.42*	11.5 ± 0.37†

The average percentage weight gain of dams from E8 to E17 and the number of live pups born per litter for each prenatal treatment group were recorded. PCOC vs. PSAL dams on average had a smaller percentage weight gain during pregnancy (*p < 0.0001) and had a lower average number of live born pups per litter († p < 0.001). All values represent the mean ± SEM.

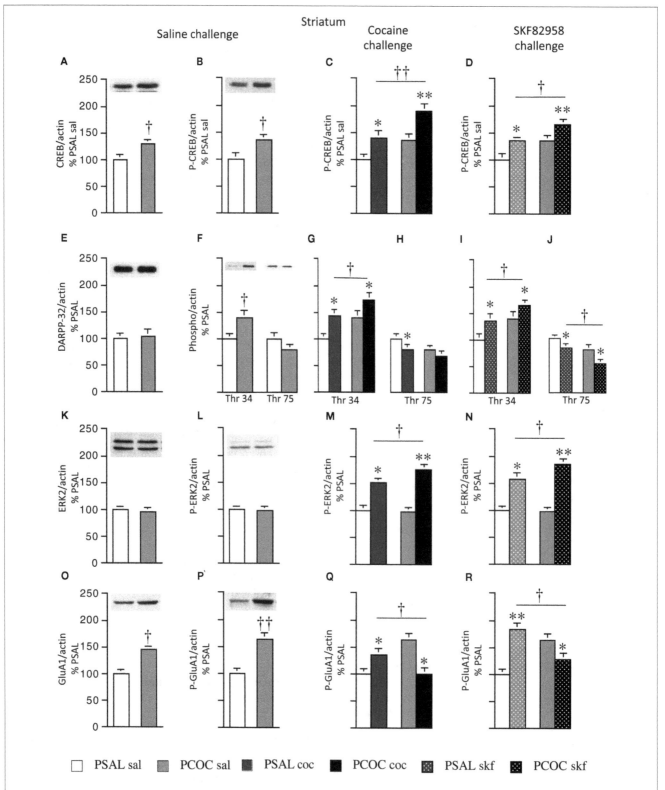

FIGURE 1 | Effect of prenatal cocaine treatment on basal, cocaine- and SKF 82958-induced protein phosphorylation in the striatum of adult mice. Representative immunoblots and quantitative analysis of protein [(A) CREB; (E) DARPP-32; (K) ERK2; (O) GluA1] and phospho-protein [(B–D) P-CREB; (F–J) Thr 34 and Thr 75 P-DARPP-32; (L–N) P-ERK2; (P–R) P-GluA1] levels normalized to actin (mean optical density ± SEM). Protein levels were measured in prenatal saline treated (PSAL) and prenatal cocaine (PCOC) treated mice administered normal saline (sal), cocaine (15 mg/kg; coc) or D1 agonist, SKF 82958 (1 mg/kg; skf) as adults. Data are represented as percentage of PSAL mice treated with saline (PSAL sal). $^{†}p < 0.05$, $^{††}p < 0.01$ PCOC pretreatment groups vs. PSAL pretreatment groups. $*p < 0.05$, $**p < 0.01$, coc or skf treated mice vs. sal treated mice within the same prenatal treatment. Error bars represent ± SEM. $N = 6–8$ mice/group.

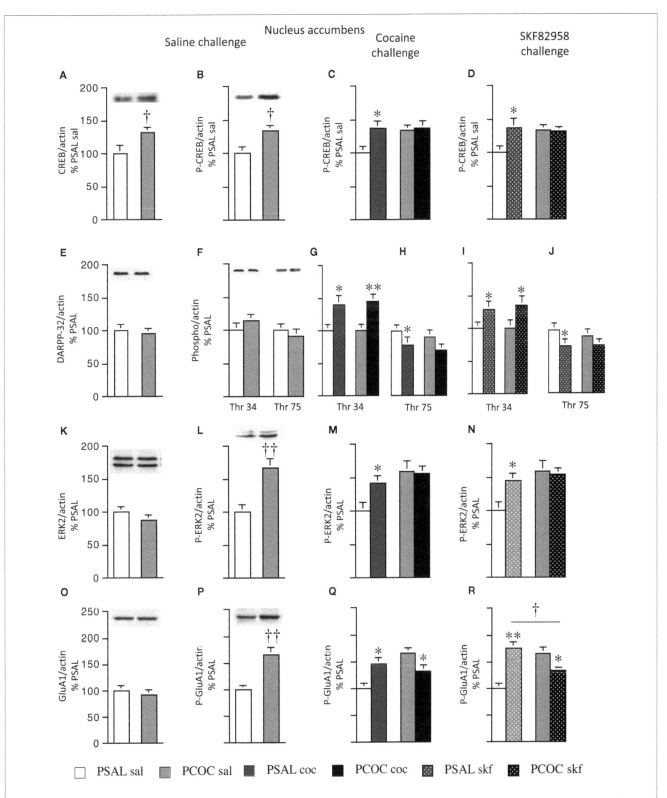

FIGURE 2 | Effect of prenatal cocaine treatment on basal, cocaine- and SKF 82958-induced protein phosphorylation in the nucleus accumbens of adult mice. Representative immunoblots and quantitative analysis of protein [**(A)** CREB; **(E)** DARPP-32; **(K)** ERK2; **(O)** GluA1] and phospho-protein [**(B–D)** P-CREB; **(F–J)** Thr 34 and Thr 75 P-DARPP-32; **(L–N)** P-ERK2; **(P–R)** P-GluA1] levels normalized to actin (mean optical density ± SEM). Protein levels were measured in prenatal saline (PSAL) treated and prenatal cocaine (PCOC) treated mice administered normal saline (sal), cocaine (15 mg/kg; coc) or D1 agonist, SKF 82958 (1 mg/kg; skf) as adults. Data are represented as percentage of PSAL mice treated with saline (PSAL sal). $^{†}p < 0.05$, $^{††}p < 0.01$ PCOC pretreatment groups vs. PSAL pretreatment groups. $*p < 0.05$, $**p < 0.01$, coc or skf treated mice vs. sal treated mice within the same prenatal treatment. Error bars represent ± SEM. $N = 6–8$ mice/group.

(**Figure 1F**) with a trend toward lower levels of Thr75 P-DARPP-32 (**Figure 1G**). Examination of ERK2 revealed no change in the basal levels of ERK2 or P-ERK2 in PCOC mice (**Figures 1K,L**, respectively). Examination of GluA1 revealed significantly higher levels of basal GluA1 and P-GluA1 in PCOC mice compared to PSAL mice (**Figures 1O,P**, respectively).

Examination of cocaine or SKF 82958-induced changes in phospho-protein levels revealed that cocaine or SKF 82958 significantly increased P-CREB in PSAL and PCOC mice compared to saline treated mice (**Figure 1C**, PSAL coc vs. PSAL sal and PCOC coc vs. PCOC sal and **Figure 1D**, PSAL skf vs. PSAL sal and PCOC skf vs. PCOC sal, respectively). Furthermore, the increase in P-CREB observed in PCOC mice was significantly augmented compared to PSAL mice (**Figure 1C**, PCOC coc vs. PSAL coc; **Figure 1D**, PCOC skf vs. PSAL skf). Similarly cocaine or SKF 82958 treatment significantly increased Thr34 P-DARPP-32 levels in PSAL and PCOC mice (**Figures 1G,I**, respectively) with significantly augmented levels evident in PCOC mice compared to that observed in PSAL mice (**Figure 1G**, PCOC coc vs. PSAL coc; **Figure 1I**, PCOC skf vs. PSAL skf). Cocaine or SKF 82958 treatment significantly decreased Thr75 P-DARPP-32 levels in PSAL mice (**Figures 1H,J**, respectively). In PCOC mice, cocaine treatment had no effect on Thr75 P-DARPP-32 levels (**Figure 1H**) whereas SKF 82958 significantly decreased Thr75 P-DARPP-32 levels (**Figure 1J**) to levels that were significantly lower than that seen in PSAL mice (**Figure 1J**, PCOC skf vs. PSAL skf). Examination of P-ERK2 levels revealed that cocaine or SKF 82958 treatment significantly increased P-ERK2 levels in both PSAL and PCOC mice (**Figures 1M,N**, respectively) with significantly augmented levels evident in PCOC mice compared to PSAL mice (**Figure 1M**, PCOC coc vs. PSAL coc; **Figure 1N**, PCOC skf vs. PSAL skf). Examination of P-GluA1 levels revealed that cocaine or SKF 82958 treatment significantly increased P-GluA1 levels in PSAL mice (**Figures 1Q,R**, respectively). However, interestingly in PCOC mice, cocaine or SKF 82958 treatment significantly decreased P-GluA1 levels (**Figures 1Q,R**, respectively), and these levels were significantly lower than that observed in PSAL mice (**Figure 1Q**, PCOC coc vs. PSAL coc; **Figure 1R**, PCOC skf vs. PSAL skf).

Nucleus accumbens
Examination of basal levels of total and phospho-proteins revealed significantly higher levels of CREB and P-CREB in the NAc of PCOC mice compared to PSAL mice (**Figures 2A,B**, respectively). Examination of basal DARPP-32 levels revealed no difference in DARPP-32, Thr34 P-DARPP-32 or Thr75 P-DARPP-32 between PSAL and PCOC mice (**Figures 2E,F**, respectively). Examination of ERK2 revealed no change in basal ERK2 in PCOC mice compared to PSAL mice (**Figure 2K**), but significantly higher P-ERK2 levels in PCOC mice compared to PSAL mice (**Figure 2L**). Similarly, examination of GluA1 levels revealed no difference in basal GluA1 levels (**Figure 2O**) between prenatal treatment groups. However, Ser 845 P-GluA1 levels were significantly higher in the NAc of PCOC mice compared to PSAL mice (**Figure 2P**).

Examination of cocaine or SKF 82958-induced changes in phospho-protein levels revealed that cocaine or SKF 82958 treatment significantly increased P-CREB levels in PSAL mice compared to saline treated mice (**Figure 2C**, PSAL coc vs. PSAL sal and **Figure 2D**, PSAL SKF vs. PSAL sal), a response that was not evident in PCOC mice (**Figures 2C,D**, respectively). Cocaine or SKF 82958 treatment significantly increased Thr34 P-DARPP-32 levels in PSAL and PCOC mice with no difference in levels between the two prenatal treatment groups (**Figures 2G,I**, respectively). Cocaine or SKF 82958 administration significantly decreased Thr75 P-DARPP-32 levels in PSAL mice, with a trend toward lower levels in PCOC mice evident (**Figures 2H,J**, respectively). Examination of P-ERK2 levels revealed that cocaine or SKF 82958 treatment significantly increased P-ERK2 levels in PSAL mice compared to saline treated mice (**Figures 2M**, PSAL coc vs. PSAL sal and **Figures 2N**, PSAL SKF vs. PSAL sal), a response that was not evident in PCOC mice (**Figures 2M,N**, respectively). Examination of P-GluA1 revealed that cocaine or SKF 82958 administration increased P-GluA1 in PSAL mice (**Figures 2Q,R**, respectively) while either cocaine or SKF 82958 treatment significantly decreased P-GluA1 in PCOC mice (**Figures 2Q,R**, respectively). SKF 82958-induced P-GluA1 levels were significantly lower in PCOC mice compared to PSAL mice (**Figure 2R**, PCOC skf vs. PSAL skf).

ALTERED BDNF IN THE Str OF PCOC MICE
We next examined levels of pro- and mature BDNF in the Str and NAc of PCOC vs. PSAL mice, along with levels in the mPFC and VTA, anatomical regions where BDNF is synthesized and transported to those targets (Conner et al., 1997; Altar and DiStefano, 1998). To identify the precise protein bands that correspond to pro- vs. mature BDNF we first compared BDNF Western blots containing striatal protein lysates with recombinant BDNF protein lysates (**Figure 3A**). A pro-BDNF protein band at 30 kDa and mature BDNF protein band at 14 kDa was used to compare levels of the two proteins in protein lysates obtained from mPFC, Str, NAc, and VTA tissue of PCOC vs. PSAL mice. Western blots revealed significantly higher levels of pro-BDNF in the Str of PCOC mice compared to PSAL mice (**Figure 3B**). No significant differences in pro-BDNF levels were observed for any other regions sampled. Examination of mature BDNF levels revealed no significant differences between PCOC and PSAL mice in any of the regions sampled (**Figure 3C**).

We next examined the effect of prenatal treatment on the levels of the BDNF receptors TrkB, p75, and NR2B in the Str and NAc of PCOC vs. PSAL mice (**Figure 4**). TrkB levels were significantly higher in the striatum of PCOC compared to PSAL mice (**Figure 4A**), while in the NAc there was no significant difference in TrkB levels between the two prenatal treatment groups. No significant differences were observed in p75 protein levels in PCOC vs. PSAL mice in the Str or NAc (**Figure 4B**). Similarly, examination of NR2B, a gene regulated by the pro-BDNF pathway (Woo et al., 2005) revealed no significant differences between PCOC and PSAL mice in either brain region (**Figure 4C**).

DISCUSSION
DA SIGNALING IN THE Str AND NAc OF PCOC MICE
We, like others, find that acute cocaine administration increases protein phosphorylation of CREB, DARPP-32, ERK2, and GluA1 in the Str and NAc of adult mice via a D1 mechanism

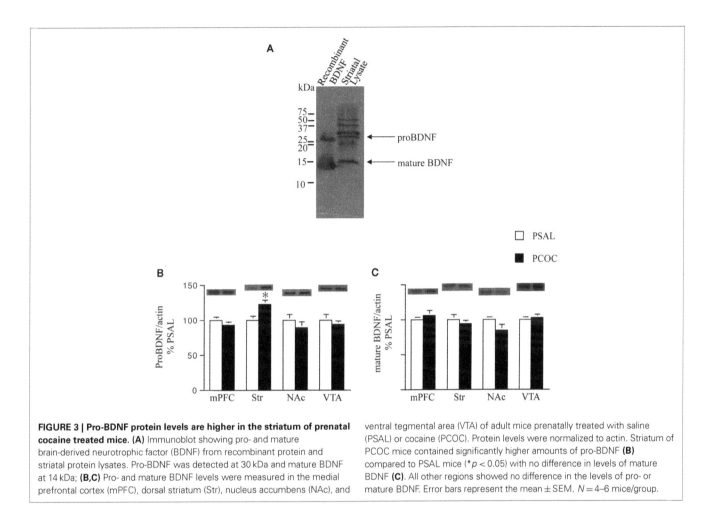

FIGURE 3 | Pro-BDNF protein levels are higher in the striatum of prenatal cocaine treated mice. (A) Immunoblot showing pro- and mature brain-derived neurotrophic factor (BDNF) from recombinant protein and striatal protein lysates. Pro-BDNF was detected at 30 kDa and mature BDNF at 14 kDa; (B,C) Pro- and mature BDNF levels were measured in the medial prefrontal cortex (mPFC), dorsal striatum (Str), nucleus accumbens (NAc), and ventral tegmental area (VTA) of adult mice prenatally treated with saline (PSAL) or cocaine (PCOC). Protein levels were normalized to actin. Striatum of PCOC mice contained significantly higher amounts of pro-BDNF (B) compared to PSAL mice ($*p < 0.05$) with no difference in levels of mature BDNF (C). All other regions showed no difference in the levels of pro- or mature BDNF. Error bars represent the mean ± SEM. $N = 4–6$ mice/group.

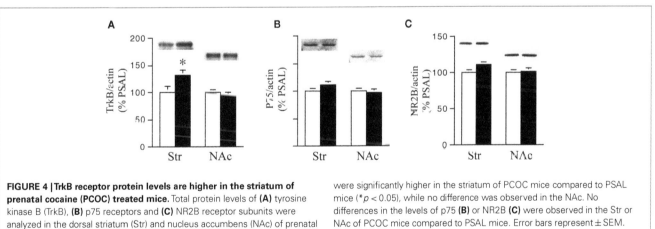

FIGURE 4 | TrkB receptor protein levels are higher in the striatum of prenatal cocaine (PCOC) treated mice. Total protein levels of (A) tyrosine kinase B (TrkB), (B) p75 receptors and (C) NR2B receptor subunits were analyzed in the dorsal striatum (Str) and nucleus accumbens (NAc) of prenatal saline (PSAL) treated vs. PCOC treated adult mice. (A) TrkB receptor levels were significantly higher in the striatum of PCOC mice compared to PSAL mice ($*p < 0.05$), while no difference was observed in the NAc. No differences in the levels of p75 (B) or NR2B (C) were observed in the Str or NAc of PCOC mice compared to PSAL mice. Error bars represent ± SEM. $N = 5–6$ mice/group.

(Fienberg et al., 1998; Zhang et al., 2002a,b; Gerfen et al., 2008; Guan et al., 2009). Specifically, following acute administration of cocaine (15 mg/kg, i.p.) or D1 agonist (SKF 82958; 1 mg/kg, i.p.) there were significantly higher levels of Ser133 P-CREB, Thr34 P-DARPP-32, Thr202/Tyr 204 P-ERK2, and Ser845 P-GluA1, as well as lower levels of Thr75 P-DARPP-32 evident in the Str and NAc of PSAL mice. Interestingly, in the Str of PCOC mice, administration of cocaine or D1 agonist further augmented the phosphorylation of CREB, DARPP-32 at Thr34, and ERK, but led to a de-phosphorylation of DARPP-32 at Thr75 and of GluA1. The augmented activation of this signaling cascade is a likely mechanism for the increased expression of both zif-268 and homer 1a mRNA observed in the striatum of PCOC mice following acute cocaine administration (see **Figure 5**), which may also be

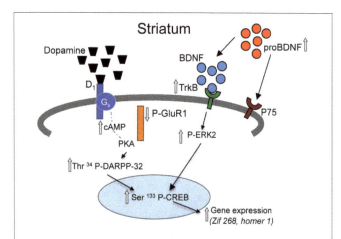

FIGURE 5 | Proposed model for adaptations in D1 receptor and BDNF signaling pathways in the striatum of prenatal cocaine treated mice. Prenatal cocaine treatment results in enhanced signaling via dopamine D1 and TrkB receptors in the striatum of adult mice via persistent adaptations in a coordinately regulated set of pre-synaptic, synaptic, and post-synaptic molecules. Gray arrows represent long-term adaptations seen in adult mice following prenatal cocaine treatment.

attributable to a persistent enhancement in the coupling of D1 with cAMP (Tropea et al., 2008a). These data are discrepant with those reported in a rabbit model of PCOC exposure, in which there is demonstration of attenuated D1 activation via uncoupling of GalphaS subunits from D1 receptors, resulting in enhanced internalization of D1 subunits (Wang et al., 1995; Jones et al., 2000; Stanwood and Levitt, 2007). While such data from rabbits suggests attenuated dopaminergic activation following PCOC exposure, this same rabbit model has additionally provided evidence of enhanced DARPP-32 phosphorylation at Thr34 (Zhen et al., 2001), data concordant with our current findings in mice. Results from different models of PCOC exposure may differ as a result of species (e.g., mice vs. rabbits), route (SC vs. IV), dose and gestational timing of cocaine exposure, or brain regions studied (e.g., Str/NAc vs. Cingulate Cortex). Further studies should be directed at elucidating the cause of such differences, and the extent to which they adequately model aspects of the clinical problem.

We also found significant differences in PCOC mice when contrasting the phosphorylation of both CREB and ERK in the Str vs. NAc following administration of cocaine or D1 agonist; there was enhanced phosphorylation of CREB and ERK evident in the Str of PCOC mice, in contrast to blunted phosphorylation of CREB and ERK in the NAc of PCOC mice. It is possible that the constitutive increase in P-ERK identified in the NAc of PCOC mice, which was not evident in the Str, prevented the subsequent phosphorylation of ERK (and perhaps CREB) in the NAc. The blunted phosphorylation of at least one of these proteins may be related to our previous observation that acute cocaine administration did not increase either zif-268 or homer 1a mRNA expression in the NAc of PCOC mice (Tropea et al., 2008a).

P-GluA1 SIGNALING IN THE Str AND NAc
In both the Str and NAc of PCOC mice, where increased constitutive expression of P-GluA1 was evident, administration of cocaine or SKF 82958 resulted in decreased GluA1 phosphorylation. This is in sharp contrast to PSAL mice, in which administration of cocaine or SKF 82958 resulted in increased expression of P-GluA1. Again, it is possible that the constitutive increase in P-GluA1 identified in both the Str and NAc of PCOC mice, prevented subsequent phosphorylation of GluA1 in both regions. Recent work has suggested that increased P-GluA1 sequesters this receptor in the cytoplasm, thereby preventing insertion of a functional receptor into the membrane, a phenomena that has been correlated with the sensitized state (for review see Mazzucchelli et al., 2002; Wolf and Ferrario, 2010). The mechanism that contributes to the constitutive increase in P-ERK evident in the Str of PCOC mice is presumably different than the mechanism that contributes to the constitutive increase in P-GluA1 evident in both the Str and NAc of PCOC mice, but both may be mediated by epigenetic mechanisms.

BDNF AND TrkB SIGNALING IN THE Str VS. NAc OF PCOC MICE
We see increases in the constitutive expression of pro-BDNF and TrkB in the Str, but not in the NAc of PCOC mice. However, we do not see changes in the expression of mature BDNF, p75, or NR2B receptor subunits, identifying a regional as well as molecular specificity in the BDNF signaling pathway that is persistently altered in PCOC mice. Work from others (Yang et al., 2009) suggests that pro-BDNF preferentially binds the p75 receptor, whereas mature BDNF preferentially binds the TrkB receptor. We are therefore pursuing additional experiments to identify the functional relevance of the increased constitutive expression of pro-BDNF and TrkB in the adult Str, which may be a result of enhanced cortico-striatal projections, which are the predominant source of striatal BDNF (Conner et al., 1997; Altar and DiStefano, 1998). Interestingly, recent data obtained from *ex vivo* cultures of embryonic mouse brains suggests that the tangential migration of GABAergic neurons from their site of origin in the ganglionic eminence to their cortical destination is delayed in the forebrain of mice prenatally exposed to cocaine, and that supplementation of those cultures with exogenous BDNF normalized this migration (McCarthy et al., 2011). Furthermore, cocaine has distinct acute and long-term effects on BDNF transcription and expression in striatum and frontal cortex (Liu et al., 2006), which is further complicated by post-transcriptional alterations in the isoforms of BDNF expressed (Jiang et al., 2009). Taken together the data suggests that perturbations in the level of BDNF at specific developmental periods can have immediate as well as long-lasting implications for neuronal migration and maturation, with impact on brain function that can persist into adulthood.

IMPLICATIONS OF OUR MOLECULAR FINDINGS ON BRAIN FUNCTION
What is unknown is whether the differential adaptations in dopaminergic signaling that persist in the Str and NAc of PCOC mice evident following acute administration of cocaine we have reported will enhance their liability for addiction following recurrent cocaine exposure as adults. Previous experiments from our group contrasting PCOC and PSAL mice have identified alterations in cocaine-induced brain stimulation reward (Malanga et al., 2008), self-administration (Rocha et al., 2002), conditioned place preference (Malanga et al., 2007), and locomotor sensitization (Crozatier et al., 2003), as well as dopamine release in the

Str and NAc during that same locomotor sensitization regimen (Malanga et al., 2009). However, in each study while the PCOC mice could be distinguished from the PSAL mice, the phenotype did not dramatically demonstrate an enhanced liability toward addiction. Such complexity could be attributable to the differential adaptations in PCOC vs. PSAL mice that we report here in the Str vs. NAc. This may preclude the progression of habit learning associated with recurrent drug exposure which is thought to require the expanded recruitment of successively more dorsal striatal circuits following the initial activation of the NAc (Everitt and Robbins, 2005; Belin and Everitt, 2008; Haber, 2008). In addition, the liability for addiction in humans is critically dependent on genetic as well as environmental factors, which may be significantly enhanced in offspring prenatally exposed to cocaine, and may be powerfully interactive with adaptations in Str and NAc neuronal function as we have described in our mouse model. As the generation of young adults prenatally exposed to cocaine initiate their own experiences with drug experimentation, they may be at greater risk for the fifth "A" – addiction.

Human imaging studies can help to identify the structural and functional correlates of the behavioral and molecular aberrations seen in animal models of PCOC exposure (reviewed in Roussotte et al., 2010). Whole brain MRI has provided evidence for reductions in parietal and occipital cortical gray matter volumes and a cocaine dose-dependant reduction in white matter of the corpus callosum in humans exposed to cocaine *in utero* (Dow-Edwards et al., 2006; Rivkin et al., 2008). Callosal volume loss was corroborated in a rodent model as well (Ma et al., 2009). Attenuated white matter integrity on DTI imaging of the left frontal callosal and right frontal projection fibers suggests suboptimal white matter development in those areas (Warner et al., 2006). Similarly, studies in opiate-exposed offspring show that white matter integrity seems to be most susceptible to damage in areas undergoing earlier CNS development (Walhovd et al., 2010). Analyses of subcortical structures have revealed a persistent decrease in caudate volume following prenatal cocaine exposure (Avants et al., 2007). Functional studies using fMRI provide evidence of a 10% reduction in cerebral blood flow most prominent in posterior and inferior brain regions of adolescents (Rao et al., 2007). Sheinkopf et al. (2009) have shown that performance in a go-no go task adolescents who were previously exposed to cocaine *in utero* showed a greater activation of right inferior frontal and striatal regions compared to controls who activated fusiform gyrus and occipital cortex more prominently, suggesting differences in cognition and attention in the PCOC-exposed group. Correlations between reduced frontal white matter and visuo-spatial and executive functioning tests (Warner et al., 2006), right parietal volume loss with visual attention, sensori-motor tasks, and syntax construction, and left occipital volume loss with poor performance in visual attention, recognition, and visuomotor tasks (Dow-Edwards et al., 2006) suggest PCOC affects visual, sensori-motor, and executive functions.

A deeper appreciation of the relevance of the persistent molecular adaptations evident in animal models, including that which we report here, to the results obtained in structural and functional imaging studies performed in humans, will require a better understanding of the mechanisms by which such molecular changes are interactive with genetic factors including common polymorphisms for genes such as BDNF, which independent of PCOC exposure may confer enhanced vulnerability vs. resilience to addiction. Such gene X (fetal) environment interactions may contribute to aspects of the PCOC phenotype demonstrated in humans by others, *including some of those reported in this monograph*. Conceptualized this way, intrauterine cocaine exposure can be thought of as a pharmacologic means of inducing a state of "fetal reprogramming" (Barker, 1995) by which molecular pathways underlying ongoing brain development are permanently altered, thereby enhancing an individual's vulnerability to subsequent disease, in this case addiction. Like with other diseases, early detection of such enhanced vulnerabilities will provide a rational starting point for behavioral and perhaps pharmacologic interventions to prevent expression of disease, which in the case of prenatal drug exposure may help prevent the problem from begetting itself.

ACKNOWLEDGMENTS

We would like to thank Dr. Francis Lee for his generous donation of recombinant BDNF protein.

REFERENCES

Accornero, V. H., Amado, A. J., Morrow, C. E., Xue, L., Anthony, J. C., and Bandstra, E. S. (2007). Impact of prenatal cocaine exposure on attention and response inhibition as assessed by continuous performance tests. *J. Dev. Behav. Pediatr.* 28, 195–205.

Alessandri, S. M., Bendersky, M., and Lewis, M. (1998). Cognitive functioning in 8- to 18-month-old drug-exposed infants. *Dev. Psychol.* 34, 565–573.

Altar, C. A., and DiStefano, P. S. (1998). Neurotrophin trafficking by anterograde transport. *Trends Neurosci.* 21, 433–437.

Avants, B. B., Hurt, H., Giannetta, J. M., Epstein, C. L., Shera, D. M., Rao, H., Wang, J., and Gee, J. C. (2007). Effects of heavy in utero cocaine exposure on adolescent caudate morphology. *Pediatr. Neurol.* 37, 275–279.

Bada, H. S., Das, A., Bauer, C. R., Shankaran, S., Lester, B., LaGasse, L., Hammond, J., Wright, L. L., and Higgins, R. (2007). Impact of prenatal cocaine exposure on child behavior problems through school age. *Pediatrics* 119, e348–e359.

Barker, D. J. (1995). Intrauterine programming of adult disease. *Mol. Med. Today* 1, 418–423.

Beeghly, M., Martin, B., Rose-Jacobs, R., Cabral, H., Heeren, T., Augustyn, M., Bellinger, D., and Frank, D. A. (2006). Prenatal cocaine exposure and children's language functioning at 6 and 9.5 years: moderating effects of child age, birthweight, and gender. *J. Pediatr. Psychol.* 31, 98–115.

Behnke, M., Eyler, F. D., Conlon, M., Casanova, O. Q., and Woods, N. S. (1997). How fetal cocaine exposure increases neonatal hospital costs. *Pediatrics* 99, 204–208.

Belin, D., and Everitt, B. J. (2008). Cocaine seeking habits depend upon dopamine-dependent serial connectivity linking the ventral with the dorsal striatum. *Neuron* 57, 432–441.

Berke, J. D., and Hyman, S. E. (2000). Addiction, dopamine, and the molecular mechanisms of memory. *Neuron* 25, 515–532.

Chao, J., and Nestler, E. J. (2004). Molecular neurobiology of drug addiction. *Annu. Rev. Med.* 55, 113–132.

Conner, J. M., Lauterborn, J. C., Yan, Q., Gall, C. M., and Varon, S. (1997). Distribution of brain-derived neurotrophic factor (BDNF) protein and mRNA in the normal adult rat CNS: evidence for anterograde axonal transport. *J. Neurosci.* 17, 2295–2313.

Crozatier, C., Guerriero, R. M., Mathieu, F., Giros, B., Nosten-Bertrand, M., and Kosofsky, B. E. (2003). Altered cocaine-induced behavioral sensitization in adult mice exposed to cocaine in utero. *Brain Res. Dev. Brain Res.* 147, 97–105.

Dow-Edwards, D. L., Benveniste, H., Behnke, M., Bandstra, E. S., Singer, L. T., Hurd, Y. L., and Stanford, L. R. (2006). Neuroimaging of prenatal drug exposure. *Neurotoxicol. Teratol.* 28, 386–402.

Drago, J., Gerfen, C. R., Westphal, H., and Steiner, H. (1996). D1 dopamine receptor-deficient mouse: cocaine-induced regulation of immediate-early gene and substance P expression in the striatum. *Neuroscience* 74, 813–823.

Everitt, B. J., and Robbins, T. W. (2005). Neural systems of reinforcement for drug addiction: from actions to habits to compulsion. *Nat. Neurosci.* 8, 1481–149.

Fienberg, A. A., Hiroi, N., Mermelstein, P. G., Song, W., Snyder, G. L., Nishi, A., Cheramy, A., O'Callaghan, J. P., Miller, D. B., Cole, D. G., Corbett, R., Haile, C. N., Cooper, D. C., Onn, S. P., Grace, A. A., Ouimet, C. C., White, F. J., Hyman, S. E., Surmeier, D. J., Girault, J., Nestler, E. J., and Greengard, P. (1998). DARPP-32: regulator of the efficacy of dopaminergic neurotransmission. *Science* 281, 838–842.

Friedman, E., and Wang, H. Y. (1998). Prenatal cocaine exposure alters signal transduction in the brain D1 dopamine receptor system. *Ann. N. Y. Acad. Sci.* 846, 238–247.

Gerfen, C. R., Paletzki, R., and Worley, P. (2008). Differences between dorsal and ventral striatum in Drd1a dopamine receptor coupling of dopamine- and cAMP-regulated phosphoprotein-32 to activation of extracellular signal-regulated kinase. *J. Neurosci.* 28, 7113–7120.

Guan, X., Tao, J., and Li, S. (2009). Dopamine D1 receptor, but not dopamine D2 receptor, is a critical regulator for acute cocaine-enhanced gene expression. *Neurol. Res.* 31, 17–22.

Haber, S. (2008). Parallel and integrative processing through the Basal Ganglia reward circuit: lessons from addiction. *Biol. Psychiatry* 64, 173–174.

Harvey, J. A. (2004). Cocaine effects on the developing brain: current status. *Neurosci. Biobehav. Rev.* 27, 751–764.

Hyman, S. E. (2005). Addiction: a disease of learning and memory. *Am. J. Psychiatry* 162, 1414–1422.

Hyman, S. E., and Malenka, R. C. (2001). Addiction and the brain: the neurobiology of compulsion and its persistence. *Nat. Rev. Neurosci.* 2, 695–703.

Jiang, X., Zhou, J., Mash, D. C., Marini, A. M., and Lipsky, R. H. (2009). Human BDNF isoforms are differentially expressed in cocaine addicts and are sorted to the regulated secretory pathway independent of the Met66 substitution. *Neuromolecular Med.* 11, 1–12.

Jones, L. B., Stanwood, G. D., Reinoso, B. S., Washington, R. A., Wang, H. Y., Friedman, E., and Levitt, P. (2000). In utero cocaine-induced dysfunction of dopamine D1 receptor signaling and abnormal differentiation of cerebral cortical neurons. *J. Neurosci.* 20, 4606–4614.

Kalivas, P. W., Pierce, R. C., Cornish, J., and Sorg, B. A. (1998). A role for sensitization in craving and relapse in cocaine addiction. *J. Psychopharmacol. (Oxford)* 12, 49–53.

Kosofsky, B. E., and Hyman, S. E. (2001). No time for complacency: the fetal brain on drugs. *J. Comp. Neurol.* 435, 259–262.

Kosofsky, B. E., Wilkins, A. S., Gressens, P., and Evrard, P. (1994). Transplacental cocaine exposure: a mouse model demonstrating neuroanatomic and behavioral abnormalities. *J. Child Neurol.* 9, 234–241.

Lester, B. M. (1998). The maternal lifestyles study. *Ann. N. Y. Acad. Sci.* 846, 296–305.

Lester, B. M., LaGasse, L. L., and Seifer, R. (1998). Cocaine exposure and children: the meaning of subtle effects. *Science* 282, 633–634.

Levine, T. P., Liu, J., Das, A., Lester, B., Lagasse, L., Shankaran, S., Bada, H. S., Bauer, C. R., and Higgins, R. (2008). Effects of prenatal cocaine exposure on special education in school-aged children. *Pediatrics* 122, e83–e91.

Lidow, M. S., and Song, Z. M. (2001). Primates exposed to cocaine in utero display reduced density and number of cerebral cortical neurons. *J. Comp. Neurol.* 435, 263–275.

Liu, Q. R., Lu, L., Zhu, X. G., Gong, J. P., Shaham, Y., and Uhl, G. R. (2006). Rodent BDNF genes, novel promoters, novel splice variants, and regulation by cocaine. *Brain Res.* 1067, 1–12.

Ma, L., Hasan, K. M., Steinberg, J. L., Narayana, P. A., Lane, S. D., Zuniga, E. A., Kramer, L. A., and Moeller, F. G. (2009). Diffusion tensor imaging in cocaine dependence: regional effects of cocaine on corpus callosum and effect of cocaine administration route. *Drug Alcohol Depend.* 104, 262–267.

Malanga, C. J. III, and Kosofsky, B. E. (1999). Mechanisms of action of drugs of abuse on the developing fetal brain. *Clin. Perinatol.* 26, 17–37, v–vi.

Malanga, C. J., and Kosofsky, B. E. (2003). Does drug abuse beget drug abuse? Behavioral analysis of addiction liability in animal models of prenatal drug exposure. *Brain Res. Dev. Brain Res.* 147, 47–57.

Malanga, C. J., Pejchal, M., and Kosofsky, B. E. (2007). Prenatal exposure to cocaine alters the development of conditioned place-preference to cocaine in adult mice. *Pharmacol. Biochem. Behav.* 87, 462–471.

Malanga, C. J., Ren, J. Q., Guerriero, R. M., and Kosofsky, B. E. (2009). Augmentation of cocaine-sensitized dopamine release in the nucleus accumbens of adult mice following prenatal cocaine exposure. *Dev. Neurosci.* 31, 76–89.

Malanga, C. J., Riday, T. T., Carlezon, W. A. Jr., and Kosofsky, B. E. (2008). Prenatal exposure to cocaine increases the rewarding potency of cocaine and selective dopaminergic agonists in adult mice. *Biol. Psychiatry* 63, 214–221.

Mayes, L. C. (2002). A behavioral teratogenic model of the impact of prenatal cocaine exposure on arousal regulatory systems. *Neurotoxicol. Teratol.* 24, 385–395.

Mayes, L. C., Grillon, C., Granger, R., and Schottenfeld, R. (1998). Regulation of arousal and attention in preschool children exposed to cocaine prenatally. *Ann. N. Y. Acad. Sci.* 846, 126–143.

Mazzucchelli, C., Vantaggiato, C., Ciamei, A., Fasano, S., Pakhotin, P., Krezel, W., Welzl, H., Wolfer, D. P., Pages, G., Valverde, O., Marowsky, A., Porrazzo, A., Orban, P. C., Maldonado, R., Ehrengruber, M. U., Cestari, V., Lipp, H. P., Chapman, P. F., Pouyssegur, J., and Brambilla, R. (2002). Knockout of ERK1 MAP kinase enhances synaptic plasticity in the striatum and facilitates striatal-mediated learning and memory. *Neuron* 34, 807–820.

McCarthy, D. M., Zhang, X., Darnell, S. B., Sangrey, G. R., Yanagawa, Y., Sadri-Vakili, G., and Bhide, P. G. (2011). Cocaine alters BDNF expression and neuronal migration in the embryonic mouse forebrain. *J. Neurosci.* 31(38), 13400–13411.

McGinty, J. F., Shi, X. D., Schwendt, M., Saylor, A., and Toda, S. (2008). Regulation of psychostimulant-induced signaling and gene expression in the striatum. *J. Neurochem.* 104, 1440–1449.

Paxinos, G., and Franklin, K. (2003). *The Mouse Brain in Stereotaxc Coordinates*, 2nd Edn. New York: Academic Press.

Rao, H., Wang, J., Giannetta, J., Korczykowski, M., Shera, D., Avants, B. B., Gee, J., Detre, J. A., and Hurt, H. (2007). Altered resting cerebral blood flow in adolescents with in utero cocaine exposure revealed by perfusion functional MRI. *Pediatrics* 120, e1245–e1254.

Renthal, W., Kumar, A., Xiao, G., Wilkinson, M., Covington, H. E. III, Maze, I., Sikder, D., Robison, A. J., LaPlant, Q., Dietz, D. M., Russo, S. J., Vialou, V., Chakravarty, S., Kodadek, T. J., Stack, A., Kabbaj, M., and Nestler, E. J. (2009). Genome-wide analysis of chromatin regulation by cocaine reveals a role for sirtuins. *Neuron* 62, 335–348.

Rivkin, M. J., Davis, P. E., Lemaster, J. L., Cabral, H. J., Warfield, S. K., Mulkern, R. V., Robson, C. D., Rose-Jacobs, R., and Frank, D. A. (2008). Volumetric MRI study of brain in children with intrauterine exposure to cocaine, alcohol, tobacco, and marijuana. *Pediatrics* 121, 741–750.

Rocha, B. A., Mead, A. N., and Kosofsky, B. E. (2002). Increased vulnerability to self-administer cocaine in mice prenatally exposed to cocaine. *Psychopharmacology (Berl.)* 163, 221–229.

Roussotte, F., Soderberg, L., and Sowell, E. (2010). Structural, metabolic, and functional brain abnormalities as a result of prenatal exposure to drugs of abuse: evidence from neuroimaging. *Neuropsychol. Rev.* 20, 376–397.

Self, D. W., Barnhart, W. J., Lehman, D. A., and Nestler, E. J. (1996). Opposite modulation of cocaine-seeking behavior by D1- and D2-like dopamine receptor agonists. *Science* 271, 1586–1589.

Sheinkopf, S. J., Lester, B. M., Sanes, J. N., Eliassen, J. C., Hutchison, E. R., Seifer, R., Lagasse, L. L., Durston, S., and Casey, B. J. (2009). Functional MRI and response inhibition in children exposed to cocaine in utero. Preliminary findings. *Dev. Neurosci.* 31, 159–166.

Spear, L. P., Silveri, M. M., Casale, M., Katovic, N. M., Campbell, J. O., and Douglas, L. A. (2002). Cocaine and development: a retrospective perspective. *Neurotoxicol. Teratol.* 24, 321–327.

Stanwood, G. D., and Levitt, P. (2007). Prenatal exposure to cocaine produces unique developmental and long-term adaptive changes in dopamine D1 receptor activity and subcellular distribution. *J. Neurosci.* 27, 152–157.

Trask, C. L., and Kosofsky, B. E. (2000). Developmental considerations of neurotoxic exposures. *Neurol. Clin.* 18, 541–562.

Tropea, T. F., Guerriero, R. M., Willuhn, I., Unterwald, E. M., Ehrlich, M. E., Steiner, H., and Kosofsky, B. E. (2008a). Augmented D1 dopamine receptor signaling and immediate-early gene induction in adult striatum after prenatal cocaine. *Biol. Psychiatry* 63, 1066–1074.

Tropea, T. F., Kosofsky, B. E., and Rajadhyaksha, A. M. (2008b). Enhanced CREB and DARPP-32 phosphorylation in the nucleus accumbens and CREB, ERK, and GluR1 phosphorylation in the dorsal hippocampus is associated with cocaine-conditioned place preference behavior. *J. Neurochem.* 106, 1780–1790.

Uhl, G. R., Hall, F. S., and Sora, I. (2002). Cocaine, reward, movement and monoamine transporters. *Mol. Psychiatry* 7, 21–26.

Unterwald, E. M., Ivkovic, S., Cuntapay, M., Stroppolo, A., Guinea, B., and Ehrlich, M. E. (2003). Prenatal exposure to cocaine decreases adenylyl cyclase activity in embryonic mouse striatum. *Brain Res. Dev. Brain Res.* 147, 67–75.

Walhovd, K. B., Westlye, L. T., Moe, V., Slinning, K., Due-Tonnessen, P., Bjornerud, A., van der Kouwe, A., Dale, A. M., and Fjell, A. M. (2010). White matter characteristics and cognition in prenatally opiate- and polysubstance-exposed children: a diffusion tensor imaging study. *AJNR Am. J. Neuroradiol.* 31, 894–900.

Wang, H. Y., Runyan, S., Yadin, E., and Friedman, E. (1995). Prenatal exposure to cocaine selectively reduces D1 dopamine receptor-mediated activation of striatal Gs proteins. *J. Pharmacol. Exp. Ther.* 273, 492–498.

Warner, T. D., Behnke, M., Eyler, F. D., Padgett, K., Leonard, C., Hou, W., Garvan, C. W., Schmalfuss, I. M., and Blackband, S. J. (2006). Diffusion tensor imaging of frontal white matter and executive functioning in cocaine-exposed children. *Pediatrics* 118, 2014–2024.

Wilkins, A. S., Genova, L. M., Posten, W., and Kosofsky, B. E. (1998). Transplacental cocaine exposure. 1; a rodent model. *Neurotoxicol. Teratol.* 20, 215–226.

Wolf, M. E., and Ferrario, C. R. (2010). AMPA receptor plasticity in the nucleus accumbens after repeated exposure to cocaine. *Neurosci. Biobehav. Rev.* 35, 185–211.

Woo, N. H., Teng, H. K., Siao, C. J., Chiaruttini, C., Pang, P. T., Milner, T. A., Hempstead, B. L., and Lu, B. (2005). Activation of p75NTR by proBDNF facilitates hippocampal long-term depression. *Nat. Neurosci.* 8, 1069–1077.

Yang, J., Siao, C. J., Nagappan, G., Marinic, T., Jing, D., McGrath, K., Chen, Z. Y., Mark, W., Tessarollo, L., Lee, F. S., Lu, B., and Hempstead, B. L. (2009). Neuronal release of proBDNF. *Nat. Neurosci.* 12, 113–115.

Zhang, D., Zhang, L., Lou, D. W., Nakabeppu, Y., Zhang, J., and Xu, M. (2002a). The dopamine D1 receptor is a critical mediator for cocaine-induced gene expression. *J. Neurochem.* 82, 1453–1464.

Zhang, J., Zhang, D., and Xu, M. (2002b). Identification of chronic cocaine-induced gene expression through dopamine d1 receptors by using cDNA microarrays. *Ann. N. Y. Acad. Sci.* 965, 1–9.

Zhen, X., Torres, C., Wang, H. Y., and Friedman, E. (2001). Prenatal exposure to cocaine disrupts D1A dopamine receptor function via selective inhibition of protein phosphatase 1 pathway in rabbit frontal cortex. *J. Neurosci.* 21, 9160–9167.

Prenatal IV cocaine: Alterations in auditory information processing

Charles F. Mactutus*, Steven B. Harrod, Lauren L. Hord, Landhing M. Moran and Rosemarie M. Booze

Behavioral Neuroscience Program, Department of Psychology, University of South Carolina, Columbia, SC, USA

*Correspondence:
Charles F. Mactutus, Behavioral Neuroscience Program, Department of Psychology, University of South Carolina, Columbia, SC 29208-0001, USA.
e-mail: mactutus@mailbox.sc.edu

One clue regarding the basis of cocaine-induced deficits in attentional processing is provided by the clinical findings of changes in the infants' startle response; observations buttressed by neurophysiological evidence of alterations in brainstem transmission time. Using the IV route of administration and doses that mimic the peak arterial levels of cocaine use in humans, the present study examined the effects of prenatal cocaine on auditory information processing via tests of the auditory startle response (ASR), habituation, and prepulse inhibition (PPI) in the offspring. Nulliparous Long–Evans female rats, implanted with an IV access port prior to breeding, were administered saline, 0.5, 1.0, or 3.0 mg/kg/injection of cocaine HCL (COC) from gestation day (GD) 8–20 (1×/day-GD8–14, 2×/day-GD15–20). COC had no significant effects on maternal/litter parameters or growth of the offspring. At 18–20 days of age, one male and one female, randomly selected from each litter displayed an increased ASR (>30% for males at 1.0 mg/kg and >30% for females at 3.0 mg/kg). When reassessed in adulthood (D90–100), a linear dose–response increase was noted on response amplitude. At both test ages, within-session habituation was retarded by prenatal cocaine treatment. Testing the females in diestrus vs. estrus did not alter the results. Prenatal cocaine altered the PPI response function across interstimulus interval and induced significant sex-dependent changes in response latency. Idazoxan, an α_2-adrenergic receptor antagonist, significantly enhanced the ASR, but less enhancement was noted with increasing doses of prenatal cocaine. Thus, *in utero* exposure to cocaine, when delivered via a protocol designed to capture prominent features of recreational usage, causes persistent, if not permanent, alterations in auditory information processing, and suggests dysfunction of the central noradrenergic circuitry modulating, if not mediating, these responses.

Keywords: prenatal cocaine, intravenous administration, auditory startle, habituation, prepulse inhibition, dose-response, norepinephrine, idazoxan

INTRODUCTION

Although a variety of data sources suggest that the years of 1979–1985 marked the height of the past epidemic of cocaine abuse in the U.S., the extraordinary levels of cocaine availability, increased purity, and the facility of smoking "crack" continue to captivate a significant segment of our population. The population of young female drug users entering childbearing age is a major concern. In 2009, an estimated 21.8 million Americans aged 12 or older were current (past month) illicit drug users, meaning they had used an illicit drug during the month prior to the survey interview (Substance Abuse and Mental Health Services Administration, 2010). This estimate represents 8.7% of the population aged 12 years old or older. Regarding cocaine usage, there are 1.6 million current cocaine users aged 12 or older, comprising 0.7% of the population (Johnston et al., 2010). These estimates are similar to the number and rate in 2008 (1.9 million or 0.7%). Clearly, illicit drug abuse, including cocaine/crack use, among young women of childbearing age remains a significant societal concern, placing future generations at risk. Comprehending the effects of prenatal drug exposure, such as cocaine/crack, on behavioral and neural development remains extremely important.

Drug use around the world is not distributed evenly and is not simply related to drug policy, as countries with more strict user-level drug policies did not have lower levels of use than countries with more liberal policies. Of the 17 countries participating in the World Health Organization's (WHO's) World Mental Health (WMH) Survey Initiative, the highest lifetime cumulative incidence of cocaine was in the United States (16.2%), followed by New Zealand, Spain, Colombia, and Mexico (range of 4.0–4.3%; Degenhardt et al., 2008). A more recent review of countries around the world has suggested high lifetime prevalence use of cocaine in Argentina (7.9%), Italy (6.6%), United Kingdom (6.5%), Chile (5.9%), and Ireland 5.3%; (Degenhardt et al., 2011). Thus, the implication of cocaine abuse for future generations appears to be far more than a U.S. health issue.

Comprehensive literature reviews providing ∼15 and ∼20 year perspectives on preschool (<6 years of age, Frank et al., 2001) and school-aged (>6 years of age, Ackerman et al., 2010) prenatal cocaine-exposed children, respectively, have failed to definitively identify any unique constellation of effects of prenatal cocaine exposure. Many findings once thought to be specific effects of *in utero* cocaine exposure are correlated with other factors, including prenatal exposure to tobacco, marijuana, or alcohol, and/or a host of social/environmental factors, such as poverty, caregiver education, placement stability, and quality of child-caregiver relationships that are known to affect a child's development. For example, among children aged 6 years or younger, across four domains (physical growth; cognition; language skills; motor skills) Frank et al. (2001) concluded there was no convincing evidence that prenatal cocaine exposure is associated with developmental toxic effects that are different in severity, scope, or kind from the sequelae of multiple other risk factors. A similar recent reaffirmation noted that studies of school-aged children have shown no long-term direct effects of prenatal cocaine exposure on children's physical growth, developmental test scores, or language outcomes (Ackerman et al., 2010).

Nevertheless, the most consistently suggested, and perhaps the most prominent, fetal cocaine effect reported to date is that of an enduring attentional dysfunction in preschool and school-aged children. Problems with attentional processes have been documented over the past 15 years with several different paradigms, including computer-controlled continuous performance tasks (Richardson et al., 1996; Heffelfinger et al., 1997, 2002; Leech et al., 1999; Bandstra et al., 2001; Noland et al., 2005; Savage et al., 2005; Accornero et al., 2007; Chiriboga et al., 2009; Carmody et al., 2011). Given the myriad of correlated factors that often characterizes this population, as discussed above, preclinical studies are important in defining and characterizing the behavioral and neural basis(es) of alterations in attentional processes. Consistent alterations in "attentionally sensitive" neurobehavioral paradigms have been reported in rodents when maternal cocaine was administered via the intravenous route and at relatively low "recreational" doses (Mactutus, 1999; Bayer et al., 2000, 2002; Garavan et al., 2000; Morgan et al., 2002; Gendle et al., 2003, 2004a,1996; Foltz et al., 2004).

One clue as to the basis for the cocaine-induced deficits in attention is provided by the clinical findings of changes in the infant's startle response as well as in neurophysiological evidence of alterations in brainstem transmission time. Initial clinical studies suggested an altered startle reactivity to a variety of stimuli (e.g., Chasnoff et al., 1985, 1989; Griffith, 1988) and impairments in auditory information processing, characterized by impaired habituation in infancy (Potter et al., 2000). Although ordinal measurement of Brazelton Behavioral Assessment Scale remains rather subjective and is a caveat of the earlier studies, reflex modification procedures also reported cocaine-exposed infants were more reactive (glabellar reflex) and more responsive to auditory stimuli, as indicated by an increased blink when the tone accompanied the tap (Anday et al., 1989). Significantly depressed startle reactivity has also been reported in prenatal cocaine-exposed children at 54 months (Mayes et al., 1998). Although there are neither striking nor consistent data across the various rodent models to corroborate the clinical *in utero* cocaine effects on the infant startle response or its plasticity (Foss and Riley, 1988, 1991a,b; Dow-Edwards and Hughes, 1995; Vorhees et al., 1995, 2000; Hughes et al., 1996; Overstreet et al., 2000), to the best of our knowledge, there is no preclinical data available with the more clinically relevant intravenous route of cocaine administration.

Neurophysiologically based clinical studies have consistently reported alterations in auditory brainstem responses (ABR, or also called brainstem auditory-evoked responses) in prenatal cocaine-exposed infants (Shih et al., 1988; Salamy et al., 1990; Cone-Wesson and Spingarn, 1993; Lester et al., 2003; Tan-Laxa et al., 2004). Prolonged interpeak latencies of the ABR of infants prenatally cocaine-exposed was reported relative to non-exposed controls (Shih et al., 1988) and replicated in both term and low-birth weight infants exposed *in utero* to cocaine (Salamy et al., 1990) as well as in infants matched for birth weight and conceptual age (Cone-Wesson and Spingarn, 1993). No increased incidence of hearing impairment was found in these early clinical studies. Further, the one report that failed to find effects of prenatal cocaine exposure on the ABR used relatively low intensity stimuli (30 dB) as the aim of that study was to ascertain if there were hearing deficits consequent to prenatal cocaine exposure (Carzoli et al., 1991). Tan-Laxa et al. (2004) reported abnormal interpeak latencies in prenatal cocaine-exposed neonates, compared with non-exposed controls, confirmed with meconium drug analysis. Lester et al. (2003) confirmed and expanded the effects of prenatal cocaine on prolonging ABR interpeak latencies at 1 month of age, and did so in a large sample in which covariate adjustments were made (other drugs, gestational age, social class); the main effects were attributable to heavy maternal cocaine use. Prolonged interpeak latencies, particularly as a function of increasing stimulation rates, may indicate that neural recovery time is slower for prenatal cocaine-exposed infants, such as attributable to neurotransmitter depletion or dysfunction. Prolongation of the I–V latency, which provides information regarding the integrity of the eighth cranial nerve to the auditory brain stem, may indicate delayed brainstem auditory system development (Salamy, 1984; Krumholz et al., 1985). In a rodent model, prolongation of the interpeak latencies was also observed as a function of prenatal cocaine exposure, but only at the highest dose (100 mg/kg/day, subcutaneous), only at 35 days of age (not at 6–10 months of age), and only at the highest stimulus intensity (Church and Overbeck, 1990). The consistent ABR evidence with *in utero* cocaine-exposed infants, in conjunction with the limited animal model data, collectively suggests an ontogenetic impairment in auditory information processing.

Auditory processing disorders are commonly thought to be the basis of some language problems. Rate of processing of brief, rapidly presented, non-linguistic auditory stimuli in infancy has been shown to the single best predictor of subsequent language development (Benasich and Tallal, 2002). Although the effects of prenatal cocaine on preschool language development are commonly referred to as equivocal and/or subtle (e.g., Singer et al., 2001; Beeghly et al., 2006; Dinehart et al., 2009), it is of particular note that significant positive associations of language decrements with prenatal cocaine are reported in covariate-controlled prospective studies by Singer's group (Singer et al., 2001; Lewis et al., 2004, 2007, 2011) and by Bandstra's group (Bandstra et al., 2002, 2004, 2011; Morrow et al., 2003, 2004). Not surprisingly, other large covariate-controlled prospective studies failed to find such effects, as documented by Hurt and colleagues (Hurt et al.,

1997, 2009; Betancourt et al., 2011), the cohort studied by Frank and colleagues (Frank et al., 2005; Beeghly et al., 2006) and by others (Delaney-Black et al., 2000; Kilbride et al., 2000, 2006). One possible mitigating factor in the disparate outcomes on language development within the larger prospective longitudinal studies is that of retention rate. Clearly, retention has been high among those studies that have reported positive associations of prenatal cocaine with language decrements (e.g., 89% of infant cohort assessed at 3 years, Morrow et al., 2004; 79% of the original cohort available for follow up at 3, 5, and 7 years, Bandstra et al., 2004; 77% of the original cohort through 10 years, Lewis et al., 2011). Although it is tempting to argue that the absence of an effect of prenatal cocaine on language may reflect low retention rates, e.g., 55%, this lowest rate was across 20 years (Betancourt et al., 2011). Perhaps most importantly, to the best of our knowledge, none of the large scale prospective studies have reported any differential effect of prenatal cocaine on retention rates. Collectively, these studies suggest that if an effect of prenatal cocaine on language is detected in a study cohort, a stable language decrement will likely be observed through to adolescence.

Because of these clinical and preclinical reports of prenatal cocaine-induced alterations in attentional processes and auditory information processing (with implications for receptive language development), and that the regulation of sensory processing serves as a gating mechanism to optimize attention, the present paper sought to investigate potential prenatal cocaine-induced alterations in auditory information processing in a rodent model within auditory startle, habituation, and reflex modification paradigms. The ASR and its plasticity [habituation, prepulse inhibition (PPI)] have much to recommend it for drug abuse studies, including its rapidity, its objectivity, its sensitivity, and its suitability for use in both humans and a variety of laboratory animals (Ison, 1984). Accordingly, the goals of the present study were fivefold. We sought to determine if prenatal cocaine, administered via the clinically relevant IV route and with doses that mimic the peak arterial levels of cocaine used by humans (cf. Evans et al., 1996; Booze et al., 1997): (1) alters the development of the ASR in preweanling rats, (2) has a long-term effect on the ASR and its habituation, (3) produces any differential effect on the ASR as a function of the sex and/or stage of the estrous cycle of the offspring, (4) alters the preattentive process of sensory gating as indexed by PPI, and (5) exerts its effects on the ASR via alterations in the noradrenergic system.

MATERIALS AND METHODS
ANIMALS
Nulliparous female Long–Evans rats were obtained from Harlan Sprague-Dawley (Indianapolis, IN, USA) at 11–12 weeks of age. The animals were pair-housed and given *ad libitum* access to both food (Purina Rat Chow) and water for 2 weeks prior to the beginning of the experiment. The animals were maintained according to NIH guidelines in AAALAC-accredited facilities. The animal facility was maintained at $21 \pm 2°C$, $50 \pm 10\%$ relative humidity, and had a 12-h light: 12-h dark cycle with lights on at 0700 h (EST). The protocols for the use of rats in this research were approved by the university IACUC.

SURGERY
Catheterization of the female rats with a vascular access port was performed as previously described in detail (Mactutus et al., 1994). Briefly, animals were anesthetized with a mixture of ketamine (100 mg/kg/ml) and xylazine (3.3 mg/kg/ml); this anesthetic mixture was chosen over pentobarbital because of the potent effect of the latter agent on cytochrome P450 activity (LaBella and Queen, 1993; Loch et al., 1995). A sterile Intracath IV catheter (22 ga., Becton/Dickinson and Co., Franklin Lakes, NJ, USA) with a Luer lock injection cap (Medex Inc., Carlsbad, CA, USA) was tunneled under the skin from the back (between the shoulder blades) and inserted into the jugular vein approximately 3 mm in the direction of the right atria. Two sutures were placed on either side of the catheter to hold the catheter in place. Both the cap and the catheter were implanted dorsally under the skin in a subcutaneous pouch. Following the surgery, animals were observed periodically and returned to the vivarium upon recovery from the anesthesia. The catheters were flushed daily with approximately 0.2 ml of 2.5% heparinized saline and the animals were observed for any signs of discomfort or behavioral distress. Body weights were recorded prior to the surgery and daily throughout recovery.

ANIMAL MATING
At 4–7 days following surgery, the females were group-housed with males overnight for breeding. Vaginal cytology and the presence of sperm were checked daily in the females. A sperm positive female was considered pregnant at gestation day (GD)0 and individually housed in plastic cages with wood-chip bedding throughout pregnancy and lactation.

EXPERIMENTAL DESIGN/DRUG TREATMENT
The pregnant catheterized female Long–Evans rats were randomly assigned to one of four treatment groups (ns = 12–13) and received 0.0 (saline), 0.5, 1.0, or 3.0 mg/kg of cocaine hydrochloride (Sigma, St. Louis, MO, USA). Cocaine and saline injections were administered in a volume of 1 ml/kg, via the intravenous access port, once per day from GD8–14 and twice per day from GD15–20. Weights of dams were taken daily. Day of birth was considered postnatal day 0 (D0). Pups were culled to four males and four females per liter. Pup body weights were obtained on D1 and thereafter at weekly intervals.

The IV injection procedure was chosen because it mimics the rapidly peaking pharmacokinetic profile following inhalation or IV injection of cocaine in humans (Isenschmid et al., 1992). The 3.0-mg/kg dose produces peak arterial plasma levels that are similar to those reported for humans IV administered 32 mg of cocaine (Evans et al., 1996; Booze et al., 1997). The acute heart rate and blood pressure responses in the late gestation pregnant rat are similar to those produced in a variety of other species (Mactutus et al., 2000). Under experimental conditions, this dose is self-administered by "users" multiple times in a 2.5-h session (Fischman and Schuster, 1982), and thus represents a low or recreational dose, highly relevant to the clinical situation being modeled. The lower doses (0.5 and 1.0 mg/kg) of cocaine in the male rat also produced peak arterial levels that reasonably approximated the peak arterial levels in humans IV administered 8 or

16 mg of cocaine (Evans et al., 1996; Booze et al., 1997). This regimen (route, dose, and rate) produces no evidence of overt maternal or fetal toxicity, no maternal seizure activity, no effect on maternal weight, and no effect on offspring growth or mortality (e.g., Mactutus et al., 1994; Mactutus, 1999; Foltz et al., 2004). Furthermore, this IV injection procedure does not reduce food intake of dams even when utilizing a cocaine dose as high as 6 mg/kg (Robinson et al., 1994), precluding the need for pair-fed controls.

APPARATUS
The commercially available startle apparatus (SR-Lab Startle Reflex System, San Diego Instruments, Inc.) was used, but with a 10-cm thick double-walled, 81-cm × 81-cm × 116-cm isolation cabinet (external dimensions; Industrial Acoustic Company, INC., Bronx, NY, USA), rather than the 1.91-cm thick ABS plastic cabinet offered with this system. The high-frequency loudspeaker of the SR-Lab system (Radio Shack model #40-1278B, frequency range of 5–16 kHz) was mounted inside the chamber, 30 cm above the perspex test cylinder, for delivery of the auditory stimuli. The perspex test cylinder varied in size with the age of the animal: 3.8 cm internal diameter (ID) for the weanling rats and 8.9 cm ID for the adult rats. The perspex test cylinder was positioned on a 12.5-cm × 20-cm perspex platform, centrally located within the test chamber. A piezoelectric accelerometer, permanently affixed to the base of each perspex cylinder, converted the deflection of the perspex cylinder produced by the animal's startle response to an analog signal. All accelerometer signals were then digitized (12 bit A–D) and saved to a hard disk on a Pentium class computer. Auditory stimulus intensities were measured and calibrated with a sound level meter (Extech Instruments, Waltham, MA, USA). Response sensitivities were calibrated using the SR-LAB startle calibration system.

GENERAL PROCEDURES
For all paradigms, each animal was tested individually in the dark. All white noise stimuli were passed as broad-band through the range possible by the horn tweeter (5–16 kHz). This broad-band white noise spans the peak sensitivity of the audiogram of the Long–Evans rat at 8 kHz (Heffner et al., 1994). For all paradigms, the dependent measures collected were peak response amplitude within a 100-ms sampling window, average response amplitude across the 100-ms sampling window, and response latency. Within the constraints of the software, response latency represents the time from the onset of the startle stimulus to the time of the peak response, rather than the more traditional definition of latency, which would be until the onset of the startle response. The error introduced by this protocol is estimated to be approximately 2–3 ms, accounting for roughly 10% of the error in response latency values.

Preweaning ASR and habituation
At 18–20 days of age, one male and one female were randomly selected for a preweaning assessment. The ASR was tested, for approximately 11 min, using the following parameters: 5 min adaptation, 70 dB(A) background, followed by 36 startle trials, 100 dB(A) white noise stimulus of 20 ms duration, and a fixed 10-s intertrial interval (ITI). The startle stimulus intensity was 120 dB(A) at 2.5 cm from the speaker, but 100 dB(A) measured inside the perspex test cylinder. Habituation across the 36 trials was examined in six-trial blocks.

Adult ASR and habituation
The adult assessment (D90+) followed the parameters as described for ASR for each animal's preweaning assessment.

Adult PPI
The animals were tested again approximately 14 days later, but with the PPI protocol. All rats were tested for approximately 18 min. Only the 3.0-mg/kg prenatal cocaine and vehicle control groups were tested in PPI. The females were tested in diestrus vs. estrus to assess any potential influence of estrous cycle. Under PPI, the animals received a 5-min adaptation period, followed by six single startle only white noise stimuli [100 dB(A), 5–16 kHz], 20 ms duration, as habituation trials with a fixed ITI of 10 s, and then 36 PPI trials [interstimulus intervals (ISIs) of 0, 8, 40, 80, 120, or 4000 ms] with a variable ITI of 20 s (range of 15–25 s), assigned by a Latin-square design. The prepulse stimulus intensity was an 85-dB(A) white noise stimulus (5–16 kHz) with a duration of 20 ms. The incorporation of a range of ISIs was fundamental to establishment of a relatively precise and defined response function, and consequently, a more accurate assessment of response inhibition. Similar ISIs have been employed in studies of the ontogeny of PPI (Parisi and Ison, 1979, 1981) as well as alterations in PPI as a function of developmental drug or toxin exposure (Ison, 1984; Fitting et al., 2006a,b,c; Lacy et al., 2011); these intervals produced clear, definable response inhibition and response latency curves. Given the constraints of the software regarding the use of any ISI intervals shorter than the prepulse stimulus duration, the ISI represented the time from the offset of the prepulse stimulus to the onset of the startle stimulus.

Adult idazoxan–ASR and habituation
The final testing of ASR of each animal occurred at approximately 120 days of age. Each animal received a subcutaneous injection of 0.5 mg/kg idazoxan (Sigma, St. Louis, MO, USA), an α_2-adrenergic receptor antagonist, immediately prior to testing. A 10-min adaptation period was the only variation to the ASR parameters stated above; a procedure implemented to permit reasonable absorption and distribution of the drug.

STATISTICAL ANALYSIS
Weight gains of dams during their gestation period were converted to a percentage of weekly and total weight gain. The litter parameters of gestation length, number of male and female pups per litter, and mean D1 body weights of male and female pups were compared based on litter means. All data were analyzed by ANOVA techniques (Statistical Solutions Ltd, 2009). Log_{10} transformations of the peak amplitude response were employed, as necessary to help provide data that were consistent with the normality assumption of ANOVA. For repeated measures factors, either orthogonal decompositions were used for those variables that classically violate compound symmetry assumptions (e.g., trials) or the Greenhouse–Geisser df correction factor was used (Greenhouse and Geisser, 1959). Tests of simple mains effects and

specific linear contrasts were also used to evaluate dose-dependent and trial-dependent effects of the cocaine treatment, respectively (Winer, 1971). An α level of $p \leq 0.05$ was the significance level set for rejection of the null hypothesis.

RESULTS
OFFSPRING GROWTH
Prenatal IV cocaine, administered from GD8–20, had no adverse effect on any of the maternal or litter parameters measured, including maternal weight gain during pregnancy, gestation length, birth weight of male or females pups, or number of male or female pups (**Table 1**; $Fs < 1.8$). No latent effects of prenatal cocaine on adult body weight were apparent (**Table 2**; $Fs < 1.0$).

ASR-PREWEANLING
The peak amplitude measure of the ASR in the preweanling rats is portrayed in **Figure 1** (36-trial mean) and **Figure 2** (habituation across six-trial blocks). Most importantly, specific

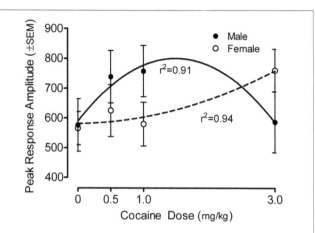

FIGURE 1 | Mean (±SEM) peak amplitude of the ASR in the preweanling rats illustrates the quadratic cocaine dose by offspring sex interaction [$F(1,78) = 5.95$, $p \leq 0.017$]. For the male offspring the best fit quadratic function accounted for 91% of the variance across dose; for the female offspring the best fit quadratic function accounted for 94% of the variance across dose. A similar finding of a quadratic cocaine dose by offspring sex interaction with the average amplitude measure was found [$F(1,78) = 5.0$, $p \leq 0.028$]; those data are not shown).

Table 1 | Prenatal treatment (mean ± SEM).

	Cocaine dose			
	0.0 mg/kg	0.5 mg/kg	1.0 mg/kg	3.0 mg/kg
N	12	13	13	13
Gest. length	22.0 ± 0.2	22.0 ± 0.1	22.1 ± 0.1	22.1 ± 0.1
% wt gain	53.5 ± 3.2	54.8 ± 2.2	60.7 ± 2.0	57.7 ± 2.1
Litter size	10.8 ± 1.0	11.4 ± 0.8	11.4 ± 0.8	11.8 ± 0.5
D1 wt (g) – males	7.9 ± 0.1	7.9 ± 0.2	8.0 ± 0.1	8.0 ± 0.2
D1 wt (g) – females	7.4 ± 0.1	7.6 ± 0.2	7.6 ± 0.1	7.4 ± 0.2
No. of males	5.1 ± 0.5	5.2 ± 0.7	6.4 ± 0.7	5.7 ± 0.5
No. of females	5.0 ± 0.7	6.2 ± 0.6	5.0 ± 0.7	6.1 ± 0.5

No significant prenatal treatment effects were present on the maternal/litter parameters examined ($Fs < 1.8$).

Table 2 | Adult body weights (g) (mean ± SEM).

	Cocaine (mg/kg)	D100	D140
Male	0.0	475.3 ± 8.9	577.2 ± 11.2
	0.5	476.1 ± 11.6	583.4 ± 14.0
	1.0	483.9 ± 9.0	600.8 ± 11.6
	3.0	469.8 ± 7.5	582.1 ± 15.4
Female	0.0	282.8 ± 3.6	324.4 ± 5.8
	0.5	277.9 ± 5.3	315.8 ± 6.0
	1.0	291.6 ± 6.4	329.4 ± 9.2
	3.0	283.7 ± 4.9	326.2 ± 6.1

A main effect of sex [$F(3,77) = 1270.7$, $p < 0.0001$], but no significant main effect of prenatal cocaine, nor interaction of cocaine with sex of the offspring, were found on the adult body weight ($Fs < 1.0$).

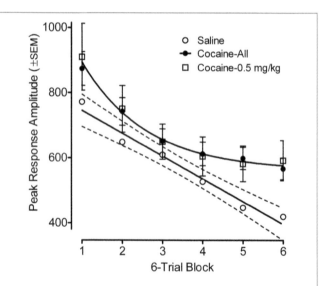

FIGURE 2 | Mean (±SEM) peak amplitude of the ASR in the preweanling rats, illustrated as a function of six-trial blocks, depicts the retarding of within-session habituation by prenatal IV cocaine. Comparison of the average prenatal cocaine group habituation with that for the saline group found a prenatal treatment by six-trial block interaction [$F(1,78) = 2.55$, $p_{GG} \leq 0.045$], with significant group differences apparent on trial blocks five and six [$F(1,82) = 5.8$, $p \leq 0.018$ and $F(1,82) = 5.1$, $p \leq 0.027$, respectively]. The best fit linear regression for the habituation curve of the saline group accounted for 97% of the variance; the best fit function for the average cocaine habituation was a quadratic that accounted for >99% of the variance. A similar pattern of differences is also illustrated when comparing the low 0.5 mg/kg cocaine dose vs. saline.

assessment of dose–response functions indicated a significant prenatal cocaine dose by offspring sex interaction [quadratic dose by sex, $F(1,78) = 5.95$, $p \leq 0.017$]. Response amplitude was increased

>18% for M > F (0.5 mg/kg), >30% for M > F (1 mg/kg) and >30% for F > M (3 mg/kg). The best fit quadratic function for males accounted for 91% of the variance ($r^2 = 0.91$), whereas the best fit quadratic fit for females accounted for 94% of the variance ($r^2 = 0.94$). A comparable pattern of results was seen with the average response amplitude measure, with a significant prenatal cocaine dose by offspring sex interaction [quadratic dose by sex, $F(1,78) = 5.0, p \leq 0.028$]; these redundant data are not illustrated. There were no statistically significant effects detectable on average response latency. The mean (±SEM) response latency across all pups was 30.6 ± 0.3 ms; all treatment/sex group means were within the range of 29.1–32.7 ms (data not illustrated).

Habituation of the ASR across six-trial blocks revealed a prominent linear decrease [$F(1,78) = 106.5, p \leq 0.001$] in peak response amplitude across trials with the contribution of a quadratic component [$F(1,78) = 10.4, p \leq 0.002$]. A comparison of the average prenatal cocaine group habituation vs. that for the saline group revealed a significant six-trial block by prenatal treatment interaction [$F(1,78) = 2.55, p_{GG} \leq 0.045$], with significant group differences apparent on trial blocks five and six [$F(1,82) = 5.8, p \leq 0.018$ and $F(1,82) = 5.1, p \leq 0.027$, respectively]. The best fit linear regression for the habituation curve of the saline group accounted for 97% of the variance; the best fit function for the average cocaine habituation was a quadratic that accounted for 99.6% of the variance. A comparison of the lowest 0.5 mg/kg cocaine dose group vs. the saline group found a very similar pattern, although the three-way interaction of six-trial block, prenatal cocaine treatment, and offspring sex was statistically significant [$F(5,190) = 3.12, p_{GG} \leq 0.021$]. The linear six-trial block by prenatal treatment interaction was prominent in males [$F(1,38) = 10.10, p \leq 0.003$], but was not evident in females. Nevertheless, significant treatment group differences (0.5 mg/kg cocaine vs. saline) were again suggested on trial blocks five and six [$F(1,38) = 3.91, p \leq 0.055$ and $F(1,38) = 5.0, p \leq 0.031$, respectively].

ASR-ADULT

The peak amplitude measure of the ASR in the adult offspring is portrayed in **Figure 3** (36-trial mean) and **Figure 4** (habituation across six-trial blocks). The peak amplitude of the ASR in the adults displayed an overall effect of prenatal dose of cocaine [$F(3,80) = 6.0, p < 0.001$], but neither of sex of the offspring nor the interaction of dose and sex approached significance ($ps > 0.10$). Trend analyses indicated the prenatal treatment factor displayed a prominent linear dose–response effect [$F(1,80) = 14.5, p \leq 0.001$] with a maximal facilitation of >75%.

The average amplitude of the ASR in the offspring as adults also indicated an augmented overall effect of prenatal dose of cocaine [$F(3,80) = 4.8, p \leq 0.004$], but neither sex of the offspring nor the interaction of dose and sex approached significance ($ps > 0.10$). Trend analyses indicated the prenatal treatment factor displayed a prominent linear dose–response effect [$F(1,80) = 11.1, p \leq 0.001$] with a maximal facilitation of ~85%; this redundant data is not illustrated.

There was no overall effect of prenatal dose of cocaine on peak response latency of the ASR in the offspring as adults [$F(3,80) = 1.5, p > 0.10$], sex of the offspring nor on the interaction of dose and sex [$Fs < 1.0$]. Further, trend analyses failed

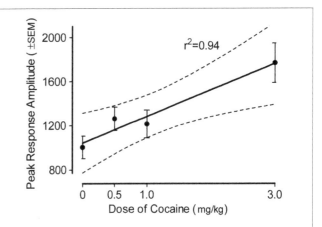

FIGURE 3 | Mean (±SEM) peak amplitude of the ASR in the offspring as adults. The effect of prenatal dose of cocaine [$F(3,80) = 6.0, p \leq 0.001$] with a prominent linear dose–response component [$F(1,80) = 14.5, p \leq 0.001$] accounted for 84% of the dose group variance. A similar prominent linear dose–response effect [$F(1,80) = 10.9, p \leq 0.0015$] was noted on the average amplitude measure (data not shown).

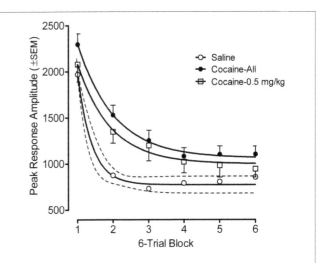

FIGURE 4 | Mean (±SEM) peak amplitude of the ASR in the offspring as adults shown as a function of six-trial blocks. The best fit function for the habituation curves of the saline group, the average cocaine group, and the 0.5-mg/kg cocaine group were each quadratic fits that accounted for >99% of the variance. Examination of habituation across all prenatal treatment dose groups revealed significant group differences were apparent on trial blocks one through six, inclusive [$Fs(3,80) \geq 2.7, p \leq 0.05$]. Thus, within-session habituation of the ASR in adulthood was also retarded by prenatal IV cocaine.

to detect any systematic relation among the treatment dose groups. The mean (±SEM) response latency across all rats was 29.1 ± 0.6 ms; all treatment group means were within the range of 28.1–31.2 ms (data not illustrated). The numeric change as a function of treatment ranged from between −3 and +8% relative to vehicle controls.

Habituation of the ASR across six-trial blocks revealed both prominent linear and quadratic components to the decrease in peak response amplitude across trials [$F(1,80) = 135.6, p \leq 0.001$

and $F(1,80) = 83.2$, $p \leq 0.001$, respectively]. The best fit function for the habituation curve of the saline group was a quadratic fit that accounted for >99% of the variance; similarly, the best fit function for the average cocaine habituation was a quadratic accounting for >99% of the variance; these curves were significantly different ($p < 0.001$). The best fit function for the 0.5-mg/kg cocaine group also accounted for >99% of the variance. Examination of habituation across all prenatal treatment dose groups revealed significant group differences were apparent on trial blocks one through six, inclusive [$F(3,80) = 2.8, p \leq 0.045$, $F(3,80) = 7.5, p \leq 0.001$, $F(3,80) = 5.6, p \leq 0.002$, $F(3,80) = 2.9$, $p \leq 0.039$, $F(3,80) = 2.8$, $p \leq 0.048$, $F(3,80) = 2.7, p \leq 0.05$]. A comparison of the average prenatal cocaine group habituation vs. that for the saline group revealed an overall prenatal cocaine effect [$F(1,84) = 5.9$, $p \leq 0.018$] with significant group differences apparent on trial blocks two and three [$F(1,84) = 10.2$, $p \leq 0.002$ and $F(1,84) = 6.2, p \leq 0.014$, respectively]. A comparison of the lowest 0.5 mg/kg cocaine dose group vs. the saline group found a very similar pattern; significant treatment group differences (0.5 mg/kg cocaine vs. saline) were again suggested on trial blocks two and three [$F(1,40) = 7.9, p \leq 0.008$ and $F(1,40) = 5.3$, $p \leq 0.026$, respectively].

ESTROUS CYCLE

Comparison of the peak response amplitude (mean ± SEM: 1227 ± 166.4 vs. 1355 ± 176.3), average response amplitude (280 ± 26.1 vs. 320 ± 30.1) and response latency (28.3 ± 0.76 vs. 29.7 ± 0.88) in the adult females as a function of stage of the estrous cycle (diestrus vs. estrus, respectively) demonstrated that there was no significant effect on any of the dependent measures [$Fs(1,20) < 1.1$].

PREPULSE INHIBITION

An overall effect of the prenatal dose of cocaine was detected on peak amplitude on the habituation trials (six-trial average) of the PPI protocol [$F(1,34) = 11.2, p \leq 0.002$], but neither sex of the offspring nor the interaction of dose and sex were significant ($ps > 0.10$). A marked facilitation was observed in both the males (65%) and females (55%) that had prenatally received the 3.0-mg/kg dose of cocaine. The average amplitude measure displayed a similar prenatal cocaine effect [$F(1,34) = 11.3$ $p \leq 0.002$], with pronounced facilitation in both males (99%) and female (82%).

The PPI peak response amplitude data from the adult offspring is illustrated in **Figure 5**, across the ISI function. The peak amplitude on the PPI trials as a function of the ISI (six-trial average/ISI) showed that the main effects of prenatal treatment and sex, as well as the interaction of treatment and sex, were not significant. The ISI function was best described by a quadratic fit [$F(1,34) = 138.1$ $p \leq 0.001$ and $F(1,34) = 75.2, p \leq 0.001$, peak and average amplitude measures, respectively]. Of greater interest, however, a significant prenatal treatment effect by prepulse ISI was observed [$F(5,170) = 4.0$, $p_{GG} \leq 0.038$, with the suggestion of linear and quadratic components $F(1,34) = 6.4, p \leq 0.016$ and $F(1,34) = 3.8, p \leq 0.059$, respectively]. The average amplitude measure similarly confirmed a significant prenatal treatment by prepulse ISI interaction [$F(5,170) = 4.7, p_{GG} \leq 0.026$], with

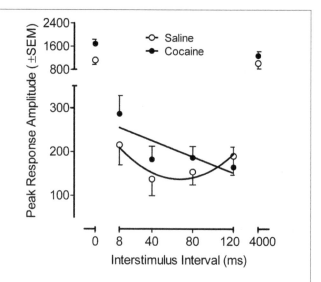

FIGURE 5 | Mean (±SEM) peak amplitude on the prepulse inhibition trials as a function of the ISI (six-trial average/ISI). A significant prenatal treatment effect by prepulse ISI was observed [$F(5,170) = 4.0$, $p_{GG} \leq 0.038$]. The characteristic quadratic function across ISIs 8–120, accounted for 88% of the variance in the control group. In contrast the progressive linear change in inhibition across ISI for the 3.0-mg/kg prenatal cocaine group accounted for 67% of the variance. A shift in the peak of inhibition from 40 to 120 ms is also apparent.

linear and quadratic components [$F(1,34) = 5.6, p \leq 0.024$, and $F(1,34) = 4.6, p \leq 0.039$, respectively]. Specific examination of the prepulse trials (ISIs 4–120) noted differential modulation of inhibition by ISI as a function of prenatal cocaine treatment. The characteristic quadratic function displayed by the saline control group account for 88% of the variance whereas a linear function accounted for 67% of the variance for the prenatal cocaine group. The different functional characterization of the inhibition curve further demonstrated a shift in the peak of inhibition from 40 to 120 ms. The evidence for an effect of prenatal cocaine treatment on the control trials (0 and 4000 ms ISI intervals) was suggested, but not consistent [peak amplitude, $F(1,34) = 3.4, p \leq 0.072$ vs. average amplitude, $F(1,34) = 4.2, p \leq 0.048$]. The calculation of a percent PPI measure, to take into account any such difference in the control trials, failed to detect any overall difference in magnitude of inhibition (prenatal saline, 87.2% vs. prenatal cocaine, 87.7%). Thus, although prenatal cocaine exposure did not alter the derived percent PPI measure, the assessment of inhibition across ISI displayed a functional alteration in modulation of inhibition by ISI, in other words, an alteration in sensorimotor gating.

The response latency measure for the PPI paradigm with the adult offspring is portrayed in **Figure 6**. An examination of response latencies across the inhibition trials (8–120 ms), where the functional alterations in response inhibition was noted above, confirmed there was a pronounced effect of ISI on response latency [$F(3,102) = 20.5, p \leq 0.001$, with a prominent linear component, $F(1,34) = 44.4, p \leq 0.001$], but ISI did not interact with prenatal treatment. Specifically, all groups generally displayed shorter latencies with the shorter ISIs. Nevertheless, a significant offspring sex effect [$F(1,34 = 4.5, p \leq 0.041$] as well as a prenatal treatment by offspring sex interaction [$F(1,34) = 5.2, p \leq 0.030$] was

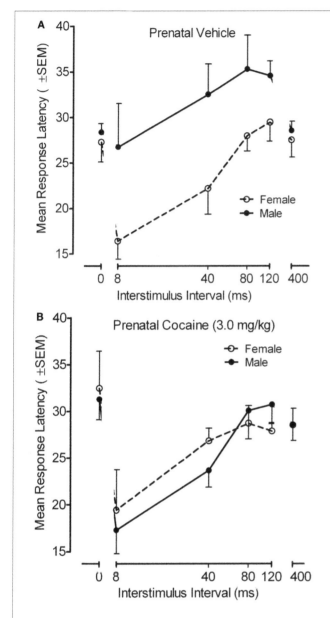

FIGURE 6 | (A) Mean (±SEM) response latency in as a function of ISI and sex of the offspring for the prenatal **(A)** vehicle- and **(B)** cocaine-treated animals. A prenatal treatment by offspring sex interaction [$F(1,34) = 5.2$, $p \leq 0.030$] was observed on the inhibition trials (ISIs of 8–120 ms). The significant sex difference in response latency for the saline control group [$F(1,34) = 9.2$, $p \leq 0.005$] was not present in the prenatal cocaine-treated adults [$F < 1.0$]. The most marked treatment group difference in response latency occurred at the 40-ms ISI [$F(1,34) = 8.0$, $p \leq 0.008$].

observed on the inhibition trials (ISIs of 8–120 ms). An examination of this interaction revealed that there was a significant sex difference in response latency for the saline control group [$F(1,34) = 9.2$, $p \leq 0.005$], which was not present in the prenatal cocaine-treated adults [$F < 1.0$]. From an alternative view, there was a significant prenatal treatment effect in the male adult offspring [$F(1,34) = 6.6$, $p \leq 0.015$], but not in the female adult offspring [$F < 1.0$]. The locus of these group differences appeared to be the attributable to the difference in response latency at the 40-ms ISI [$F(1,34) = 8.0$, $p \leq 0.008$].

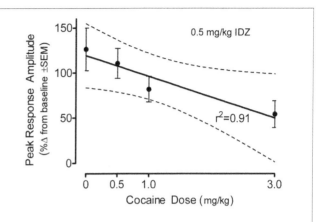

FIGURE 7 | Mean (±SEM) percent change in the peak amplitude of the ASR following idazoxan (0.5 mg/kg) administration in the adult offspring shown as a function of prenatal cocaine dose. There was a significant prenatal treatment effect [$F(3,79) = 3.1$, $p \leq 0.03$] which was characterized by a prominent linear trend [$F(1,79) = 8.9$, $p \leq 0.004$]. A similar linear trend was shown by the average amplitude response data [$F(1,79) = 4.2$, $p \leq 0.043$] (not shown).

IDAZOXAN

The percent change in the peak amplitude of the ASR following idazoxan administration in the adult offspring is displayed as a function of prenatal cocaine dose in **Figure 7**. There was a significant prenatal treatment effect [$F(3,79) = 3.1$, $p \leq 0.031$] which was characterized by a prominent linear trend [$F(1,79) = 8.9$, $p \leq 0.004$]. Although an effect of offspring sex approached significance [$F(1,79) = 3.6$, $p \leq 0.062$], there was little evidence for an interaction of prenatal cocaine dose and sex of the offspring was [$F(1,79) = 1.3$]. An evaluation of the percent change in the average amplitude of the ASR confirmed the major finding of a differential sensitivity to idazoxan as a linear function of prenatal cocaine dose [$F(1,79) = 4.2$, $p \leq 0.043$]. The evidence for idazoxan-induced changes in response latency [$F(3,79) = 3.5$, $p < 0.019$] displayed a prominent quadratic component across increasing prenatal cocaine dose [$F(1,79) = 9.3$, $p < 0.003$] having no obvious association with the response amplitude effects of idazoxan. The response latency data (mean ± SEM), across increasing prenatal cocaine dose, were 3.0 ± 3.1, 8.7 ± 3.7, 6.4 ± 4.5, and $-10.3 \pm 7.0\%$, respectively.

DISCUSSION

Administration of cocaine to pregnant rats from the time of implantation until parturition produced significant alterations in auditory information processing in the Long–Evans rat within auditory startle, habituation, and reflex modification paradigms. Three prominent effects observed were: (1) the magnitude of the ASR, as indexed by waveform amplitude, was significantly increased as a function of prenatal dose of cocaine; (2) decreased rates of within-session habituation were observed at even the lowest maternally administered dose; and (3) differential sensitivity to PPI was noted as a function of prenatal cocaine with manipulation of the ISI function; this differential sensitivity of the preattentive process of sensorimotor gating was observed for both response amplitude and response latency measures. Perhaps more importantly, (4) significant alterations in each of the three paradigms were found in adulthood, regardless of whether or not there was evidence available for the persistence, as opposed to a latent emergence, of the effects. Further, (5) an alteration in the function of the noradrenergic system in adulthood was suggested by the prenatal cocaine dose-dependent attenuation of the ability of 0.5 mg/kg idazoxan to enhance the ASR. Finally, these alterations in auditory information processing were observed with cocaine being delivered by the clinically relevant IV route and at physiologically relevant doses; conditions under which no adverse effects on maternal/litter parameters were significantly altered.

Early clinical data suggested an altered startle reactivity to a variety of stimuli (e.g., Chasnoff et al., 1985, 1989; Griffith, 1988) may be observed in prenatal cocaine-exposed infants. Subsequent experimental data reported increased responsiveness to auditory stimuli (Anday et al., 1989); but depressed startle reactivity has also been noted (Mayes et al., 1998). The increased ASR response presently reported during the preweaning period ($\sim$30%) and in adulthood (>75%) was particularly notable in light of the relatively modest, if any, changes available in the literature with rodent models (Foss and Riley, 1988, 1991a,b; Dow-Edwards and Hughes, 1995; Vorhees et al., 1995, 2000; Hughes et al., 1996). In the initial, preliminary study, the ASR of prenatal cocaine rats (60 mg/kg/day, peroral (PO) route, GD14–21) was enhanced at 90, but not at 60, days of age (Foss and Riley, 1988). However, a very systematic replication study by the same laboratory, with the addition of pair-fed controls, and a second set of rats administered cocaine via the subcutaneous (SC) route (40 mg/kg/day, GD8–21) failed to find any significant changes in the ASR, in startle habituation, or in reflex modification tests that could be attributed to prenatal exposure to cocaine (Foss and Riley, 1991a). Not surprisingly, prenatal cocaine during a more restricted period of gestation (GD14–21, SC route) also failed to significantly affect the peak ASR in adult rats (Foss and Riley, 1991b). Repeated daily dosing (five doses/day × 20 mg/kg/dose) on GD7–12 or GD13–18, failed to affect the ASR on D50–52 (Vorhees et al., 1995). In the one "positive" peer-reviewed prenatal study, cocaine administered intragastric (IG; GD8–22) failed to affect the peak ASR at 60 days of age, although there was a small, statistically significant decrease in the ASR of females (Hughes et al., 1996). Even the neonatal rat model, promoted to more specifically mimic fetal brain exposure to cocaine during the third trimester of human pregnancy (Dobbing and Sands, 1979), has provided, at best, equivocal results (Dow-Edwards and Hughes, 1995; Vorhees et al., 2000). Comparing D1–10 vs. D11–20 treatment with cocaine revealed no significant alteration in the ASR on an initial test at 60–65 days of age (Dow-Edwards and Hughes, 1995). In the "positive" study, neonatal cocaine-treated rats (60 mg/kg, SC, PND 1–10) showed a significantly augmented ($\sim$30%) peak ASR at D50–52; however, an analysis of covariance adjusting for significant cocaine-induced decreases in body weight, reduced the augmentation to a statistically non-significant level (Vorhees et al., 2000). Clearly, there are neither striking nor consistent positive data within the extant rodent models to corroborate the clinical *in utero* cocaine effects on the infant ASR.

Dose-dependent alterations in the ASR characterized by prenatal cocaine treatment were apparent during both the preweaning period and in adulthood. The early alterations in the ASR were differently expressed dependent upon the sex of the offspring. Prenatal cocaine-exposed males were most adversely affected by the low and middle doses of cocaine, as reflected in a quadratic dose–response fit, whereas the females were most adversely affected by the high-dose of cocaine, as reflected in a growth curve fit. In adulthood, a linear dose–response function, independent of offspring sex, captured 94% of the variance in ASR amplitude. The presence of a sex-dependent effect of cocaine well before puberty, but not in adulthood, on the same dependent measure suggests the likelihood of an organizational effect on the brain (Gorski et al., 1975). The consequences of such an organizational effect are not readily revealed as a function of ASR testing of the adult females in estrus vs. diestrus vs. males. Nevertheless, as discussed in detail below, the pronounced prenatal cocaine by sex interaction on response latency in the PPI paradigm is wholly consistent with such an effect on early brain development.

Deficits in auditory information processing, characterized by impaired habituation in prenatal cocaine-exposed neonates, were reported using habituation and recovery of head-turning toward an auditory stimulus (Potter et al., 2000). The response pattern of the prenatal cocaine-exposed infants was consistent with a slower speed on auditory information processing. Cocaine-exposed newborns showed inferior performance on the habituation cluster of the Brazelton scale, requiring more trials than controls to habituate to auditory (as well as visual and tactile) stimuli (Eisen et al., 1991). The presently reported alterations in within-session habituation detected during the preweaning period as well as in adulthood were also especially notable in light of the paucity of such information in the preclinical literature. No differences were seen as a function of prenatal cocaine in rate of habituation to a pulsing tone in assessment of the heart rate orienting response in preweanling rats (Heyser et al., 1994). Impaired between-session habituation at 60–65 days of age was found following neonatal cocaine exposure on D1–10; ASR amplitude was higher throughout session 2 than session 1, however, the polynomial fit across startle trials did not differentiate the prenatal treatments (Dow-Edwards and Hughes, 1995).

The use of the relatively short ITI, to facilitate within-session habituation, was able to differentiate habituation between prenatal cocaine vs. vehicle controls in the preweaning period. The linear habituation in controls contrasts sharply with the best fit quadratic function in prenatal cocaine animals, reflecting their failure to show progressive habituation throughout the ASR session. In adulthood a similar differentiation of within-session habituation was apparent. The very rapid decrease in response amplitude to a plateau after the first six-trial block in controls is markedly distinct from the gradual curvilinear process observed with the prenatal cocaine-exposed adults. Perhaps of greater note, at both test ages, the overall cocaine effect was readily apparent with the lowest administered dose. It will be of great interest to ascertain the generality of this impaired habituation with tactile startling stimuli, such as with an air-puff.

Reflex modification procedures have much to recommend it for drug abuse studies in both humans and a variety of laboratory animals (Ison, 1984). The preattentive processes underlying reflex modification procedures, such as PPI, are presumed to protect encoding by gating out other stimulation that occurs in close temporal proximity to the initial stimulus; i.e., attenuated PPI would suggest less efficient gating mechanisms (Hoffman and Ison, 1980; Ison and Hoffman, 1983). In the only clinical reflex modification study of which we are aware, prenatal cocaine-exposed infants displayed an exaggerated glabellar reflex when the tap was accompanied by a tone (Anday et al., 1989). Although more reflex modification studies are available in the preclinical literature, they have consistently failed to find significant alterations in PPI.

Presently, the differential sensitivity to PPI observed as a function of prenatal cocaine was revealed by systematic manipulation of the ISI function; this differential sensitivity of the preattentive process of sensorimotor gating was observed for both response amplitude and response latency measures. It is of interest that the commonly reported metric for response amplitude, percentage PPI, was not altered by the prenatal cocaine treatment when tested in adulthood. However, the incorporation of a reasonably complete ISI function was sensitive to revealing alterations in sensorimotor gating. In contrast to the characteristic curvilinear function relating PPI to ISI, as seen with other stimulants or toxic proteins (e.g., Ison, 1984; Fitting et al., 2006a,b,c; Lacy et al., 2011), the prenatal cocaine-exposed adults displayed a progressive increase in PPI as the ISI increased throughout the range examined (8–120 ms). Thus, the temporal process of sensorimotor gating, as revealed by manipulation of ISI, appeared adversely affected by the prenatal cocaine treatment.

Alterations in response latencies during PPI were striking, particularly in light of the alterations in the brainstem evoked potential alteration reported in human infants (Shih et al., 1988; Salamy et al., 1990; Cone-Wesson and Spingarn, 1993; Lester et al., 2003; Tan-Laxa et al., 2004). The response latencies on PPI latency trials of the saline animals demonstrated a clear sex-dependent pattern whereas those of the prenatal IV cocaine-exposed males and females failed to display any significant variation as a function of sex. Again, of the limited prior rodent studies, either no significant alterations were observed in prenatal cocaine-exposed animals on any measure of PPI (Foss and Riley, 1991a; Vorhees et al., 1995, 2000), or a small, albeit statistically significant increase in the magnitude of PPI was reported compared to controls (relative difference of 8%) at 50–60 days of age (30 mg/kg/day cocaine on GD1–20; Hughes et al., 1996).

One factor that differed between the present and prior studies is that the cocaine was delivered to the dam by different routes of administration, IV vs. SC or PO. IV injection is one of the most clinically relevant routes; stimulant abuse liability is a function of the rapidity with which the drug reaches the brain (e.g., Russell and Feyerabend, 1978; Henningfield and Keenan, 1993; Abreu et al., 2001); a consequence not unexpected given that rate of IV drug delivery is well-established to increase maximum arterial drug concentration (Gibaldi, 1991). Furthermore, IV maternal administration of cocaine not only results in significant fetal plasma levels of cocaine (3 mg/kg – 300 ng/ml; 6 mg/kg – 500 ng/ml – Robinson et al., 1994), but also an appreciable tissue uptake of cocaine by fetal brain (at least under a repeated daily dosing regimen; Robinson et al., 1994). Moreover, unlike the SC and PO routes of administration (Spear et al., 1989a; Dow-Edwards, 1990), the IV route is associated with a rapid elimination of cocaine from fetal brain (Robinson et al., 1994). Thus, the fetus is rapidly and transiently exposed to significant amounts of cocaine using the IV dosing model.

The pharmacokinetic profile of near instantaneous distribution and short half-life for IV cocaine in rats closely mimics that observed in humans following inhalation or IV injection of cocaine (Evans et al., 1996; Booze et al., 1997). In contrast, the pharmacokinetics of cocaine delivered by the SC route involves a prolonged absorption process as well as a protracted elimination half-life (Collins et al., 1999). Second, the doses of cocaine employed in the current study are not only 1–2 orders of magnitude less than that employed with SC or PO dosing, but are known to produce arterial plasma levels of cocaine comparable to that of humans provided recreational doses of cocaine (Evans et al., 1996). Furthermore, the IV model precludes the potential confounds of cocaine-induced necrotic lesions characteristic of other routes of administration (e.g., intranasal, SC, Bruckner et al., 1982) and the possibility of extraplacental fetal absorption of cocaine (SC, Lipton et al., 1998). Third, the animals in the present study were tested beginning at 90 days of age vs. 50–60 used in many of the prior studies. Although there have been clear ontogenetic drifts in physiological profiles, at least historically, vaginal opening of LE female rats occurred at approximately D72 with maximum fertility achieved at D100–D300 (Farris, 1949); it may be prudent to refrain from labeling 50 to 60-day-old LE rats as adults.

Pretreatment with an acute low dose of idazoxan at 120 days of age significantly enhanced the magnitude of the ASR, but as the dose of prenatal IV cocaine increased, less enhancement of the ASR was observed. The enhancement of the ASR by idazoxan, an α_2-adrenergic receptor antagonist, was expected based upon the well-characterized anatomy and pharmacology of the ASR (Davis, 1984; Yeomans and Frankland, 1996). Idazoxan may affect noradrenergic activity via pre-synaptic and/or postsynaptic actions, since α_2-receptors (the drug's binding site) are localized both pre- and post-synaptically (Nicholas et al., 1996; Docherty, 1998). Idazoxan blockade of pre-synaptic α_2-receptors increases NE release due to a reduction in NE-mediated negative feedback, whereas idazoxan's blockade of postsynaptic α_2-receptors antagonizes the effects of released NE at synapses with post-junctional α_2-receptors. The marked stimulation of the ASR in control animals (>225%) is consistent with a pre-synaptic "stimulatory" effect and an increase in LC firing and release of NE (Freedman and Aghajanian, 1984; Dennis et al., 1987). Moreover, previous work suggests that idazoxan specifically altered selective attention in a distraction task that also revealed altered selective attention in rats exposed to cocaine prenatally (Bunsey and Strupp, 1995; Bayer et al., 2002). Prenatal IV cocaine exposure results in a persistent alteration in forebrain NE systems as indicated by alterations in receptor density in adolescent (D35; Booze et al., 2006) and adult (D395) rats (Ferris et al., 2007). The sex-dependent nature of these alterations in receptor proteins is of note, particularly given the striking sex-dependent alterations in PPI response latencies, as discussed above. Collectively, the above findings suggest that the enduring changes produced by prenatal cocaine in the ASR and its plasticity may be due to underlying changes in the ceruleocortical NE system. These data are important as they suggest that the increased reactivity seen in the prenatal cocaine-exposed animals was attributable to dysfunction in the descending NE system.

Specific effects of idazoxan in a distraction task have been previously shown in adult offspring, following maternal IV cocaine, without similarly affecting vigilance implicating endogenous norepinephrine influences on distractibility and/or selective attention (Bayer et al., 2002). The pattern of results and the specificity of the IDZ dose effect rules out non-specific alterations in performance (Bunsey and Strupp, 1995). Given that the noradrenergic system appears to be involved in the focusing of attention, possibly by attenuating distraction caused by irrelevant stimuli (Coull, 1994; Aston-Jones and Cohen, 2005), these data suggest alterations in the ascending noradrenergic system provide the basis for this "distracting" effect.

Traditionally, the actions of cocaine have been attributed to non-selective inhibition of catecholaminergic neurotransmitter reuptake systems. However, emerging evidence supports the view that cocaine may have non-traditional mechanisms for its effects on neuron function (Snow et al., 2001, 2004; Dey et al., 2006). In both *in vitro* and *in vivo* studies noradrenergic neurons of the locus coeruleus were exposed to cocaine at a physiologically relevant concentration, and for the *in vivo* studies via the clinically relevant IV route of administration (Evans et al., 1996; Booze et al., 1997). Following 7 days of *in vitro* administration, cocaine decreased cell survival as well as neurite elongation in comparison to vehicle controls (Snow et al., 2001, 2004). In subsequent studies, cocaine exposure *in vitro* induced apoptosis in fetal LC neurons putatively regulated by Bax, via activation of caspases and their downstream target proteins (Dey et al., 2006; Dey and Snow, 2007). The results were obtained from 7 days of cocaine administration (*in vitro*); a longer term exposure might augment the adverse neuronal effects. These data suggest a decreased ability of LC neurons to network with target cells through both ascending (attention/distraction task with idazoxan challenge, Bayer et al., 2002) and descending (present auditory startle and idazoxan challenge studies) NE pathways, where damage to the NE cell bodies of the LC might provide a unifying mechanism underlying these widespread effects.

Importantly, our evidence for an alteration in the cocaine-exposed offspring's processing of novel auditory information was detected in the absence of any support for the contribution of indirect effects on maternal growth and nutrition. The IV administration of cocaine to pregnant rats during the last 2 weeks of gestation produced no detectable evidence of toxicity in either the dams or the offspring. A similar failure to find evidence of maternal or fetal toxicity attributable to cocaine, when delivered via the IV route, was previously reported (Mactutus et al., 1994; Mactutus, 1999; Foltz et al., 2004). This negative finding is also consonant with several other studies in rats, mice, and rabbits, all of which have employed IV cocaine doses greater than or equal to those employed here (Mehanny et al., 1991; Kunko et al., 1993; Robinson et al., 1994; Murphy et al., 1997). Together, these observations argue that the IV route of exposure does not require the use of pair-fed nutritional controls as, unlike the SC (Church et al., 1988; Spear et al., 1989b) or PO (Dow-Edwards et al., 1989; Hutchings et al., 1989) models, there appear to be no detectable effects on pregnancy weight gain, putatively the most sensitive routine measure of maternal health. Thus, it is tempting to speculate that the effects of maternal IV cocaine may satisfy the conditions of a pure neurobehavioral teratogen. Nevertheless, higher IV doses of cocaine, as typically delivered to pregnant rabbits (4 mg/kg 2× day, Harvey, 2004) causes a loss of approximately half of the kits within the first postnatal week (Murphy et al., 1997); no such effects have ever been reported with the 3-mg/kg 2× dose as employed by others that use the IV rabbit model (e.g., Stanwood and Levitt, 2007).

Despite the growing and converging evidence for a primary effect of prenatal IV cocaine on the LC and noradrenergic system, alterations in dopaminergic systems may also be contributing to the pattern of observed results, i.e., idazoxan may conceivably be altering norepinephrine-modulated release of dopamine from the ventral tegmental area and/or substantia nigra (Gresch et al., 1995; Devoto et al., 2004). Nevertheless, such an effect would remain consistent with a primary effect of prenatal IV cocaine on the noradrenergic system. When a direct comparison of potential noradrenergic vs. dopaminergic system alterations has been made, dissociations of the effects on prenatal IV cocaine on noradrenergic vs. dopaminergic systems are observed, e.g., on neurite outgrowth (Dey et al., 2006) and apoptotic signaling (Dey et al., 2007). Future studies that manipulate the timing of gestational cocaine exposure may permit further dissociation of the effects on noradrenergic vs. dopaminergic systems.

Finally, while there is very good reason to believe that the reported alterations are attributable to direct effects of cocaine on the developing fetus, one must acknowledge the possibility that there was also some contribution of altered maternal care that may have contributed to the alterations noted in the offspring, i.e., the offspring were not fostered to non-exposed dams at birth. However, we have purposely used a low dose of cocaine in our research program to preclude effects on maternal nutrition and pregnancy weight gain, and on fetal growth. We have never been interested in a high-dose model which would confound nutritional effects with other direct effects of cocaine. Across the studies of the past 15 years in which we have performed research with prenatal cocaine, we have never seen an adverse effect of prenatal cocaine on offspring growth (often touted as one of the most sensitive variables one can measure) implicating any impairment in maternal care. Further, in light of the half-life of cocaine in the rat when delivered via the IV route (Booze et al., 1997), one would not expect the presence of cocaine in the maternal compartment on the day the animals gave birth. Finally, the dosage regimen employed has no detectable effects on maternal retrieval in newborn pups (unpublished observations), again suggesting the low dosages of cocaine employed with the IV route are not consistent with any impairment in maternal care.

In sum, the ASR and its plasticity (habituation, PPI) were sensitive to revealing teratogenic effects of cocaine when delivered by the clinically relevant IV route and at physiologically relevant doses. These conditions produced no detectable adverse effects on maternal/litter parameters. Significant alterations in each of the three paradigms were found in adulthood, regardless of whether or not there was evidence available for the persistence, as opposed to a latent emergence, of the effects. Functional alteration of the noradrenergic system in adulthood was suggested by the prenatal cocaine dose-dependent attenuation of the ability of 0.5 mg/kg idazoxan to enhance the ASR. Thus, *in utero* exposure to cocaine, when delivered via a protocol designed to capture prominent features of recreational usage, causes persistent, if not permanent, alterations in auditory information processing, and suggests dysfunction of the central noradrenergic circuitry modulating, if not mediating, these responses.

ACKNOWLEDGMENTS

This research was supported, in part, by grants from the National Institutes of Health: National Institute on Drug Abuse, DA 009160 (Charles F. Mactutus), DA013137 (Rosemarie M. Booze), and DA 021287 (Steven B. Harrod), and National Institute of Child Health and Human Development, HD 043680 (Charles F. Mactutus). The authors gratefully acknowledge the efforts of M. A. Welch for her technical assistance in the conduct of this research. Graduate students Lauren L. Hord and Landhing M. Moran contributed equally to the research; their authorship position was determined by a coin toss. The authors also gratefully acknowledge the input of the referees for their comments and suggestions during the review process.

REFERENCES

Abreu, M. E., Bigelow, G. E., Fleisher, L., and Walsh, S. L. (2001). Effect of intravenous injection speed on responses to cocaine and hydromorphone in humans. *Psychopharmacology (Berl.)* 154, 76–84.

Accornero, V. H., Amado, A. J., Morrow, C. E., Xue, L., Anthony, J. C., and Bandstra, E. S. (2007). Impact of prenatal cocaine exposure on attention and response inhibition as assessed by continuous performance tests. *J. Dev. Behav. Pediatr.* 28, 195–205.

Ackerman, J. P., Riggins, T., and Black, M. M. (2010). A review of the effects of prenatal cocaine exposure among school-aged children. *Pediatrics* 125, 554–565.

Anday, E., Cohen, M., Kelley, N., and Leitner, D. (1989). Effect of in utero cocaine exposure on startle and its modification. *Dev. Pharmacol. Ther.* 12, 137–145.

Aston-Jones, G., and Cohen, J. D. (2005). An integrative theory of locus coeruleus-norepinephrine function: adaptive gain and optimal performance. *Annu. Rev. Neurosci.* 28, 403–450.

Bandstra, E. S., Morrow, C. F., Accornero, V. H., Mansoor, E., Xue, L., and Anthony, J. C. (2011). Estimated effects of in utero cocaine exposure on language development through early adolescence. *Neurotoxicol. Teratol.* 33, 25–35.

Bandstra, E. S., Vogel, A. L., Morrow, C. E., Xue, L., and Anthony, J. C. (2004). Severity of prenatal cocaine exposure and child language functioning through age seven years: a longitudinal latent growth curve analysis. *Subst. Use. Misuse* 39, 25–59.

Bandstra, E. S., Morrow, C. E., Vogel, A. L., Fifer, R. C., Ofir, A. Y., Dausa, A. T., Xue, L., and Anthony, J. C. (2002). Longitudinal influence of prenatal cocaine exposure on child language functioning. *Neurotoxicol. Teratol.* 24, 297–308.

Bandstra, E. S., Morrow, C. E., Anthony, J. C., Accornero, V. H., and Fried, P. A. (2001). Longitudinal investigation of task persistence and sustained attention in children with prenatal cocaine exposure. *Neurotoxicol. Teratol.* 23, 545–559.

Bayer, L. E., Brown, A., Mactutus, C. F., Booze, R. M., and Strupp, B. J. (2000). Prenatal cocaine exposure increases sensitivity to the attentional effects of the dopamine D1 agonist SKF81297. *J. Neurosci.* 20, 8902–8908.

Bayer, L. E., Kakumanu, S., Mactutus, C. F., Booze, R. M., and Strupp, B. J. (2002). Prenatal cocaine exposure alters sensitivity to the effects of idazoxan in a distraction task. *Behav. Brain Res.* 133, 185–196.

Beeghly, M., Martin, B., Rose-Jacobs, R., Cabral, H., Heeren, T., Augustyn, M., Bellinger, D., and Frank, D. A. (2006). Prenatal cocaine exposure and children's language functioning at 6 and 9.5 years: moderating effects of child age, birthweight, and gender. *J. Pediatr. Psychol.* 31, 98–115.

Benasich, A. A., and Tallal, P. (2002). Infant discrimination of rapid auditory cues predicts later language impairment. *Behav. Brain Res.* 136, 31–49.

Betancourt, L. M., Yang, W., Brodsky, N. L., Gallagher, P. R., Malmud, E. K., Giannetta, J. M., Farah, M. J., and Hurt, H. (2011). Adolescents with and without gestational cocaine exposure: longitudinal analysis of inhibitory control, memory and receptive language. *Neurotoxicol. Teratol.* 33, 36–46.

Booze, R. M., Lehner, A. F., Wallace, D. R., Welch, M. A., and Mactutus, C. F. (1997). Dose-response cocaine pharmacokinetics and metabolite profile following intravenous administration and arterial sampling in unanesthetized, freely moving male rats. *Neurotoxicol. Teratol.* 19, 7–15.

Booze, R. M., Wallace, D. R., Silvers, J. M., Strupp, B. J., Snow, D. M., and Mactutus, C. F. (2006). Prenatal cocaine exposure alters alpha2 receptor expression in adolescent rats. *BMC Neurosci.* 7, 33. doi: 10.1186/1471-2202-7-33

Bruckner, J. V., Jiang, W. D., Ho, B. T., and Levy, B. M. (1982). Histopathological evaluation of cocaine-induced skin lesions in the rat. *J. Cutan. Pathol.* 9, 83–95.

Bunsey, M. D., and Strupp, B. J. (1995). Specific effects of idazoxan in a distraction task: evidence that endogenous norepinephrine plays a role in selective attention in rats. *Behav. Neurosci.* 109, 903–911.

Carmody, D. P., Bennett, D. S., and Lewis, M. (2011). The effects of prenatal cocaine exposure and gender on inhibitory control and attention. *Neurotoxicol. Teratol.* 33, 61–68.

Carzoli, R. P., Murphy, S. P., Hammer-Knisely, J., and Houy, J. (1991). Evaluation of auditory brain-stem response in full-term infants of cocaine-abusing mothers. *Am. J. Dis. Child.* 145, 1013–1016.

Chasnoff, I. J., Burns, W. J., Schnoll, S. H., and Burns, K. A. (1985). Cocaine use in pregnancy. *N. Engl. J. Med.* 313, 666–669.

Chasnoff, I. J., Griffith, D. R., MacGregor, S., Dirkes, K., and Burns, K. A. (1989). Temporal patterns of cocaine use in pregnancy. Perinatal outcome. *J. Am. Med. Assoc.* 261, 1741–1744.

Chiriboga, C. A., Starr, D., Kuhn, L., and Wasserman, G. A. (2009). Prenatal cocaine exposure and prolonged focus attention. Poor infant information processing ability or precocious maturation of attentional systems? *Dev. Neurosci.* 31, 149–158.

Church, M. W., Dintcheff, B. A., and Gessner, P. K. (1988). Dose dependent consequences of cocaine on pregnancy outcome in the Long–Evans rat. *Neurotoxicol. Teratol.* 10, 51–58.

Church, M. W., and Overbeck, G. W. (1990). Prenatal cocaine exposure in the Long-Evans rat: III. Developmental effects on the brainstem auditory-evoked potential. *Neurotoxicol. Teratol.* 12, 345–351.

Collins, L. M., Pahl, J. A., and Meyer, J. S. (1999). Distribution of cocaine and metabolites in the pregnant rat and fetus in a chronic subcutaneous injection model. *Neurotoxicol. Teratol.* 21, 639–646.

Cone-Wesson, B., and Spingarn, A. (1993). Effects of maternal cocaine abuse on neonatal auditory brainstem responses. *Am. J. Audiol.* 2, 48–54.

Coull, J. T. (1994). Pharmacological manipulation of the α2-noradrenergic system. Effects on cognition. *Drugs Aging* 5, 116–126.

Davis, M. (1984). "The mammalian startle response," in *Neural Mechanisms of Startle Behavior*, ed. R. C. Eaton (New York, NY: Plenum Press), 287–351.

Degenhardt, L., Bucello, C., Calabria, B., Nelson, P., Roberts, A., Hall, W., Lynskey, M., Wiessing, L., and The GBD Illicit Drug Use Writing Group. (2011). What data are available on the extent of illicit drug use and dependence globally? Results of four systematic reviews. *Drug Alcohol Depend.* doi: 10.1016/j.drugalcdep.2010.11.032. [Epub ahead of print].

Degenhardt, L., Chiu, W. T., Sampson, N., Kessler, R. C., Anthony, J. C., Angermeyer, M., Bruffaerts, R., de Girolamo, G., Gureje, O., Huang, Y., Karam, A., Kostyuchenko, S., Lepine, J. P., Mora, M. E., Neumark, Y., Ormel, J. H., Pinto-Meza, A., Posada-Villa, J., Stein, D. J., Takeshima, T., and Wells, J. E. (2008). Toward a global view of alcohol, tobacco, cannabis, and cocaine use: findings from the WHO World Mental Health Surveys. *PLoS Med.* 5, e141. doi: 10.1371/journal.pmed.0050141

Delaney-Black, V., Covington, C., Templin, T., Kershaw, T., Nordstrom-Klee, B., Ager, J., Clark, N., Surendran, A., Martier, S., and Sokol, R. J. (2000). Expressive language development of children exposed to cocaine prenatally: literature review and report of a prospective cohort study. *J. Commun. Disord.* 33, 463–480.

Dennis, T., L'Heureux, R., Carter, C., and Scatton, B. (1987). Presynaptic alpha-2 adrenoceptors play a major role in the effects of idazoxan on cortical noradrenaline release (as measured by in vivo dialysis) in the rat. *J. Pharmacol. Exp. Ther.* 241, 642–649.

Devoto, P., Flore, G., Pira, L., Longu, G., and Gessa, G. L. (2004). Alpha2-adrenoceptor mediated co-release of dopamine and noradrenaline from noradrenergic neurons in the cerebral cortex. *J. Neurochem.* 88, 1003–1009.

Dey, S., Mactutus, C. F., Booze, R. M., and Snow, D. M. (2006). Specificity of prenatal cocaine on inhibition of locus coeruleus neurite outgrowth. *Neuroscience* 139, 899–907.

Dey, S., Mactutus, C. F., Booze, R. M., and Snow, D. M. (2007). Cocaine exposure in vitro induces apoptosis in fetal locus coeruleus neurons by altering the Bax/Bcl-2 ratio and through caspase-3 apoptotic signaling. *Neuroscience* 144, 509–521.

Dey, S., and Snow, D. M. (2007). Cocaine exposure in vitro induces apoptosis in fetal locus coeruleus neurons through TNF-alpha-mediated induction of Bax and phosphorylated c-Jun NH(2)-terminal kinase. *J. Neurochem.* 103, 542–556.

Dinehart, L. H. B., Kaiser, M. Y., and Hughes, C. (2009). Language delay and elicitation intervention in children born cocaine exposed: a pilot study. *J. Dev. Phys. Disabil.* 21, 9–22.

Dobbing, J., and Sands, J. (1979). Comparative aspects of the brain growth spurt. *Early Hum. Dev.* 3, 79–83.

Docherty, J. R. (1998). Subtypes of functional alpha1- and alpha2-adrenoceptors. *Eur. J. Pharmacol.* 361, 1–15.

Dow-Edwards, D. L., Fico, T. A., Osman, M., Gamagaris, Z., and Hutchings, D. E. (1989). Comparison of oral and subcutaneous routes of cocaine administration on behavior, plasma drug concentration and toxicity in female rats. *Pharmacol. Biochem. Behav.* 33, 167 173.

Dow-Edwards, D. (1990). Fetal and maternal cocaine levels peak rapidly following intragastric administration in the rat. *J. Subst. Abuse* 2, 427–437.

Dow-Edwards, D., and Hughes, H. (1995). Adult reactivity in rats exposed to cocaine during two early postnatal periods. *Neurotoxicol. Teratol.* 17, 553–557.

Eisen, L. N., Field, T. M., Bandstra, E. S., Roberts, J. P., Morrow, C., Larson, S. K., and Steele, B. M. (1991). Perinatal cocaine effects on neonatal stress behavior and performance on the Brazelton Scale. *Pediatrics* 88, 477–480.

Evans, S. M., Cone, E. J., and Henningfeld, J. E. (1996). Arterial and venous cocaine plasma concentrations in humans: relationship to route of administration, cardiovascular effects and subjective effects. *J. Pharmacol. Exp. Ther.* 279, 1345–1356.

Farris, E. J. (1949). "Breeding of the rat," in *The Rat in Laboratory Investigation*, 2nd edn. eds E. J. Farris and J. Q. Griffith, Jr. (New York, NY: Hafner Publishing Co.), 1–18.

Ferris, M. J., Mactutus, C. F., Silvers, J. M., Hasselrot, U., Beaudin, S. A., Strupp, B. J., and Booze, R. M. (2007). Sex mediates dopamine and adrenergic receptor expression in adult rats exposed prenatally to cocaine. *Int. J. Dev. Neurosci.* 25, 445–454.

Fischman, M. W., and Schuster, C. R. (1982). Cocaine self-administration in humans. *Fed. Proc.* 41, 241–246.

Fitting, S., Booze, R. M., Hasselrot, U., and Mactutus, C. F. (2006a). Intrahippocampal injections of Tat: effects on prepulse inhibition of the auditory startle response in adult male rats. *Pharmacol. Biochem. Behav.* 84, 189–196.

Fitting, S., Booze, R. M., and Mactutus, C. F. (2006b). Neonatal intrahippocampal glycoprotein 120 injection: the role of dopaminergic alterations in prepulse inhibition in adult rats. *J. Pharmacol. Exp. Ther.* 318, 1352–1358.

Fitting, S., Booze, R. M., and Mactutus, C. F. (2006c). Neonatal hippocampal Tat injections: developmental effects on prepulse inhibition (PPI) of the auditory startle response. *Int. J. Dev. Neurosci.* 24, 275–283.

Foltz, T. L., Snow, D. M., Strupp, B. J., Booze, R. M., and Mactutus, C. F. (2004). Prenatal intravenous cocaine and the heart rate-orienting response: a dose-response study. *Int. J. Dev. Neurosci.* 22, 285–296.

Foss, J. A., and Riley, E. (1988). Behavioral evaluation of animals exposed prenatally to cocaine. *Teratology* 37, 517.

Foss, J. A., and Riley, E. (1991a). Elicitation and modification of the acoustic startle reflex in animals prenatally exposed to cocaine. *Neurotoxicol. Teratol.* 13, 541–546.

Foss, J. A., and Riley, E. (1991b). Failure of acute cocaine administration to differentially affect acoustic startle and activity in rats prenatally exposed to cocaine. *Neurotoxicol. Teratol.* 13, 547–551.

Frank, D. A., Augustyn, M., Knight, W. G., Pell, T., and Zuckerman, B. (2001). Growth, development, and behavior in early childhood following prenatal cocaine exposure: a systematic review. *J. Am. Med. Assoc.* 285, 1613–1625.

Frank, D. A., Rose-Jacobs, R., Beeghly, M., Wilbur, M., Bellinger, D., and Cabral, H. (2005). Level of prenatal cocaine exposure and 48-month IQ: importance of preschool enrichment. *Neurotoxicol. Teratol.* 27, 15–28.

Freedman, J. E., and Aghajanian, G. K. (1984). Idazoxan (RX 781094) selectively antagonizes alpha 2-adrenoceptors on rat central neurons. *Eur. J. Pharmacol.* 105, 265–272.

Garavan, H., Morgan, R. E., Mactutus, C. F., Levitsky, D. A., Booze, R. M., and Strupp, B. J. (2000). Prenatal cocaine exposure impairs selective attention: evidence from serial reversal and extradimensional shift tasks. *Behav. Neurosci.* 114, 725–738.

Gendle, M. H., Strawderman, M. S., Mactutus, C. F., Booze, R. M., Levitsky, D. A., and Strupp, B. J. (2003). Impaired sustained attention and altered reactivity to errors in an animal model of prenatal cocaine exposure. *Brain Res. Dev. Brain Res.* 147, 85–96.

Gendle, M. H., White, T. L., Strawderman, M., Mactutus, C. F., Booze, R. M., Levitsky, D. A., and Strupp, B. J. (2004a). Enduring effects of prenatal cocaine exposure on selective attention and reactivity to errors: evidence from an animal model. *Behav. Neurosci.* 118, 290–297.

Gendle, M. H., Strawderman, M. S., Mactutus, C. F., Booze, R. M., Levitsky, D. A., and Strupp, B. J. (2004b). Prenatal cocaine exposure does not alter working memory in adult rats. *Neurotoxicol. Teratol.* 26, 319–329.

Gibaldi, M. (1991). *Biopharmaceutics and Clinical Pharmacokinetics*, 4th Edn. Philadelphia, PA: Lea & Febiger.

Gorski, R. A., Mennin, S. P., and Kubo, K. (1975). The neural and hormonal bases of the reproductive cycle of the rat. *Adv. Exp. Med. Biol.* 54, 115–153.

Greenhouse, S. W., and Geisser, S. (1959). On methods in the analysis of profile data. *Psychometrika* 24, 95–112.

Gresch, P. J., Sved, A. F., Zigmond, M. J., and Finlay, J. M. (1995). Local influence of endogenous norepinephrine on extracellular dopamine in rat medial prefrontal cortex. *J. Neurochem.* 65, 111–116.

Griffith, D. R. (1988). "The effects of perinatal cocaine exposure on infant neurobehavior and early maternal-infant interactions," in *Drugs, Alcohol, Pregnancy and Parenting*, ed. I. J. Chasnoff (Dordrecht: Kluwer Academic Publishers), 105–113.

Harvey, J. A. (2004). Cocaine effects on the developing brain: current status. *Neurosci. Biobehav. Rev.* 27, 751–764.

Heffelfinger, A., Craft, S., and Shyken, J. (1997). Visual attention in children with prenatal cocaine exposure. *J. Int. Neuropsychol. Soc.* 3, 237–245.

Heffelfinger, A. K., Craft, S., White, D. A., and Shyken, J. (2002). Visual attention in preschool children prenatally exposed to cocaine: implications for behavioral regulation. *J. Int. Neuropsychol. Soc.* 8, 12–21.

Heffner, H. E., Heffner, R. S., Contos, C., and Ott, T. (1994). Audiogram of the hooded Norway rat. *Hear. Res.* 73, 244–247.

Henningfield, J., and Keenan, R. (1993). Nicotine delivery kinetics and abuse liability. *J. Consult. Clin. Psychol.* 61, 743–750.

Heyser, C. J., McKinzie, D. L., Athalie, F., Spear, N. E., and Spear, L. P. (1994). Effects of prenatal exposure to cocaine on heart rate and nonassociative learning and retention in infant rats. *Teratology* 49, 470–478.

Hoffman, H. S., and Ison, J. R. (1980). Reflex modification in the domain of startle: I. Some empirical findings and their implications for how the nervous system processes sensory input. *Psychol. Rev.* 87, 175–189.

Hughes, H. E., Donohue, L. M., and Dow-Edwards, D. L. (1996). Prenatal cocaine exposure affects the acoustic startle response in adult rats. *Behav. Brain Res.* 75, 83–90.

Hurt, H., Betancourt, L. M., Malmud, E. K., Shera, D. M., Giannetta, J. M., Brodsky, N. L., and Farah, M. J. (2009). Children with and without gestational cocaine exposure: a neurocognitive systems analysis. *Neurotoxicol. Teratol.* 31, 334–341.

Hurt, H., Malmud, E., Betancourt, L., Brodsky, N. L., and Giannetta, J. (1997). A prospective evaluation of early language development in children with in utero cocaine exposure and in control subjects. *J. Pediatr.* 130, 310–312.

Hutchings, D. E., Fico, T. A., and Dow-Edwards, D. L. (1989). Prenatal cocaine: maternal toxicity, fetal effects and locomotor activity in rat offspring. *Neurotoxicol. Teratol.* 11, 65–69.

Isenschmid, D. S., Fischman, M. W., Foltin, R. W., and Caplan, Y. H. (1992). Concentration of cocaine and metabolites in plasma of humans following intravenous administration and smoking of cocaine. *J. Anal. Toxicol.* 16, 311–314.

Ison, J. R. (1984). Reflex modification as an objective test for sensory processing following toxicant exposure. *Neurobehav. Toxicol. Teratol.* 6, 437–445.

Ison, J. R., and Hoffman, H. S. (1983). Reflex modification in the domain of startle: II. The anomalous history of a robust and ubiquitous phenomenon. *Psychol. Bull.* 94, 3–17.

Johnston, L. D., O'Malley, P. M., Bachman, J. G., and Schulenberg, J. E. (2010). *Monitoring the Future National Survey Results on Drug Use, 1975-2009. Volume I: Secondary School Students (NIH Publication No. 10-7584)*. Bethesda, MD: National Institute on Drug Abuse, 734.

Kilbride, H., Castor, C., Hoffman, E., and Fuger, K. L. (2000). Thirty-six month outcome of prenatal cocaine exposure for term or near-term infants: impact of early case management. *J. Dev. Behav. Pediatr.* 21, 19–26.

Kilbride, H. W., Castor, C. A., and Fuger, K. L. (2006). School-age outcome of children with prenatal cocaine exposure following early case management. *J. Dev. Behav. Pediatr.* 27, 181–187.

Krumholz, A., Felix, J. K., Goldstein, P. J., and McKenzie, E. (1985). Maturation of the brainstem auditory evoked potential in premature infants. *Electroencephalogr. Clin. Neurophysiol.* 62, 124–134.

Kunko, P. M., Moyer, D., and Robinson, S. E. (1993). Intravenous gestational cocaine in rats: effects on offspring development and weanling behavior. *Neurotoxicol. Teratol.* 15, 335–344.

LaBella, F. S., and Queen, G. (1993). General anesthetics inhibit cytochrome P450 monoxygenases and arachidonic acid metabolism. *Can. J. Physiol. Pharmacol.* 71, 48–53.

Lacy, R. T., Mactutus, C. F., and Harrod, S. B. (2011). Prenatal IV nicotine exposure produces a sex difference in sensorimotor gating of the auditory startle reflex in adult rats. *Int. J. Dev. Neurosci.* 29, 153–161.

Leech, S. L., Richardson, G. A., Goldschmidt, L., and Day, N. L. (1999). Prenatal substance exposure: effects on attention and impulsivity of 6-year-olds. *Neurotoxicol. Teratol.* 21, 109–118.

Lester, B. M., Lagasse, L., Seifer, R., Tronick, E. Z., Bauer, C. R., Shankaran, S., Bada, H. S., Wright, L. L., Smeriglio, V. L., Liu, J., Finnegan, L. P., and Maza, P. L. (2003). The Maternal Lifestyle Study (MLS): effects of prenatal cocaine and/or opiate exposure on auditory brain response at one month. *J. Pediatr.* 142, 279–285.

Lewis, B. A., Kirchner, H. L., Short, E. J., Minnes, S., Weishampel, P., Satayathum, S., and Singer, L. T. (2007). Prenatal cocaine and tobacco effects on children's language trajectories. *Pediatrics* 120, 78–85.

Lewis, B. A., Minnes, S., Short, E. J., Weishampel, P., Satayathum, S., Min, M. O., Nelson, S., and Singer, L. T. (2011). The effects of prenatal cocaine on language development at 10 years of age. *Neurotoxicol. Teratol.* 33, 17–24.

Lewis, B. A., Singer, L. T., Short, E. J., Minnes, S., Arendt, R., Weishampel, P., Klein, N., and Min, M. O. (2004). Four-year language outcomes of children exposed to cocaine in utero. *Neurotoxicol. Teratol.* 26, 617–627.

Lipton, J. W., Robie, H. C., Ling, Z., Weese-Mayer, D. E., and Carvey, P. M. (1998). The magnitude of brain dopamine depletion from prenatal cocaine exposure is a function of uterine position. *Neurotoxicol. Teratol.* 20, 373–382.

Loch, J. M., Potter, J., and Bachmann, K. A. (1995). The influence of anesthetic agents on rat hepatic cytochromes P450 in vivo. *Pharmacology* 50, 146–153.

Mactutus, C. F. (1999). Prenatal intravenous cocaine adversely affects attentional processing in preweanling rats. *Neurotoxicol. Teratol.* 21, 539–550.

Mactutus, C. F., Booze, R. M., and Dowell, R. T. (2000). The influence of route of administration on the acute cardiovascular effects of cocaine in conscious unrestrained pregnant rats. *Neurotoxicol. Teratol.* 22, 357–368.

Mactutus, C. F., Herman, A. S., and Booze, R. M. (1994). Chronic intravenous model for studies of drug abuse in the pregnant and/or group-housed rat: an initial study with cocaine. *Neurotoxicol. Teratol.* 16, 183–191.

Mayes, L. C., Grillon, C., Granger, R., and Schottenfeld, R. (1998). Regulation of arousal and attention in preschool children exposed to cocaine prenatally. *Ann. N. Y. Acad. Sci.* 846, 126–143.

Mehanny, S. Z., Abdel-Rahman, M. S., and Ahmed, Y. Y. (1991). Teratogenic effect of cocaine and diazepam in CF1 mice. *Teratology* 43, 11–17.

Morgan, R. E., Garavan, H. P., Mactutus, C. F., Levitsky, D. A., Booze, R. M., and Strupp, B. J. (2002). Enduring effects of prenatal cocaine exposure on attention and reaction to errors. *Behav. Neurosci.* 116, 624–633.

Morrow, C. E., Bandstra, E. S., Anthony, J. C., Ofir, A. Y., Xue, L., and Reyes, M. B. (2003). Influence of prenatal cocaine exposure on early language development: longitudinal findings from four months to three years of age. *J. Dev. Behav. Pediatr.* 24, 39–50.

Morrow, C. E., Vogel, A. L., Anthony, J. C., Ofir, A. Y., Dausa, A. T., and Bandstra, E. S. (2004). Expressive and receptive language functioning in preschool children with prenatal cocaine exposure. *J. Pediatr. Psychol.* 7, 543–554.

Murphy, E. H., Fischer, I., Friedman, E., Grayson, D., Jones, L., Levitt, P., O'Brien-Jenkins, A., Wang, H. Y., and Wang, X. H. (1997). Cocaine administration in pregnant rabbits alters cortical structure and function in their progeny in the absence of maternal seizures. *Exp. Brain Res.* 114, 433–441.

Nicholas, A. P., Hökfelt, T., and Pieribone, V. A. (1996). The distribution and significance of CNS adrenoceptors examined with in situ hybridization. *Trends Pharmacol. Sci.* 17, 245–255.

Noland, J. S., Singer, L. T., Short, E. J., Minnes, S., Arendt, R. E., Kirchner, H. L., and Bearer, C. (2005). Prenatal drug exposure and selective attention in preschoolers. *Neurotoxicol. Teratol.* 27, 429–438.

Overstreet, D. H., Moy, S. S., Lubin, D. A., Gause, L. R., Lieberman, J. A., and Johns, J. M. (2000). Enduring effects of prenatal cocaine administration on emotional behavior in rats. *Physiol. Behav.* 70, 149–156.

Parisi, T., and Ison, J. R. (1979). Development of the acoustic startle response in the rat: ontogenetic changes in the magnitude of inhibition by prepulse stimulation. *Dev. Psychobiol.* 12, 219–230.

Parisi, T., and Ison, J. R. (1981). Ontogeny of control over the acoustic startle reflex by visual prestimulation in the rat. *Dev. Psychobiol.* 14, 311–316.

Potter, S. M., Zelazo, P. R., Stack, D. M., and Papageorgiou, A. N. (2000). Adverse effects of fetal cocaine exposure on neonatal auditory information processing. *Pediatrics* 105, E40.

Richardson, G. A., Conroy, M. L., and Day, N. L. (1996). Prenatal cocaine exposure: effects on the development of school-age children. *Neurotoxicol. Teratol.* 18, 627–634.

Robinson, S. E., Enters, E. K., Jackson, G. F., Chinchilli, V. M., Maher, J. R., McDowell, K. P., Allen, H. M., and Guo, H. (1994). Maternal and fetal brain and plasma levels of cocaine and benzoylecgonine after acute or chronic maternal intravenous administration of cocaine. *J. Pharmacol. Exp. Ther.* 271, 1234–1239.

Russell, M. A., and Feyerabend, C. (1978). Cigarette smoking: a dependence on high-nicotine boli. *Drug Metab. Rev.* 8, 29–57.

Salamy, A. (1984). Maturation of the auditory brainstem response from birth through early childhood. *J. Clin. Neurophysiol.* 1, 293–329.

Salamy, A., Eldredge, L., Anderson, J., and Bull, D. (1990). Brain-stem transmission time in infants exposed to cocaine in utero. *J. Pediatr.* 117, 627–629.

Savage, J., Brodsky, N. L., Malmud, E., Giannetta, J. M., and Hurt, H. (2005). Attentional functioning and impulse control in cocaine-exposed and control children at age ten years. *J. Dev. Behav. Pediatr.* 26, 42–47.

Shih, L., Cone-Wesson, B., and Reddix, B. (1988). Effects of maternal cocaine abuse on the neonatal auditory system. *Int. J. Pediatr. Otorhinolaryngol.* 15, 245–251.

Singer, L. T., Arendt, R., Minnes, S., Salvator, A., Siegel, A. C., and Lewis, B. A. (2001). Developing language skills of cocaine-exposed infants. *Pediatrics* 107, 1057–1064.

Snow, D. M., Carman, H. M., Smith, J. D., Booze, R. M., Welch, M. A., and Mactutus, C. F. (2004). Cocaine-induced inhibition of process outgrowth in locus coeruleus neurons: role of gestational exposure period and offspring sex. *Int. J. Dev. Neurosci.* 22, 297–308.

Snow, D. M., Smith, J. D., Booze, R. M., Welch, M. A., and Mactutus, C. F. (2001). Cocaine decreases cell survival and inhibits neurite extension of rat locus coeruleus neurons. *Neurotoxicol. Teratol.* 23, 225–234.

Spear, L. P., Frambes, N. A., and Kirstein, C. L. (1989a). Fetal and maternal brain and plasma levels of cocaine and benzoylecgonine following chronic subcutaneous administration of cocaine during gestation in rats. *Psychopharmacology (Berl.)* 97, 427–431.

Spear, L. P., Kirstein, C. L., Bell, J., Yoottanasumpun, V., Greenbaum, R., Oshea, J., Hoffmann, H., and Spear, N. E. (1989b). Effects of prenatal cocaine exposure on behavior during the early postnatal period. *Neurotoxicol. Teratol.* 11, 57–63.

Stanwood, G. D., and Levitt, P. (2007). Prenatal exposure to cocaine produces unique developmental and long-term adaptive changes in dopamine D1 receptor activity and subcellular distribution. *J. Neurosci.* 27, 152–157.

Statistical Solutions Ltd. (2009). *BMDP 2009*. Cork: Statistical Solutions.

Substance Abuse and Mental Health Services Administration. (2010). *Results from the 2009 National Survey on Drug Use and Health: Volume I. Summary of National Findings (Office of Applied Studies, NSDUH Series H-38A, HHS Publication No. SMA 10-4586 Findings)*. Rockville, MD.

Tan-Laxa, M. A., Sison-Switala, C., Rintelman, W., and Ostrea, E. M. Jr. (2004). Abnormal auditory brainstem response among infants with prenatal cocaine exposure. *Pediatrics* 113, 357–360.

Vorhees, C., Wood, S., Morford, L., Reed, T., Moran, M., Pu, C., and Cappon, G. (2000). Evaluation of neonatal exposure to cocaine on learning, activity, startle, scent marking, immobility, and plasma cocaine concentrations. *Neurotoxicol. Teratol.* 22, 255–265.

Vorhees, C. V., Reed, T. M., Acuff-Smith, K. D., Schilling, M. A., Cappon, G. D., Fisher, J. E., and Pu, C. (1995). Long-term learning deficits and changes in unlearned behaviors following in utero exposure to multiple daily doses of cocaine during different exposure periods and maternal plasma cocaine concentrations. *Neurotoxicol. Teratol.* 17, 253–264.

Winer, B. J. (1971). *Statistical Principles in Experimental Design*, 2nd Edn. New York: McGraw-Hill.

Yeomans, J., and Frankland, P. (1996). The acoustic startle reflex: neurons and connections. *Brain Res. Rev.* 21, 301–314.

Litter gender composition and sex affect maternal behavior and DNA methylation levels of the *Oprm1* gene in rat offspring

*Yanli Hao[1,2], Wen Huang[1,2], David A. Nielsen[1,2] and Therese A. Kosten[1,2]**

[1] Menninger Department of Psychiatry and Behavioral Sciences, Baylor College of Medicine, Houston, TX, USA
[2] Michael E Debakey Veterans Administration Medical Center, Houston, TX, USA

***Correspondence:**
Therese A. Kosten, Menninger Department of Psychiatry and Behavioral Sciences, Baylor College of Medicine, 2002 Holcombe Boulevard, Houston, TX 77030, USA.
e-mail: tkosten@bcm.edu

The mu-opioid receptor is encoded by the *Oprm1* gene and contributes to mother–infant behaviors. Rodent dams lick male pups more than female pups in the anogenital region. This behavior is linked to stress responsivity in the offspring that may be mediated by epigenetic changes. We hypothesized that maternal behavior may affect DNA methylation levels of the *Oprm1* gene and show sex differences. To further explore sex differences in mother–pup behaviors and DNA methylation levels, we altered the litter gender composition (LGC) of rats. Litters were culled to eight all male, all female, or four male/four female pups on postnatal (PN) day 1. On PN4, 7, and 10, a dam was placed in a test cage with a pup for a 10-min period. Latency to pup contact was determined as were times spent licking the anogenital and other body regions of the pup. Frequencies of other behaviors were tabulated. On PN35, samples from various brain regions were obtained. DNA methylation at specific CpG sites in the *Oprm1* promoter region were measured by direct sequencing of bisulfite-treated DNA. LGC and sex interacted with day for latency to pup contact. Latencies were longest on PN4 for single-sex males and on PN10 for single-sex females. Dams licked male pups more than female pups in both the anogenital and other body areas. Sex differences were seen in other behaviors. LGC altered DNA methylation at specific CpG's of *Oprm1* in hippocampus with higher levels in single-sex rats. In nucleus accumbens, single-sex males showed hypermethylation levels, a trend seen in caudate–putamen. Results confirm and extend sex differences in maternal care with modest LGC effects. That both LGC and sex have enduring effects on DNA methylation of the *Oprm1* gene in brain regions associated with addiction, stress regulation, motivation, and cognition may suggest one factor that contributes to gender differences in these behaviors.

Keywords: mu-opioid, epigenetics, CREB, female, attachment behavior

INTRODUCTION

Males and females differ in incidences of several behavioral disorders. Autism, antisocial personality and addictive disorders are more common in men, whereas depressive and anxiety disorders are more common in women (Fombonne, 2003; Grant et al., 2009; Vigod and Stewart, 2009). Although alcoholism and drug addiction are more common in men, women progress more quickly from initial use to abuse and dependence (Greenfield et al., 2010). Further, women are just as likely as men to use or abuse prescription opiate drugs (McCabe et al., 2005). In addition, stress exposure, that can precipitate behavioral disorders (Sinha, 2001; Caspi et al., 2003), has greater effects in women than men (Kudielka and Kirschbaum, 2005).

Stress exposure activates the hypothalamic–pituitary–adrenal (HPA) axis. A cascade of events occurs in which corticotrophin-releasing factor release from the paraventricular nucleus of the hypothalamus stimulates the pituitary to cleave proopiomelanocortin into adrenocorticotropic hormone (ACTH) and the endogenous opioid, beta-endorphin as well as other peptides. ACTH is released into the blood stream causing secretion of the glucocorticoid, corticosterone, from the adrenal cortex (Rivier and Plotsky, 1986; Dunn and Berridge, 1990). Beta-endorphins interact with opioid receptors, particularly mu-type receptors, both centrally and in the periphery.

Sex differences are seen in stress responsivity and in the behavioral responses to opioids in rats. Female rats show larger stress hormone and behavioral responses to foot shock compared to male rats (Beatty and Beatty, 1970; Kosten et al., 2006) and greater analgesic responses to various opioids (Craft, 2003). There are also sex differences in the reinforcing effects of opioids. In most cases, female rats show greater operant self-administration (Lynch and Carroll, 1999; Carroll et al., 2002; Cicero et al., 2003) and place conditioning effects of opioids (Cicero et al., 2000) although not in all cases (Stewart et al., 1996). These sex differences may reflect activational or organization effects of gonadal hormones (Kitay, 1961; Viau and Meaney, 1991; Cicero et al., 2002; McCormick et al., 2002) and may relate to the higher density or binding of mu-opioid receptors in female rats and humans relative to males (Hammer, 1990; Zubieta et al., 1999).

Mu-opioid receptors are involved with mother–infant attachment (Nelson and Panksepp, 1998). Administration of morphine or other opioid agonists reduces the rat pups' ultrasonic vocalizations (USV; Kehoe and Blass, 1986; Carden et al., 1991) provoked by isolation from the dam and decrease vocalizations of the infant non-human primate after separation from its mother (Kalin et al., 1988). Although this neuropharmacological relationship was called into question (Winslow and Insel, 1991), recent molecular genetic work confirms the role of mu-opioid receptors in attachment behavior in both rodents and non-human primates. After separation from their dam, mice lacking the mu-opioid receptor gene, *Oprm1*, emit fewer USVs (Moles et al., 2004). Maternal separation-induced vocalizations in infant primates associates with a polymorphism of the *OPRM1* gene (Barr et al., 2008). These studies not only reaffirm the role of the mu-opioid receptor in mother–infant attachment but also suggest a genetic basis for variations in maternal behaviors. However, it is possible that manipulating maternal behavior may affect this gene expression.

Emerging evidence suggests that changes in gene expression resulting in stable phenotypic alterations can be induced by early life manipulations. Genes may be silenced during development through DNA methylation (Jones and Taylor, 1980). Once a methyl group is attached to DNA, transcriptional factors cannot access the gene and it is silenced (Razin, 1998). The methylation status of the $Gr1_7$ promoter in hippocampus was found to be associated with variations in the maternal behavior of anogenital licking and binding of the transcription factor nerve growth factor-inducible factor A (Ngfi-a) in the offspring (Champagne et al., 2003; Weaver et al., 2004). Further, this altered gene expression associates with hormonal and behavioral responses to stress in the adult offspring. Other early life manipulations, such as limited nesting material or high-fat diet, affect DNA methylation of other genes (Roth et al., 2009; Vucetic et al., 2010, 2011). Thus, the structure of DNA can be modified by early life manipulations resulting in a change in the phenotype of the offspring.

Maternal behavior differs by sex of the pup. Dams spend more time in active nursing, nest-building, and licking male pups in the anogenital region compared to female pups (Moore and Morelli, 1979; Richmond and Sachs, 1984; Moore and Chadwick-Dias, 1986; Alleva et al., 1989; Cirulli et al., 1997). Licking the anogenital area stimulates urine and feces elimination of the pup (Gubernick and Alberts, 1983) and helps suppress HPA activity (Stanton et al., 1988; Suchecki et al., 1995; Levine, 2001). Suppression of the HPA axis and the ensuing increase in corticosterone levels may be particularly important for a pup because it can prevent glucocorticoid and mineralocorticoid receptor stimulation in hippocampus. Stimulation of these receptors could have deleterious effects (Sapolsky and Meaney, 1986) on the developing hippocampus (Rice and Barone, 2000; Dumas, 2005), a region that is important for modulating stress responses (Chrousos and Gold, 1992), and also for learning, memory (Scoville and Milner, 1957; McGaugh, 2000), and emotion (Gray, 1982; McHugh et al., 2004; Barkus et al., 2010).

The sex-dependent effects of maternal behavior can be altered by modifying the litter gender composition (LGC) in which offspring of single-sex litters are compared to offspring of mixed-sex litters (Moore and Morelli, 1979; Alleva et al., 1989; Cirulli et al., 1997; Laviola et al., 1999). LGC affects various behaviors of the offspring including analgesic responses to morphine in juvenile male mice with mixed-sex males showing longer response latencies than single-sex males (Alleva et al., 1986). In the present study, we further examined if LGC affects the sex dependency of mother–pup behaviors assessed after a short separation. At 7-weeks of age (PN35), brain tissue samples were obtained from hippocampus, nucleus accumbens (NAc), and other areas to test for DNA methylation levels of the *Oprm1* gene.

MATERIALS AND METHODS
SUBJECTS AND HOUSING

Male and female rats (Sprague-Dawley, Charles River, MA, USA) were housed in polypropylene cages in a temperature- and humidity-controlled vivarium maintained on a 12:12 light/dark cycle (lights on at 0700 hours). Food and water were available *ad libitum*. All procedures were approved by the Baylor College of Medicine Institutional Animal Care and Use Committee (IACUC) in strict accordance with guidelines set forth by the National Institutes of Health.

Sets of one male and two females were paired for breeding. When pregnancy was suspected, females were transferred to individual cages. Litters found before 1700 hours were considered born on that day (Postnatal Day 0; PN0). On PN1, litters were weighed and culled to eight pups. Pups that were not needed for the study were euthanized humanely at this time.

GROUPS

Litter gender composition was manipulated by cross-fostering litters to either single-sex (male or female) or mixed-sex (half male and half female). A total of 42 litters were studied including 10 single male, 12 single female, and 20 mixed-sex litters. Only one pup per litter was sampled. Half of the mixed-sex litters were used to sample a male pup and the other half were used to study the female pup in the mother–pup behavior study. However, in the DNA methylation study, tissue samples were obtained from one male and one female in each of the mixed-sex litters (i.e., *n*'s = 20) and one pup was chosen from each single-sex litter. One of the single male litters was lost so for this analysis, there were nine single male litters.

MOTHER–PUP BEHAVIOR PROCEDURE

Ratings of mother–pup behaviors were performed between 0900 and 1200 in the following manner. The dam was removed from the home cage and placed in a glass observation tank (13′ H × 20′ L × 16.5′ W) contained in a sound-attenuating cubicle equipped with a video camera for 30-min. One of her pups was then removed from the home cage and placed in the observation tank for 10-min. The remaining pups in the litter were kept in the home cage and placed under a heat lamp during the observation period. Video was recorded as soon as the pup was placed in the tank. Video files were coded so that the rater would be blind to litter condition, sex of pup, and postnatal day. This procedure was performed at three time points, PN4, PN7, and PN10, to allow for ontogenetic effects based on previous work (Richmond and Sachs, 1984). The pup was weighed prior to placing it in the observation tank with the exception of the first four litters (one from each condition).

Video files were rated by tabulating the frequency of various behaviors using a time sampling procedure. The rater listened to a recording that beeped every 30-s at which time she would record which behaviors were occurring. The behaviors tabulated are listed and defined in **Table 1**. Data on frequencies of each behavior were summed across the entire 10-min session on each of the three test days (PN4, PN7, PN10) in order to examine the effects of LGC and sex on each behavior. In addition to rating these behaviors, latency to the initial contact with the pup and the total times spent licking

Table 1 | List and definitions of mother–pup behaviors that were either rated for frequency of occurrence or timed during the 10-min observation sessions conducted on PN4, PN7, and PN10.

Variable	Definition	Analysis
Carry	Dam picks up pup by dorsal skin with her incisors and carries it to another place	Rate frequency
Blanket nursing	Dam engages in blanket nursing in which she is over the pup in a bilaterally symmetrical manner and is relatively immobile with or without limb support	Rate frequency
Burrowing	Dam displaces cage bedding with nose or paws	Rate frequency
Climbing	Dam places one or both forepaws on wall of cage	Rate frequency
Rearing	Dam stands on hindlimbs without touching cage wall	Rate frequency
Grooming	Dam licks, scratches, or chews any part of own body	Rate frequency
Latency	Time it takes for the dam to touch the pup with forepaws or nose	Time (s)
Anogenital licking	Time dam spends licking the pup's anogenital region exclusively	Time (s)
Body licking	Time dam spends licking the pup's body except for anogenital region	Time (s)

the anogenital region and other parts of the body were recorded in seconds over the entire 10-min session each day. These behaviors are defined in **Table 1**.

DNA METHYLATION

Tissue samples of hippocampus, NAc, caudate–putamen (CP), and cerebellum were obtained from one rat per condition and sex on PN35 with the purpose of measuring DNA methylation levels of the *Oprm1* gene. We chose this age because it allows enough post-weaning time to test if potential effects on DNA methylation are long-lasting. Rats were anesthetized (Ketamine) then decapitated. Tissue samples were rapidly dissected in slices of 1.5-mm using a Rodent Brain Matrix (RBM-4000C, ASI Instruments, Warren, MI, USA) and immediately placed on dry ice. Samples were stored at −80°C until they were processed for DNA. DNA was isolated from the tissue using the Gentra Purgene DNA isolation method (Qiagen, Valencia, CA, USA) according to manufacturer's protocol.

DNA methylation levels were quantified using the methods detailed previously (Nielsen et al., 2009). Nucleotide sequence of the rat *Oprm1* gene promoter region [chr1:37533440-37536440, Rat Nov. 2004 (Baylor 3,4/rn4)] was downloaded from the UCSC Genome Browser website (genome.ucsc.edu). The predicted bisulfite-treated sequence was determined using the Methyl Primer Express 1.0 software (Applied Biosystems, Foster City, CA, USA) and exported to Vector NTI Advance 11 (Invitrogen, Carlsbad, CA, USA). Primers for amplification of the bisulfite-treated DNA were designed with Vector NTI Advance 11, and synthesized (Midland Reagent Co., Midland, TX, USA).

To determine percent cytosine methylation, genomic DNA (300 ng) was sodium bisulfite-treated using the EZ-96 DNA Methylation Kit D5004 (Zymo Research, Orange, CA, USA) and amplified with primers M-RATOPRM1-1F (5′-TTTTGGTTTTATTAGGGTTG-3′) and M-RATOPRM1-1R (5′-ACCAAAAACCAAATACTAAA-3′). Amplification was performed with 2 μl bisulfite-treated DNA, 1 μM of each primer, 200 μM each of dATP, dCTP, dGTP, and TTP, 18 mM ammonium sulfate, 2 mM $MgSO_4$, 0.5 units Platinum® Taq DNA Polymerase High Fidelity (Invitrogen), and 60 mM $Tris–SO_4$ (pH 8.9) in 25 μl. Amplification consisted of 1 min at 94°C, 3 cycles of 15 s at 94°C, 15 s at 55°C, and 15 s at 68°C, 3 cycles of 15 s at 94°C, 15 s at 52°C, and 15 s at 68°C, 3 cycles of 15 s at 94°C, 15 s at 49°C, and 15 s at 68°C, 3 cycles of 15 s at 94°C, 15 s at 46°C, and 15 s at 68°C, 3 cycles of 15 s at 94°C, 15 s at 43°C, and 15 s at 68°C, followed by a final elongation step at 68°C for 7 min. Unincorporated nucleotides and primers were degraded by mixing 4 μl of the final PCR reaction mixture with 1 μl ExoSAP-IT (USB Corp., Cleveland, OH, USA) followed by incubation at 37°C for 30 min and 80°C for 15 min. For sequencing, 1 μl ExoSAP-IT-treated DNA was added to 11 μl 8 pM primer M-RATOPRM1-1F or M-RATOPRM1-1R. Sequencing was performed at GENEWIZ, Inc. (South Plainfield, NJ, USA) on an ABI 3730 XL sequencer using the ABI 3730POP7SR basecaller (Applied Biosystems). Trace files (.ab1) were analyzed using the ESME version 3.2.1 software from Epigenomics AG (Berlin, Germany; Lewin et al., 2004). Nucleotides are numbered relative to the A of the ATG of the *Oprm1* translation start site. The rat *Oprm1* promoter region was analyzed for predicted transcription factor binding sites using TESS: Transcription Element Search System (Schug and Overton, 1977).

DATA ANALYSIS

The sums of the frequencies of each behavior on each day were analyzed in separate 2 × 2 × 3 ANOVAs using litter as the experimental unit for analysis. This represents the between group factors of LGC (single-sex or mixed-sex litter) and sex (male or female) with repeated measures on postnatal day. Total times (seconds) spent licking (anogenital region and other body regions) were analyzed in the same manner. Body weight was analyzed using weight on PN1 as a co-variate although there was no difference in body weights across litter conditions on this day. DNA methylation levels were analyzed using separate 2 × 2 × 7 ANOVAs by brain region. This represents the same between group factors with repeated measure on CpG site. *Post hoc* univariate tests were used to follow-up on significant effects. Significance was set at 0.05 and trend toward significance was set at 0.10.

RESULTS
BODY WEIGHT

Body weight was measured on PN1, 4, 7, and 10. These data are shown in **Figure 1**. As seen in the figure, body weight increased over days as supported by the Day effect, $F(3,114) = 1,144.48$; $P < 0.0001$. Neither LGC nor Sex affected body weight (P's > 0.10).

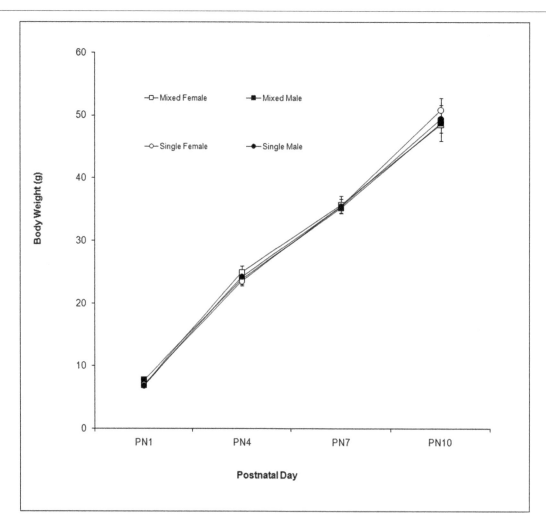

FIGURE 1 | Mean (±SEM) body weight (g) is presented for mixed- (squares) and single- (circles) sex litters for female (open symbols) and male (closed symbols) rats over postnatal days. All groups gained weight over this period with no effect of LGC or Sex seen.

FREQUENCIES OF BEHAVIORS

The effects of LGC and sex on these behaviors on PN4, 7, and 10 are shown in **Tables 2–4**, respectively. None of these behaviors supported significant main effects of LGC or Sex or their interaction (Ps > 0.10). However, some behaviors show Day or Sex × Day effects. There is a significant interaction of Sex × Day for Carry, $F(2,76) = 3.83$; $P < 0.05$. As seen in **Tables 2–4**, this interaction likely reflects that the dam increased carrying male pups over days and decreased carrying female pups over days. Burrowing also shows a significant Sex × Day interaction, $F(2,76) = 3.50$; $P < 0.05$. Dams with female pups show decreases in burrowing over days whereas dams with male pups burrow about the same amount over days. There is a trend for a significant effect of Day for Climbing, $F(2,76) = 2.41$; $P < 0.10$. The data in **Tables 2–4** suggest that this reflects a tendency to increase on PN7 over what is seen on PN4 and then decrease on PN10. The dam's behavior of grooming herself shows a trend toward significance for the Sex × Day interaction, $F(2,76) = 2.38$; $P < 0.10$ and this likely reflects that her grooming tends to decrease over days with male pups but tends to increase over days with female pups. There are no significant effects of Day or its interactions with LGC or Sex for blanket nursing or for rearing (Ps > 0.10).

Table 2 | Mean (±SEM) total frequencies of each behavior across 10-min sessions conducted on PN4.

Variable	Mixed-sex litters		Same-sex litters	
	Male	Female	Male	Female
Carry	1.9 (1.1)	1.3 (0.4)	2.0 (0.6)	1.6 (0.4)
Blanket	2.8 (1.3)	2.9 (1.1)	1.2 (0.6)	0.1 (0.01)
Burrowing	3.9 (1.4)	6.7 (1.2)	5.7 (1.3)	6.9 (1.3)
Climbing	7.9 (1.3)	7.8 (1.0)	8.8 (1.2)	9.2 (1.1)
Rearing	5.8 (1.0)	4.2 (1.0)	5.0 (1.0)	5.0 (1.4)
Grooming	6.8 (1.2)	3.0 (0.7)	5.4 (1.1)	4.5 (0.9)

LATENCY TO PUP CONTACT

The latencies to contact the pup over days are shown in **Figure 2**. There is a trend for dams to contact male pups more quickly than female pups as supported by the trend toward significance for the Sex effect, $F(1,76) = 3.21$; $P < 0.10$. Although the main effects of LGC and Day are not significant (Ps > 0.10), there is a significant

Table 3 | Mean (±SEM) total frequencies of each behavior across 10-min sessions conducted on PN7.

Variable	Mixed-sex litters		Same-sex litters	
	Male	Female	Male	Female
Carry	2.3 (0.9)	2.4 (0.9)	2.0 (0.7)	1.9 (0.5)
Blanket	1.8 (1.1)	1.4 (0.6)	1.0 (0.6)	2.0 (1.2)
Burrowing	4.6 (1.1)	5.6 (0.9)	7.6 (1.6)	4.5 (1.0)
Climbing	10.2 (1.7)	6.7 (1.2)	9.3 (2.8)	9.0 (4.7)
Rearing	4.9 (1.2)	4.0 (0.9)	4.3 (1.1)	5.1 (1.3)
Grooming	4.0 (0.8)	3.7 (0.8)	5.9 (1.0)	6.8 (1.3)

Table 4 | Mean (±SEM) total frequencies of each behavior across 10-min sessions conducted on PN10.

Variable	Mixed-sex litters		Same-sex litters	
	Male	Female	Male	Female
Carry	3.0 (0.8)	1.0 (0.5)	2.4 (0.5)	0.6 (0.4)
Blanket	2.0 (1.0)	3.0 (1.3)	1.5 (1.0)	2.2 (1.1)
Burrowing	4.2 (1.5)	6.1 (1.5)	2.3 (1.2)	6.3 (1.2)
Climbing	7.0 (1.6)	7.3 (1.5)	5.9 (1.7)	8.0 (1.4)
Rearing	4.0 (1.5)	3.9 (3.2)	4.6 (1.7)	3.5 (0.9)
Grooming	4.3 (1.0)	3.9 (0.8)	3.8 (1.0)	4.3 (0.7)

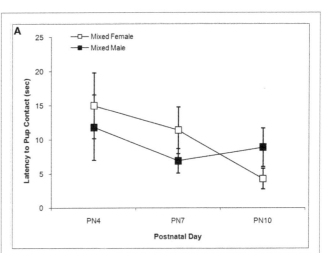
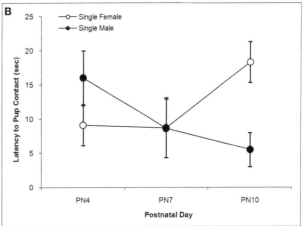

FIGURE 2 | Mean (±SEM) latencies (s) for the dam to contact the pup are presented for mixed- [squares; (A)] and single- [circles; (B)] sex litters for male (closed symbols) and female (open symbols) rats over postnatal days. Dams with single-sex litters took longer to contact their male pups on PN4 and their female pups on PN10 relative to other days and to dams of mixed-sex litters. Dams tended to take longer to contact female vs. male pups. See text for statistics.

LGC × Sex × Day effect, $F(2,76) = 8.14$; $P < 0.001$. Post hoc univariate statistics revealed significant LGC × Sex effects on PN4 and PN10 (P's < 0.01). As seen in **Figure 2A**, dams with mixed-sex male pups take less time to contact their pup compared to dams with mixed-sex female pups. and this LGC effect is not seen on PN7 or PN10. In contrast, as seen in **Figure 2B**, dams with single-sex male pups take longer to contact their pup on PN4 compared to dams with single-sex female pups. However, latencies decrease on PN10 for dams with single-sex male pups and increase for dams of mixed sex female pups.

ANOGENITAL AND BODY LICKING

The total times spent licking the pup in the anogenital region and in other body regions are shown in **Figures 3 and 4** respectively. Anogenital licking times differ by Sex, $F(1,38) = 4.76$; $P < 0.05$, but not by LGC and do not change over Days (P's > 0.10). Dams lick their male pups more than female pups as shown in **Figure 3A** for mixed-sex litters and in **Figure 3B** for single-sex litters. Dams also lick other body parts of their male pups more than of their female pups as seen in **Figure 4**. This is supported by the significant effect of Sex, $F(1, 38) = 4.85$; $P < 0.05$ and can be seen for mixed-sex litters in **Figure 4A** and for single-sex litters in **Figure 4B**. There are no significant effects of LGC or Day or their interactions for body licking (P's > 0.10).

DNA METHYLATION OF THE *OPRM1* GENE

DNA methylation of the *Oprm1* gene promoter region in hippocampus is greater in single-sex litters compared to mixed-sex litters as supported by the significant LGC effect, $F(1,57) = 8.81$; $P < 0.005$, but did not differ by Sex ($P > 0.10$). Methylation levels also differ significantly by CpG site, $F(6,342) = 4.90$; $P < 0.001$. Post hoc univariate comparisons reveals significant LGC effects at CpG sites −59, −20, and 33 (P's < 0.05). Compared to mixed-sex litters seen in **Figure 5A**, hypermethylation at most CpG sites can be seen in **Figure 5B** for single-sex litters. For ease of presentation, **Figure 5C** shows the means across CpG sites by LGC and Sex in Hippocampus.

In NAc, single-sex males have the highest mean DNA methylation level over the *Oprm1* gene promoter region and this is supported by the significant LGC × Sex interaction, $F(1,57) = 4.33$; $P < 0.05$. Neither the LGC nor Sex main effect is significant (P's > 0.10) but methylation levels differ significantly by CpG site, $F(6,342) = 4.33$; $P < 0.001$. Post hoc univariate comparisons reveal a significant LGC × Sex effect at CpG site −107 ($P < 0.05$). This is shown in **Figure 6A** for mixed-sex litters and in **Figure 6B** for single-sex litters. The means across CpG sites for all four groups are shown in **Figure 6C**.

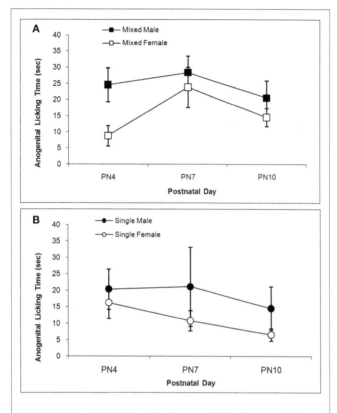

FIGURE 3 | Mean (±SEM) times the dam spent licking the anogenital region of her pup are presented for mixed- [squares; (A)] and single- [circles; (B)] sex litters for male (closed symbols) and female (open symbols) rats over postnatal days. Dams lick the anogenital region of male pups more than female pups. See text for statistics.

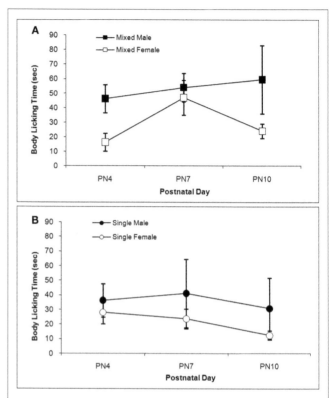

FIGURE 4 | Mean (±SEM) times the dam spent licking the body of her pup except in the anogenital region are presented for mixed- [squares; (A)] and single- [circles; (B)] sex litters for male (closed symbols) and female (open symbols) rats over postnatal days. Dams lick the body of male pups more than female pups. See text for statistics.

Single-sex males tend to have the highest mean DNA methylation level over the *Oprm1* gene promoter region in CP. This statement is supported by the trends toward significance of the main effect of Sex, $F(1,57) = 3.77$; $P < 0.10$ and the interaction of LGC × Sex, $F(1,57) = 3.07$; $P < 0.10$. The CpG effect was not significant, $P > 0.10$, in this brain region. These data are shown in **Figures 7A–C**. We find no significant effects on DNA methylation in cerebellum for LGC or Sex or CpG site or any significant interactions (P's > 0.10; data not shown).

DISCUSSION

These experiments provide important new data on epigenetic alterations linked to the subtle early life manipulation of modifying LGC as well as to sex differences both of which affected maternal behavior. Results from the present study confirm and extend prior work showing sex differences and modest LGC effects on mother–pup behaviors as well as support for the involvement of the mu-opioid system in these behaviors. We demonstrate that dams provide more maternal care to their male pups than to their female pups and that LGC interacts with sex of pup and postnatal day to alter latency to pup contact. Further, both sex of pup and LGC had significant effects on DNA methylation levels of the *Oprm1* gene promoter region. Male rats raised in single-sex litters show *Oprm1* hypermethylation, particularly in NAc and CP, and rats of both sexes raised in single-sex litters show hypermethylation in hippocampus compared to rats raised in mixed-sex litters. It is unlikely that these effects can be explained by gross developmental differences because we found that neither sex nor LGC altered body weight gain. These data are the first to demonstrate that sex and composition of the family unit is associated with epigenetic alterations in the DNA methylation of *Oprm1* gene promoter region. These levels of methylation may reflect differences in the levels of maternal care received.

The present study confirms and extends prior work because we demonstrated sex dependency of some mother–pup behaviors. As others reported (Moore and Morelli, 1979; Richmond and Sachs, 1984; Moore and Chadwick-Dias, 1986), we showed that dams licked their male pups more in the anogenital region compared to their female pups. We also found that dams with male pups licked other regions of the body more than dams with female pups. Sex differences were seen in the behavior of carrying or handling the pup. Moore and Morelli (1979) reported that introducing a new male pup to the litter increased the dam's handling pups with her forepaws. We saw that dams with male pups showed increasing times carrying them over postnatal days compared to dams with female pups that showed decreasing carrying times over days. Latency to contact a pup tended to be shorter for male pups than for female pups in our study although Moore and Morelli (1979) found no sex differences in this measure.

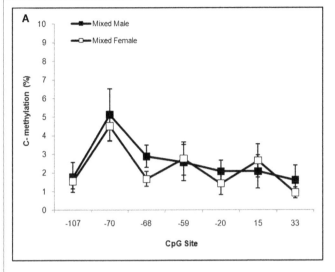
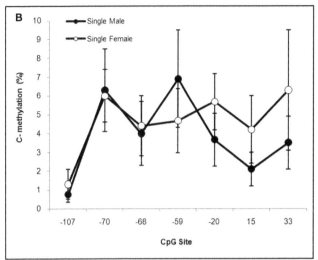
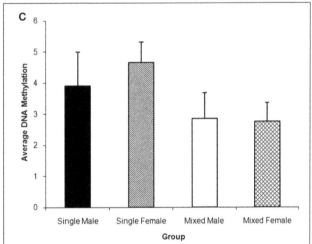

FIGURE 5 | Mean (±SEM) DNA methylation levels of the *Oprm1* gene promoter region in hippocampus are presented for mixed- [squares; (A)] and single- [circles; (B)] sex litters for male (closed symbols) and female (open symbols) rats over CpG site. Mean DNA methylation levels across CpG sites are shown in (C). Levels are higher in single- vs. mixed-sex litters and differ by CpG site. *Post hoc* analyses reveal significant effects at −59, −20, and 33 sites. See text for statistics.

Similar to previous work (Moore and Morelli, 1979; Alleva et al., 1989; Cirulli et al., 1997), we found that LGC had modest effects on mother–pup behaviors. Dams of male mice raised in single-sex litters spent more time engaged in nest-building and in arched-back or active nursing compared to dams of single-sex females or mixed-sex litters (Alleva et al., 1989; Cirulli et al., 1997). We did not see active nursing in our 10-min sessions although we rated blanket nursing and found no significant LGC or Sex effects. In fact, only one measure showed an LGC effect in the present study and it interacted with Sex and Day. Dams of male pups in mixed-sex litters showed the lowest latencies to pup contact and it remained low across the 3 postnatal days assessed. However, if the dams' male pups were in single-sex litters, then the latency to contact was high on PN4 and not unlike the levels seen for dams of female pups. On subsequent days, single-sex male pups were then contacted in a short time frame not unlike the times seen for mixed-sex male pups. In contrast, the dams' latencies to retrieve female pups from single-sex litters increased on PN10 whereas latencies decreased on this day for dams of mixed-sex females. The day effect seen for male pups is similar to findings from Moore and Morelli (1979). In their procedure, the litter remained with the dam and a new pup (male or female) was introduced. If a male pup was introduced to dam with all male pups, the latency to retrieve was very high on PN3 and decreased to very low levels on PN10. We can speculate that the dam's ability to discriminate the sex of her pups may be facilitated by the presence of pups of both sexes so that if she has only males in her litter, it may take a few days for her to retrieve or contact male pups as efficiently as dams with mixed-sex litters.

There are some methodological differences in procedures used to assess sex or LGC effects on maternal behavior between our study and those of others. Observations of mother–pup interactions were made in the home cage in the previous studies whereas in the present study, observations were made in a separate test room with dam and one pup placed in a test cage after a short

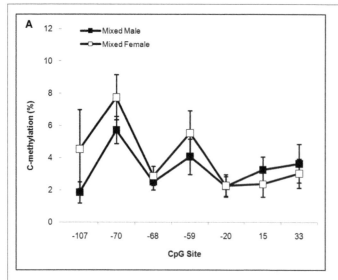
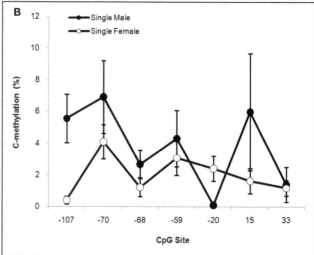
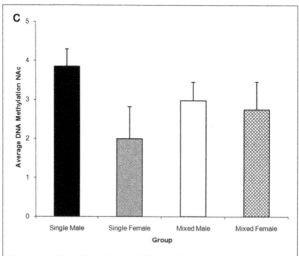

FIGURE 6 | Mean (±SEM) DNA methylation levels of the *Oprm1* gene promoter region in nucleus accumbens are presented for mixed- [squares; (A)] and single- [circles; (B)] sex litters for male (closed symbols) and female (open symbols) rats over CpG site. Mean DNA methylation levels across CpG sites are shown in (C). Levels are highest in males of single-sex litters and differ by CpG site. *Post hoc* analyses reveal a significant LGC × Sex effect at 107. See text for statistics.

separation period. The former procedure allowed assessing behavior under natural and undisturbed conditions whereas the latter procedure was likely disruptive to the dam and pup. However, such a disruption can stimulate a bout of maternal behavior that may enhance the ability to find significant effects of the experimental manipulations. Also, the dam, and possibly the pup, may habituate to these effects over subsequent test days (Kosten and Kehoe, 2010). The reason we chose to use this procedure is that, unlike previous studies, it allowed us to study sex and LGC independently. That is, we employed twice as many mixed-sex litters and used half to sample a pup of each sex. The previous studies had only one mixed-sex group to compare to single-sex female and single-sex male litters and thus could not assess the effect of sex alone or its interaction with LGC.

Both LGC and sex affected DNA methylation levels of the *Oprm1* gene promoter region in the present study. We found hypermethylation in single-sex litters in hippocampus with no changes seen in cerebellum. In NAc single-sex male litters showed hypermethylation, an effect that trended toward significance in the CP. The *Oprm1* gene codes for the mu-opioid receptor that is widespread in the central nervous system. It is the site of action of beta-endorphins as well as for several opioid drugs such as morphine and heroin. This system is involved in many physiological and behavioral functions most notably in analgesia, drug addiction, and motivation to seek natural rewards (Kreek et al., 2005; Koob and Le Moal, 2008). The contribution of the mu-opioid system to attachment behavior is particularly relevant to the present study. Early pharmacological studies suggested that endogenous opioids are released in the infant during caretaking and that this serves to motivate it to seek out and maintain closeness to its caregiver (Kehoe and Blass, 1986; Kalin et al., 1988; Carden et al., 1991; Nelson and Panksepp, 1998).

More recent molecular genetic studies support the contribution of the mu-opioid system in infant–mother attachment. Mice lacking the *Oprm1* gene emit fewer USVs after separation from

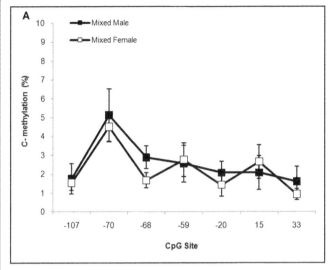
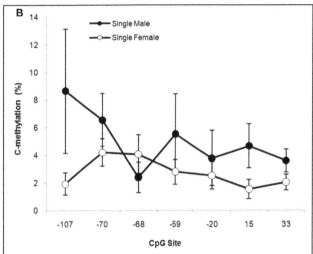
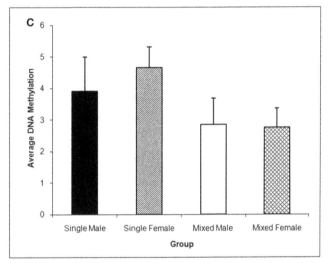

FIGURE 7 | Mean (±SEM) DNA methylation levels of the *Oprm1* gene promoter region in caudate–putamen are presented for mixed- [squares; (A)] and single- [circles; (B)] sex litters for male (closed symbols) and female (open symbols) rats over transcription site. Mean DNA methylation levels across CpG sites are shown in **(C)**. Levels tend to be highest in males, particularly those from single-sex litters. See text for statistics.

their dam, a behavior that is not modulated by morphine in the knock-out as it is in the wild-type mouse (Moles et al., 2004). Further, a polymorphism of the *OPRM1* gene in infant primates (C77G) associates with vocalizations and expression of attachment behaviors (e.g., clinging behavior; Barr et al., 2008). That is, infants with a G allele show persistence in vocalization emissions and increasing social contact after repeated separations from the mother whereas infant primates with the C/C genotype do not (Barr et al., 2008). In humans, the G allele of the *OPRM1* A118G variant has been shown to relate to lower potency of analgesic effects of opioids and greater pain experiences as well as greater distress after social rejection (Chou et al., 2006; Way et al., 2009). The G allele of the *OPRM1* gene is associated with reduced levels of mu-opioid receptor mRNA and protein compared to the A allele (Kroslak et al., 2007). Among children living in disruptive family environments, the 118G allele is associated with greater quality of parental relationship and fewer parental arguments (Copeland et al., 2011). Perhaps this reflects that these children expressed greater attachment behaviors as infants as suggested by the non-human primate study.

In general, DNA methylation means that transcriptional factors are not accessed and less gene promoter is expressed (Razin, 1998). In the case of the *Oprm1* gene, DNA hypomethylation associates with increased *OPRM1* transcription (Andria and Simon, 1999; Hwang et al., 2009). In fact, another early life manipulation, exposure to a high-fat diet, also increased methylation of the *Oprm1* gene and this is associated with decreased mRNA expression of the mu-opioid receptor in reward regions of the brains of mice (Vucetic et al., 2011). The increase in *Oprm1* DNA methylation seen in male rats in the present study, particularly those raised in single-sex litters, suggests that they too have lower mu-opioid receptor availability. Such rats would be predicted to have lower analgesic effects of morphine. Indeed, morphine is less effective in male mice raised in same-sex litters compared to male mice raised in mixed-sex litters (Alleva et al., 1986). Further, our findings that LGC altered DNA methylation of the *Oprm1* gene promoter region in brain regions that contribute to drug reward (NAc, hippocampus, CP) but not in a region not involved with this effect (cerebellum), suggest that this early life manipulation may also affect vulnerability to addiction. The lack of significant effects of LGC or sex on global DNA methylation levels in these regions of interest (data not shown) supports our finding that changes in the *Oprm1* DNA methylation levels are specific. These brain regions are also involved in stress responsivity (Chrousos and Gold, 1992), memory (Scoville and Milner, 1957; McGaugh, 2000), and emotion (Gray, 1982; McHugh et al., 2004; Barkus et al., 2010). Phenotypes related to these constructs may also be modified by LGC or sex via a DNA methylation-induced alteration in the *Oprm1* gene.

DNA methylation of CpGs in transcription factor binding sites reduces the binding affinity of cognate transcription factors and their ability to transactivate gene expression. In hippocampus, we find that LGC affected the +33 CpG site specifically increasing methylation in rats from single-sex litters (see **Figure 5**). This CpG site is located in an E2F binding site (TESS R08845; Schug and Overton, 1977). E2Fs are a family of transcription factors that have been shown to regulate the cell cycle and DNA biosynthesis and play a central role in the development of the central nervous system (Swiss and Casaccia, 2010). No mammalian transcription factor binding sites have been identified that contain the −59 and −20 CpG sites (TESS; Schug and Overton, 1977). The −107 CpG site is significantly altered in NAc by LGC in a sex-dependent manner. That is, male pups raised in single-sex litters show greater methylation at this site compared to male pups raised in mixed-sex litters. In contrast, females raised in single-sex litters show lower methylation at this site compared to their mixed-sex litter counterparts (see **Figure 6**). The −107 CpG site is located in overlapping CREB (TESS R02710) and activator protein-1 (AP-1; TESS R00368) transcription factor binding sites. CREB, in addition to its role in intracellular signaling of the cAMP/PKA pathway, is essential for survival and expansion of neural progenitor cells, while both CREB and activator protein-1 (AP-1), a dimer of c-fos and Jun family members, appears to control synaptic plasticity (Flavell and Greenberg, 2008; Dworkin et al., 2009). CREB levels in NAc are related to the rewarding and aversive effects of drugs of abuse, including opiates, as well as to chronic effects of drug exposure, such as tolerance, dependence, and withdrawal (Carlezon et al., 2005). Further, both depression and anxiety are linked to CREB activity in NAc (Carlezon et al., 2005). Interestingly, there are gender differences in the rates of all of these disorders (see Introduction) raising the possibility that sexual dimorphism in DNA methylation of the CREB CpG site of the *OPRM1* gene in humans may exist and may contribute to the differential risk or resiliency to develop these disorders.

The present study adds to the literature demonstrating that epigenetic modification of gene expression and resulting changes in phenotypic expression may be mediated via maternal care (Weaver et al., 2004; Roth et al., 2009). Further, these effects may be transmitted to future generations (Meaney, 2001; Roth et al., 2009) through non-genomic transmission of maternal behavior (Francis et al., 1999; Champagne and Meaney, 2001) or perhaps via imprinting the effects from parent to daughter cells.

ACKNOWLEDGMENTS

This research was supported by grant DA 020117 (Therese A. Kosten). We greatly acknowledge the technical assistance provided by A. Aruffo, M. Kosten, P. O'Malley, M. Rengasamy, J. Taylor, X. Xiang, and A. Yarnall.

REFERENCES

Alleva, E., Caprioli, A., and Laviola, G. (1986). Postnatal social environment affects morphine analgesia in male mice. *Physiol. Behav.* 36, 779–781.

Alleva, E., Caprioli, A., and Laviola, G. (1989). Litter gender composition affects maternal behavior of the primiparous mouse dam (*Mus musculus*). *J. Comp. Psychol.* 103, 83–87.

Andria, M. L., and Simon, E. J. (1999). Localization of promoter elements in the human mu-opioid receptor gene and regulation by DNA methylation. *Brain Res. Mol. Brain Res.* 70, 54–65.

Barkus, C., McHugh, S. B., Sprengel, R., Seeburg, P. H., Rawlins, J. N. P., and Bannerman, D. M. (2010). Hippocampal NMDA receptors and anxiety: at the interface between cognition and emotion. *Eur. J. Pharmacol.* 626, 49–56.

Barr, C. S., Schwandt, M. L., Lindell, S. G., Higley, J. D., Mestripieri, D., Goldman, D., Suomi, S. J., and Heilig, M. (2008). Variation at the mu-opioid receptor gene (OPRM1) influences attachment behavior in infant primates. *Proc. Natl. Acad. Sci. U.S.A.* 105, 5277–5281.

Beatty, W. W., and Beatty, P. A. (1970). Hormonal determinants of sex differences in avoidance behavior and reactivity to electric shock in the rat. *J. Comp. Physiol. Psychol.* 73, 446–455.

Carden, S. E., Barr, G. A., and Hofer, M. A. (1991). Differential effects of specific opioid receptor agonists on rat pup isolation calls. *Brain Res. Dev. Brain Res.* 62, 17–22.

Carlezon, W. A., Duman, R. S., and Nestler, E. J. (2005). The many faces of CREB. *Trends Neurosci.* 28, 436–445.

Carroll, M. E., Morgan, A. D., Campbell, U. C., Lynch, W. J., and Dess, N. K. (2002). Cocaine and heroin i.v. self-administration in rats selectively bred for differential saccharin intake: phenotype and sex differences. *Psychopharmacology* 161, 304–313.

Caspi, A., Sugden, K., Moffitt, T. E., Taylor, A., Craig, I. W., Harrington, H., Mccaly, J., Mill, J., Martin, J., Braithwaite, A., and Pouton, R. (2003). Influence of life stress on depression: moderation by a polymorphism in the 5-HTT gene. *Science* 301, 386–389.

Champagne, F., and Meaney, M. J. (2001). Like mother, like daughter: evidence for non-genomic transmission of parental behavior and stress responsivity. *Prog. Brain Res.* 133, 287–302.

Champagne, F. A., Francis, D. D., Mar, A., and Meaney, M. J. (2003). Variations in maternal care in the rat as a mediating influence for the effects of environment on development. *Physiol. Behav.* 79, 359–371.

Chou, W.-Y., Wang, C.-H., Liu, P.-H., Liu, C.-C., Tseng, C.-C., and Jawan, B. (2006). Human opioid receptor A118G polymorphism affects intravenous patient-controlled analgesia morphine consumption after total abdominal hysterectomy. *Anesthesiology* 105, 334–337.

Chrousos, G. P., and Gold, P. W. (1992). The concepts of stress and stress system disorders. Overview of physical and behavioral homeostasis. *J. Am. Med. Assoc.* 267, 1244–1252.

Cicero, T. J., Aylward, S. C., and Meyer, E. R. (2003). Gender differences in the intravenous self-administration of mu opiate agonists. *Pharmacol. Biochem. Behav.* 74, 541–549.

Cicero, T. J., Ennis, T., Ogden, J., and Meyer, E. R. (2000). Gender differences in the reinforcing properties of morphine. *Pharmacol. Biochem. Behav.* 65, 91–96.

Cicero, T. J., Nock, B., O'connor, L., and Meyer, E. R. (2002). Role of steroids in sex differences in morphine-induced analgesia: activational and organizational effects. *J. Pharmacol. Exp. Ther.* 300, 695–701.

Cirulli, F., Adriani, W., and Laviola, G. (1997). Sexual segregation in infant mice: behavioural and neuroendocrine responses to D-amphetamine administration. *Psychopharmacology (Berl.)* 134, 140–152.

Copeland, W. E., Sun, H., Costello, E. J., Angold, A., Heilig, M. A., and Barr, C. S. (2011). Child m-opioid receptor gene variant influences parent-child relations. *Neuropsychopharmacology* 36, 1165–1172.

Craft, R. M. (2003). Sex differences in opioid analgesia: "from mouse to man". *Clin. J. Pain* 19, 175–186.

Dumas, T. C. (2005). Late postnatal maturation of excitatory synaptic transmission permits adult-like expression of hippocampal behaviors. *Hippocampus* 15, 562–578.

Dunn, A. J., and Berridge, C. W. (1990). Physiological and behavioral responses to corticotropin-releasing factor administration: is CRF a mediator of anxiety or stress responses? *Brain Res. Rev.* 15, 71–100.

Dworkin, S. J., Malaterre, J., Hollande, F., Darcy, P. K., Ramsay, R. G., and Mantamadiotis, T. (2009). cAMP response element binding protein is required for mouse neural progenitor cell survival and expansion. *Stem Cells* 27, 1347–1357.

Flavell, S. W., and Greenberg, M. E. (2008). Signaling mechanisms linking neuronal activity to gene expression and plasticity of the nervous system. *Annu. Rev. Neurosci.* 31, 563–590.

Fombonne, E. (2003). Epidemiological surveys of autism and other pervasive developmental disorders: an update. *J. Autism Dev. Disord.* 33, 365–382.

Francis, D. D., Diorio, J., Liu, D., and Meaney, M. J. (1999). Nongenomic transmission across generations of maternal behavior and stress responses in the rat. *Science* 286, 1155–1158.

Grant, B. F., Goldstein, R. B., Chou, S. P., Huang, B., Stinson, F. S., Dawson, D. A., Saha, T. D., Smith, S. M., Pulay, A. J., Pickering, R. P., Ruan, W. J., and Compton, W. M. (2009). Sociodemographic and psychopathologic predictors of first incidence of DSM IV substance use, mood and anxiety disorders: results from the Wave 2 National Epidemiologic Survey on Alcohol and Related Conditions. *Mol. Psychiatry* 14, 1051–1066.

Gray, J. A. (1982). *The Neuropsychology of Anxiety: An Enquiry into the Functions of the Septo-Hippocampal System.* Oxford: Oxford University Press.

Greenfield, S. F., Back, S. E., Lawson, K., and Brady, K. T. (2010). Substance abuse in women. *Psychiatr. Clin. North Am.* 33, 339–355.

Gubernick, D. J., and Alberts, J. R. (1983). Maternal licking of young: resource exchange and proximate controls. *Physiol. Behav.* 31, 593–601.

Hammer, R. P. (1990). m-Opiate receptor binding in the medial preoptic area is cyclical and sexually dimorphic. *Brain Res.* 515, 187–192.

Hwang, C. K., Song, K. Y., Kim, C. S., Choi, H. S., Guo, X. H., Law, P. Y., Wei, L. N., and Loh, H. H. (2009). Epigenetic programming of mu-opioid receptor gene in mouse brain is regulated by MeCP2 and Brg1 chromatin remodelling factor. *J. Cell. Mol. Med.* 13, 3591–3615.

Jones, P. A., and Taylor, S. M. (1980). Cellular differentiation, cytidine analogs and DNA methylation. *Cell* 20, 85–93.

Kalin, N. H., Shelton, S. E., and Barksdale, C. M. (1988). Opiate modulation of separation-induced distress in non-human primates. *Brain Res.* 440, 285–292.

Kehoe, P., and Blass, E. M. (1986). Opioid-mediation of separation distress in 10-day-old rats: reversal of stress with maternal stimuli. *Dev. Psychobiol.* 19, 385–398.

Kitay, J. I. (1961). Sex differences in adrenal cortical secretion in the rat. *Endocrinology* 68, 818–824.

Koob, G. F., and Le Moal, M. (2008). Addiction and the brain antireward system. *Annu. Rev. Psychol.* 59, 29–53.

Kosten, T. A., and Kehoe, P. (2010). The immediate and enduring effects of neonatal isolation on maternal behavior in rats. *Int. J. Dev. Neurosci.* 28, 53–61.

Kosten, T. A., Lee, H. J., and Kim, J. J. (2006). Early life stress impairs fear conditioning in adult male and female rats. *Brain Res.* 1087, 142–150.

Kreek, M. J., Nielsen, D. A., Butelman, E. R., and Laforge, K. S. (2005). Genetic influences on impulsivity, risk taking, stress responsivity, and vulnerability to drug abuse and addiction. *Nat. Neurosci.* 8, 1450–1457.

Kroslak, T., Laforge, K. S., Ho, A., Nielsen, D. A., and Kreek, M. J. (2007). The single nucleotide polymorphism A118G alters functional properties of the human mu opioid receptor. *J. Neurochem.* 103, 77–87.

Kudielka, B. M., and Kirschbaum, C. (2005). Sex differences in HPA axis responses to stress: a review. *Biol. Psychiatry* 69, 113–132.

Laviola, G., Adriani, W., Terranova, M. L., and Gerra, G. (1999). Psychobiological risk factors for vulnerability to psychostimulants in human adolescents and animal models. *Neurosci. Biobehav. Rev.* 23, 993–1010.

Levine, S. (2001). Primary social relationships influence the development of the hypothalamic-pituitary-adrenal axis in the rat. *Physiol. Behav.* 73, 255–260.

Lewin, J., Schmitt, A. O., Adorjan, P., Hildmann, T., and Piepenbrock, C. (2004). Quantitative DNA methylation analysis based on four-dye trace data from direct sequencing of PCR amplifications. *Bioinformatics* 20, 3005–3012.

Lynch, W. J., and Carroll, M. E. (1999). Sex differences in the acquisition of intravenously self-administered cocaine and heroin in rats. *Psychopharmacology (Berl.)* 144, 77–82.

McCabe, S. E., Teter, C. J., Boyd, C. J., Knight, J. R., and Wechsler, H. (2005). Nonmedical use of prescription opioids among U.S. college students: prevalence and correlates from a national survey. *Addict. Behav.* 30, 879–805.

McCormick, C. M., Linkroum, W., Sallinen, B. J., and Miller, N. W. (2002). Peripheral and central sex steroids have differential effects on the HPA axis of male and female rats. *Stress* 5, 235–247.

McGaugh, J. L. (2000). Memory – a century of consolidation. *Science* 287, 248–251.

McHugh, S. B., Deacon, R. M., Rawlins, H. N., and Bannerman, D. M. (2004). Amygdala and ventral hippocampus contribute differentially to mechanisms of fear and anxiety. *Behav. Neurosci.* 118, 63–78.

Meaney, M. J. (2001). Maternal care, gene expression, and the transmission of individual differences in stress reactivity across generations. *Annu. Rev. Neurosci.* 24, 1161–1192.

Moles, A., Kieffer, B. L., and D'amato, F. R. (2004). Deficit in attachment behavior in mice lacking the mu-opioid receptor gene. *Science* 304, 1983–1986.

Moore, C. L., and Chadwick-Dias, A. M. (1986). Behavioral responses of infant rats to maternal licking: variations with age and sex. *Dev. Psychobiol.* 19, 427–438.

Moore, C. L., and Morelli, G. A. (1979). Mother rats interact differently with male and female offspring. *J. Comp. Physiol. Psychol.* 93, 667–684.

Nelson, E. E., and Panksepp, J. (1998). Brain substrates of infant-mother attachment: contributions of opioids, oxytocin, and norepinephrine. *Neurosci. Biobehav. Rev.* 22, 437–452.

Nielsen, D. A., Yuferov, V., Hamon, S., Jackson, C., Ho, A., Ott, J., and Kreek, M. J. (2009). Increased OPRM1 DNA methylation in lymphocytes of methadone-maintained former heroin addicts. *Neuropsychopharmacology* 34, 867–873.

Razin, A. (1998). CpG methylation, chromatin structure and gene silencing-a three-way connection. *EMBO J.* 17, 4905–4908.

Rice, D., and Barone, S. (2000). Critical periods of vulnerability for the developing nervous system: evidence from human and animal models. *Environ. Health Perspect.* 108, 511–533.

Richmond, G., and Sachs, B. D. (1984). Maternal discrimination of pup sex in rats. *Dev. Psychobiol.* 17, 87–89.

Rivier, C. L., and Plotsky, P. M. (1986). Mediation by corticotropin releasing factor (CRF) of adrenohypophysial hormone secretion. *Annu. Rev. Physiol.* 48, 475–494.

Roth, T. L., Lubin, F. D., Funk, A. J., and Sweatt, J. D. (2009). Lasting epigenetic influence of early-life adversity on the BDNF gene. *Biol. Psychiatry* 65, 760–769.

Sapolsky, R. M., and Meaney, M. J. (1986). Maturation of the adrenocortical stress response: neuroendocrine control mechanisms and the stress hyporesponsive period. *Brain Res. Rev.* 11, 65–76.

Schug, J., and Overton, G. C. (1977). *TESS: Transcription Element Search Software on the WWW.* [http://www.cbil.upenn.edu/cgi-bin/tess/tess]. University of Pennsylvania. [accessed February 7, 2011].

Scoville, W. B., and Milner, B. (1957). Loss of recent memory after bilateral hippocampal lesions. *J. Neurol. Neurosurg. Psychiatr.* 20, 11–21.

Sinha, R. (2001). How does stress increase risk of drug abuse and relapse? *Psychopharmacology* 158, 343–359.

Stanton, M. E., Gutierrez, Y. R., and Levine, S. (1988). Maternal deprivation potentiates pituitary-adrenal stress responses in infant rats. *Behav. Neurosci.* 102, 692–700.

Stewart, J., Woodside, B., and Shaham, Y. (1996). Ovarian hormones do not affect the initiation and maintenance of intravenous self-administration of heroin in the female rat. *Psychobiology* 24, 154–159.

Suchecki, D., Nelson, D. Y., Vanoers, H., and Levine, S. (1995). Activation and inhibition of the hypothalamic-pituitary-adrenal axis of the neonatal rat: effects of maternal deprivation. *Psychoneuroendocrinology* 20, 169–182.

Swiss, V. A., and Casaccia, P. (2010). Cell-context specific role of the E2F/Rb pathway in development and disease. *Glia* 58, 377–390.

Viau, V., and Meaney, M. J. (1991). Variations in the hypothalamic-pituitary-adrenal response to stress during the estrous cycle in the rat. *Endocrinology* 129, 2503–2511.

Vigod, S. N., and Stewart, D. E. (2009). Emergent research in the cause of mental illness in women across the lifespan. *Curr Opin Psychiatry* 22, 396–400.

Vucetic, Z., Kimmel, J., and Reyes, T. M. (2011). Chronic high-fat diet drives postnatal epigenetic regulation of μ-opioid receptor in brain. *Neuropsychopharmacology* 36, 1199–1206.

Vucetic, Z., Kimmel, J., Totoki, K., Hollenbeck, E., and Reyes, T. M. (2010). Maternal high-fat diet alters methylation and gene expression of dopamine and opioid-related genes. *Endocrinology* 151, 4756–4764.

Way, B. M., Taylor, S. E., and Eisenberger, N. I. (2009). Variation in the m-opioid receptor gene (OPRM1) is associated with dispositional and neural sensitivity to social rejection. *Proc. Natl. Acad. Sci. U.S.A.* 106, 15079–15084.

Weaver, I. C., Cervoni, N., Champagne, F. A., D'alessio, A. C., Sharma, S., Seckl, J. R., Dymov, S., Szyf, M., and Meaney, M. J. (2004). Epigenetic programming by maternal behavior. *Nat. Neurosci.* 7, 847–854.

Winslow, J. T., and Insel, T. R. (1991). Endogenous opioids: do they modulate the rat pup's response to social isolation? *Behav. Neurosci.* 105, 253–263.

Zubieta, J.-K., Dannals, R. F., and Frost, J. J. (1999). Gender and age influences on human brain mu-opioid receptor binding measured by PET. *Am. J. Psychiatry* 156, 842–848.

Are behavioral effects of early experience mediated by oxytocin?

Karen L. Bales[1]*, Ericka Boone[2], Pamela Epperson[2], Gloria Hoffman[3] and C. Sue Carter[2]

[1] Department of Psychology, University of California, Davis, CA, USA
[2] Brain-Body Center, Department of Psychiatry, University of Illinois, Chicago, IL, USA
[3] Department of Biology, Morgan State University, Baltimore, MD, USA

*Correspondence:
Karen L. Bales, Department of Psychology, University of California, 135 Young Hall, Davis, CA 95616, USA.
e-mail: klbales@ucdavis.edu

Early experiences can alter adaptive emotional responses necessary for social behavior as well as physiological reactivity in the face of challenge. In the highly social prairie vole (*Microtus ochrogaster*), manipulations in early life or hormonal treatments specifically targeted at the neuropeptides oxytocin (OT) and arginine vasopressin (AVP), have long-lasting, often sexually dimorphic, consequences for social behavior. Here we examine the hypothesis that behavioral changes associated with differential early experience, in this case handling the family during the first week of life, may be mediated by changes in OT or AVP or their brain receptors. Four early treatment groups were used, differing only in the amount of manipulation received during the first week of life. MAN1 animals were handled once on post-natal day 1; MAN1 treatment produces a pattern of behavior usually considered typical of this species, against which other groups were compared. MAN1–7 animals were handled once a day for post-natal days 1–7, MAN 7 animals were handled once on post-natal day 7, and MAN0 animals received no handling during the first week of life. When tested following weaning, males in groups that had received manipulation during the first few days of life (MAN1 and MAN1–7) displayed higher alloparenting than other groups. Neuroendocrine measures, including OT receptor binding and OT and AVP immunoreactivity, varied by early treatment. In brain areas including the nucleus accumbens, bed nucleus of stria terminalis and lateral septum, MAN0 females showed increased OT receptor binding. MAN1 animals also displayed higher numbers of immunoreactive OT cell bodies in the supraoptic nucleus. Taken together these findings support the broader hypothesis that experiences in the first few days of life, mediated in part by sexually dimorphic changes in neuropeptides, especially in the receptor for OT, may have adaptive consequences for sociality and emotion regulation.

Keywords: oxytocin, vasopressin, monogamy, parental care, anxiety

INTRODUCTION

The role of early experience in the development of adult behavior and psychopathology has been of considerable interest to neurobiologists for decades (Harlow, 1961, 1964; Harlow and Suomi, 1971; Hofer, 1978, 2006; Plotsky, 1997, 2002; Levine, 2002a). Early neglect or traumatic experiences may increase vulnerability in later life, contributing to the symptoms associated with depression, anxiety disorders, substance abuse, and post-traumatic stress disorder (Heim et al., 1997; Henry and Wang, 1998; Plotsky et al., 1998; Sanchez et al., 2001; Gilmer and McKinney, 2003; Advani et al., 2007; Francis and Kuhar, 2008). In contrast, early experiences can have positive consequences for later sociality (Carter et al., 2009) and emotion regulation (Francis et al., 2002a), disease resistance (Nithiantharajah and Hannan, 2006), and memory (Berardi et al., 2007; Herring et al., 2008), among other variables.

A rich literature chronicles the behavioral and physiological effects of early handling in rodents (Levine, 1957; Levine and Lewis, 1959b; Denenberg et al., 1962; Denenberg and Whimbey, 1963), particularly focused on stress reactivity of the offspring (Levine, 2002b). Short separations from the mother tend to produce offspring that display improved capacities to manage a social or physical challenge (Levine, 2005; Aguilar, 2010; Zanettini et al., 2010), though this was not true in every study (Todeschin et al., 2009); while either drastically reduced handling or long separations tend to produce offspring that are hyper-responsive to stressors (Levine, 2002a). It is often hypothesized that this effect is maternally mediated, possibly due to increases in maternal attention to infants upon reunion, although alternative hypotheses have also been suggested (Denenberg et al., 1962; Denenberg and Whimbey, 1963; Smotherman and Bell, 1980; Boccia and Pedersen, 2001; Tang, 2001; Tang et al., 2006; Macri et al., 2008). Sex differences in the response to early handling are also a consistent finding, although these differences are not always in the same direction (Eklund and Arborelius, 2006; Slotten et al., 2006; Bales et al., 2007a; Renard et al., 2007; Aisa et al., 2008; Desbonnet et al., 2008).

Other studies have also linked changes in mothering behavior in rats, whether spontaneously occurring or induced by an intervention, to changes in the oxytocin (OT) and arginine vasopressin (AVP) systems (Francis et al., 2000, 2002b; Champagne et al., 2001; Pedersen and Boccia, 2002). In adults, OT and AVP have been implicated in social behaviors, including pair-bonding (Winslow et al., 1993; Williams et al., 1994; Cho et al., 1999; Lim et al., 2004), parental behavior (Pedersen et al., 1982; Wang et al., 1994; Bales et al., 2004b), and also measures of anxiety (Neumann, 2002). Increases in oxytocin receptors (OTR) in the central amygdala and bed nucleus of the stria terminalis (BNST) in female offspring, and AVP V1a receptor (V1aR) binding in the central amygdala in male offspring (Francis et al., 2002b), have also been associated with increased maternal licking.

Prairie voles are small rodents, native to the midwestern United States. Members of this species show high levels of social behavior and display a monogamous social system, characterized by biparental care and a strong preference for a pair-mate, measured both in the field and in the laboratory (Getz et al., 1981; Carter et al., 1995). These species-typical traits can be influenced by apparently small differences in experience during the first few days of life (Bales et al., 2007a). Animals from families that were manipulated, by picking up the family for a few minutes during the first day of post-natal life (MAN1) were compared to prairie voles in which external manipulations of the family were minimized by not disturbing the family during the first few days of life (termed MAN0). Behavioral differences in later life were striking and in some cases sexually dimorphic. When tested with pups following weaning, MAN0 males showed low levels of alloparenting (i.e., spontaneous display of parenting-like behavior by juveniles). Tested in adulthood, selective social behaviors indicative of pair-bonding were disrupted; in this case the effect was especially obvious in females. Female prairie voles that received reduced early handling (MAN0) did not exhibit selective preferences for a familiar male, even when given six times the amount of exposure to a male that is typically sufficient to induce a preference. In addition, in both sexes tested in adulthood, MAN0 animals showed increased anxiety-like behaviors when tested in an elevated plus-maze (EPM). We hypothesize that these differences are due primarily to an early environment that is for MAN0 offspring less enriched or even impoverished. We further hypothesize even a small amount of handling (which typically occurs during cage change in most animal facilities) is sufficient to produce changes in the parental-infant interactions, which in turn leads to species-typical levels of behaviors in the offspring in later life. The effects of this manipulation were discovered serendipitously. However, the MAN1 versus MAN0 model for the effects of early experience is advantageous in some ways, in that this comparison is based on a subtle manipulation of early experience and one in which other variables (e.g., time away from the parents or temperature) are held relatively constant. Because young voles have milk-teeth and are attached to the mother during the handling manipulation, direct contact with the pups is avoided and we hypothesize that observed group differences are due to changes in the behavior of the parents (Tyler et al., 2005).

Evidence from other rodent species suggests that the effects of early experience can be time dependent and especially potent during the first week of life. However, responses to early handling may differ by species or even within the same strains of a given species (Holmes et al., 2005; Enthoven et al., 2008). Although early work in this field, primarily done in rats, tended to emphasize direct effects of handling on the offspring, more recent evidence suggests that individual differences in maternal behavior or maternal responses to disruption may significantly influence subsequent behavioral outcomes.

Consistent with our own findings in voles (Carter et al., 2009), and earlier work in rats (Champagne et al., 2001; Francis et al., 2002b; Todeschin et al., 2009), we hypothesized here that the effects of parental stimulation or its absence in post-natal life might be mediated by alterations in the OT or AVP systems. One purpose of the present study was to use the vole manipulation model to examine the effects of differential early experience on OT and AVP systems, measured in later life; here we have measured indices of central peptide synthesis, as well as receptor binding for the OTR and the AVP V1aR. We also examined the hypothesis that the age at which manipulations occurred and the frequency of handling might influence behavior or endocrine outcomes. Based on the outcome of earlier studies we predicted that groups receiving reduced stimulation in the first days of life would be less likely to be alloparental and more likely to show indices of anxiety, such as reduced exploration of or autogrooming in an EPM, and to show associated changes in the release of the adrenal steroid, corticosterone (CORT). We further predicted that changes in behavior would be associated with the parallel changes in the endogenous OT system, indexed by measures of OT synthesis or receptor binding. Also measured were possible experience-induced changes in cells synthesizing AVP and receptor binding in the AVP V1aR. Here we chose to examine outcome measures in juveniles due to our previous finding of low alloparenting in juvenile males (Bales et al., 2007a); future work will examine the same measures in adults.

MATERIALS AND METHODS
EARLY MANIPULATIONS

Subjects were laboratory-bred male and female prairie voles (*Microtus ochrogaster*), descendants of a wild stock originally caught near Champaign, IL, USA. Stock was systematically outbred. Animals were maintained on a 14-h light: 10-h dark cycle and given food (high-fiber Purina rabbit chow) and water *ad libitum*. Breeding pairs were maintained in large polycarbonate cages (44 cm × 22 cm × 16 cm) and provided with cotton for nesting material. Litters varied from 4 to 6 offspring and were not culled to avoid any additional handling. At 20 days of age offspring were removed and housed in same-sexed sibling pairs in smaller (27 cm × 16 cm × 13 cm) cages. The goal was 10 animals of each sex for each handling group; actual numbers of animals varied by outcome variable.

Sixteen multiparous pairs were used as breeders. The first treatment was assigned randomly for each pair. For the next litter, each pair received a different treatment (no pair received the same treatment more than once). There were four early handling treatments, here referred to as MAN0, MAN1, MAN1–7, and MAN7. MAN1 litter handling involved lifting the parents by the scruff of the neck with a hand covered in a thick leather glove. Pups were attached to the mother by milk-teeth and therefore were not touched (if pups were not attached, researchers waited to perform the manipulation). MAN1–7 received an identical manipulation once a day for 7 days postpartum, while MAN7 received this manipulation once on day 7. MAN0 litters were lifted briefly in a clear plastic cup. Sitting animals were scooped into the cup. If the animal was moving, the cup was maneuvered in front of the animal as it walked into it. In this manipulation, infants would be supported by the cup while being moved, rather than dangling from the mother's nipples. Cages were changed in the day preceding birth (almost always the day after the previous litter was weaned). Thereafter, cages were changed on day 7 and cage-changing was kept constant across groups. During subsequent cage changes, all animals were moved to the new cage in a cup. MAN0 litters were therefore manipulated in the cup three times (one for the early manipulation, two other times for cage-cleaning). The other groups received their described early manipulation (cup or hand) and all subsequent cage changes were performed by cup.

On day 20 postpartum, the infants were weaned and housed in same-sex pairs throughout testing. In order to utilize all of the offspring from each litter two experimental groups were formed, as described here.

Experimental group 1
On day 21–25, this group was tested in an alloparental care test (see methods below). The following day, they received an EPM test. The day following that, they were anesthetized with ketamine and xylazine, received an eyebleed, and were euthanized by cervical dislocation under deep anesthesia. Brains were flash-frozen for use in receptor autoradiography.

Experimental group 2
On day 21–25, these animals were removed from their cage, immediately anesthetized with ketamine and xylazine, received an eyebleed (data not presented here), and were euthanized by cervical dislocation under deep anesthesia. Brains were passively perfused for use in immunohistochemistry (methods detailed below), and sliced at 40 μm thickness on a sliding microtome.

All studies were approved by the Animal Care and Use Committee of the University of Illinois, Chicago, IL, USA and complied with National Institutes of Health ethical guidelines as set forth in the Guide for Lab Animal Care.

BEHAVIORAL TESTING
All behavioral testing was performed between 08:00 and 12:00 h.

Alloparental care testing
Animals were always weaned before the birth of the next litter in their home cage, thus ensuring that previous exposure to neonates had not occurred. Test animals were introduced into an apparatus which consisted of two cages connected by a 5 cm clear tube, and given 45 min to acclimate. Two pups (1–3 days old) were then introduced into one cage. The test animal was exposed to the pups for 10 min (methods based on (Roberts et al., 1998). If the test animal showed any pup-directed aggression, the test was stopped immediately and the pups removed and treated as necessary. Aggression displayed by 21-day olds rarely results in significant injury to the infant. Behaviors were scored from videotape by an observer blind to experimental treatment on behavioral software (Behavior Tracker, www.behaviortracker.com) for sniffing, huddling, non-huddling contact (any contact with pups not covered by another category), retrievals, licking/grooming, and aggression.

ANALYSIS STRATEGY
Data analysis was carried out by ANOVA. Residuals were checked for normality. All significance levels were set at $p < 0.05$ and all tests were two-tailed. We also conducted planned comparisons between MAN1 and MAN0 animals, to determine replicability of earlier findings with these groups, and to specifically examine possible neuroendocrine correlates of behavioral changes between these groups. In some cases, we also combined groups that received manipulations during the first week (MAN1 and MAN1–7) and groups that did not receive manipulation during the first week (MAN0 and MAN7).

Elevated Plus-maze testing
This test examines responses to nonsocial stimuli associated with a novel environment, and also has been used as a form of mild stressor (Insel et al., 1995; Ramos and Mormede, 1998). Time spent in the closed arm of the EPM is considered a measure of anxiety or fear response, due to the fact that presumably most rodents find open spaces aversive. Behavior in the EPM is responsive to both anxiolytic and anxiogenic drugs, and fear responses in the EPM have been found to be fairly resistant to environmental conditions (Ramos and Mormede, 1998). Prairie voles may find open areas less aversive than do other rodents such as meadow voles, a closely related polygynous species (Stowe et al., 2005), but EPM behavior in prairie voles has been shown to be responsive to manipulations such as injection of vasopressin (Dharmadhikari et al., 1997) and early handling (Bales et al., 2007a).

The EPM consisted of two open and two closed, opaque arms, each 67-cm long and 5.5-cm wide (Insel et al., 1995), elevated 1 m above the floor. Each vole was placed in the neutral area in the center of the EPM and its behavior scored for five minutes using Behavior Tracker. Plus-maze activity was indexed as time spent in the open arm/(time spent in the open arm + time spent in the closed arm). Data were analyzed by mixed model ANOVAs (Littell et al., 1996) in SAS 9.2 (SAS Institute, Cary, NC, USA). All significance levels were set at $p < 0.05$ and all tests were two-tailed.

HORMONE ASSAYS
Plasma OT was assayed using a commercial enzyme immunoassay (Assay Designs, Ann Arbor, MI, USA, now Enzo Life Sciences), validated for use in the prairie vole (Kramer et al., 2004). Non-extracted samples were diluted at 1:8 for OT (40 μl of plasma) and 1:12 for AVP (25 μl of plasma) and assayed according to kit instructions. Intra-assay c.v. for OT was 1.5% and inter-assay c.v. was 13.5%. For AVP intra-assay c.v. was 1.2% and inter-assay c.v. was 2.9%.

Corticosterone was assayed using a radioimmunoassay (MP Biomedicals, Irvine, CA, USA) previously validated for the prairie vole (Taymans et al., 1997). Non-extracted samples were assayed at 1:2000 dilution in order to insure that all samples fell on the standard curve. Intra-assay c.v.s averaged 3.7% and inter-assay c.v. was 4.3%.

RECEPTOR AUTORADIOGRAPHY
Following sacrifice, brains were quickly removed, flash-frozen on dry ice and stored at −80°C. Brains were sectioned at 20-μm thickness, mounted onto Super-frost slides, and stored at −80°C until the time of assay. Sections were allowed to thaw to room temperature and then immersed in 0.1% paraformaldehyde for 2 min to optimize tissue integrity. Sections then were rinsed three times in 50 mM Tris–HCl (pH 7.4) at room temperature

for 5 min and incubated for 60 min at room temperature in a solution of 50 mM Tris–HCl (pH 7.4) with 10 mM $MgCl_2$, 0.1% bovine serum albumin, and 50 pM of radiotracer. For OTR binding, [^{125}I]-ornithine vasotocin analog [(^{125}I)OVTA] was employed [vasotocin, d(CH_2)$_5$[Tyr(Me)^2,Thr^4,Orn^8, (^{125}I)Tyr^9–NH_2]; 2200 Ci/mmol]; (NEN Nuclear, Boston, MA, USA). For V1aR binding, ^{125}I–lin–vasopressin [^{125}I–phenylacetyl–D–Tyr(ME)–Phe–Gln–Asn–Arg–Pro–Arg–Tyr–NH_2]; (NEN Nuclear) was used. Nonspecific binding was determined by incubating adjacent sections with the radioactive specific ligand as well as with 50 µM of unlabeled Thr^4, Gly^7 OT, a selective OT ligand (Peninsula Laboratories, Belmont, CA, USA) or 50 µM of unlabeled [1-(-mercapto-,-cyclopentamethylene propionic acid),2-(O-methyl)-tyrosine]-arg^8-vasopressin, selective for the V1aR. Following incubation, sections were washed four times at 5 min each in 50 mm Tris–HCl (pH 7.4) with 10 mM $MgCl_2$ at 4°C, followed by a final rinse in this same buffer for 30 min while stirred with a magnetic bar. Slides then were quickly dipped in cold dH_2O and rapidly dried with a stream of cold air. Sections were apposed to Kodak BioMaxMR film (Kodak, Rochester, NY, USA). Autoradiographic ^{125}I-receptor binding was quantified from film using the NIH Image program to measure uncalibrated optical density. Background was quantified for each slide from a cortical area lacking receptors. The number of slides scored for each area varied, but averaged approximately nine sections per area. Both sides of each area were quantified separately, compared for any differences according to hemisphere (which were not found), then a mean obtained for each slice. A mean for the area for each animal was then calculated, which was the value used in analyses.

IMMUNOHISTOCHEMISTRY

Free-floating tissue sections were rinsed in 0.05 M KPBS. To block endogenous peroxidase activity, sections were incubated for 15 min in 0.014% phenylhydrazine and then rinsed in KPBS. Next, sections were incubated in rabbit OT antisera (generously provided by Dr. Mariana Morris) at 1:150,000 or rabbit anti-AVP (MP Biomedicals, Irvine, CA, USA) at 1:100,000 dilution in 0.05 M KPBS-0.4% Triton X-100 (1 h at room temperature and then 48 h at 4°C).

Sections were rinsed in KPBS before being incubated for 1 h at room temperature in biotinylated goat, anti-rabbit IgG (1:600 dilution in KPBS-0.4% Triton X-100; H + L, BA-1000; Vector Laboratories, Burlingame, CA, USA). Sections were rinsed in KPBS and then incubated in an avidin–biotin peroxidase complex (4.5 A and 4.5 µl B per 1 ml KPBS–0.4% Triton X-100; Vectastain ABC kit-elite pk-6100 standard; Vector Laboratories) for 1 h at room temperature. Sections were rinsed in KPBS and then rinsed in 0.175 M sodium acetate. Finally, OT-immunoreactivity (OT-IR) and AVP-IR were visualized by incubation in a nickel sulfate–diaminobenzidine chromogen solution (250 mg Nickel II Sulfate, 2 mg DAB, 8.3 µl 3% H_2O_2 per 10 ml 0.175 M sodium acetate) for 15 min, then rinsed in sodium acetate followed by KPBS rinses. Following labeling for OT or AVP, sections were mounted onto subbed glass slides and air-dried overnight. Sections then were dehydrated in ascending ethanol solutions, cleared in Histoclear (National Diagnostics, Atlanta, GA, USA), and the slides were coverslipped with Histomount (National Diagnostics).

Images were captured using a Nikon Eclipse E 800 microscope, Sensi-cam camera, and IP Lab Software®. Pictures for analysis were taken at 100× magnification. Analysis was performed using Image J software (National Institutes of Health, Bethesda, MD, USA). Density of staining within each nucleus was quantified using the threshold function to separate stained cells and fibers from the background. Within the PVN and SON, a standardized sampling area was used to determine the number of pixels labeled using the thresholding function. This was done to ensure that differences were not a result of variability in defining the borders of a nucleus. Density was calculated as the percentage of threshold labeled pixels versus non-labeled pixels within the entire sampling area. Similar methods have been used to determine differences in OT and AVP cell and fiber staining in other studies (Wang et al., 1996; Bester-Meredith and Marler, 2003; Ruscio et al., 2007). Density measurements from each nucleus were taken from sections matched in rostral–caudal orientation to minimize variability. In all cases, density measures were taken by two observers blind to the condition of the subject and the average was calculated. Due to the high concentration of cells and fibers within certain nuclei, we felt that cell counts would not be accurate as it was often not possible to discern exact cell numbers (due to overlapping cells) and cells from fibers within the central portions of densely stained nuclei.

Arginine vasopressin and OT densities were measured in the PVN and SON. Measurements within the PVN were taken in a caudal section of the nucleus where the stained cells and fibers take a characteristic shape and branching pattern, as demonstrated in previous studies (Wang et al., 1996). This section is further characterized by the medial–lateral position of the fornix (relative to the third ventricle) and medial and dorsal location of the optic tract (relative to more central and ventral position in more rostral sections). It is approximate to Figure 49 in Paxinos and Watson (2005). Two density measures within each section were taken; one in the center (sampling area: 125 µm × 125 µm) measuring both cells and fibers, and another in the periphery (sampling area: 375 µm × 250 µm) measuring projecting fibers from the PVN. AVP and OT density measurements in the SON were taken at the same rostral–caudal level as the PVN. Because of the SON's curved shape and location, we used two areas to ensure that the optic tract was not included in the thresholding function. Both measures (sampling areas: horizontal, 282 µm × 375 µm and vertical 225 µm × 440 µm) were within the SON (cells and fibers) and the density was the sum of stained fibers and cells with both areas.

RESULTS

ALLOPARENTAL BEHAVIOR

When groups that were manipulated before day 7 (MAN1 and MAN1–7) were combined and compared to groups that were not manipulated before day 7 (MAN0 and MAN7), they differed significantly in alloparental behavior. Males that were manipulated before day 7 displayed a significantly longer duration of non-huddling contact ($n = 42$, $F_1 = 4.95$, $p = 0.035$; **Figure 1**) and total time spent in alloparental behavior (including sniffing, licking/grooming, non-huddling contact, and huddling; $F_1 = 4.24$, $p = 0.046$). When only MAN0 and MAN1 males were compared directly, there was a trend for a difference in non-huddling contact ($n = 20$, $F_1 = 3.79$, $p = 0.067$) and other behaviors were non-significant (**Table 1**). In a one-tailed test (justified by *a priori* expectation of direction), the difference between MAN0 and MAN1 in non-huddling contact is significant ($p = 0.033$).

No female alloparental behaviors varied significantly by early treatment (**Table 1**). When MAN0 and MAN1 females were compared directly, there were also no significant differences in alloparental behaviors.

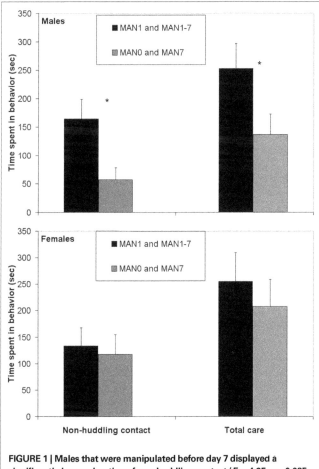

FIGURE 1 | Males that were manipulated before day 7 displayed a significantly longer duration of non-huddling contact ($F_1 = 4.95, p = 0.035$; Table 1) and total time spent in alloparental behavior ($F_1 = 4.24, p = 0.046$).

ELEVATED PLUS-MAZE

Autogrooming in the EPM differed by treatment for females ($n = 39$, $F_3 = 4.38$, $p = 0.012$; **Figure 2**) but not for males ($n = 38$, $F_3 = 0.98$, $p = 0.414$). While time spent in the open arm, and the ratio of time spent in the open arm over time spent in both arms did not differ for either sex, in females there was a trend (Kruskal–Wallis test, $\chi^2 = 7.14$, $p = 0.067$; **Figure 2**) for treatment to influence time spent in the closed arms, with MAN7 and MAN1–7 spending the most time there.

When only MAN1 and MAN0 groups were compared, no significant differences for males were seen; however MAN1 females autogroomed significantly more than MAN0 females ($n = 19$, $F_1 = 4.87$, $p = 0.041$; note though, that this was opposite the predicted direction) and tended to spend more time in the closed arms ($F_1 = 3.38$, $p = 0.084$).

OXYTOCIN AND ARGININE VASOPRESSIN (V1A) RECEPTOR BINDING

Oxytocin receptor binding differed in several areas in females, with MAN0 females having significantly higher OTR binding than other groups (**Figures 3 and 4**). Treatment differences were significant in the BNST ($n = 26$, $F_3 = 3.37$, $p = 0.032$) and the nucleus accumbens (NAcc; $F_3 = 2.96$, $p = 0.048$). OTR binding in females was also marginally significant in the same direction in the cingulate cortex ($F_3 = 2.89$, $p = 0.051$; optical densities, MAN1 = 0.107 ± 0.03, MAN1–7 = 0.115 ± 0.02, MAN7 = 0.126 ± 0.3, MAN0 = 0.248 ± 0.06) and the lateral septum (LS; $F_3 = 2.97$, $p = 0.054$; optical densities, MAN1 = 0.114 ± 0.03, MAN1–7 = 0.15 ± 0.02, MAN7 = 0.181 ± 0.7, MAN0 = 0.289 ± 0.09). OTR binding in males differed significantly in the BNST ($n = 34$, $F_3 = 3.85$, $p = 0.018$; **Figure 5**), and tended to differ in the NAcc ($F_3 = 2.65$, $p = 0.065$). These differences were in the same direction as females (MAN0 and MAN7 higher than MAN1), with even higher levels in some groups.

When comparing across the four groups there were no significant treatment group differences in either males or females in V1aR binding (**Tables 2 and 3**). Pre-planned comparisons of MAN1 and MAN0 groups did not reveal any significant differences in V1aR, when compared in separate brain areas. Though non-significant, it may be important to note that the levels of V1a binding in each of the brain areas studied was higher in MAN0 males versus MAN1 males. This pattern was not seen in females.

Table 1 | Alloparental behaviors in a pup test, including time spent in infant care and contact (non-huddling) were more common in prairie voles that were handled at least once in the first few days of life (MAN1 and MAN1–7) versus those that received no handling until at least PND 7 (MAN0 and MAN7).

	MALE: Manipulation in the first week (MAN1 and MAN1–7; $n = 21$)	MALE: No early manipulation (MAN0 and MAN 7; $n = 21$)	Statistic	p-value	FEMALE: Manipulation in the first week (MAN1 and MAN1–7; $n = 20$)	FEMALE: No early manipulation (MAN0 and MAN 7; $n = 20$)	Statistic	p-value
Sniff	31.52 ± 4.13	37.86 ± 6.86	$F = 0.21$	0.653	17.85 ± 3.2	24.36 ± 4.79	$F = 0.38$	0.768
Lick	56.0 ± 18.67	36.86 ± 15.58	$\chi^2 = 2.01$	0.156	70.05 ± 37.32	49.47 ± 18.68	$\chi^2 = 2.33$	0.507
Retrievals	2.67 ± 0.72	1.81 ± 0.60	$\chi^2 = 1.99$	0.158	1.55 ± 0.47	4.47 ± 1.77	$\chi^2 = 3.33$	0.344
Huddling	1.24 ± 0.86	5.71 ± 4.15	$\chi^2 = 1.11$	0.737	33.9 ± 23.22	16.32 ± 9.23	$\chi^2 = 5.04$	0.169

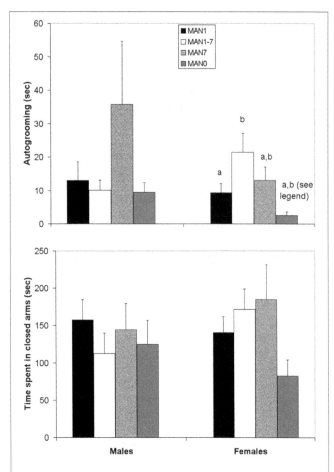

FIGURE 2 | Time spent autogrooming in the elevated plus-maze differed among treatment groups in females ($F_3 = 4.38$, $p = 0.012$). There was a trend for time spent in the closed arms to differ (Kruskal–Wallis test, $\chi^2 = 7.14$, $p = 0.067$). Groups which differ significantly from each other in the overall ANOVA are indicated by different letters. When MAN1 and MAN0 females were compared directly in pre-planned comparisons, MAN1 females autogroomed significantly more than MAN0 females ($F_1 = 4.87$, $p = 0.041$) and MAN1 females tended to spend more time in the closed arms than MAN0 females ($F_1 = 3.38$, $p = 0.084$).

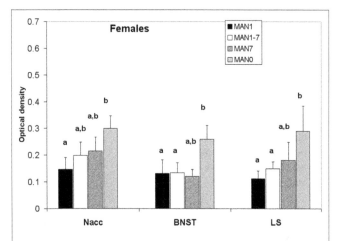

FIGURE 3 | Oxytocin receptor binding (optical density), females. Bars with different letters indicate groups that are significantly different in *post hoc* testing.

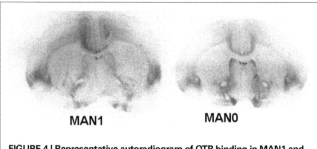

FIGURE 4 | Representative autoradiogram of OTR binding in MAN1 and MAN0 females.

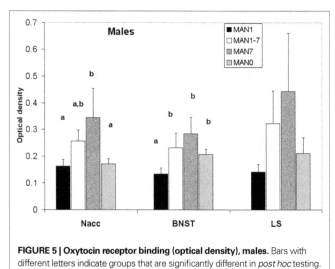

FIGURE 5 | Oxytocin receptor binding (optical density), males. Bars with different letters indicate groups that are significantly different in *post hoc* testing.

CENTRAL OT AND AVP PRODUCTION (IMMUNOHISTOCHEMISTRY)

The density of OT cell bodies in the SON differed significantly by treatment for males ($n = 33$, $F_3 = 4.12$, $p = 0.018$; **Figures 6 and 7**), but not for females ($n = 27$, $F_3 = 1.9$, $p = 0.157$), although results were in the same direction in both sexes with MAN1 higher than other groups.

The density of OT fibers in the SON did not differ by treatment, and neither the density of OT cell bodies, nor the density of OT fibers, differed significantly in the PVN. No measures of AVP production (SON cell bodies, SON fibers, PVN cell bodies, PVN fibers) differed significantly by treatment (**Tables 4 and 5**). However, planned comparisons between MAN0 and MAN1 groups revealed that the differences in density of AVP immunoreactive cell bodies approached significance ($F_1 = 4.34$, $p = 0.056$) with high levels of AVP in MAN0 versus MAN1 males. This difference was not observed in females; however, in females there was a trend for MAN0 females to have higher OT cell bodies in the PVN than MAN1 females ($F_1 = 3.41$, $p = 0.088$).

PLASMA HORMONES

There was a trend for CORT to differ in females ($n = 36$, $F_3 = 2.41$, $p = 0.085$; **Figure 8**) but not in males ($n = 40$, $F_3 = 0.68$, $p = 0.569$) following the EPM test, a mild stressor. MAN0 females had significantly higher CORT than MAN1 females ($t_1 = 2.66$, $p = 0.012$).

Table 2 | Radiolabeled ligand binding for AVP V1a receptors (optical density) for males (means ± SD). Groups also did not differ in V1a receptor binding.

	MAN1 ($n = 6$)	MAN1-7 ($n = 10$)	MAN7 ($n = 10$)	MAN0 ($n = 9$)	Statistic (F)	p-value
Lateral septum	0.263 ± 0.04	0.255 ± 0.01	0.289 ± 0.03	0.356 ± 0.06	1.56	0.229
Ventral pallidum	0.502 ± 0.08	0.738 ± 0.14	0.727 ± 0.14	0.701 ± 0.13	0.57	0.641
BNST	0.266 ± 0.02	0.291 ± 0.01	0.308 ± 0.03	0.338 ± 0.03	1.15	0.347
Medial amygdala	0.303 ± 0.01	0.368 ± 0.06	0.337 ± 0.03	0.427 ± 0.08	0.77	0.518
Posterior cingulate cortex	0.251 ± 0.03	0.285 ± 0.03	0.331 ± 0.06	0.305 ± 0.03	0.48	0.696

Table 3 | Radiolabeled ligand binding for AVP V1a receptors (optical density) for females (means ± SD).

	MAN1 ($n = 8$)	MAN1-7 ($n = 7$)	MAN7 ($n = 3$)	MAN0 ($n = 10$)	Statistic (F)	p-value
Lateral septum	0.285 ± 0.04	0.239 ± 0.01	0.299 ± 0.01	0.282 ± 0.04	0.22	0.880
Ventral pallidum	0.717 ± 0.12	0.596 ± 0.15	0.882 ± 0.22	0.564 ± 0.09	0.91	0.454
BNST	0.297 ± 0.03	0.302 ± 0.02	0.280 ± 0.02	0.291 ± 0.03	0.07	0.976
Medial amygdala	0.326 ± 0.04	0.419 ± 0.06	0.307 ± 0.02	0.348 ± 0.08	0.45	0.721
Posterior cingulate cortex	0.339 ± 0.05	0.285 ± 0.03	0.301 ± 0.04	0.323 ± 0.05	0.27	0.847

Groups also did not differ in V1a receptor binding.

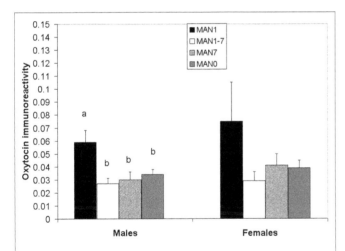

FIGURE 6 | The number of OT cell bodies in the SON differed significantly by treatment for males ($F_3 = 5.46$, $p = 0.005$). Although the overall ANOVA for females was not significant ($F_3 = 1.9$, $p = 0.157$), there was a trend for a difference between MAN0 and MAN1 ($t_1 = -1.73$, $p = 0.096$).

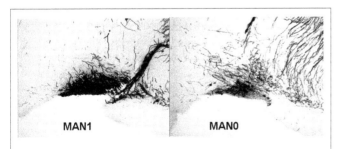

FIGURE 7 | Representative photographs of OT immunoreactivity in the SON in MAN1 and MAN0 animals.

Plasma AVP did not differ significantly by treatment following the EPM test in males ($n = 31$, $F_3 = 0.33$, $p = 0.802$; **Figure 9**) or females ($n = 32$, $F_3 = 0.07$, $p = 0.977$). OT also did not differ significantly by treatment in males ($F_3 = 1.63$, $p = 0.199$; **Figure 10**) or females ($F_3 = 1.23$, $p = 0.316$). Comparisons of MAN0 and MAN1 groups did not reveal significant effects in either sex.

DISCUSSION

The results of this study replicate earlier findings in prairie voles showing that alloparental behavior, tested in the postweaning period, can be influenced by handling during the first week of life (Bales et al., 2007a). Findings from our studies in prairie voles are consistent with literature from other mammals indicating that behavioral patterns and emotional reactions may undergo long-lasting adaptations based on early experience, and possibly moderated by parental stimulation in early life. The present findings also suggest that these effects are sexually dimorphic, possibly based in part on neuroendocrine differences between the sexes in the consequences of differential early experiences.

Research in rats strongly supports the importance of early experience in determining later social and emotional responses. For example, individual differences in maternal stimulation, including licking, may influence the later expression of parental behavior by the offspring (Meaney, 2001; Pedersen and Boccia, 2002; Champagne and Meaney, 2007). In addition, in rats offspring that received moderate amounts of stimulation in early life, either by an investigator or by the mother rat, generally were more adaptable in later life, at least as measured by changes in hormones of the hypothalamic–pituitary–adrenal axis, in comparison to offspring that were deliberately left undisturbed (Levine, 1957, 2002a). Research in rats also has suggested that young animals may be particularly sensitive in the first week of life to the effects of the presence or absence of parental stimulation (Levine and Lewis, 1959a).

Table 4 | Immunohistochemistry results for OT and AVP measures in males.

	MAN1 ($n = 6$)	MAN1–7 ($n = 7$)	MAN7 ($n = 10$)	MAN0 ($n = 10$)	Statistic (F)	p-value
OT cell body density – PVN	0.170 ± 0.04	0.150 ± 0.03	0.137 ± 0.02	0.178 ± 0.01	0.96	0.429
AVP cell body density – PVN	0.112 ± 0.03	0.119 ± 0.02	0.172 ± 0.06	0.189 ± 0.02	1.44	0.254
AVP cell body density – SON	0.118 ± 0.02	0.159 ± 0.02	0.109 ± 0.02	0.123 ± 0.01	1.64	0.205

Table 5 | Immunohistochemistry results for OT and AVP measures in females.

	MAN1 ($n = 5$)	MAN1–7 ($n = 7$)	MAN7 ($n = 5$)	MAN0 ($n = 10$)	Statistic (F)	p-value
OT cell body density – PVN	0.124 ± 0.02	0.141 ± 0.01	0.148 ± 0.02	0.171 ± 0.02	1.21	0.328
AVP cell body density – PVN	0.274 ± 0.04	0.161 ± 0.05	0.191 ± 0.02	0.192 ± 0.04	1.63	0.215
AVP cell body density – SON	0.137 ± 0.03	0.087 ± 0.02	0.127 ± 0.01	0.139 ± 0.03	1.32	0.296

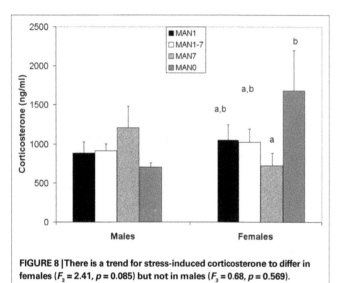

FIGURE 8 | There is a trend for stress-induced corticosterone to differ in females ($F_3 = 2.41$, $p = 0.085$) but not in males ($F_3 = 0.68$, $p = 0.569$).

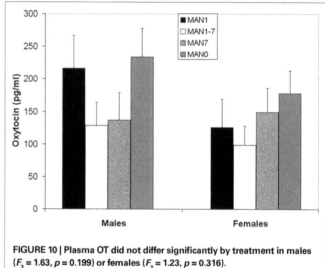

FIGURE 10 | Plasma OT did not differ significantly by treatment in males ($F_3 = 1.63$, $p = 0.199$) or females ($F_3 = 1.23$, $p = 0.316$).

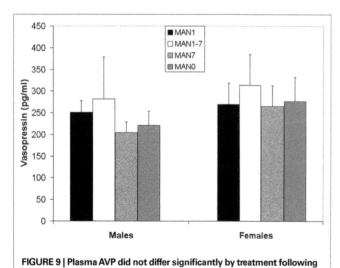

FIGURE 9 | Plasma AVP did not differ significantly by treatment following the EPM test in males ($F_3 = 0.33$, $p = 0.802$) or females ($F_3 = 0.07$, $p = 0.977$).

The present design included animals that were deliberately manipulated within the first day of post-natal life (MAN1) and those that were left undisturbed for at least one week (MAN0) with minimal disturbance through out the rest of the pre-weaning period. As in previous studies the male offspring of the manipulated group (MAN1) showed higher levels of later alloparenting compared to the MAN0 males (Bales et al., 2007a). However, when the first experience of manipulation was postponed until post-natal day 7 (MAN7), the male offspring showed an alloparenting pattern more similar to that seen in animals that were not handled (MAN0). We also examined the hypothesis that more frequent manipulation, daily during the first week of life (MAN1–7), would further increase alloparenting. However, no difference in alloparenting was observed between MAN1 and MAN1–7 males; a high proportion of both MAN1 (67%) and MAN1–7 (75%) showed alloparental behavior. In contrast, the proportion of alloparental males was much lower in the MAN0 (33%) and MAN7 (20%) groups. Female alloparenting did not vary significantly with early manipulation, as was also found in the previous study (Bales et al., 2007a); 54% of MAN0 females and 38% of MAN7 females showed alloparental behavior, with 40% of MAN1 and 60% of MAN1–7 females displaying alloparenting.

In the present study, because the full family including both parents and their infants were manipulated, it was not possible to determine whether the observed changes were due to direct stimulation of the young or mediated through differential parenting. However, immediately following handling we observed that both parents, and especially mothers, directed increased levels of stimulation toward their pups, including licking and grooming (Tyler et al., 2005). In contrast, undisturbed families were less interactive with pups, especially on the first day of life. More recently, we have also examined the consequences in prairie voles of repeated handling, three times at 3–4 h intervals on post-natal day. Immediately following the third episode of handling, parents showed reductions in interactions with their infants. As in the MAN0 treatment, the male offspring from this repeated handling group showed low levels of alloparenting in later life (Boone et al., 2009). Taken together with the results of the present study, these findings suggest that in male prairie voles reduced parental stimulation, especially in the immediate post-natal period, may contribute to the deficits in later alloparenting observed after either reduced or repeated handling.

Both MAN0 and MAN7 males (which displayed low alloparenting) also produced less OT in the SON than MAN1 males. In contrast, MAN1–7 males displayed both high alloparenting and low OT. One hypothesis for future studies is that MAN1–7 males might compensate for low OT production with higher AVP production. While MAN1–7 had low OT in the SON, their AVP in the SON was relatively high (**Table 4**). We did not present *post hoc* comparisons in the table due to the non-significant findings in the main ANOVA, but if performed, MAN1–7 males did have significantly higher AVP cell bodies in the SON than MAN7 males ($p = 0.05$) and displayed a non-significant trend for higher values than MAN0 males ($p = 0.11$). Previous research has shown that male prairie voles can facilitate alloparenting through either the OT or AVP system (Bales et al., 2004b).

As in our previous study, we found sex differences in the effects of handling treatments. While in females we found no difference in alloparenting, we did find differences in behaviors that may reflect anxiety. Our previous study comparing MAN1 and MAN0 (Bales et al., 2007a) showed higher levels of anxiety-like behaviors in MAN0 animals, as measured in the EPM, which we did not detect here. In fact, we found the opposite: MAN0 females tended to spend less time in the closed arms of the EPM than MAN1 females. This could be due to the age of testing, as the previous study tested animals at 60 days of age while in the present study animals were tested at 22 days (directly after weaning). In animal models, changes of anxiety with age are a common finding although the direction is not always consistent (Lynn and Brown, 2010). In the current study, changes in gonadal hormones are an unlikely mechanism for age-related changes in anxiety because prairie voles are induced ovulators (Carter et al., 1980). However, changes in peptide systems could be a possibility; we are not aware of any studies directly comparing adolescent and adult production of OT or AVP in prairie voles. A second possibility is that time since receiving other tests could have affected the outcome of the EPM. In Bales et al. (2007a, 2007b) the adult voles had not received another behavioral test for approximately 38 days; while in the present study, the juvenile voles had received the alloparenting test the day before they received the EPM. It is therefore possible that in this study, the alloparenting test was residually affecting the EPM in some fashion.

In females, we did observe significant treatment differences in autogrooming in the EPM. Interestingly, the two groups in the present study which received reduced manipulation in the first week of life (MAN0 and MAN7), displayed very different autogrooming behavior in the EPM; this suggests that there may not be a critical period for handling effects on this particular behavior, or at least that it is longer than one week. MAN0 females autogroomed the least of all groups (**Figure 2**). MAN0 females may be displaying a more passive coping style, with higher levels of CORT released during stress and lower autogrooming in response to stress; MAN7 females, on the other hand, display an active response (autogrooming) resulting in lower CORT levels. The same patterns were not seen in males. These findings are consistent with the hypothesis that coping strategies in the face of challenge differ between males and females (Koolhaas et al., 2001, 2007), especially when these challenges occur in early life (Carter et al., 2009). However, the experiential factors that differentiate the MAN0 and MAN7 paradigms remain to be described. There might be age-related differences in the dependence of the offspring on parental stimulation. Alternatively, parents of pups of different ages may differ in their reactions to experiences (or the absence of experiences).

The MAN1–7 group in particular presents several challenges of interpretation. Above, we discussed the possible role of increased AVP in the SON in normalizing alloparenting behavior in MAN1–7 males. MAN1–7 females were similar to MAN1 females on almost every measure except for autogrooming in the EPM, where they showed increased autogrooming compared to all other groups, perhaps suggestive of increased anxiety. In females, we did not do *post hoc* comparisons between groups due to non-significance of the overall ANOVA for OT in the SON. However, a direct comparison between MAN1 and MAN1–7 females does suggest lower OT-IR in the SON in MAN1–7 females ($p = 0.025$).

One purpose of this study was to examine the hypothesis that changes in central neuropeptide systems might mediate the long-term consequences of early experience. In the present study, the OT system, and especially the OTR, responded to variations in early experiences, whereas changes were less obvious in the V1aR system. In contrast, a series of studies of the effects of exposure to exogenous OT on post-natal day 1 (Bales and Carter, 2003a, 2003b; Bales et al., 2004a, 2004c), revealed changes in the V1aR, but with no detectable differences in OTRs or dopamine D2 receptors (Bales et al., 2007b). The source of these differences has not been identified. However, exogenous OT, possibly given at a pharmacological dose, might have produced secondary binding to V1aRs (Gimpl and Fahrenholz, 2001). In addition, the age of the animals at the time of sacrifice differed between the two studies.

The effects most apparent in females from the MAN0 group were increased OTR binding in the NAcc, the BNST, and LS. The higher availability of OTR may be related to the lower anxiety displayed by MAN0 females at this age. OT is generally anxiolytic (Neumann, 2002; Labuschagne et al., 2010). It is possible that the elevated OTRs in these brain regions are a response to lower OT peptide availability, either during development (due to decreased stimulation by parents) or during adulthood (**Figure 5**). We would hypothesize that lower OT during development is more likely, given that MAN0 females actually had higher OT production in the PVN in this study than MAN1 females. Although the SON is unlikely to be the major source of OT peptide to these areas, recent studies have shown that the SON in prairie voles does have oxytocinergic projections to the NAcc (Ross et al., 2009).

Variations in early handling were associated with later changes in neuropeptide production and binding, although these relationships differed for males and females. MAN0 males displayed elevated OTR in the BNST, lower OT production in the SON, and elevated AVP production in the PVN when compared to MAN1 males. Previous literature has suggested that male prairie voles can facilitate alloparenting behavior through either the OT or the AVP system (Bales et al., 2004b). It is possible that extensive dysregulation, rather than changes in one particular neuropeptide or neuropeptide receptor, may have affected alloparenting behavior in this paradigm.

The results of this study are also consistent with preliminary data on methylation in a CpG island in the promoter region of the OTR gene. In these studies animals from a MAN1 group demonstrated higher levels of methylation in tissue from the NAcc compared to MAN0 animals in which methylation was low (Connelly and Carter, unpublished data). Low levels of methylation would be expected to permit increased expression of the OTR, which was the outcome seen in females in the MAN0 group in the present study (**Figure 3**). Other preliminary studies from our group suggest that OT may increase methylation of the OTR gene (Connelly and Carter, unpublished data). At the time of sampling in the present study, PND 22, OT synthesis in the SON (indexed by immunohistochemical staining) was higher in MAN1 animals than in any other group. This effect was seen in both sexes, although was only significant in males. It is still unknown whether OT levels at the time of the handling treatment were enhanced in MAN1 animals, but that would be consistent with other findings.

Oxytocin production in the SON also may occur in response to chronic stress (Neumann, 2002; Grippo et al., 2007); stress in turn might increase subsequent synthesis or release of AVP (Neumann et al., 2006). It is possible that the higher levels of SON OT available to MAN1 animals may impact on their stress systems (perhaps by other measures than those shown here), and in prairie voles stress is well-known to affect social behavior (DeVries et al., 1995, 1996; Bales et al., 2006). In rats, maternal separation resulted in an increase in AVP immunoreactivity in SON (Veenema et al., 2006). In the present study, there are preliminary indications that AVP, especially in males, might be upregulated in the MAN0 group, which might also be receiving less parental stimulation.

CONCLUSIONS

Differential early handling experiences in prairie voles were associated with long-term, sexually dimorphic changes in social and anxiety-related behaviors, as well as neuroendocrine parameters. As a whole, these measures indicate that subtle variations in early experience, perhaps mediated by changes in the behavior of the parents following disruptions of the family (Tyler et al., 2005) can have long-term effects on social behaviors in prairie voles. The disruptive effects on alloparental behavior of reduced manipulation during the first few days of life (MAN0), when compared to those of animals that were handled (MAN1), were similar to those observed in previous studies (Bales et al., 2007a). In males, daily manipulations of the family (MAN1–7) also produced effects on alloparenting that were similar to those seen in MAN1 and when manipulations were delayed until post-natal day 7 (MAN7), the consequences for subsequent alloparental behavior were similar to MAN0. However, the neuroendocrine effects of MAN1–7 versus MAN1 and the effects of MAN7 versus MAN0 were not always similar. These results suggest that different amounts of handling and manipulations during different time periods have behavioral effects that are not identical to those for neuroendocrine systems.

The present findings yielded complex group differences in behavior and neuroendocrine measures. These findings do not allow strong conclusions regarding the causal roles of OT or AVP in alloparental- or anxiety-related behaviors. However, we cannot exclude the possibly that the behavioral results obtained here reflect interactions between the OT and AVP systems, and that both show adaptive changes adjusting the expression of social behavior and responsivity to novel environments.

While we did not measure changes in OT at the time of the early experience we did find long-term treatment effects on the OT system, with increases in the OTR in females. In general, changes in AVP were less obvious.

ACKNOWLEDGMENTS

We are grateful for research support from NIMH (RO1 073022 to C. Sue Carter and Karen L. Bales), the National Alliance for Autism Research (to C. Sue Carter), and NSF (0437523 to Karen L. Bales). We thank the following for help in performing these studies: Antoniah Lewis-Reese, Lisa Sanzenbacher, Amber Tyler, Julie Van Westerhuyzen, Alex Kowalczyk, Thinh Hoang, Julie Hazelton, Nathaniel Grotte, and Soraya Foutouhi. We also thank Drs. Terry Hewett and Jim Artwohl for veterinary care.

REFERENCES

Advani, T., Hensler, J. G., and Koek, W. (2007). Effects of early rearing conditions on alcohol drinking and 5-HT$_{1a}$ receptor function in C57BL/6J mice. *Int. J. Neuropsychopharmacol.* 10, 595–607.

Aguilar, R. (2010). Infantile experience and play motivation. *Soc. Neurosci.* 5, 422–440.

Aisa, B., Tordera, R., Lasheras, B., Del Rio, J., and Ramirez, M. J. (2008). Effects of maternal separation on hypothalamic-pituitary-adrenal responses, cognition, and vulnerability to stress in adult female rats. *Neuroscience* 154, 1218–1226.

Bales, K. L., Abdelnabi, M., Cushing, B. S., Ottinger, M. A., and Carter, C. S. (2004a). Effects of neonatal oxytocin manipulations on male reproductive potential in prairie voles. *Physiol. Behav.* 81, 519–526.

Bales, K. L., Kim, A. J., Lewis-Reese, A. D., and Carter, C. S. (2004b). Both oxytocin and vasopressin may influence alloparental behavior in male prairie voles. *Horm. Behav.* 45, 354–361.

Bales, K. L., Pfeifer, L. A., and Carter, C. S. (2004c). Sex differences and effects of manipulations of oxytocin on alloparenting and anxiety in prairie voles. *Dev. Psychobiol.* 44, 123–131.

Bales, K. L., and Carter, C. S. (2003a). Developmental exposure to oxytocin facilitates partner preferences in male prairie voles (*Microtus ochrogaster*). *Behav. Neurosci.* 117, 854–859.

Bales, K. L., and Carter, C. S. (2003b). Sex differences and developmental effects of oxytocin on aggression and social behavior in prairie voles (*Microtus ochrogaster*). *Horm. Behav.* 44, 178–184.

Bales, K. L., Kramer, K. M., Lewis-Reese, A. D., and Carter, C. S. (2006). Effects of stress on parental care are sexually dimorphic in prairie voles. *Physiol. Behav.* 87, 424–429.

Bales, K. L., Lewis-Reese, A. D., Pfeifer, L. A., Kramer, K. M., and Carter, C. S. (2007a). Early experience affects the traits of monogamy in a sexually dimorphic manner. *Dev. Psychobiol.* 49, 335–342.

Bales, K. L., Plotsky, P. M., Young, L. J., Lim, M. M., Grotte, N. D., Ferrer, E., and Carter, C. S. (2007b). Neonatal oxytocin manipulations have long-lasting, sexually dimorphic effects on vasopressin receptors. *Neuroscience* 144, 38–45.

Berardi, N., Braschi, C., Capsoni, S., Cattaneo, A., and Maffei, L. (2007). Environmental enrichment delays the onset of memory deficits and reduces neuropathological hallmarks in a mouse model of Alzheimer-like neurodegeneration. *J. Alz. Dis.* 11, 359–370.

Bester-Meredith, J. K., and Marler, C. A. (2003). Vasopressin and the transmission of paternal behavior across generations in mated, cross-fostered Peromyscus mice. *Behav. Neurosci.* 117, 455–463.

Boccia, M. L., and Pedersen, C. A. (2001). Brief vs. long maternal separations in infancy: contrasting relationships with adult maternal behavior and lactation levels of aggression and anxiety. *Psychoneuroendocrinology* 26, 657–672.

Boone, E. M., Sanzenbacher, L. L., Stanfill, S. D., Bales, K. L., and Carter, C. S. (2009). Oxytocin injections in early life reversed negative behavioral effects of repeated handling. *Soc. Neurosci. Abstr.* 468.12.

Carter, C. S., Boone, E. M., Pournajafi-Nazarloo, H., and Bales, K. L. (2009). Consequences of early experience and exposure to oxytocin and vasopressin are sexually dimorphic. *Dev. Neurosci.* 31, 332–341.

Carter, C. S., DeVries, A. C., and Getz, L. L. (1995). Physiological substrates of mammalian monogamy: the prairie vole model. *Neurosci. Biobehav. Rev.* 19, 303–314.

Carter, C. S., Getz, L. L., Gavish, L., McDermott, J. L., and Arnold, P. (1980). Male-related pheromones and the activation of female reproduction in the prairie vole (*Microtus ochrogaster*). *Biol. Repro.* 23, 1038–1045.

Champagne, F., Diorio, J., Sharma, S., and Meaney, M. J. (2001). Naturally occurring variations in maternal behavior in the rat are associated with differences in estrogen-inducible central oxytocin receptors. *Proc. Natl. Acad. Sci. U.S.A.* 98, 12736–12741.

Champagne, F. A., and Meaney, M. J. (2007). Transgenerational effects of social environment on variations in maternal care and behavioral response to novelty. *Behav. Neurosci.* 121, 1353–1363.

Cho, M. M., DeVries, A. C., Williams, J. R., and Carter, C. S. (1999). The effects of oxytocin and vasopressin on partner preferences in male and female prairie voles (*Microtus ochrogaster*). *Behav. Neurosci.* 113, 1071–1079.

Denenberg, V. H., Ottinger, D. R., and Stephans, M. W. (1962). Effects of maternal factors upon growth and behavior of the rat. *Child Dev.* 33, 65–71.

Denenberg, V. H., and Whimbey, A. E. (1963). Infantile stimulation and animal husbandry: a methodological study. *J. Comp. Physiol. Psych.* 56, 877–878.

Desbonnet, L., Garrett, L., Daly, E., McDermott, K. W., and Dinan, T. G. (2008). Sexually dimorphic effects of maternal separation stress on corticotrophin-releasing factor and vasopressin systems in the adult rat brain. *Int. J. Dev. Neurosci.* 26, 259–268.

DeVries, A. C., DeVries, M. B., Taymans, S., and Carter, C. S. (1995). The modulation of pair bonding by corticosterone in female prairie voles (*Microtus ochrogaster*). *Proc. Natl. Acad. Sci. U.S.A.* 92, 7744–7748.

DeVries, A. C., DeVries, M. B., Taymans, S. E., and Carter, C. S. (1996). The effects of stress on social preferences are sexually dimorphic in prairie voles. *Proc. Natl. Acad. Sci. U.S.A.* 93, 11980–11984.

Dharmadhikari, A., Lee, Y. S., Roberts, R. L., and Carter, C. S. (1997). Exploratory behavior correlates with social organization and is responsive to peptide injections in prairie voles. *Ann. N. Y. Acad. Sci.* 807, 610–612.

Eklund, M. B., and Arborelius, L. (2006). Twice daily long maternal separations in Wistar rats decreases anxiety-like behaviour in feamles but does not affect males. *Behav. Brain Res.* 172, 278–285.

Enthoven, L., de Kloet, E. R., and Oitzl, M. S. (2008). Differential development of stress system (re)activity at weaning dependent on disruption of maternal care. *Brain Res.* 1217, 62–69.

Francis, D. D., Diorio, J., Plotsky, P. M., and Meaney, M. J. (2002a). Environmental enrichment reverses the effects of maternal separation on stress reactivity. *J. Neurosci.* 22, 7840–7843.

Francis, D. D., Young, L. J., Meaney, M. J., and Insel, T. R. (2002b). Naturally occurring differences in maternal care are associated with the expression of oxytocin and vasopressin (V1a) receptors: gender differences. *J. Neuroendocrin.* 14, 349–353.

Francis, D. D., and Kuhar, M. J. (2008). Frequency of maternal licking and grooming correlates negatively with vulnerability to cocaine and alcohol use in rats. *Pharmacol. Biochem. Behav.* 90, 497–500.

Francis, D. D., Young, L. J., Meaney, M. J., and Insel, T. R. (2000). Variations in maternal behavior are associated with differences in oxytocin receptors levels in the rat. *J. Neuroendocrin.* 12, 1145–1148.

Getz, L. L., Carter, C. S., and Gavish, L. (1981). The mating system of the prairie vole *Microtus ochrogaster*: field and laboratory evidence for pair-bonding. *Behav. Ecol. Sociobiol.* 8, 189–194.

Gilmer, W. S., and McKinney, W. T. (2003). Early experience and depressive disorders: human and non-human primate studies. *J. Aff. Dis.* 75, 97–113.

Gimpl, G., and Fahrenholz, F. (2001). The oxytocin receptor system: structure, function, and regulation. *Physiol. Rev.* 81, 629–683.

Grippo, A. J., Gerena, D., Huang, J., Kumar, N., Shah, M., Ughreja, R., and Carter, C. S. (2007). Social isolation induces behavioral and neuroendocrine disturbances relevant to depression in female and male prairie voles. *Psychoneuroendocrinology* 32, 966–980.

Harlow, H. F. (1961). "The development of affectional patterns in infant monkeys," in *Determinants of Infant Behavior*, ed. B. M. Foss (New York: Wiley), 75–97.

Harlow, H. F. (1964). "Early social deprivation and later behavior in the monkey," in *Unfinished Tasks in the Behavioral Sciences*, eds A. Abrams, H. H. Garner, and J. E. P. Tomal (Baltimore, MD: Williams & Wilkins), 154–173.

Harlow, H. F., and Suomi, S. J. (1971). Social recovery of isolation-reared monkeys. *Proc. Natl. Acad. Sci. U.S.A.* 68, 1534–1538.

Heim, C., Owens, M. J., Plotsky, P. M., and Nemeroff, C. B. (1997). The role of early adverse life events in the etiology of depression and posttraumatic stress disorder – focus on corticotropin-releasing factor. *Psychobiol. Posttraum. Stress Disord.* 821, 194–207.

Henry, J. P., and Wang, S. (1998). Effects of early stress on adult affiliative behavior. *Psychoneuroendocrinology* 23, 863–875.

Herring, A., Yasin, H., Ambree, O., Sachser, N., Paulus, W., and Keyvani, K. (2008). Environmental enrichment counteracts Alzheimer's neurovascular dysfunction in TgCRND8 mice. *Brain Path.* 18, 32–39.

Hofer, M. A. (1978). "Hidden regulatory processes in early social relationships," in *Perspectives in Ethology*, Vol. 3, eds P. P. G. Bateson and P. H. Klopfer (New York: Plenum Press), 135–166.

Hofer, M. A. (2006). Psychobiological roots of early attachment. *Curr. Dir. Psychol. Sci.* 15, 84–88.

Holmes, A., le Guisquet, A. M., Vogel, E., Millstein, R. A., Leman, S., and Belzung, C. (2005). Early life genetic, epigenetic, and environmental factors shaping emotionality in rodents. *Neurosci. Biobehav. Rev.* 29, 1335–1346.

Insel, T. R., Preston, S., and Winslow, J. T. (1995). Mating in the monogamous male: Behavioral consequences. *Physiol. Behav.* 57, 615–627.

Koolhaas, J. M., de Boer, S. F., Buwalda, B., and van Reenen, K. (2007). Individual variation in coping with stress: a multidimensional approach of ultimate and proximate mechanisms. *Brain Behav. Evol.* 70, 218–226.

Koolhaas, J. M., de Boer, S. F., Buwalda, B., van der Vegt, B. N., Carere, C., Groothuis, A. G. G. (2001). "How and why coping systems vary among individuals," in *Coping With Challenge: Welfare in Animals Including Humans*, ed. D. M. Broom (Dahlem Workshop Report #87), 197–209.

Kramer, K. M., Cushing, B. S., Carter, C. S., Wu, J., and Ottinger, M. A. (2004). Sex and species differences in plasma oxytocin using an enzyme immunoassay. *Can. J. Zool.* 82, 1194–1200.

Labuschagne, I., Phan, K. L., Wood, A., Angstadt, M., Chua, P., Heinrichs, M., Stout, J. C., and Nathan, P. J. (2010). Oxytocin attenuates amygdala reactivity to fear in generalized social anxiety disorder. *Neuropsychopharmacology* 35, 2403–2413.

Levine, S. (1957). Infantile experience and resistance to physiological stress. *Science* 126, 405.

Levine, S. (2002a). "Enduring effects of early experience on adult behavior," in *Hormones, Brain and Behavior*, eds D. W. Pfaff, A. P. Arnold, A. M. Etgen, S. E. Fahrbach, and R. T. Rubin (New York: Academic Press), 535–542.

Levine, S. (2002b). Regulation of the hypothalamic-pituitary-adrenal axis in the neonatal rat: the role of maternal behavior. *Neurotox. Res.* 4, 557–564.

Levine, S. (2005). Developmental determinants of sensitivity and resistance to stress. *Psychoneuroendocrinology* 30, 939–946.

Levine, S., and Lewis, G. W. (1959a). Critical period for effects of infantile experience on maturation of stress. *Science* 129, 42–43.

Levine, S., and Lewis, G. W. (1959b). The relative importance of experimenter contact in an effect produced by extra-stimulation in infancy. *J. Comp. Physiol. Psychol.* 52, 368–369.

Lim, M. M., Hammock, E. A. D., and Young, L. J. (2004). The role of vasopressin in the genetic and neural regulation of monogamy. *J. Neuroendocrin.* 16, 325–332.

Littell, R., Milliken, G. A., Stroup, W. W., and Wolfinger, R. D. (1996). *SAS System for Mixed Models*. Cary, NC: SAS Institute Inc.

Lynn, D. A., and Brown, G. R. (2010). The ontogeny of anxiety-like behavior in rats from adolescence to adulthood. *Dev. Psychobiol.* 52, 731–739.

Macri, S., Chiarotti, F., and Wurbel, H. (2008). Maternal separation and maternal care act independently on the development of HPA responses in male rats. *Beh. Brain Res.* 191, 227–234.

Meaney, M. J. (2001). Maternal care, gene expression, and the transmission of individual differences in stress reactivity across generations. *Ann. Rev. Neurosci.* 24, 1161–1192.

Neumann, I. D. (2002). Involvement of the brain oxytocin system in stress coping: interactions with the hypothalamo-pituitary-adrenal axis. *Prog. Brain Res.* 139, 147–162.

Neumann, I. D., Torner, L., Toschi, N., and Veenema, A. H. (2006). Oxytocin actions within the supraoptic and paraventricular nuclei: differential effects on intranuclear and peripheral vasopressin release. *Am. J. Physiol. Integr. Comp. Physiol.* 291, R29–R36.

Nithianantharajah, J., and Hannan, A. J. (2006). Enriched environments, experience-dependent plasticity and disorders of the nervous system. *Nat. Rev. Neurosci.* 7, 697–709.

Paxinos, G., and Watson, C. (2005). *Rat Brain in Stereotaxic Coordinates*, 5th Edn. New York: Elsevier.

Pedersen, C. A., Ascher, J. A., Monroe, Y. L., and Prange, A. J. Jr. (1982). Oxytocin induces maternal behavior in virgin female rats. *Science* 216, 648–650.

Pedersen, C. A., and Boccia, M. L. (2002). Oxytocin links mothering received, mothering bestowed, and adult stress responses. *Stress* 5, 267.

Plotsky, P. M. (1997). Long-term consequences of adverse early experience: a rodent model. *Biol. Psychiat.* 41, 262.

Plotsky, P. M. (2002). Altering the developmental trajectory of the brain: Short and long term consequences of early experience in animal models. *Biol. Psychiat.* 51, 100S.

Plotsky, P. M., Owens, M. J., and Nemeroff, C. B. (1998). Psychoneuroendocrinology of depression – Hypothalamic-pituitary-adrenal axis. *Psychiatr. Clin. North Am.* 21, 293–307.

Ramos, A., and Mormede, P. (1998). Stress and emotionality: a multidimentional and genetic approach. *Neurosci. Biobehav. Rev.* 22, 33–57.

Renard, G. M., Rivarola, M. A., and Suarez, M. M. (2007). Sexual dimorphism in rats: effects of early maternal separation and variable chronic stress on pituitary-adrenal axis and behavior. *Int. J. Dev. Neurosci.* 25, 373–379.

Roberts, R. L., Williams, J. R., Wang, A. K., and Carter, C. S. (1998). Cooperative breeding and monogamy in prairie voles: influence of the sire and geographical variation. *Anim. Behav.* 55, 1131–1140.

Ross, H. E., Cole, C. D., Smith, Y., Neumann, I. D., Landgraf, R., Murphy, A. Z., and Young, L. J. (2009). Characterization of the oxytocin system regulating affiliative behavior in female prairie voles. *Neuroscience* 162, 892–903.

Ruscio, M. G., Sweeny, T., Hazelton, J. L., Suppatkul, P., and Carter, C. S. (2007). Social environment regulates corticotropin releasing factor, corticosterone and vasopressin in juvenile prairie voles. *Horm. Behav.* 51, 54–61.

Sanchez, M. M., Ladd, C. O., and Plotsky, P. M. (2001). Early adverse experience as a developmental risk factor for later psychopathology: Evidence from rodent and primate models. *Dev. Psychopathol.* 13, 419–449.

Slotten, H. A., Kalinichev, M., Hagan, J. J., Marsden, C. A., and Fone, K. C. F. (2006). Long-lasting changes in behavioural and neuroendocrine indices in the rat following neonatal maternal separation: gender-dependent effects. *Brain Res.* 1097, 125–132.

Smotherman, W. P., and Bell, R. W. (1980). "Maternal mediation of early experience," in *Maternal Influence and Early Behavior*, eds W. P. Smotherman, and R. W. Bell (New York: Spectrum Publishing).

Stowe, J. R., Liu, Y., Curtis, J. T., Freeman, M. E., and Wang, Z. X. (2005). Species differences in anxiety-related responses in male prairie and meadow voles: The effects of social isolation. *Physiol. Behav.* 86, 369–378.

Tang, A. C. (2001). Neonatal exposure to novel environment enhances hippocampal-dependent memory function during infancy and adulthood. *Learn. Mem.* 8, 257–264.

Tang, A. C., Akers, K. G., Reeb, B. C., Romeo, R. D., and McEwen, B. S. (2006). Programming social, cognitive, and neuroendocrine development by early exposure to novelty. *Proc. Natl. Acad. Sci. U.S.A.* 103, 15716–15721.

Taymans, S. E., DeVries, A. C., DeVries, M. B., Nelson, R. J., Friedman, T. C., Detera-Wadleigh, S., Carter, C. S., and Chrousos, G. P. (1997). The hypothalamic-pituitary-adrenal axis of prairie voles (*Microtus ochrogaster*): evidence for target tissue glucocorticoid resistance. *Gen. Comp. Endocrinol.* 106, 48–61.

Todeschin, A. S., Winkelmann-Duarte, E. C., Jacob, M. H. V., Aranda, B. C. C., Jacobs, S., Fernandes, M. C., Ribeiro, M. F. M., Sanvitto, G. L., and Lucion, A. B. (2009). Effects of neonatal handling on social memory, social interaction, and number of oxytocin and vasopressin neurons in rats. *Horm. Behav.* 56, 93–100.

Tyler, A. N., Michel, G. F., Bales, K. L., and Carter, C. S. (2005). Do brief early disturbances of parents affect parental care in the bi-parental prairie vole (*Microtus ochrogaster*)? *Dev. Psychobiol.* 47, 451.

Veenema, A. H., Blume, A., Niederle, D., Buwalda, B., and Neumann, I. D. (2006). Effects of early life stress on adult male aggression and hypothalamic vasopressin and serotonin. *Eur. J. Neurosci.* 24, 1711–1720.

Wang, Z. X., Ferris, C. F., and Devries, G. J. (1994). Role of septal vasopressin innervation in paternal behavior in prairie voles (*Microtus ochrogaster*). *Proc. Natl. Acad. Sci. U.S.A.* 91, 400–404.

Wang, Z. X., Zhou, L., Hulihan, T. J., and Insel, T. R. (1996). Immunoreactivity of central vasopressin and oxytocin pathways in microtine rodents: a quantitative comparative study. *J. Comp. Neurol.* 366, 726–737.

Williams, J. R., Insel, T. R., Harbaugh, C. R., and Carter, C. S. (1994). Oxytocin centrally administered facilitates formation of a partner preference in female prairie voles (*Microtus ochrogaster*). *J. Neuroendocrin.* 6, 247–250.

Winslow, J. T., Hastings, N., Carter, C. S., Harbaugh, C. R., and Insel, T. R. (1993). A role for central vasopressin in pair bonding in monogamous prairie voles. *Nature* 365, 545–548.

Zanettini, C., Carola, V., Lo Iacona, L., Moles, A., Gross, C., and d'Amato, F. R. (2010). Postnatal handling reverses social anxiety in serotonin receptor 1A knockout mice. *Genes Brain Behav.* 9, 26–32.

Technical and conceptual considerations for performing and interpreting functional MRI studies in awake rats

Marcelo Febo[1,2]*

[1] Department of Psychiatry, The McKnight Brain Institute, University of Florida College of Medicine, Gainesville, FL, USA
[2] Department of Neuroscience, The McKnight Brain Institute, University of Florida College of Medicine, Gainesville, FL, USA

*Correspondence:
Marcelo Febo, Department of Psychiatry, University of Florida College of Medicine, P.O. Box 100256, Gainesville, FL 32610-0256, USA.
e-mail: febo@ufl.edu

Functional neuroimaging studies in rodents have the potential to provide insight into neurodevelopmental and psychiatric conditions. The strength of the technique lies in its non-invasive nature that can permit longitudinal functional studies in the same animal over its adult life. The relatively good spatial and temporal resolution and the ever-growing database on the biological and biophysical basis of the blood oxygen level dependent (BOLD) signal make it a unique technique in preclinical neuroscience research. Our laboratory has used imaging to investigate brain activation in awake rats following cocaine administration and during the presentation of lactation-associated sensory stimuli. Factors that deserve attention when planning functional magnetic resonance imaging studies in rats include technical issues, animal physiology and interpretability of the resulting data. The present review discusses the pros and cons of animal imaging with a particular focus on the technical aspects of studies with awake rats. Overall, the benefits of the technique outweigh its limitations and the rapidly evolving methods will open the way for more laboratories to employ the technique in neuroscience research.

Keywords: fMRI, rats, anesthesia, neural circuits, awake rat imaging, motion artifact, stress, neuroimaging

INTRODUCTION

For over two decades functional magnetic resonance imaging (fMRI) has been used to investigate human and animal brain function using a variety of experimental paradigms. The most popular functional imaging technique relies on the blood oxygen level dependent (BOLD) contrast mechanism first reported in the anesthetized rat by Ogawa et al. (1990). Rodent fMRI studies have evolved from experiments focused on developing new MR imaging methods to recent work that employs the technique to investigate specific neurobiological mechanisms. A significant advantage of fMRI is that it allows a functional characterization of the awake rodent brain under different treatment and pharmacological conditions (Peeters et al., 2001; Sachdev et al., 2003; Febo et al., 2004b, 2005a,b; Ferris et al., 2005, 2006, 2008; Chin et al., 2006, 2011; Chen et al., 2009; Liang et al., 2011; Zhang et al., 2011). Rather than providing a direct window into neuronal activity, the BOLD fMRI signal depends on the brain's blood supply and cellular oxidative metabolism. However, it supersedes previous *in vitro* techniques that were used to examine cerebral blood flow (CBF) and glucose utilization in the rat brain using injectable radiolabeled tracers because of its measurement of neural signals in real-time (Porrino et al., 1988; Stein and Fuller, 1992, 1993).

Thanks to a growing number of studies on the nature of the BOLD signal, there is improved knowledge about the relationship between BOLD and neuronal activity (Fox and Raichle, 1986; Fox et al., 1988; Davis et al., 1998; Logothetis et al., 2001; Shmuel et al., 2002, 2006; Kennerley et al., 2005; Tian et al., 2011). The BOLD signal arises from changes in the oxy-to-deoxyhemoglobin ratio in tissue and thus is primarily a hemodynamic signal restricted by the biophysical properties of the local neurovasculature. This should be kept in mind when interpreting neuroimaging data. The use of *in vivo* single-unit, multi-unit, and local field potential (LFP) recordings and optical imaging methods to investigate changes in neural activity and vascular reactivity at sub-anatomical levels can strengthen the interpretability of fMRI data. We have performed fMRI of the neural actions of cocaine and the lactation stimulus in the unanesthetized maternal rat (Febo et al., 2004b, 2008). The present review will use these studies as methodological examples of fMRI in awake animals. Parallel preclinical and clinical imaging studies can provide a basis for direct translational research that could aid discoveries in different fields of neuropsychiatry. For instance, there have been significant human imaging studies that have investigated the neural actions of cocaine (Breiter et al., 1997; Gollub et al., 1998; Li et al., 2000), whereas there have been a separate series of imaging experiments on human maternal care (Bartels and Zeki, 2004; Nitschke et al., 2004; Strathearn et al., 2008). Collectively, these and other imaging studies have been in partial agreement with several animal studies on the brain regions that are involved in responding to cocaine or infant sensory cues. Animal studies have the design flexibility to verify results with a multiplicity of invasive brain methods that can inform human work and aid in data interpretations. Despite the advantages, there are also challenges to awake animal imaging that are different from those in anesthetized preparations. Several of these have been addressed in past studies (Lahti et al., 1998, 1999; Ludwig et al., 2004; King et al., 2005; Ferris et al., 2008). These include hardware issues (Lahti et al., 1998; Ludwig et al., 2004), animal stress (King et al., 2005), data processing and artifacts (Ferris et al., 2005, 2008). This review provides a summary of the methods used for functional MRI experiments in rats with a special focus on awake imaging methods that are used in our laboratory. This includes information on technical and conceptual aspects of fMRI in awake rats, starting with the physiological basis of the BOLD fMRI signal, describing the hardware and methods used to image awake as opposed to anesthetized rats and concluding with a detailed examination of data interpretations.

PHYSIOLOGY OF THE BOLD CONTRAST MECHANISM
THE BOLD SIGNAL

The nuclear magnetic resonance mechanism that provides the basis for generating contrast in MR images depends on the behavior of hydrogen nuclei (protons) in water within the main tissue compartments of the brain. Unpaired protons contain a net positive charge and can act as tiny magnetic dipoles that align along the longitudinal axis (z-axis) of the external magnetic field (B_0). Protons possess an angular moment (ω_0), or precession, that is directly proportional to B_0 and is described by the Larmor equation $\omega_0 = \gamma B_0$, where γ is the gyromagnetic ratio (in the case of H^1 42.6 MHz/T). Precession along the longitudinal z-axis is manipulated during typical MR experiments. Combinations of radiofrequency (RF) excitation pulses and switching of magnetic field gradients ultimately result in the recovery of tissue RF signals from different areas of the brain. RF pulses excite protons away from their steady state position imposed by the surrounding B_0 field. Relaxation back to the steady state position is governed by two time constants termed T_1 and T_2. The time constants are associated with the intrinsic properties of specific tissue types (cerebrospinal fluid, white matter, gray matter) and thus allow the generation of contrast through the experimenter-mediated adjustment of echo times (TE) and repetition times (TR). The excitation and relaxation processes result in the emission of RF signals from tissue compartments of the brain. These are detected using coils that localize signals from the tissue of interest (in reality the MR signal is an "echo" of the original relaxation signal). The RF excitation and detection mechanism is accompanied by a series of slice selective, read-out and phase encoding gradient variations that allow the encoding of brain spatial information.

A variant of T_2, known as T_2^* ("T-2-star"), is produced by inhomogeneities in the magnetic field that cause reductions in T_2 (faster transverse relaxation rate). Deoxyhemoglobin (dHb) in plasma red blood cells (RBCs) is paramagnetic while oxyhemoglobin (HbO_2) is diamagnetic (Pauling and Coryell, 1936) and the intravascular difference between the two provides for an endogenous contrast mechanism (Ogawa et al., 1990). Ogawa et al. (1990) provided evidence that a decreased T_2^* signal in blood vessels, particularly veins of the rat cortex, is due to blood oxygenation state. Darker veins in the cortex were distinguishable in rats inhaling low O_2 concentrations in inspired air (more dHb) while increased O_2 saturation (significantly less dHb) increased the brightness of images. The T_2^* contrast was observed to be dependent on blood oxygenation. Therefore the BOLD signal arises from changes in the tissue concentrations of dHb. Seminal publications followed that provided support for task-dependent changes in the BOLD signal that occurs in T_2^* weighted images of the human somatosensory, motor and visual cortices (Bandettini et al., 1992; Ogawa et al., 1992).

RELATION BETWEEN CEREBRAL HEMODYNAMICS AND NEURONAL ACTIVITY

Oxidative and non-oxidative metabolism supports neurons and glial cells (Kasischke et al., 2004). Elevations in arterial blood flow supply glucose and O_2, which serve as fuel to generate the cellular energy substrates ATP and lactate. Most of the neuronal ATP expenditure is used to restore the equilibrium of the electrochemical potential for Na^+, K^+ and Ca^{2+} at synapses (Attwell and Iadecola, 2002). During conditions of high neuronal and metabolic activity, O_2 diffuses down a steep concentration gradient from plasma RBCs across the capillary walls into the surrounding parenchymal tissue. This leads to dHb accumulation in the venous compartment. The paramagnetic effect of dHb is "felt" by local water protons in the intra and extravascular compartments, and this increases the relaxation rate of protons, decreasing the signal intensity in T_2^* weighted MR images. This is a transient effect, however, as the BOLD signal increases (increased T_2^*) within a few seconds of stimulus delivery. The supply of oxygenated blood is associated with increased delivery to metabolically active regions of the brain. Fractional increases in plasma HbO_2 saturation from baseline levels therefore increase the T_2^* signal. Indeed, visual and somatosensory evoked changes in O_2 metabolism was estimated to be 5% above baseline levels, but there is nearly a 30–50% increase in blood flow to the active cortical regions (Fox and Raichle, 1986; Fox et al., 1988). Therefore, increased CBF is several orders of magnitude above the O_2 demand of the tissue. The over-compensatory mechanism is instrumental in generating the BOLD response observed in many studies.

There have been thorough investigations of the possible neurovascular mechanisms contributing to the BOLD signal as well as the relation between the BOLD signal and neuronal activity. Knowledge from these studies contributes to the understanding of fMRI data. Stimulus-dependent increases in O_2 consumption in the rat brain are associated with presynaptic action potential firing and ATPase-dependent movement of ions against their electrochemical gradients across the cell membrane (Attwell and Iadecola, 2002). Techniques to measure microscopic changes in tissue oxygenation and perfusion have been instrumental in understanding the underlying dynamics of the BOLD signal. Using intrinsic optical imaging and laser Doppler flowmetry, Malonek and Grinvald (1996) investigated the dynamics of the hemodynamic response in the cat visual cortex. It was shown that an increase in HbO_2 and CBF response near single cortical columns occurs within several seconds (2–3 s) of visual stimulus presentation (Malonek and Grinvald, 1996; Malonek et al., 1997). At the single neuron level, it appears that there is an initial decrease in tissue O_2 content due to a greater oxygen extraction fraction immediately after increasing firing activity (Thompson et al., 2003). This is followed by increases in O_2 that may be due to the elevated CBF (Thompson et al., 2003). Simultaneous fMRI and neurophysiological recordings taken from the anesthetized rhesus macacque's visual cortex demonstrated a near linear relation between BOLD and LFP, but this may not be the case for single-unit activity (Logothetis et al., 2001). The closer correspondence between BOLD and LFP's may be helpful in understanding the "type" of neural processing and "computational level" contributing the most to fMRI results. Estimates of the primate cortex indicate that each 1 mm^3 (which is about the size of a single volume element or "voxel" in human studies) contains approximately 50,000 neurons (Douglas et al., 2004). LFPs reflect larger scale electrical activity as a result of the cooperative interactions between populations of perhaps thousands of neurons rather than spike input or output at the single neuron level (Nadasdy et al., 1998). This is perhaps one of the most critical aspects of neural processing that should be carefully considered when interpreting BOLD data.

To sum, the above data describe biological correlates of the mechanisms involved in generating the BOLD responses observed in fMRI studies. It appears, at the microscopic level (measured by intrinsic optical techniques), that there is evidence of a tight coupling between single neuron activity and oxygen metabolism that contributes to generating the BOLD signal, but larger scale electrical oscillations at a macroscopic level may contribute to a larger extent. Regardless the specific neural mechanism, the steps between neuronal activity and BOLD involves coupling cellular metabolism and cerebrovascular reactivity (Davis et al., 1998; Lee et al., 2001; Sheth et al., 2004). fMRI signals are ultimately an indirect reflection of neural activity that cannot offer details on specific neuronal firing patterns as measured by electrophysiological techniques (Buzsaki et al., 2007; Logothetis, 2008). On the other hand, the measurement and mapping of neural signals over extended regions of the rat brain is unmatched by these techniques.

HARDWARE
MR SCANNER

The high field MR scanner produces the external B_0 field and contains the spatial encoding gradient coils that are oriented along the longitudinal z and transverse x–y axes. The use of 4.7 and 7 T horizontal bore systems for rodent applications have been optimal both because of the high signal-to-noise ratio (SNR) and good T_2/T_2^* contrast for functional studies. Scanners with high quality spatial encoding gradients, automated shimming (for correcting small field variations around the brain), and pre-installed pulse sequence routines that run on user-friendly console software are of choice for many applications-driven laboratories. At higher fields it is possible to obtain an in-plane voxel resolution for functional scans of about 390 × 469 μm^2 with 12–20 coronal slices (1–1.2 mm slice thickness). This covers most of the rat brain from the olfactory bulb to the cerebellum using T_2 weighted fast spin echo (FSE) sequences with minimal anatomical distortions (**Figure 1**). For localized rat brain studies with fewer slices, focusing on the coordinated activity of a few subsets of areas, the in-plane resolution can be increased to 100–250 μm^2. An advantage of having higher resolution images is that they can create voxels that better localize activity in the cortex (see columnar level resolution studies in Kim et al., 2000). However, the smaller voxel size results in lower SNR especially at lower field strengths.

Many fMRI studies have been performed using gradient echo echo planar imaging (GE EPI) because of its greater sensitivity to magnetic susceptibility and the BOLD effect. Gradient echo sequences use rapidly changing MR gradients to excite protons into the transverse plane (rather than using RF pulses). However, because of the same susceptibility effects, the GE EPI is highly vulnerable to signal loss at air-tissue interfaces in the temporal and paranasal regions. This leads to loss of data in important

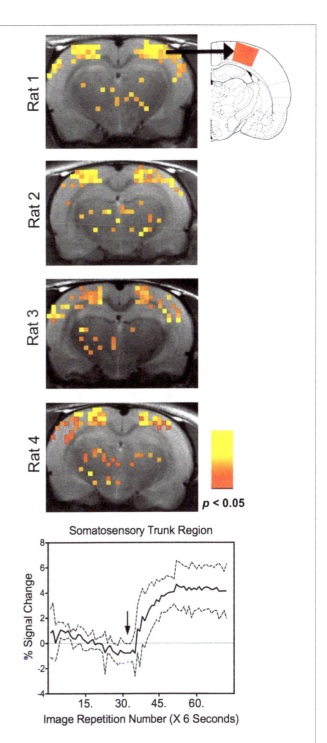

FIGURE 1 | Consistent somatosensory activation with ventrum trunk stimulation across awake fMRI studies. Top images show four representative rat coronal brain slices with significant increases in BOLD bilaterally in the cortical representation ventrum. Colored pixels overlaid onto high-resolution anatomical scans indicate significant differences from baseline ($p < 0.05$, corrected using false-detection rate (Genovese et al., 2002)). Atlas map to the right shows the somatosensory trunk region (Paxinos and Watson, 1997). Bottom panel shows the temporal profile of the BOLD signal response to ventrum stimulation (mean ± SD). Arrows shows onset of stimulus. Data were acquired using a T_2 weighted fast spin echo sequence at 4.7T (effective TE = 53 ms and TR = 8.3 s).

areas such as the ventral hippocampus, amygdala, and medial prefrontal cortex (Febo et al., 2004b; Ludwig et al., 2004). GE EPI has a high sensitivity to physiological noise and shows anatomical distortions (spatial warping) that can produce alignment and registration errors. Most modern MR console software contains built-in algorithms that correct these distortions. However, to correct the spatial warping, additional scan time must be added to acquire field maps that aid in unwarping reconstructed images. Finally, GE EPI sequences are more sensitive to intravascular and extravascular large vein signals that are distant from the actual foci of activity (Duong et al., 2003). Spin echo EPI (SE EPI) at high fields are more sensitive to intra and extravascular compartments closer to the capillaries and therefore are commonly used for fMRI studies at higher field strengths (Duong et al., 2003).

At high fields, T_2 weighted spin echo sequences appear to suffer less from the aforementioned issues (Duong et al., 2003; Goense and Logothetis, 2006; Poser and Norris, 2007; Ye et al., 2011). Single shot spin echo sequences (SE EPI) and multi-segmented T_2 weighted FSE can be used successfully with rats. The latter has been the sequence of choice for many of our experiments in awake rats. There is support in the literature for the use of FSE and SE EPI sequences for BOLD imaging (Duong et al., 2003; Goense and Logothetis, 2006; Poser and Norris, 2007; Ye et al., 2011). **Figure 1** illustrates the results from a study of the rat somatosensory cortex (Febo et al., 2008). In the study, awake female rats were stimulated on the ventrum skin while being imaged at 4.7 T using a T_2 weighted FSE sequence (TR = 8 s and TE = 53 ms). We observed increased BOLD signal intensity in areas that correspond to the trunk region of the primary somatosensory cortex (**Figure 1**). This was observed in all the tested animals. Temporal profiles of the BOLD signal are shown for seven individual rats just to give an idea of the variability between subjects. **Figure 2** further supports the notion that T_2 FSE sequences provide BOLD weighting. Awake rats were provided with 5% CO_2 in inspired air during functional scanning. A rise in signal intensity is observed at the specific times in which animals are exposed to hypercapnia. Switching back to normocapnic conditions results in a return to baseline signal intensity. This global cerebrovascular reactivity is due to changes in CBF in the absence of alterations in neuronal activity. These two studies indicate that BOLD signal changes may be of neural (**Figure 1**) and also of vascular origin (**Figure 2**).

RF COILS AND ACCESSORY EQUIPMENT

Studies of the rat brain using MR scanners require the use of RF coils that serve as the source of the B_1 field (the 90 and 180 degree pulses) that excite water protons in tissue to the transverse planes. The RF coils also serve to detect longitudinal and transverse signal relaxation. There are varieties of coils that are used for neuro-applications. Many laboratories construct their own RF coils (Ugurbil et al., 2003; Doty et al., 2007). These are usually single copper wire loop tuned to the magnet frequency (4.7–7 T or 200–300 MHz range, respectively). The coil is aligned over the area of interest, such as over the head overlying the cortex. The loop coil configuration, however, has less spatial coverage and usually results in signal drop from dorsal to ventral areas of the brain that makes this type of configuration less favorable for developmental studies. The configuration prohibits coverage of signals from brain structures such as the hypothalamus and midbrain that are farthest in distance from the coil. This can be overcome by using a dual RF coil system built into an MR compatible restrainer of the head and body (Ludwig et al., 2004), or a quadrature coil system with improved B_1 coverage of the brain (EkamImaging Inc., Shrewsbury, MA, USA; **Figure 3**).

In addition to the main electronics that are needed to run functional brain scanning in rats there are also other useful accessory devices. For anesthetized preps, beds with integrated head and/or body holders are important to place animals correctly inside the bore of the magnet. Typically these are necessary to align animals correctly within the isocenter of the MR spectrometer prior to image acquisition. Physiological monitoring devices are also an essential part of the animal imaging setup. This includes MR compatible temperature probes, pulse oximeters, capnometers, electroencephalographic (EEG) and electromyographic (EMG) recorders, respiratory pillows and transducers, and other devices according to the needs of the investigator. The physiological measures are used to "gate" the image acquisitions to remove respiratory and cardiac pulsations that can appears as low frequency artifacts (Purdon and Weisskoff, 1998; Peeters and Van Der Linden, 2002; Bhattacharyya and Lowe, 2004). Stimulation devices may be needed when evoking sensory responses, such as for whisker and forepaw stimulations. The stimuli for sensory evoked responses can be timed to the functional image acquisitions for accurate correlations with BOLD signal responses during block design studies.

ANIMAL EXPERIMENTAL PREPARATIONS
ANESTHETIZED PREPARATION

Anesthetized preparations are used extensively for fMRI studies in rats. The methods used generally are not suitable for longitudinal studies in the same population of animals. In many applications

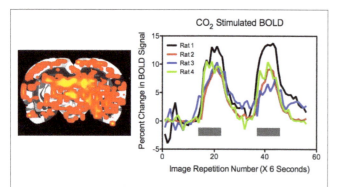

FIGURE 2 | Vascular reactivity contributes to BOLD signal changes. The figure illustrates how hypercapnic conditions can elevate the BOLD signal in the absence of any neural stimulus. The activation map on the left shows dramatic increases in BOLD with 5% CO_2 inhalation during functional image acquisition. Plot on the right shows the timecourse of BOLD signal intensity changes over the course of the scanning. Plots are shown for four individual rats, each showing a similar pattern of BOLD signal change. The gray bars below indicate the interleaved epochs of normocapnia and CO_2 exposure. Data were acquired using a T_2 weighted fast spin echo sequence at 4.7T (effective TE = 53 ms and TR = 8.3 s).

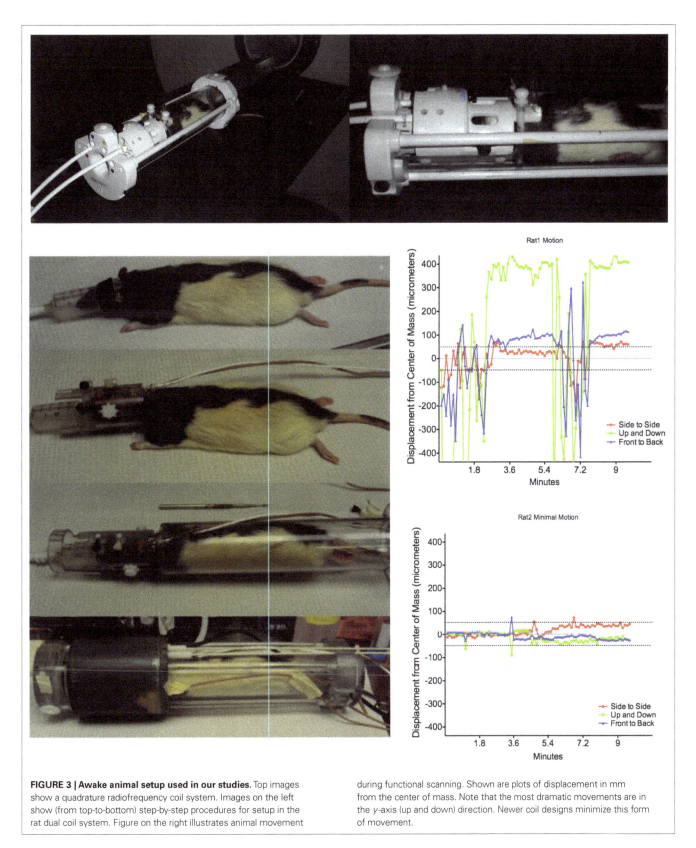

FIGURE 3 | Awake animal setup used in our studies. Top images show a quadrature radiofrequency coil system. Images on the left show (from top-to-bottom) step-by-step procedures for setup in the rat dual coil system. Figure on the right illustrates animal movement during functional scanning. Shown are plots of displacement in mm from the center of mass. Note that the most dramatic movements are in the y-axis (up and down) direction. Newer coil designs minimize this form of movement.

the femoral artery of the rat is catheterized to allow the sampling of arterial blood gases and a close monitoring of arterial blood pressure and pH during scanning. Changes in the partial pressures of blood gases may be indicative of alterations of basal conditions that can alter the magnitude of the BOLD signal. This is important since hypoxia and hypercapnia modulate baseline

BOLD signal in the rat, perhaps independently of basal neural activity and metabolism (Bandettini and Wong, 1997; Cohen et al., 2002). **Figure 2** shows an example of this. Controlling for movement is also important and some laboratories use chemical agents that can suppress muscle contractility during scanning. Marota et al. (2000) used the paralyzing agent pancuronium to eliminate unwanted respiratory pulsations in the anesthetized rat. Others have used the muscle relaxant gallamine to paralyze animals during MR scanning (Xi et al., 2004). The animals in the cited studies were tracheostomized and mechanically ventilated during experiments (Marota et al., 2000). The experimenter-controlled activity facilitates "gating" procedures to remove artifacts without significant spontaneous variations in breathing rate. From a strict engineering approach, this rigorous methodology is ideal given the tenuous quality of the BOLD signal. Despite some of these advantages, however, the invasive procedure precludes long-term developmental studies in rats. Alternatively, arterial blood pressure and respiration rates can be measured non-invasively using a pulse oximetry over the tail of the rat and a respiratory pillow placed just underneath the animals' chest.

AWAKE SETUP

Our laboratory has utilized methods to image awake rats as an alternative to imaging under anesthesia. Before this is done, however, animals must be acclimated to the restraint conditions and MR pulse sequence noise. The procedures for acclimation are carried out for 5 days prior to collection of imaging data. Both acclimation and actual imaging experimental setup procedures are done under similar conditions. Rats are first anesthetized under 2–4% isoflurane gas to enable placement into a head restrainer (**Figure 3**). There is evidence that isoflurane anesthetized animals regain motor function and coordination within minutes (Eger and Johnson, 1987), and thus, volatile anesthetics such as isoflurane are useful when quick setup and awakening are desired. An important part of the restraint setup are the ear bars that allow the proper orientation of the head (**Figure 3**). A semi-circular plastic headpiece containing blunted ear bars are first placed over the animal's head and fitted into the ear canals. These are non-invasive (requiring no surgery) and are not made of abrasive or harmful material. Their placement is the same as standard stereotaxic ear bars. Other laboratories have taken another approach, that is, to bolt or permanently affix the holders to the skull of the animals to ensure that the animals will not be able to move during scanning (Miller et al., 2003; Sachdev et al., 2003; Desai et al., 2011). We have not found that this approach is necessary. The animal is then guided through the center of the coil/head holder unit and the incisors placed over a bite bar. A plastic latch locks down over the nose with a screw. The lateral ear bars contain outer grooves that accommodate lateral screws that are used to align the animal in the holder and fix its position in the restrainer. The body is placed into a tube that has shoulder bars and an overlying square plastic peg that prevents up-and-down movement during scanning. The entire system is placed into a chassis that fits the bore of the magnet and can be fastened inside of it. In the experience of the author, the setup time is quite short (∼10 min). The system has plenty of room to accommodate accessory equipment for stimulus delivery or physiological monitoring (see above). The above system allows the rodent to remain in a semi-crouched position while being scanned (forelimb movement is more restricted). **Figure 3** shows movement along the z and x–y directions inside the scanner. As may be observed, most movement comes from the y direction (up and down movements). The rats seldom move in the back-and-forth (z) and side-to-side (x) if positioned correctly. The design of the newer coil system used in our laboratory (Febo and Pira, 2011) minimizes the y direction movement. Other groups have used positioning screws that are affixed to the skull and have obtained good results. For example, Desai et al. (2011) carried out fMRI-optogenetic experiments in awake restrained mice. The mice had miniature plastic screws affixed to the skull. They used a short (3-day) acclimatization period and provided animals with "treats" after restraint sessions. It is possible that both approaches will yield good results, and perhaps using cranial fixtures to prevent movement may be preferable for methods that include additional invasive procedures during fMRI scanning.

POTENTIAL EFFECTS OF ANESTHETICS AND RESTRAINT STRESS
EFFECTS OF ANESTHETICS ON BASAL NEURONAL FIRING

Motion must be minimize during MR scanning (**Figure 3**). Both gross movements (for example, slow shifts in head position, sustained or transient leg motion, chewing, vocalizations) and physiological motion (pulsations due to cardiac and respiratory cycles) can significantly degrade multi-repetitions MR scans. It can also contribute to false activation patterns that correlate motion with stimulus presentations (Freire and Mangin, 2001). In our laboratory, we prescreen and process data for motion artifact and signal drift that may arise from different sources. Images with minor artifacts are realigned using in house software or Statistical Parametric Mapping software (SPM8; http://www.fil.ion.ucl.ac.uk/spm/). Of course, anesthetizing animals during scanning also minimizes motion artifacts but this reduces the magnitude of the BOLD signal in the rat brain (Lahti et al., 1999; Peeters et al., 2001).

There are significant lines of evidence suggesting that agents typically used for anesthetizing animals can suppress certain forms of neuronal activity and modify specific patterns of neuronal activity and metabolism. For instance, there are differences in basal and stimulated brain glucose utilization (cerebral metabolic rate for glucose, or, CMR_{glu}) and CBF in awake vs. anesthetized rats (Nakao et al., 2001). Stimulation of the whisker-to-barrel cortex pathway resulted in differential CBF and CMR_{glu} across regions when rats were anesthetized with halothane (Nakao et al., 2001). The results of the latter study suggest that although the barrel cortex is active in the anesthetized state, other regions along the pathway arising from the stimulation of peripheral sensory receptors are suppressed and may thus require a conscious state (Nakao et al., 2001). Evoked potentials in the barrel field cortex have been shown to vary between anesthetic conditions (Martin et al., 2006). The amplitudes of field potential responses to graded levels of repetitive electrical stimulation to the whisker pads are reduced to a greater degree in anesthetized vs. awake rats (Martin et al., 2006). Firing of action potentials over localized regions of the awake rat visual cortex showed higher frequencies and bursting but lower pair-wise correlations between single units than ketamine-anesthetized rats (Greenberg et al., 2008), suggesting that the propagation of actions potential in localized networks is modified by the induction of an anesthetized state. Halothane, isoflurane, and desflurane can differentially affect gamma band oscillations in the rat cortex (Imas et al., 2004, 2005). This is important because field potential activity is believed to correlate well with BOLD signal changes. Graded levels of isoflurane (1.8–2.2%) also suppress EEG bursts measured in the primary sensory cortical area representing the forelimb of the rat and also reduced spontaneous variations in CBF (Liu et al., 2011). These levels of isoflurane are within the range that causes suppression of bursting in sensory cortical EEG patterns (Hartikainen et al., 1995). Research on the role of anesthetic agents in modulating neuronal activity raises concerns about the use of deep levels of anesthesia for rat brain imaging experiments (Austin et al., 2005; Masamoto et al., 2009; Angenstein et al., 2011). Variations in the pattern and magnitude of neuronal activity will vary according to anesthesia type and concentration. This underscores the importance of parsimony when interpreting data from studies with anesthetized animals. It is impossible to infer the animal's baseline state and unwarranted to assume that functionally interconnected regions respond similarly in awake and anesthetized conditions (Nakao et al., 2001).

EFFECTS OF ANESTHETICS ON CEREBRAL HEMODYNAMICS
In addition to the cited neural actions, anesthesia can influence global cerebrovascular reactivity. The choice of anesthetic and calibration of the depth of anesthesia are therefore important. The effects of volatile anesthetics on the BOLD signal, CBF, and CBV have been investigated. Hypercapnia-induced BOLD signal changes, which occur in the absence of neuronal activity, are of much greater magnitude in awake rats (Brevard et al., 2003). This suggests that cerebrovascular reactivity is affected by anesthesia. It is also important to note that basal levels of O_2 metabolism and neuronal spiking frequency in the cortex are reduced by deep levels of alpha-chloralose (Hyder et al., 2002). The results of the latter study provide evidence that basal conditions might be associated with the magnitude BOLD signal changes. Larger magnitude changes in BOLD may reflect lower basal firing of neurons in animals that are deeply anesthetized whereas lighter levels of anesthesia allow for smaller magnitude changes in BOLD in the face of higher basal activity (Hyder et al., 2002). Thus, the absence of neuronal recording methods or imaging methods to assess CBF may lead to incorrect interpretation of the magnitude of the BOLD signal.

Basal CBF levels in 2% isoflurane anesthetized rats were observed to be greater than in the awake state (Sicard et al., 2003). Isoflurane anesthesia can act as a vasodilating agent that increases blood flow. The percent change in CBF and BOLD in response to CO_2, however, is lower in anesthetized rats (Sicard et al., 2003). The lower magnitude response could be due to higher basal levels of blood flow (Sicard et al., 2003). Thus, in isoflurane anesthetized animals there seems to be direct modulation of CBF that is independent of the effects on neuronal activity (Masamoto et al., 2009). Isoflurane reportedly increases CBF globally due to its vasodilating actions (Liu et al., 2011). Spontaneous CBF changes are suppressed by increasing levels of isoflurane from 1.8 to 2.2% (Liu et al., 2011). Thus, light sedation with isoflurane (<1.8% in inspired air) might minimize the above-described effects. It has also been reported that alpha-chloralose specific parameters for forepaw stimulated BOLD activity in the somatosensory cortex do not work under isoflurane anesthesia (Masamoto et al., 2009). The accumulating evidence underscores the importance of considering the effects of anesthetics on both neuronal activity and cerebrovascular reactivity when designing fMRI studies and interpreting the data.

Finally, a fundamental concern of anesthetized preparations is that, as a preference of choice or perhaps based in published data, different laboratories vary their use of specific types of anesthetic agents. These include volatile anesthetics, such as isoflurane, desflurane, halothane, urethane, and injectable agents, such as medetomidine, ketamine, alpha-chloralose, and others. There is growing evidence that the different agents may have varying effects on BOLD signal and neuronal activity, and this could potentially lead to variations in findings between laboratories. Austin et al. (2005) compared the effects of halothane levels and alpha-chloralose on cortical stimulation evoked BOLD activity and found that the amplitude responses with varying levels of halothane were unchanged, whereas deepening anesthesia levels with alpha-chloralose lead to greater amplitude evoked responses (Austin et al., 2005). Indeed, a similar finding is reported by Masamoto et al. (2009), however, the latter study seems to show greater variability in peak CBF and summed field potential responses with alpha-chloralose than with isoflurane (Masamoto et al., 2009). BOLD functional connectivity (FC) analysis during resting state is also hindered by variations of the type of anesthetic chemical used. Medetomidine anesthesia allows better-localized correlations between seed voxel regions (higher specificity of correlated regions) and isoflurane has the opposite effect on FC analysis (Williams et al., 2011). It appears that FC analysis works optimally under isoflurane with concentrations in the range of 0.5–1.0% but fails at higher levels (2.9%; Wang et al., 2011). Frequency-dependent changes in amplitude BOLD and field potential responses to forepaw stimulation were observed over a wider range of stimulation frequencies under urethane (1–15 Hz) than under alpha-chloralose (1–3 Hz; Huttunen et al., 2008). Therefore, two laboratories implementing different types of anesthetics, say urethane in one and alpha-chloralose in the other, may result in disparate results. There are no optimal anesthetic types that can be used that will produce entirely reproducible findings across laboratories that carry out discovery-oriented research. The development of the technique, given the above-summarized data, should be to employ the technique in awake conditions wherever possible.

RESTRAINT STRESS
Stress is one of the biggest factors that present challenges to designing and interpreting fMRI data in awake animals. One of the concerns of acclimation is that it may produce chronic stress exposure to the animals. Is the type of restraint used for imaging equivalent to the form of restraint used in studies investigating the chronic effects of immobilization stress? The latter usually uses a wire mesh that restricts total movement while the imaging setup only involves restraint of the head while the limbs

and torso are not restrained. Thus, the imaging setup seems to involve intermittent stress that may have transient and not chronic effects. Do any residual chronic stress effects during acclimation have a permanent impact on brain physiology and behavior? This question really attends to the permanent changes that have been reported using other chronic stress models such as the social defeat stress model (Tornatzky and Miczek, 1993) that may result in animal groups that are in an overall depressed state or a state of behavioral despair (Krishnan and Nestler, 2008). Whether or not stress is present in restraint-acclimated rats is not a matter of debate. The aim is to determine whether the effects of stress are at tolerable levels.

King et al. (2005) reported that various physiological variables (e.g., respiratory rates, blood pressure, corticosterone levels) of Sprague-Dawley rats are reduced following 5–8 days of restraint. Most measures are reduced near to pre-stress baseline levels on day 4–5. An important outcome however was that there was a significant increase in contrast to noise while no changes in basal CBF values were noted. This could signify that the lower gross movement and physiological rhythms improve image quality. At the same time it points to the brains autoregulatory capacity in awake rats that remains intact regardless of whether or not they are acclimated (King et al., 2005). The data are consistent with reports indicating that rats habituate to repeated daily 1–2 h restraint for 4–9 days (Melia et al., 1994; Dhabhar et al., 1997). Rats show normal patterns of food intake and heart rate following habituation to restraint (Haleem, 1996; Stamp and Herbert, 2001). Importantly, habituation to repeated daily sessions of restraint is not necessarily indicative of impaired hypothalamic–pituitary–adrenal (HPA) axis function, since rats acclimated to restraint stress still show increased c-fos activation and corticosterone levels to a novel stressor (Melia et al., 1994). Recent unpublished work from my laboratory provides evidence that 22 kHz ultrasonic "distress" calls are reduced by day 4 and 5 of acclimatization in comparison to day 1 (**Figure 4**, unpublished results by Michael Reed and Marcelo Febo). At the same time struggle movements diminish in these animals when tested on a forced swim assay (**Figure 4**). One interpretation might be that animals are in a state of behavioral despair and are therefore not struggling. However, when viewed collectively the tests point to signs of physical and behavioral adaptations to the restraint conditions. The results support less struggle movements reported previously in Sprague-Dawley rats (King et al., 2005). Therefore rats seem to be fully capable of adapting to the head restraint conditions.

A central question is whether animals adapt to stress and is this adaptation indicative of learning or an overall impairment of the HPA axis and a resultant depressed behavioral state. There is partial support in the literature against the latter assertions. Parry and Mcelligott (1993) devised a method for head immobilization in awake rats in order to study central regulation of cardiovascular function. They reported that side-by-side acclimatization of rats to restraint reduced the stress of individual animals that are being acclimated. We have used a similar acclimatization procedure in our studies in which groups of animals are simultaneously exposed to daily sessions of restraint. Heart rate and blood pressure normalized after initial exposure to restraint indicating that the procedure was minimally stressful (Parry and Mcelligott, 1993). Barnum et al. (2007) investigated the hyperthermia effects of chronic restraint stress and compared these to other forms of stress such as the social defeat model and isolated cage confinement (Barnum et al., 2007). They observed that corticosterone and stress-induced hyperthermic responses to restraint stress adapted after 5–6 days of repeated exposure. However, this was not observed for the social defeat stress model indicating that the two forms of stress have different outcomes. There have been reports of the differential reactivity of the HPA axis to stress and immunological challenge across various strains of rats. Our initial experiments were all in Sprague-Dawley (SD) rats while the more recent work is performed in Long Evans. Dhabhar et al. (1997) investigated the chronic effects of stress on adaptation of the HPA axis in SD, Lewis and F344 rats (Dhabhar et al., 1997). SD and Lewis rats showed adaptations over the course of the 4-h immobilization stress paradigm as well as during the 10-day chronic regime of stress whereas F344 rats did not in either case (Dhabhar et al., 1997). Despite the reported evidence of adaptations to stress, there are important long-term effects that should not be

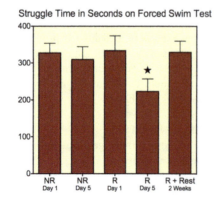
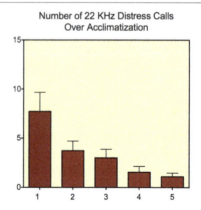

FIGURE 4 | Effects of restraint over the course of 5 days on struggling time in a forced swim test and on the emission of 22 KHz ultrasonic vocalizations. R, restraint; NR, no restraint; NR + Rest, no restraint and re-test after 2 weeks of rest. Star indicates significant difference between R Day 1 and R Day 5 conditions ($p < 0.05$ paired t-test).

overlooked. Naert et al. (2011) report a "depressed-like state" in rats chronically exposed to repeated restraint stress. This included behavioral changes while in the elevated plus maze indicative of higher anxiety levels, changes in hedonic state as measured by the sucrose preference test, depressed locomotion and a reduction in body weight by 17% (Naert et al., 2011). The adaptation was accompanied by HPA associated changes in brain derived neurotrophic factor (BNDF) expression, corticotropic releasing hormone (CRH) and arginine vasopressin (AVP) levels suggesting several biological markers for plasticity within the stress axis (Naert et al., 2011).

It is important to keep in mind, however, that these studies use very intensive stress exposure schedules. Most studies looking at immobilization stress restrain animals for 90–120 min a day or more. King et al. (2005) reported a maximum time spent under restraint of 90 min. Ferris et al. (2008) have had success with 60-min daily sessions over the course of 4–5 days. Animals are imaged the day after the last acclimatization session or several days later. Our laboratory has had success as well with incremental steps in restraint duration (20, 40, up to 60 min). Success is measured by the proportion of animals that are imaged without gross motion and physiological artifact. **Figure 4** shows the significant reduction in 22 kHz ultrasonic "distress" calls during 60-min sessions over 5 days. In the above-cited study, the authors employed 3 h daily sessions for 3 weeks (Naert et al., 2011). In addition to being stressful, an extended stress paradigm imposes a physical challenge to animals that can reduce overall activity (see results in **Figure 4**). Results from an unpublished study in **Figure 4** show that there is reduction in time spent struggling on the fifth day of restraint in comparison to the first restraint and FST session. The reduced struggle time, or a curtailed effort to escape, may be considered a sign of learned helplessness. However, an alternative explanation is that the effort to escape on the first day of restraint and FST is reduced on day 5 because of physical fatigue. Evidence for this comes from a group in **Figure 4** showing data for rats restrained for 5 days and then re-tested 2 weeks later (R + Rest). These animals recover their levels of struggle time to levels observed in the first day of testing. This result, in addition to supporting an adaptive behavioral mechanism, also suggests that experiments should ideally be carried out immediately after day 5 of restraint acclimation procedures. Animals may again increase movement if not imaged before 2 weeks (**Figure 4**). Reduced exposure time to intermittent daily sessions may therefore minimize the effects seen with longer chronic restraint sessions.

Evidence indicates that intensity of a stressor may have more of an impact than the duration on the subsequent stress responsiveness of the animal (Garcia et al., 2000). However, there is residual impairment of HPA ACTH responses with immobilization stress (Garcia et al., 2000). The question remains whether all stressors are equal and whether immobility stress as classically studied has the same neurobiological and behavioral impact as the head restraint used in functional neuroimaging studies. There have been a host of other studies seeking to understand adaptations to restraint stress and whether the changes involved permanent modifications of the rodents brain (causing long-term changes in the behavioral and neural responses; Kant et al., 1985; Briski and Sylvester, 1987; Pierzchala and Van Loon, 1990; Girotti et al., 2006). This latter effect may not be entirely avoidable. Indeed, even single exposure to immobility stress can have long-term effects on behavior, such as cross-sensitization of responses to stressors (Belda et al., 2008).

EXPERIMENTS IN AWAKE RATS AND DATA INTERPRETATIONS

The methodology for imaging awake animals is recent enough that it has not yet been used across a broad spectrum of applications. The work in our laboratory has focused on studies of the effects of psychoactive substances, aggressive motivation, and the neural basis of maternal behavior during lactation. In both cases the methods employed can be of great use for studies seeking to understand neurodevelopmental changes during distinct reproductive stages of rats. The guidelines described apply to any investigation in which BOLD fMRI data are acquired. There have been significant studies employing *in vitro* methods assessing cerebral glucose metabolism following acute and repeated cocaine exposure (Porrino et al., 1988; Stein and Fuller, 1992, 1993; Hammer et al., 1993). Since the rewarding and psychomotor properties of cocaine are attributed to changes in neuronal and synaptic activity within mesocortical and mesolimbic systems (Einhorn et al., 1988; Chang et al., 1998), we used fMRI to investigate the neural actions of cocaine in awake animals (Febo et al., 2004b). Prior to this experiment there were several human functional imaging experiments investigating changes in brain activation following intravenous cocaine administration (Breiter et al., 1997; Kaufman et al., 1998; Li et al., 2000), however, experiments seeking to understand the developmental events leading to an addicted state cannot be studied in humans. Animal studies carried out in anesthetized rats are hampered by the use of general anesthetics for the reasons cited above (Marota et al., 2000; Mandeville et al., 2001). We used spin EPI in unconscious rats at 4.7 T following an intracerebroventricular injection of cocaine (20 μg) in artificial cerebrospinal fluid (10 μL). Within 5 min of injection, there was a significant increase in BOLD signal intensity in the substantia nigra, ventral tegmental area, nucleus accumbens, dorsal striatum and prefrontal cortex, as compared to vehicle controls (**Figure 5**). Minimal negative BOLD signal changes were observed in response to cocaine and no significant perturbations in normal cardiovascular and respiratory function. The findings demonstrated the technical feasibility of studying psychostimulant-induced brain activity using functional MRI in conscious rats. The results using BOLD fMRI corroborate findings from previous animal studies. Metabolic mapping with radiolabelled deoxyglucose showed cocaine-induced, site-specific glucose utilization in the multiple areas of the brain (London et al., 1986; Porrino et al., 1988). In a follow up study the repeated effects of cocaine were examined using the same methods. Seven days of pretreatment with cocaine significantly reduced the BOLD response to the drug. Although the lower BOLD response to cocaine appeared to be a generalized and non-specific effect, several brain areas of acutely and repeatedly treated rats did not show differences in BOLD signal intensity (namely, the dorsal prefrontal cortex, cingulate, and somatosensory cortex). In addition, the lower BOLD response was not associated with differences in cerebrovascular reactivity between the two treatment groups, as measured by brief exposure to

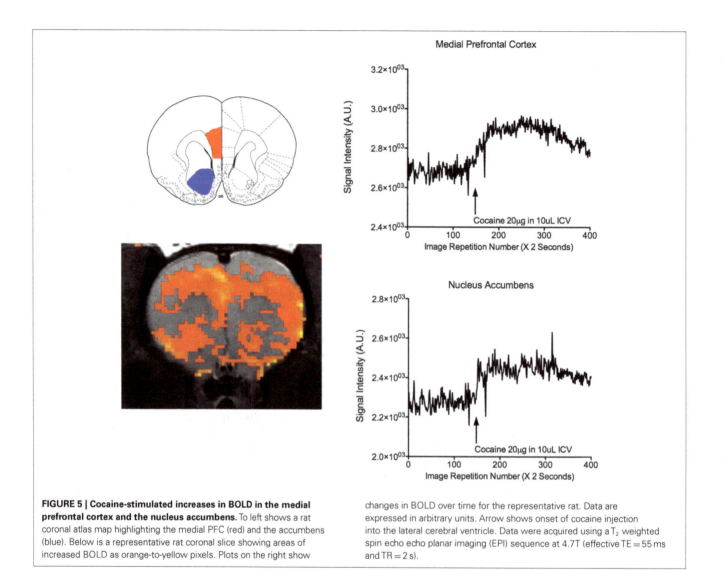

FIGURE 5 | Cocaine-stimulated increases in BOLD in the medial prefrontal cortex and the nucleus accumbens. To left shows a rat coronal atlas map highlighting the medial PFC (red) and the accumbens (blue). Below is a representative rat coronal slice showing areas of increased BOLD as orange-to-yellow pixels. Plots on the right show changes in BOLD over time for the representative rat. Data are expressed in arbitrary units. Arrow shows onset of cocaine injection into the lateral cerebral ventricle. Data were acquired using a T_2 weighted spin echo echo planar imaging (EPI) sequence at 4.7T (effective TE = 55 ms and TR = 2 s).

hypercapnia. One explanation proposed for the decreased BOLD response observed is that it might be associated with the previously observed decreases in glucose metabolism (Hammer et al., 1993) and could also be related to reductions in basal and cocaine-stimulated synaptic monoamine concentrations (Imperato et al., 1992; Kalivas and Duffy, 1993; Parsons et al., 1996). Alternatively, the reduced BOLD response could be due to differences in basal cerebrovascular reactivity.

A series of experiments in awake lactating rats have been carried out using the methods described above. Many of these have focused on the neural processing of the natural suckling stimulus from pups (Febo et al., 2005b, 2008; Ferris et al., 2005; Febo and Ferris, 2007). It has been reported that suckling stimulation from pups modulates the expression of maternal behaviors in rats by promoting arched back nursing postures (Stern and Johnson, 1990; Stern et al., 2002) and slow-wave sleep (Lincoln et al., 1980; Blyton et al., 2002). The fMRI technique was used to map the cortical pattern of activity during suckling, and the stimulus was compared to artificial suction in the absence of pups and mechanical stimulation on the ventrum skin (Febo et al., 2008). During the processing of somatosensory stimuli, information coming from the landscape of peripheral sensory receptors underlying body skin surface is relayed to the cortex through the spinothalamic pathway and topographically represented in the cerebrum. In the case of the mammillae, primary afferent fibers terminate in the ipsilateral dorsal root ganglia between spinal segments C5 and L6 (Tasker et al., 1986), with afferent relays along the lateral cervical nucleus, the dorsal column nuclei and the sensory and spinal portions of the trigeminal complex (Dubois-Dauphin et al., 1985; Stern et al., 2002). In contrast with studies using c-fos assays that provide exquisite cellular spatial detail (Walsh et al., 1996; Lonstein and Stern, 1997; Lin et al., 1998; Lonstein et al., 1998; Lee et al., 1999), the detection of real-time brain activity during the actual act of nursing is limited by the very wide temporal window (usually taken 60–120 min post-stimulus). Findings from electrophysiological recordings taken from neurons in the somatosensory cortex of the anesthetized rat indicate that the receptive field for the ventrum skin surrounding the nipple area doubles in size during the lactation period (Xerri et al., 1994). It was found in the fMRI study that wide areas of the postpartum rat cerebrum exhibit an increase in the fMRI BOLD signal during suckling stimulation, suggesting that neural activity is modified over wide areas of the cerebral cortex in response to a rather specific stimulus (Febo et al., 2008). The artificial suckling stimulus caused a similar degree of cortical activation. Therefore, although auditory, olfactory, and non-suckling tactile stimulation from pups may contribute to cortical activity, the suckling itself is fully capable of causing a widespread cortical response. There have been experiments examining the patterns of brain activity in mothers presented with infant sensory cues, but as yet, none have investigated the effects of the lactational stimulus. Our rat studies suggest that there would be significant cortical activation not only in limbic cortical divisions, as reported previously (Lorberbaum et al., 2002), but in areas that might correspond to long-term memory storage. These are cortical representations of the suckling stimulus that might be important for the maternal–infant bond during the early lactational period. This remains to be tested in primates, including humans.

One should be cognizant of the biological underpinnings contributing to the BOLD signal in order to interpret fMRI results. A few concepts, which are based on the literature across several fields of research, have been presented in Section "Physiology of the BOLD Contrast Mechanism". The simplistic designation of "activation" or "deactivation" is often used to refer to increases in BOLD or statistically significant interactions between variables of an fMRI study. The terminology has allowed an easy interpretation of fMRI findings across many human and animal studies. However, one cannot infer neuronal excitation and inhibition without direct neurophysiological measurements. If the ultimate goal of the study is to identify and/or attribute a general role for a brain region in a task or in responding to a stimulus, then the simple terminology can be helpful. If, on the other hand, the goal is to investigate and infer complex neuronal processing then it is really not. Whatever the case, the prudent MR imager needs to keep in mind the multiple factors that play key roles in generating the BOLD signal and the statistical maps that are present in many research studies (see **Figure 6**). Shown in **Figure 6** are several factors that underlie or influence the BOLD signal and that have been briefly discussed in the preceding sections. The cooperative synaptic activity of clusters of neurons generates neural signal changes that can be measured by LFPs. These arise to a large extent from somato-dendritic fields, with large net changes in extracellular electrical sources (current leaving cells) and sinks (current entering cells). The metabolic demand generated by such activity is "more than" balanced by the delivery of energy substrates in the bloodstream (**Figure 6**). Concepts of neuronal and vascular mechanisms should therefore be significantly relied upon during data interpretations. This should be accompanied by a clear understanding of the nature of the stimulus (whether simple or complicated) presented to the animal during fMRI scanning. What cannot be assumed is that BOLD signal maps are maps for receptor or protein distribution, as in autoradiographic, immunohistochemical and cellular c-fos assays, or that fMRI data show functional neuroanatomical connectivity (as would be observed in studies using orthodromic stimulation of a synaptic terminal region to record spike activity from a soma in a distant site). At the backdrop of the biological underpinnings are the principles of nuclear magnetic resonance, signal processing, and statistical mapping, which are at the heart of fMRI studies. The nuclear magnetic resonance phenomenon is so disconnected from the neurophysiological underpinnings that it can make the understanding of functional neuroimaging data difficult. However, the biological link is, as stated above (See Physiology of the BOLD Contrast Mechanism), the hemodynamic mechanism that directly influences the MR signal, and that is, the ratio between HbO_2 and dHb in the vascular and capillary bed surrounding areas of increased or decreased neuronal activity and metabolism (**Figure 6**). A greater value of HbO_2/dHb (if one were to measure these variables directly) during stimulation vs. baseline periods is indicative of increased O_2 in response to metabolic activation. As in the original Ogawa et al. (1990) work, a greater O_2 tension resulted in increased local signal intensity, which is what is measured in most fMRI studies. This is most likely due to the lowered paramagnetic effects of dHb. Statistical mapping is also a very important area in animal imaging experiments and this will not be discussed here. Suffice it to say that there are significant differences between human and animal imaging both in terms of the software used and study design that absolutely have to be taken into account. It is of the author's awareness that this is a source of great confusion to those that are not closely following the field of neuroimaging and that still find it difficult to trust the reliability of the MR methods compared with traditional techniques.

In both the cocaine experiment and the lactation study cited above one assumes that the BOLD signal changes are predominantly related to changes in neuronal activity and not only due to increased blood flow (as in the case of **Figure 2** where CO_2 produces increases in BOLD without expected changes in neuronal activity because of the vasodilatory effects of CO_2). Differences in percent changes in BOLD between the different experimental conditions are expected to represent differences in neuronal activity of comparable magnitude. Therefore, if one were to carry out the same experiments using similar procedures (e.g., restraint, acclimation, stimulus delivery) but instead record synaptic activity within the regions of interest, there would be comparable differences, for example, for changes in field potential activity. There are many reasons for considering that this is the case and these were discussed above. The direct action of cocaine, for example, on preventing the reuptake of dopamine and other catecholamines stimulates synaptic activity through increased firing and neurotransmitter metabolism. Suckling stimulation and mechanical stimulation on the ventrum increases intra-cortical processing of the sensory stimulus through net changes in synaptic firing with accompanying increases in metabolism (see **Figure 1**). However, as stated previously one cautiously interprets fMRI data in this direction since other biological mechanisms take effect and can alter the magnitude changes in BOLD. This could include effects on cerebrovascular reactivity for instance with drug treatments or with endogenous variations in hormones (Febo et al., 2004a, 2005a). Addressing changes in CBF can be performed by using arterial spin labeling methods as in Schmidt et al. (2006) or testing cerebrovascular reactivity between groups through CO_2 challenges as in Febo et al. (2004a). These procedures can provide the investigator with direct and indirect assessments of basal hemodynamics.

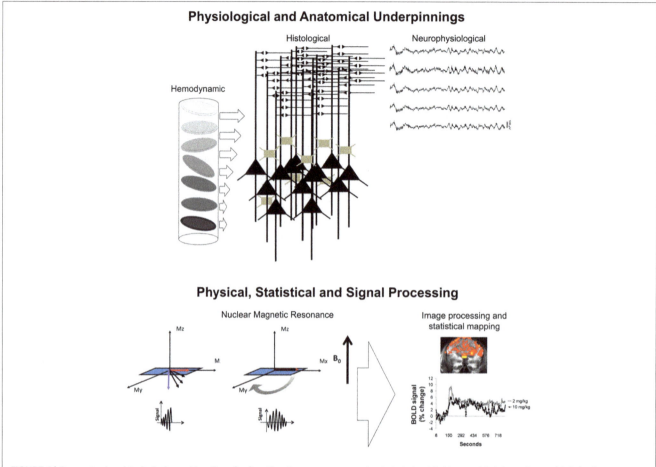

FIGURE 6 | Conceptual and technical considerations for functional magnetic resonance imaging of animals. The top images show several physiological and neuroanatomical factors that are important for data interpretations. These include knowledge of the tissue histological properties (e.g., layer specific organization of the cortex vs. heterogenous organization of other subcortical regions such as the striatum). For example, here in the middle are populations of neuronal soma typically found in layer 5 of the neocortex with overlying dendritic fields, which process incoming synaptic inputs. Electrophysiological correlates of this neural processing include local field potentials (shown in top right) that have been associated with BOLD signal changes. The BOLD signal is also associated with vascular-level changes such as tissue-capillary O_2 exchange and changes in oxy-to-deoxyhemoglobin concentrations in red blood cells (shown in left). In the background, shown in the lower portion of the figure, are other technical and conceptual factors associated with the physical principles of nuclear magnetic resonance, image processing, and statistical mapping (see text Experiments in Awake Rats and Data Interpretations for details).

There has been other significant research in awake animals that have primarily focused on investigating the neural actions of pharmacological agents (Chin et al., 2011), investigations of the differences in the hemodynamic response function in awake vs. anesthetized rats (Martin et al., 2006), cerebellar dependent motor learning though eye-blink conditioning in the rabbit (Miller et al., 2003), FC studies of the awake rat brain (Liang et al., 2011; Zhang et al., 2011), combined examination of sensory neural processing in specific circuits using fMRI and optogenetics in awake mice (Desai et al., 2011), and awake Rhesus macaques and marmoset monkeys (Ferris et al., 2001, 2004; Brevard et al., 2006; Goense and Logothetis, 2008). The studies support the use of awake fMRI methods in neuroscience research and have been performed using a variety of elegant and creative custom procedures that will not be discussed here. In general, all involve head restraint and many of these used some form of training of animals prior to studies. Miller et al. (2003) used the rabbit model in their studies of eye-blink conditioning. These animals are resilient to restraint stress and thus provide an interesting model for awake imaging. There were changes in cerebellar BOLD signal responses during progressive conditioning trials that closely matched patterns of electrical activity during learning (Miller et al., 2003). Desai et al. (2011) recently used optogenetic methods that pair the virally mediated expression of photorhodopsin in glutamatergic neurons of the barrel field cortex to study light-stimulated increases in neuronal activity in the somatosensory cortex of the awake mouse during fMRI. Light induced increases in neuronal activity produced BOLD signal responses in the barrel field region that were comparable to activation evoked by whisker deflection (Desai et al., 2011). This is an interesting study since it provides data on the role of excitatory activity on generation of the BOLD response but also because postsynaptic activity of pyramidal cells is considered to produce less energy expenditure compared to presynaptic activity. Therefore the BOLD responses here could correspond to local somatodendritic activity with the channel-rhodopsin mediated increase in activity. The combined use of fMRI and optogenetics may be an important future venue to those that are interesting in delving into the functional roles of specific neural circuits. To sum, interpretability of fMRI data is strong when used in conjunction with additional methods assessing neuroanatomy and neurophysiology and using multiple imaging modalities (BOLD and CBF). However, when the technique is used on its own it still provides important information on neural mechanisms particularly the responses to a variety of sensory stimuli. Interpretations should consider the methods employed (anesthetized vs. awake) and also the underlying assumptions of the BOLD signal as it relates to neuronal activity.

ADDITIONAL CONSIDERATIONS, FUTURE DIRECTIONS, AND ALTERNATIVE APPLICATIONS

Awake rat imaging can be used to investigate brain function and the actions of drugs in the brain, perhaps developmental processes as well. However it is important to keep in mind the underlying mechanisms of the BOLD fMRI technique when interpreting data. There are limitations to the use of the technique that mostly stem from the restriction of head movement in both anesthetized and awake preparations. This imposes an upper limit on the questions that can be asked regarding the relation of brain activity to behavior. Consider for instance the fact that motivational systems, such as the mesolimbic dopamine system, are involved in interfacing limbic and motor responses (Mogenson and Yang, 1991). Therefore, a limiting factor is that the technique lacks the ability to establish links between brain activity and many forms of motivational behavior and this is especially confounded in anesthetized rat preparations. Another factor to consider is the baseline hemodynamic state. When there are differences in the magnitude of the BOLD signal change this could originate from underlying neural mechanisms but may also be associated with changes in basal state of the cerebrovasculature. Methods are available to circumvent this latter issue using direct CBF measurements that quantitatively examine basal arterial flow and this can shed light on neuroadaptive changes contributing to differences among experimental groups.

The field of MR see's an ever-growing expansion of applications, conceptual considerations, and technical advances that will surely impact the use of animal imaging methods in the future. For example, BOLD signal decreases have not been mentioned here, although negative BOLD responses are pervasive in fMRI studies. There is empirical evidence for correlations between negative BOLD responses and decreased neuronal firing (Shmuel et al., 2006). The estimates from this latter study find that almost 60% of negative BOLD signal changes may correspond to reductions in multi-unit and field potential activity (Shmuel et al., 2006). However, there are also significant experiments that indicate that the negative BOLD responses are associated with "vascular-steal" (Harel et al., 2002). That is, areas adjacent to the site of activity lose blood to areas that are most active. Under normal circumstances, one of these two scenarios may explain negative BOLD responses. In other instances, high temporal resolution scans at high fields can resolve initial transient negative BOLD responses that are related to immediate increases in O_2 metabolism and extraction from plasma (Kim et al., 2000). However, most fMRI studies do not report this effect since it is overridden by dramatic increases in CBF after the onset of neural activity. There are two other scenarios that relate to the negative BOLD response, these include the post-stimulus undershoot (Buxton, 2002) and conditions which result in uncoupling between CBF and $CMRO_2$ (the latter exceeding CBF changes; Schridde et al., 2008). An example of this latter case is given by Schridde et al. (2008), which observed long-lasting BOLD signal reductions while at the same time measured CBF increases during bicuculline-induced seizures in rats. Interestingly, this was region specific since the mismatches were most prominent for the hippocampus rather than the cortex. Therefore, exceedingly high levels of $CMRO_2$ may have occurred during seizure activity that could have resulted in negative signal responses. The negative BOLD responses that are observed in most studies that do not intend to modulate inhibitory activity are difficult to explain. More data are needed in order to understand and perhaps even modulate negative BOLD responses rather than positive BOLD responses (Desalvo et al., 2011). Finally, as discussed in Section "Physiology of the BOLD Contrast Mechanism," the Larmor equation establishes a relationship between precessional frequency and field strength. Based upon this relationship it may be possible that increasing field strength could increase signal to noise and better spatial resolution in functional images. There are several experiments that are pursuing this direction, which should be of great importance in future work employing murine models (Silva and Koretsky, 2002; Seehafer et al., 2011).

Other techniques that have not been discussed can significantly contribute to investigations in different fields of neuroscience and animal imaging. These include techniques such as manganese enhanced MRI (MEMRI), FC analysis and fiber tracking using diffusion tensor imaging (DTI). For example, in MEMRI manganese chloride is used as an intracellular contrast agent that enhances T_1 signal intensity on high-resolution MR images. The Mn^{2+} ion is taken up by actively firing neurons through calcium channels and reflects synaptic activity more directly and in a quantitative manner (Aoki et al., 2002; Pautler et al., 2003). There is substantial experimental validation of the technique in its different variations. For example, one study showed a comparable match between BOLD signal and T_1 enhanced signal intensity due to Mn^{2+} uptake in the somatosensory cortex (Duong et al., 2000). There have been many more applications of the technique (Saleem et al., 2002; Yu et al., 2005; Nairismagi et al., 2006; Chen et al., 2007). Therefore, when used correctly the technique can provide accurate information regarding the functional neuroanatomical organization of the brain. The temporal resolution is very sluggish compared to fMRI, taking several hours rather than seconds, but can still be used to examine correlations between synaptic activity and behavior (Lu et al., 2007) and to investigate functional neural circuits (Saleem et al., 2002). MRI and fMRI techniques are invaluable in many neuroscience fields.

Many issues regarding anesthetized and awake animal imaging have been discussed here and continue to be investigated further. As we understand the effects of restraint, anesthetics and as more tools for preprocessing and analyzing data become available, applications of the technology in animal studies will prove to be an even more powerful tool for brain research. Ultimately this requires close collaborations between neuroscientists in different disciplines and engineers at academic imaging laboratories.

ACKNOWLEDGMENTS

The author would like to thank Dr. Josephine Todrank and Martha Caffrey for the helpful comments and suggestions. Support is provided by NIH grant DA019946.

REFERENCES

Angenstein, F., Krautwald, K., and Scheich, H. (2011). The current functional state of local neuronal circuits controls the magnitude of a BOLD response to incoming stimuli. *Neuroimage* 50, 1364–1375.

Aoki, I., Tanaka, C., Takegami, T., Ebisu, T., Umeda, M., Fukunaga, M., Fukuda, K., Silva, A. C., Koretsky, A. P., and Naruse, S. (2002). Dynamic activity-induced manganese-dependent contrast magnetic resonance imaging (DAIM MRI). *Magn. Reson. Med.* 48, 927–933.

Attwell, D., and Iadecola, C. (2002). The neural basis of functional brain imaging signals. *Trends Neurosci.* 25, 621–625.

Austin, V. C., Blamire, A. M., Allers, K. A., Sharp, T., Styles, P., Matthews, P. M., and Sibson, N. R. (2005). Confounding effects of anesthesia on functional activation in rodent brain: a study of halothane and alpha-chloralose anesthesia. *Neuroimage* 24, 92–100.

Bandettini, P. A., and Wong, E. C. (1997). A hypercapnia-based normalization method for improved spatial localization of human brain activation with fMRI. *NMR Biomed.* 10, 197–203.

Bandettini, P. A., Wong, E. C., Hinks, R. S., Tikofsky, R. S., and Hyde, J. S. (1992). Time course EPI of human brain function during task activation. *Magn. Reson. Med.* 25, 390–397.

Barnum, C. J., Blandino, P. Jr., and Deak, T. (2007). Adaptation in the corticosterone and hyperthermic responses to stress following repeated stressor exposure. *J. Neuroendocrinol.* 19, 632–642.

Bartels, A., and Zeki, S. (2004). The neural correlates of maternal and romantic love. *Neuroimage* 21, 1155–1166.

Belda, X., Fuentes, S., Nadal, R., and Armario, A. (2008). A single exposure to immobilization causes long-lasting pituitary-adrenal and behavioral sensitization to mild stressors. *Horm. Behav.* 54, 654–661.

Bhattacharyya, P. K., and Lowe, M. J. (2004). Cardiac-induced physiologic noise in tissue is a direct observation of cardiac-induced fluctuations. *Magn. Reson. Imaging* 22, 9–13.

Blyton, D. M., Sullivan, C. E., and Edwards, N. (2002). Lactation is associated with an increase in slow-wave sleep in women. *J. Sleep Res.* 11, 297–303.

Breiter, H. C., Gollub, R. L., Weisskoff, R. M., Kennedy, D. N., Makris, N., Berke, J. D., Goodman, J. M., Kantor, H. L., Gastfriend, D. R., Riorden, J. P., Mathew, R. T., Rosen, B. R., and Hyman, S. E. (1997). Acute effects of cocaine on human brain activity and emotion. *Neuron* 19, 591–611.

Brevard, M. E., Duong, T. Q., King, J. A., and Ferris, C. F. (2003). Changes in MRI signal intensity during hypercapnic challenge under conscious and anesthetized conditions. *Magn. Reson. Imaging* 21, 995–1001.

Brevard, M. E., Meyer, J. S., Harder, J. A., and Ferris, C. F. (2006). Imaging brain activity in conscious monkeys following oral MDMA ("ecstasy"). *Magn. Reson. Imaging* 24, 707–714.

Briski, K. P., and Sylvester, P. W. (1987). Effects of repetitive daily acute stress on pituitary LH and prolactin release during exposure to the same stressor or a second novel stress. *Psychoneuroendocrinology* 12, 429–437.

Buxton, R. B. (2002). *Introduction to Functional Magnetic Resonance Imaging: Principles and Techniques.* New York: Cambridge University Press.

Buzsaki, G., Kaila, K., and Raichle, M. (2007). Inhibition and brain work. *Neuron* 56, 771–783.

Chang, J. Y., Janak, P. H., and Woodward, D. J. (1998). Comparison of mesocorticolimbic neuronal responses during cocaine and heroin self-administration in freely moving rats. *J. Neurosci.* 18, 3098–3115.

Chen, W., Shields, J., Huang, W., and King, J. A. (2009). Female fear: influence of estrus cycle on behavioral response and neuronal activation. *Behav. Brain Res.* 201, 8–13.

Chen, W., Tenney, J., Kulkarni, P., and King, J. A. (2007). Imaging unconditioned fear response with manganese-enhanced MRI (MEMRI). *Neuroimage* 37, 221–229.

Chin, C. L., Fox, G. B., Hradil, V. P., Osinski, M. A., Mcgaraughty, S. P., Skoubis, P. D., Cox, B. F., and Luo, Y. (2006). Pharmacological MRI in awake rats reveals neural activity in area postrema and nucleus tractus solitarius: relevance as a potential biomarker for detecting drug-induced emesis. *Neuroimage* 33, 1152–1160.

Chin, C. L., Upadhyay, J., Marek, G. J., Baker, S. J., Zhang, M., Mezler, M., Fox, G. B., and Day, M. (2011). Awake rat pharmacological magnetic resonance imaging as a translational pharmacodynamic biomarker: metabotropic glutamate 2/3 agonist modulation of ketamine-induced blood oxygenation level dependence signals. *J. Pharmacol. Exp. Ther.* 336, 709–715.

Cohen, E. R., Ugurbil, K., and Kim, S. G. (2002). Effect of basal conditions on the magnitude and dynamics of the blood oxygenation level-dependent fMRI response. *J. Cereb. Blood Flow Metab.* 22, 1042–1053.

Davis, T. L., Kwong, K. K., Weisskoff, R. M., and Rosen, B. R. (1998). Calibrated functional MRI: mapping the dynamics of oxidative metabolism. *Proc. Natl. Acad. Sci. U.S.A.* 95, 1834–1839.

Desai, M., Kahn, I., Knoblich, U., Bernstein, J., Atallah, H., Yang, A., Kopell, N., Buckner, R. L., Graybiel, A. M., Moore, C. I., and Boyden, E. S. (2011). Mapping brain networks in awake mice using combined optical neural control and fMRI. *J. Neurophysiol.* 105, 1393–1405.

Desalvo, M. N., Schridde, U., Mishra, A. M., Motelow, J. E., Purcaro, M. J., Danielson, N., Bai, X., Hyder, F., and Blumenfeld, H. (2011). Focal BOLD fMRI changes in bicuculline-induced tonic-clonic seizures in the rat. *Neuroimage* 50, 902–909.

Dhabhar, F. S., Mcewen, B. S., and Spencer, R. L. (1997). Adaptation to prolonged or repeated stress – comparison between rat strains showing intrinsic differences in reactivity to acute stress. *Neuroendocrinology* 65, 360–368.

Doty, F. D., Entzminger, G., Kulkarni, J., Pamarthy, K., and Staab, J. P. (2007). Radio frequency coil technology for small-animal MRI. *NMR Biomed.* 20, 304–325.

Douglas, R., Markram, H., and Martin, K. (2004). "Neocortex," in *The Synaptic Organization of the Brain*, ed. G. M. Sheperd, 5th Edn (New York: Oxford University Press), 499–558.

Dubois-Dauphin, M., Armstrong, W. E., Tribollet, E., and Dreifuss, J. (1985). Somatosensory systems and the milk-ejection reflex in the rat. II. The effects of lesions in the ventroposterior thalamic complex, dorsal columns and lateral cervical nucleus-dorsolateral funiculus. *Neuroscience* 15, 1131–1140.

Duong, T. Q., Silva, A. C., Lee, S. P., and Kim, S. G. (2000). Functional MRI of calcium-dependent synaptic activity: cross correlation with CBF and BOLD measurements. *Magn. Reson. Med.* 43, 383–392.

Duong, T. Q., Yacoub, E., Adriany, G., Hu, X., Ugurbil, K., and Kim, S. G. (2003). Microvascular BOLD contribution at 4 and 7 T in the human brain: gradient-echo and spin-echo fMRI with suppression of blood effects. *Magn. Reson. Med.* 49, 1019–1027.

Eger, E. I. II, and Johnson, B. H. (1987). Rates of awakening from anesthesia with I-653, halothane, isoflurane, and sevoflurane: a test of the effect of anesthetic concentration and duration in rats. *Anesth. Analg.* 66, 977–982.

Einhorn, L. C., Johansen, P. A., and White, F. J. (1988). Electrophysiological effects of cocaine in the mesoaccumbens dopamine system: studies in the ventral tegmental area. *J. Neurosci.* 8, 100–112.

Febo, M., and Ferris, C. F. (2007). Development of cocaine sensitization before pregnancy affects subsequent maternal retrieval of pups and prefrontal cortical activity during nursing. *Neuroscience* 148, 400–412.

Febo, M., Ferris, C. F., and Segarra, A. C. (2005a). Estrogen influences cocaine-induced blood oxygen level-dependent signal changes in female rats. *J. Neurosci.* 25, 1132–1136.

Febo, M., Numan, M., and Ferris, C. F. (2005b). Functional magnetic resonance imaging shows oxytocin activates brain regions associated with mother-pup bonding during suckling. *J. Neurosci.* 25, 11637–11644.

Febo, M., and Pira, A. S. (2011). Increased BOLD activation to predator stressor in subiculum and midbrain of amphetamine-sensitized maternal rats. *Brain Res.* 1382, 118–127.

Febo, M., Segarra, A. C., Nair, G., Schmidt, K., Duong, T. Q., and Ferris, C. F. (2004a). The neural consequences of repeated cocaine exposure revealed by functional MRI in awake rats. *Neuropsychopharmacology* 30, 936–943.

Febo, M., Segarra, A. C., Tenney, J. R., Brevard, M. E., Duong, T. Q., and Ferris, C. F. (2004b). Imaging cocaine-induced changes in the mesocorticolimbic dopaminergic system of conscious rats. *J. Neurosci. Methods* 139, 167–176.

Febo, M., Stolberg, T. L., Numan, M., Bridges, R. S., Kulkarni, P., and Ferris, C. F. (2008). Nursing stimulation is more than tactile sensation: it is a multisensory experience. *Horm. Behav.* 54, 330–339.

Ferris, C. F., Febo, M., Luo, F., Schmidt, K., Brevard, M., Harder, J. A., Kulkarni, P., Messenger, T., and King, J. A. (2006). Functional magnetic resonance imaging in conscious animals: a new tool in behavioural neuroscience research. *J. Neuroendocrinol.* 18, 307–318.

Ferris, C. F., Kulkarni, P., Sullivan, J. M. Jr., Harder, J. A., Messenger, T. L., and Febo, M. (2005). Pup suckling is more rewarding than cocaine: evidence from functional magnetic resonance imaging and three-dimensional computational analysis. *J. Neurosci.* 25, 149–156.

Ferris, C. F., Snowdon, C. T., King, J. A., Duong, T. Q., Ziegler, T. E., Ugurbil, K., Ludwig, R., Schultz-Darken, N. J., Wu, Z., Olson, D. P., Sullivan Jr, J. M., Tannenbaum, P. L., and Vaughan, J. T. (2001). Functional imaging of brain activity in conscious monkeys responding to sexually arousing cues. *Neuroreport* 12, 2231–2236.

Ferris, C. F., Snowdon, C. T., King, J. A., Sullivan, J. M. Jr., Ziegler, T. E., Olson, D. P., Schultz Darken, N. J., Tannenbaum, P. L., Ludwig, R., Wu, Z., Einspanier, A., Vaughan, J. T., and Duong, T. Q. (2004). Activation of neural pathways associated with sexual arousal in non-human primates. *J. Magn. Reson. Imaging* 19, 168–175.

Ferris, C. F., Stolberg, T., Kulkarni, P., Murugavel, M., Blanchard, R., Blanchard, D. C., Febo, M., Brevard, M., and Simon, N. G. (2008). Imaging the neural circuitry and chemical control of aggressive motivation. *BMC Neurosci.* 9, 111. doi: 10.1186/1471-2202-9-111

Fox, P. T., and Raichle, M. E. (1986). Focal physiological uncoupling of cerebral blood flow and oxidative metabolism during somatosensory stimulation in human subjects. *Proc. Natl. Acad. Sci. U.S.A.* 83, 1140–1144.

Fox, P. T., Raichle, M. E., Mintun, M. A., and Dence, C. (1988). Nonoxidative glucose consumption during focal physiologic neural activity. *Science* 241, 462–464.

Freire, L., and Mangin, J. F. (2001). Motion correction algorithms may create spurious brain activations in the absence of subject motion. *Neuroimage* 14, 709–722.

Garcia, A., Marti, O., Valles, A., DalZotto, S., and Armario, A. (2000). Recovery of the hypothalamic-pituitary-adrenal response to stress. Effect of stress intensity, stress duration and previous stress exposure. *Neuroendocrinology* 72, 114–125.

Genovese, C. R., Lazar, N. A., and Nichols, T. (2002). Thresholding of statistical maps in functional neuroimaging using the false discovery rate. *Neuroimage* 15, 870–878.

Girotti, M., Pace, T. W., Gaylord, R. I., Rubin, B. A., Herman, J. P., and Spencer, R. L. (2006). Habituation to repeated restraint stress is associated with lack of stress-induced c-fos expression in primary sensory processing areas of the rat brain. *Neuroscience* 138, 1067–1081.

Goense, J. B., and Logothetis, N. K. (2006). Laminar specificity in monkey V1 using high-resolution SE-fMRI. *Magn. Reson. Imaging* 24, 381–392.

Goense, J. B., and Logothetis, N. K. (2008). Neurophysiology of the BOLD fMRI signal in awake monkeys. *Curr. Biol.* 18, 631–640.

Gollub, R. L., Breiter, H. C., Kantor, H., Kennedy, D., Gastfriend, D., Mathew, R. T., Makris, N., Guimaraes, A., Riorden, J., Campbell, T., Foley, M., Hyman, S. E., Rosen, B., and Weisskoff, R. (1998). Cocaine decreases cortical cerebral blood flow but does not obscure regional activation in functional magnetic resonance imaging in human subjects. *J. Cereb. Blood Flow Metab.* 18, 724–734.

Greenberg, D. S., Houweling, A. R., and Kerr, J. N. (2008). Population imaging of ongoing neuronal activity in the visual cortex of awake rats. *Nat. Neurosci.* 11, 749–751.

Haleem, D. J. (1996). Adaptation to repeated restraint stress in rats: failure of ethanol-treated rats to adapt in the stress schedule. *Alcohol Alcohol.* 31, 471–477.

Hammer, R. P. Jr., Pires, W. S., Markou, A., and Koob, G. F. (1993). Withdrawal following cocaine self-administration decreases regional cerebral metabolic rate in critical brain reward regions. *Synapse* 14, 73–80.

Harel, N., Lee, S. P., Nagaoka, T., Kim, D. S., and Kim, S. G. (2002). Origin of negative blood oxygenation level-dependent fMRI signals. *J. Cereb. Blood Flow Metab.* 22, 908–917.

Hartikainen, K. M., Rorarius, M., Perakyla, J. J., Laippala, P. J., and Jantti, V. (1995). Cortical reactivity during isoflurane burst-suppression anesthesia. *Anesth. Analg.* 81, 1223–1228.

Huttunen, J. K., Grohn, O., and Penttonen, M. (2008). Coupling between simultaneously recorded BOLD response and neuronal activity in the rat somatosensory cortex. *Neuroimage* 39, 775–785.

Hyder, F., Rothman, D. L., and Shulman, R. G. (2002). Total neuroenergetics support localized brain activity: implications for the interpretation of fMRI. *Proc. Natl. Acad. Sci. U.S.A.* 99, 10771–10776.

Imas, O. A., Ropella, K. M., Ward, B. D., Wood, J. D., and Hudetz, A. G. (2005). Volatile anesthetics enhance flash-induced gamma oscillations in rat visual cortex. *Anesthesiology* 102, 937–947.

Imas, O. A., Ropella, K. M., Wood, J. D., and Hudetz, A. G. (2004). Halothane augments event-related gamma oscillations in rat visual cortex. *Neuroscience* 123, 269–278.

Imperato, A., Mele, A., Scrocco, M. G., and Puglisi-Allegra, S. (1992). Chronic cocaine alters limbic extracellular dopamine. Neurochemical basis for addiction. *Eur. J. Pharmacol.* 212, 299–300.

Kalivas, P. W., and Duffy, P. (1993). Time course of extracellular dopamine and behavioral sensitization to cocaine. I. Dopamine axon terminals. *J. Neurosci.* 13, 266–275.

Kant, G. J., Eggleston, T., Landman-Roberts, L., Kenion, C. C., Driver, G. C., and Meyerhoff, J. L. (1985). Habituation to repeated stress is stressor specific. *Pharmacol. Biochem. Behav.* 22, 631–634.

Kasischke, K. A., Vishwasrao, H. D., Fisher, P. J., Zipfel, W. R., and Webb, W. W. (2004). Neural activity triggers neuronal oxidative metabolism followed by astrocytic glycolysis. *Science* 305, 99–103.

Kaufman, M. J., Levin, J. M., Maas, L. C., Rose, S. L., Lukas, S. E., Mendelson, J. H., Cohen, B. M., and Renshaw, P. F. (1998). Cocaine decreases relative cerebral blood volume in humans: a dynamic susceptibility contrast magnetic resonance imaging study. *Psychopharmacology (Berl.)* 138, 76–81.

Kennerley, A. J., Berwick, J., Martindale, J., Johnston, D., Papadakis, N., and Mayhew, J. E. (2005). Concurrent fMRI and optical measures for the investigation of the hemodynamic response function. *Magn. Reson. Med.* 54, 354–365.

Kim, D. S., Duong, T. Q., and Kim, S. G. (2000). High-resolution mapping of iso-orientation columns by fMRI. *Nat. Neurosci.* 3, 164–169.

King, J. A., Garelick, T. S., Brevard, M. E., Chen, W., Messenger, T. L., Duong, T. Q., and Ferris, C. F. (2005). Procedure for minimizing stress for fMRI studies in conscious rats. *J. Neurosci. Methods* 148, 154–160.

Krishnan, V., and Nestler, E. J. (2008). The molecular neurobiology of depression. *Nature* 455, 894–902.

Lahti, K. M., Ferris, C. F., Li, F., Sotak, C. H., and King, J. A. (1998). Imaging brain activity in conscious animals using functional MRI. *J. Neurosci. Methods* 82, 75–83.

Lahti, K. M., Ferris, C. F., Li, F., Sotak, C. H., and King, J. A. (1999). Comparison of evoked cortical activity in conscious and propofol-anesthetized rats using functional MRI. *Magn. Reson. Med.* 41, 412–416.

Lee, A., Li, M., Watchus, J., and Fleming, A. S. (1999). Neuroanatomical basis of maternal memory in postpartum rats: selective role for the nucleus accumbens. *Behav. Neurosci.* 113, 523–538.

Lee, S. P., Duong, T. Q., Yang, G., Iadecola, C., and Kim, S. G. (2001). Relative changes of cerebral arterial and venous blood volumes during increased cerebral blood flow: implications for BOLD fMRI. *Magn. Reson. Med.* 45, 791–800.

Li, S. J., Biswal, B., Li, Z., Risinger, R., Rainey, C., Cho, J. K., Salmeron, B. J., and Stein, E. A. (2000). Cocaine administration decreases functional connectivity in human primary visual and motor cortex as detected by functional MRI. *Magn. Reson. Med.* 43, 45–51.

Liang, Z., King, J., and Zhang, N. Uncovering intrinsic connectional architecture of functional networks in awake rat brain. (2011). *J. Neurosci.* 31, 3776–3783.

Lin, S. H., Miyata, S., Matsunaga, W., Kawarabayashi, T., Nakashima, T., and Kiyohara, T. (1998). Metabolic mapping of the brain in pregnant, parturient and lactating rats using fos immunohistochemistry. *Brain Res.* 787, 226–236.

Lincoln, D. W., Hentzen, K., Hin, T., Van Der Schoot, P., Clarke, G., and Summerlee, A. J. (1980). Sleep: a prerequisite for reflex milk ejection in the rat. *Exp. Brain Res.* 38, 151–162.

Liu, X., Zhu, X. H., Zhang, Y., and Chen, W. (2011). Neural origin of spontaneous hemodynamic fluctuations in rats under burst-suppression anesthesia condition. *Cereb. Cortex* 21, 374–384.

Logothetis, N. K. (2008). What we can do and what we cannot do with fMRI. *Nature* 453, 869–878.

Logothetis, N. K., Pauls, J., Augath, M., Trinath, T., and Oeltermann, A. (2001). Neurophysiological investigation of the basis of the fMRI signal. *Nature* 412, 150–157.

London, E. D., Wilkerson, G., Goldberg, S. R., and Risner, M. E. (1986). Effects of L-cocaine on local cerebral glucose utilization in the rat. *Neurosci. Lett.* 68, 73–78.

Lonstein, J. S., Simmons, D. A., Swann, J. M., and Stern, J. M. (1998). Forebrain expression of c-fos due to active maternal behaviour in lactating rats. *Neuroscience* 82, 267–281.

Lonstein, J. S., and Stern, J. M. (1997). Somatosensory contributions to c-fos activation within the caudal periaqueductal gray of lactating rats: effects of perioral, rooting, and suckling stimuli from pups. *Horm. Behav.* 32, 155–166.

Lorberbaum, J. P., Newman, J. D., Horwitz, A. R., Dubno, J. R., Lydiard, R. B., Hamner, M. B., Bohning, D. E., and George, M. S. (2002). A potential role for thalamocingulate circuitry in human maternal behavior. *Biol. Psychiatry* 51, 431–445.

Lu, H., Xi, Z. X., Gitajn, L., Rea, W., Yang, Y., and Stein, E. A. (2007). Cocaine-induced brain activation detected by dynamic manganese-enhanced magnetic resonance imaging (MEMRI). *Proc. Natl. Acad. Sci. U.S.A.* 104, 2489–2494.

Ludwig, R., Bodgdanov, G., King, J., Allard, A., and Ferris, C. F. (2004). A dual RF resonator system for high-field functional magnetic resonance imaging of small animals. *J. Neurosci. Methods* 132, 125–135.

Malonek, D., Dirnagl, U., Lindauer, U., Yamada, K., Kanno, I., and Grinvald, A. (1997). Vascular imprints of neuronal activity: relationships between the dynamics of cortical blood flow, oxygenation, and volume changes following sensory stimulation. *Proc. Natl. Acad. Sci. U.S.A.* 94, 14826–14831.

Malonek, D., and Grinvald, A. (1996). Interactions between electrical activity and cortical microcirculation revealed by imaging spectroscopy: implications for functional brain mapping. *Science* 272, 551–554.

Mandeville, J. B., Jenkins, B. G., Kosofsky, B. E., Moskowitz, M. A., Rosen, B. R., and Marota, J. J. (2001). Regional sensitivity and coupling of BOLD and CBV changes during stimulation of rat brain. *Magn. Reson. Med.* 45, 443–447.

Marota, J. J., Mandeville, J. B., Weisskoff, R. M., Moskowitz, M. A., Rosen, B. R., and Kosofsky, B. E. (2000). Cocaine activation discriminates dopaminergic projections by temporal response: an fMRI study in Rat. *Neuroimage* 11, 13–23.

Martin, C., Martindale, J., Berwick, J., and Mayhew, J. (2006). Investigating neural-hemodynamic coupling and the hemodynamic response function in the awake rat. *Neuroimage* 32, 33–48.

Masamoto, K., Fukuda, M., Vazquez, A., and Kim, S. G. (2009). Dose-dependent effect of isoflurane on neurovascular coupling in rat cerebral cortex. *Eur. J. Neurosci.* 30, 242–250.

Melia, K. R., Ryabinin, A. E., Schroeder, R., Bloom, F. E., and Wilson, M. C. (1994). Induction and habituation of immediate early gene expression in rat brain by acute and repeated restraint stress. *J. Neurosci.* 14, 5929–5938.

Miller, M. J., Chen, N. K., Li, L., Tom, B., Weiss, C., Disterhoft, J. F., and Wyrwicz, A. M. (2003). fMRI of the conscious rabbit during unilateral classical eyeblink conditioning reveals bilateral cerebellar activation. *J. Neurosci.* 23, 11753–11758.

Mogenson, G. J., and Yang, C. R. (1991). The contribution of basal forebrain to limbic-motor integration and the mediation of motivation to action. *Adv. Exp. Med. Biol.* 295, 267–290.

Nadasdy, Z., Csicsvari, J., Penttonen, M., Hetke, J., Wise, K., and Buzsaki, G. (1998). "Extracellular recording and analysis of neuronal activity: from single cells to ensembles," in *Neuronal Ensembles: Strategies for Recording and Decoding*, 1st Edn, eds H. Eichenbaum and J. L. Davis (New York: Wiley-Liss), 17–56.

Naert, G., Ixart, G., Maurice, T., Tapia-Arancibia, L., and Givalois, L. (2011). Brain-derived neurotrophic factor and hypothalamic-pituitary-adrenal axis adaptation processes in a depressive-like state induced by chronic restraint stress. *Mol. Cell. Neurosci.* 46, 55–66.

Nairismagi, J., Pitkanen, A., Narkilahti, S., Huttunen, J., Kauppinen, R. A., and Grohn, O. H. (2006). Manganese-enhanced magnetic resonance imaging of mossy fiber plasticity in vivo. *Neuroimage* 30, 130–135.

Nakao, Y., Itoh, Y., Kuang, T. Y., Cook, M., Jehle, J., and Sokoloff, L. (2001). Effects of anesthesia on functional activation of cerebral blood flow and metabolism. *Proc. Natl. Acad. Sci. U.S.A.* 98, 7593–7598.

Nitschke, J. B., Nelson, E. E., Rusch, B. D., Fox, A. S., Oakes, T. R., and Davidson, R. J. (2004). Orbitofrontal cortex tracks positive mood in mothers viewing pictures of their newborn infants. *Neuroimage* 21, 583–592.

Ogawa, S., Lee, T. M., Kay, A. R., and Tank, D. W. (1990). Brain magnetic resonance imaging with contrast dependent on blood oxygenation. *Proc. Natl. Acad. Sci. U.S.A.* 87, 9868–9872.

Ogawa, S., Tank, D. W., Menon, R., Ellermann, J. M., Kim, S. G., Merkle, H., and Ugurbil, K. (1992). Intrinsic signal changes accompanying sensory stimulation: functional brain mapping with magnetic resonance imaging. *Proc. Natl. Acad. Sci. U.S.A.* 89, 5951–5955.

Parry, T. J., and Mcelligott, J. G. (1993). A method for restraining awake rats using head immobilization. *Physiol. Behav.* 53, 1011–1015.

Parsons, L. H., Koob, G. F., and Weiss, F. (1996). Extracellular serotonin is decreased in the nucleus accumbens during withdrawal from cocaine self-administration. *Behav. Brain Res.* 73, 225–228.

Pauling, L., and Coryell, C. D. (1936). The magnetic properties and structure of hemoglobin, oxyhemoglobin and carbonmonoxyhemoglobin. *Proc. Natl. Acad. Sci.* 22, 210–216.

Pautler, R. G., Mongeau, R., and Jacobs, R. E. (2003). In vivo trans-synaptic tract tracing from the murine striatum and amygdala utilizing manganese enhanced MRI (MEMRI). *Magn. Reson. Med.* 50, 33–39.

Paxinos, G., and Watson, C. (1997). *The Rat Brain in Stereotaxic Coordinates.* Boston: Academic Press.

Peeters, R. R., Tindemans, I., De Schutter, E., and Van Der Linden, A. (2001). Comparing BOLD fMRI signal changes in the awake and anesthetized rat during electrical forepaw stimulation. *Magn. Reson. Imaging* 19, 821–826.

Peeters, R. R., and Van Der Linden, A. (2002). A data post-processing protocol for dynamic MRI data to discriminate brain activity from global physiological effects. *Magn. Reson. Imaging* 20, 503–510.

Pierzchala, K., and Van Loon, G. R. (1990). Plasma native and peptidase-derivable Met-enkephalin responses to restraint stress in rats. Adaptation to repeated restraint. *J. Clin. Invest.* 85, 861–873.

Porrino, L. J., Domer, F. R., Crane, A. M., and Sokoloff, L. (1988). Selective alterations in cerebral metabolism within the mesocorticolimbic dopaminergic system produced by acute cocaine administration in rats. *Neuropsychopharmacology* 1, 109–118.

Poser, B. A., and Norris, D. G. (2007). Fast spin echo sequences for BOLD functional MRI. *MAGMA* 20, 11–17.

Purdon, P. L., and Weisskoff, R. M. (1998). Effect of temporal autocorrelation due to physiological noise and stimulus paradigm on voxel-level false-positive rates in fMRI. *Hum. Brain Mapp.* 6, 239–249.

Sachdev, R. N., Champney, G. C., Lee, H., Price, R. R., Pickens, D. R. III, Morgan, V. L., Stefansic, J. D., Melzer, P., and Ebner, F. F. (2003). Experimental model for functional magnetic resonance imaging of somatic sensory cortex in the unanesthetized rat. *Neuroimage* 19, 742–750.

Saleem, K. S., Pauls, J. M., Augath, M., Trinath, T., Prause, B. A., Hashikawa, T., and Logothetis, N. K. (2002). Magnetic resonance imaging of neuronal connections in the macaque monkey. *Neuron* 34, 685–700.

Schmidt, K. F., Febo, M., Shen, Q., Luo, F., Sicard, K. M., Ferris, C. F., Stein, E. A., and Duong, T. Q. (2006). Hemodynamic and metabolic changes induced by cocaine in anesthetized rat observed with multimodal functional MRI. *Psychopharmacology (Berl.)* 185, 479–486.

Schridde, U., Khubchandani, M., Motelow, J. E., Sanganahalli, B. G., Hyder, F., and Blumenfeld, H. (2008). Negative BOLD with large increases in neuronal activity. *Cereb. Cortex* 18, 1814–1827.

Seehafer, J. U., Kalthoff, D., Farr, T. D., Wiedermann, D., and Hoehn, M. (2011). No increase of the blood oxygenation level-dependent functional magnetic resonance imaging signal with higher field strength: implications for brain activation studies. *J. Neurosci.* 30, 5234–5241.

Sheth, S. A., Nemoto, M., Guiou, M., Walker, M., Pouratian, N., and Toga, A. W. (2004). Linear and nonlinear relationships between neuronal activity, oxygen metabolism, and hemodynamic responses. *Neuron* 42, 347–355.

Shmuel, A., Augath, M., Oeltermann, A., and Logothetis, N. K. (2006). Negative functional MRI response correlates with decreases in neuronal activity in monkey visual area V1. *Nat. Neurosci.* 9, 569–577.

Shmuel, A., Yacoub, E., Pfeuffer, J., Van De Moortele, P. F., Adriany, G., Hu, X., and Ugurbil, K. (2002). Sustained negative BOLD, blood flow and oxygen consumption response and its coupling to the positive response in the human brain. *Neuron* 36, 1195–1210.

Sicard, K., Shen, Q., Brevard, M. E., Sullivan, R., Ferris, C. F., King, J. A., and Duong, T. Q. (2003). Regional cerebral blood flow and BOLD responses in conscious and anesthetized rats under basal and hypercapnic conditions: implications for functional MRI studies. *J. Cereb. Blood Flow Metab.* 23, 472–481.

Silva, A. C., and Koretsky, A. P. (2002). Laminar specificity of functional MRI onset times during somatosensory stimulation in rat. *Proc. Natl. Acad. Sci. U.S.A.* 99, 15182–15187.

Stamp, J., and Herbert, J. (2001). Corticosterone modulates autonomic responses and adaptation of central immediate-early gene expression to repeated restraint stress. *Neuroscience* 107, 465–479.

Stein, E. A., and Fuller, S. A. (1992). Selective effects of cocaine on regional cerebral blood flow in the rat. *J. Pharmacol. Exp. Ther.* 262, 327–334.

Stein, E. A., and Fuller, S. A. (1993). Cocaine's time action profile on regional cerebral blood flow in the rat. *Brain Res.* 626, 117–126.

Stern, J. M., and Johnson, S. K. (1990). Ventral somatosensory determinants of nursing behavior in Norway rats. I. Effects of variations in the quality and quantity of pup stimuli. *Physiol. Behav.* 47, 993–1011.

Stern, J. M., Yu, Y. L., and Crockett, D. P. (2002). Dorsolateral columns of the spinal cord are necessary for both suckling-induced neuroendocrine reflexes and the kyphotic nursing posture in lactating rats. *Brain Res.* 947, 110–121.

Strathearn, L., Li, J., Fonagy, P., and Montague, P. R. (2008). What's in a smile? Maternal brain responses to infant facial cues. *Pediatrics* 122, 40–51.

Tasker, J. G., Theodosis, D. T., and Poulain, D. A. (1986). Afferent projections from the mammary glands to the spinal cord in the lactating rat – I. A neuroanatomical study using the transganglionic transport of horseradish peroxidase-wheatgerm agglutinin. *Neuroscience* 19, 495–509.

Thompson, J. K., Peterson, M. R., and Freeman, R. D. (2003). Single-neuron activity and tissue oxygenation in the cerebral cortex. *Science* 299, 1070–1072.

Tian, P., Teng, I. C., May, L. D., Kurz, R., Lu, K., Scadeng, M., Hillman, E. M., De Crespigny, A. J., D'arceuil, H. E., Mandeville, J. B., Marota, J. J., Rosen, B. R., Liu, T. T., Boas, D. A., Buxton, R. B., Dale, A. M., and Devor, A. (2011). Cortical depth-specific microvascular dilation underlies laminar differences in blood oxygenation level-dependent functional MRI signal. *Proc. Natl. Acad. Sci. U.S.A.* 107, 15246–15251.

Tornatzky, W., and Miczek, K. A. (1993). Long-term impairment of autonomic circadian rhythms after brief intermittent social stress. *Physiol. Behav.* 53, 983–993.

Ugurbil, K., Adriany, G., Andersen, P., Chen, W., Garwood, M., Gruetter, R., Henry, P. G., Kim, S. G., Lieu, H., Tkac, I., Vaughan, T., Van De Moortele, P. F., Yacoub, E., and Zhu, X. H. (2003). Ultrahigh field magnetic resonance imaging and spectroscopy. *Magn. Reson. Imaging* 21, 1263–1281.

Walsh, C. J., Fleming, A. S., Lee, A., and Magnusson, J. E. (1996). The effects of olfactory and somatosensory desensitization on Fos-like immunoreactivity in the brains of pup-exposed postpartum rats. *Behav. Neurosci.* 110, 134–153.

Wang, K., Van Meer, M. P., Van Der Marel, K., Van Der Toorn, A., Xu, L., Liu, Y., Viergever, M. A., Jiang, T., and Dijkhuizen, R. M. (2011). Temporal scaling properties and spatial synchronization of spontaneous blood oxygenation level-dependent (BOLD) signal fluctuations in rat sensorimotor network at different levels of isoflurane anesthesia. *NMR Biomed.* 24, 61–67.

Williams, K. A., Magnuson, M., Majeed, W., Laconte, S. M., Peltier, S. J., Hu, X., and Keilholz, S. D. (2011). Comparison of alpha-chloralose, medetomidine and isoflurane anesthesia for functional connectivity mapping in the rat. *Magn. Reson. Imaging* 28, 995–1003.

Xerri, C., Stern, J. M., and Merzenich, M. M. (1994). Alterations of the cortical representation of the rat ventrum induced by nursing behavior. *J. Neurosci.* 14, 1710–1721.

Xi, Z. X., Wu, G., Stein, E. A., and Li, S. J. (2004). Opiate tolerance by heroin self-administration: an fMRI study in rat. *Magn. Reson. Med.* 52, 108–114.

Ye, Y., Zhuo, Y., Xue, R., and Zhou, X. J. (2011). BOLD fMRI using a modified HASTE sequence. *Neuroimage* 49, 457–466.

Yu, X., Wadghiri, Y. Z., Sanes, D. H., and Turnbull, D. H. (2005). In vivo auditory brain mapping in mice with Mn-enhanced MRI. *Nat. Neurosci.* 8, 961–968.

Zhang, N., Rane, P., Huang, W., Liang, Z., Kennedy, D., Frazier, J. A., and King, J. (2011). Mapping resting-state brain networks in conscious animals. *J. Neurosci. Methods* 189, 186–196.

Using animal models to disentangle the role of genetic, epigenetic, and environmental influences on behavioral outcomes associated with maternal anxiety and depression

Lisa M. Tarantino[1]*, Patrick F. Sullivan[1,2] and Samantha Meltzer-Brody[1]

[1] Department of Psychiatry, University of North Carolina, Chapel Hill, NC, USA
[2] Department of Genetics, University of North Carolina, Chapel Hill, NC, USA

Correspondence:
Lisa M. Tarantino, Department of Psychiatry, University of North Carolina, 1012 Genetic Medicine Building, CB#7361, 120 Mason Farm Road, Chapel Hill, NC 27599, USA.
e-mail: lisat@med.unc.edu

The etiology of complex psychiatric disorders results from both genetics and the environment. No definitive environmental factor has been implicated, but studies suggest that deficits in maternal care and bonding may be an important contributing factor in the development of anxiety and depression. Perinatal mood disorders such as postpartum depression occur in approximately 10% of pregnant women and can result in detriments in infant care and bonding. The consequences of impaired maternal–infant attachment during critical early brain development may lead to adverse effects on socioemotional and neurocognitive development in infants resulting in long-term behavioral and emotional problems, including increased vulnerability for mental illness. The exact mechanisms by which environmental stressors such as poor maternal care increase the risk for psychiatric disorders are not known and studies in humans have proven challenging. Two inbred mouse strains may prove useful for studying the interaction between maternal care and mood disorders. BALB/c (BALB) mice are considered an anxious strain in comparison to C57BL/6 (B6) mice in behavioral models of anxiety. These strain differences are most often attributed to genetics but may also be due to environment and gene by environment interactions. For example, BALB mice are described as poor mothers and B6 mice as good mothers and mothering behavior in rodents has been reported to affect both anxiety and stress behaviors in offspring. Changes in gene methylation patterns in response to maternal care have also been reported, providing evidence for epigenetic mechanisms. Characterization of these two mouse inbred strains over the course of pregnancy and in the postpartum period for behavioral and neuroendocrine changes may provide useful information by which to inform human studies, leading to advances in our understanding of the etiology of anxiety and depression and the role of genetics and the environment.

Keywords: perinatal, anxiety, depression, mothering, bonding, genetic, epigenetic, mice

INTRODUCTION

Maternal psychiatric illness during pregnancy and following childbirth (the perinatal period) is both common and morbid; if untreated, it can result in potentially devastating consequences to the mother and her baby. Both antenatal and postpartum maternal anxiety and depression have been shown to have adverse effects on the offspring (O'Hara and Swain, 1996; Bennett et al., 2004; Flynn et al., 2004; Marmorstein et al., 2004; Gavin et al., 2005; Gaynes et al., 2005; Feldman et al., 2009; Ross and Dennis, 2009; Field, 2010) and increase vulnerability to psychiatric disorders in adulthood (Gluckman et al., 2008). Increased risk for psychiatric disorders in offspring may be due, in part, to genetic predisposition. However, mothering behavior has also been shown to be an important factor. Maternal anxiety and depression may lead to unresponsive or inconsistent care by the mother toward the child leading to insecure attachment (NECCR, 1999; Campbell et al., 2004) which has been linked to increased risk for anxiety and depression in offspring (Wan and Green, 2009; Brumariu and Kerns, 2010a,b). Recent studies in rodents support these findings (Francis et al., 1999b; Champagne et al., 2003; Weaver et al., 2004). Studies indicate that perinatal maternal stress, which often manifests clinically as anxiety and depression, may also mediate these persistent effects on health in offspring (Talge et al., 2007). The biological mechanisms underlying maternal anxiety and depression have been difficult to define. Furthermore, identifying the means by which maternal anxiety and depression impact the health of the offspring has been even more challenging.

Efforts to identify biomarkers that explain the pathophysiology of early adverse life events are complicated by a variety of factors including ethical considerations, lack of experimental control over the subject's environment and genetic background and inaccessibility of primary tissues required for analysis. Therefore, the use of animal models provides a complementary approach for understanding the processes by which maternal behavior during pregnancy and the postpartum period influences the physiological and psychological health of offspring, resulting in the development of behavioral and emotional disorders. Clearly, this is a highly complex area of study, as there are a multitude of psychosocial, environmental and biological processes involved in parenting behavior. Furthermore, it is likely that a combination of genetic, epigenetic, and environmental processes will most accurately explain the link between insecure mother–infant attachment and the development of psychiatric disorders in offspring.

The overarching goal of this review is to examine the usefulness of animal models to disentangle the role of genetics, epigenetics, and the environment on maternal anxiety and depression with regard to maternal care and its effects on offspring. We examine the similarities between humans and rodent models in this vulnerable period of development and discuss how these similarities present an opportunity to inform human research and result in clinically relevant and translational discoveries. We will briefly review the epidemiology, presentation, and pathogenesis of perinatal mood disorders, clinical syndromes that encompass both anxiety and depression in humans, and describe their putative role on impaired mothering behaviors and the resulting adverse effects in offspring. Finally, we discuss specific inbred mouse strains that may serve as a model for the complex genetic, environmental, and epigenetic mechanisms that mediate maternal mental illness during the perinatal period including the subsequent influence on maternal behavior and infant outcomes.

PERINATAL MOOD AND ANXIETY DISORDERS: EPIDEMIOLOGY, CLINICAL PRESENTATION, AND PATHOGENESIS

Maternal behavior during pregnancy and the postpartum period is influenced by many factors. However, it is important to consider the contributions of perinatal depression on maternal behavior during this vulnerable time. Perinatal depression is an episode of major depressive disorder (MDD) occurring during pregnancy or within the first 6 months postpartum (Gavin et al., 2005; Gaynes et al., 2005). Perinatal depression is common, has a prevalence of 10–15% in women of childbearing age and is associated with significant morbidity and mortality including increased risk for maternal suicide and infanticide (Lindahl et al., 2005). Perinatal depression and anxiety have been linked to poor childbirth outcomes such as preterm delivery and low birth weight (Rahman et al., 2004; Smith et al., 2011), adverse effects on maternal sensitivity in the postpartum period (NECCR, 1999; Campbell et al., 2004), decreased maternal engagement with the infant (Weinberg and Tronick, 1998; NECCR, 1999; Campbell et al., 2004) and a decrease in healthy child development behaviors (Paulson et al., 2006).

The literature shows that maternal antenatal stress is associated with adverse neurobehavioral outcomes in offspring including both social/emotional and cognitive functioning during childhood and later in life (Talge et al., 2007) and may be a mechanism by which perinatal anxiety and depression results in increased risk for mood disorders in offspring. One working hypothesis suggests that negative maternal emotions during pregnancy can be considered behavioral teratogens; in other words, high levels of maternal stress, anxiety, or depression can trigger a cascade of physiological events in the mother, the placenta, and the fetus that lead to deleterious affects on fetal and postnatal neurobehavioral development (Van den Bergh and Marcoen, 2004). Support for this hypothesis is illustrated by examples in the literature. Infants of mothers reporting higher levels of depression and anxiety during pregnancy show increased levels of negative affect and motor activity when presented with novel toys (Davis et al., 2004) and this infant behavioral profile may continue into later childhood and is manifested by shyness and anxiety disorders (Kagan et al., 1987). Prospective studies document increased rates of ADHD and other anxiety disorders persisting into later childhood and early adulthood in children exposed to maternal antenatal stress (O'Connor et al., 2002a,b; Van den Bergh and Marcoen, 2004; Van den Bergh et al., 2005). In sum, these studies suggest that children who are exposed to maternal antenatal stress and anxiety suffer from a range of adverse outcomes although they can be quite variable. Other maternal/child effects may contribute to these associations including severity of or length of exposure to stress, genetic influences, and other indirect mechanisms.

Although the pathogenesis of perinatal depression is unknown, it is an active area of research. The transition from pregnancy to the postpartum period is characterized by an enormous state of hormonal flux (Mastorakos and Ilias, 2003). In humans, the third trimester of pregnancy is characterized by high estrogen and progesterone levels and a hyperactive hypothalamic–pituitary adrenal (HPA) axis with resulting high plasma cortisol (Nolten et al., 1980) that is stimulated in part by the high levels of estrogen and progesterone (Bloch et al., 2003). At childbirth and during the transition to the postpartum period, levels of estrogen and progesterone fall rapidly and there is blunted HPA axis activity due to suppressed hypothalamic corticotrophin-releasing hormone secretion (Magiakou et al., 1996). Estrogen and progesterone have profound interactions with the HPA axis and may trigger HPA axis abnormalities in susceptible women. Despite normal levels of reproductive hormones, women with postpartum depression (PPD) have an abnormal response to changes in estrogen and progesterone (Bloch et al., 2000, 2005).

RATIONALE FOR USE OF ANIMAL MODELS: A COMPLEMENTARY APPROACH

Currently, reliable biomarkers for human PPD do not exist and efforts to elucidate state biomarkers for MDD have proven difficult and frustrating (Rich-Edwards et al., 2008; Meltzer-Brody et al., 2011). Human studies to identify biomarkers for reproductive mood disorders are complicated by a variety of factors including lack of experimental control over the subject's environment and genetic background and inaccessibility of brain tissue required for analysis. The use of animal models, and particularly rodents, has been helpful in this regard. Animal models provide a complementary approach for understanding the processes by which maternal behavior during pregnancy and the postpartum period influences the physiological and psychological health of offspring, resulting in the development of behavioral and emotional disorders that may persist into adulthood. Identification of discrete genetic or pathophysiological pathways in animal models can serve to narrow the genomic search space, resulting in a more directed approach to gene identification and the effects of environmental factors in human studies.

Obviously, rodent gestation is substantially different from human pregnancy – the gestation period is shorter and regularly results in a litter of two or more offspring rather than a single infant. In addition, mouse pups are less developed at birth than human infants – the developmental changes that occur from birth to weaning in mice are roughly equivalent to development occurring in the third trimester in humans (Clancy et al., 2001). However, the endocrine changes throughout pregnancy and immediately postpartum are similar with one deviation – withdrawal of progesterone from the maternal circulation in rodents is necessary to induce parturition while in humans, plasma progesterone remains high throughout the latter part of pregnancy and decreases sharply after parturition (Mitchell and Taggart, 2009). Regardless of these differences, however, rodents recapitulate many of the endocrinological and HPA axis changes observed in humans during pregnancy including, for example, increasing estrogen and progesterone throughout gestation and high basal HPA activity in mid to late pregnancy. In addition, many of the same neuropeptides and hormones that promote maternal care and behavior in humans serve the same function in rodents (Brunton and Russell, 2010).

USING MICE TO MODEL ANXIETY AND DEPRESSION

Complex neuropsychiatric syndromes like MDD and PPD are multifactorial, and result from a combination of genetic and nongenetic factors. Their complex nature, along with the obvious ethical and logistical impediments to research in humans, has impacted the ability to identify the specific genetic and environmental components that predispose individuals to develop these disorders. While it will never be possible to mimic all facets of a complex human psychiatric syndrome in a rodent model, specific features can be modeled. Historically, rodent models of psychiatric endophenotypes have focused on models with good predictive validity, that responded to commonly used anxiolytics or antidepressants. However, recent commentary has recommended modeling the underlying pathophysiology and neurobiology of the disease rather than using behavioral models based on specific clinical symptoms or response to current pharmacotherapies (Insel et al., 2010; Nestler and Hyman, 2010; Cuthbert and Insel, 2011).

Functional MRI studies have implicated neural circuitry and brain regions involved in postpartum anxiety and depression and maternal bonding (Silverman et al., 2007; Swain et al., 2007; Swain, 2008). Many of the same brain regions and neurotransmitter systems have been implicated in rodents (Tarantino and Bucan, 2000; O'Mahony et al., 2010a,b; Krishnan and Nestler, 2011). Hormonally mediated behavioral changes in animal models of anxiety and depression also mimic those seen in humans (Yan et al., 2010; Krishnan and Nestler, 2011; O'Mahony et al., 2011) indicating that animal models of anxiety, depression, and maternal behavior may share common etiology with human disorders. Therefore, animal model research has the potential to provide information that can be directly translated to humans and, eventually, result in improvements in both the diagnosis and treatment of these devastating disorders.

C57BL/6 AND BALB/c INBRED STRAINS AS MODELS OF MATERNAL CARE, ANXIETY, AND DEPRESSION

Inbred mice have recently emerged as the primary model for studying genetic and genomic aspects of human disease (Cryan et al., 2005). This is due, in large part, to the availability of a vast array of resources for such endeavors in the mouse. The power of the mouse as a genetic model lies in the availability of hundreds of inbred strains, millions of cataloged genetic variants (e.g., single nucleotide polymorphisms, SNPs), inexpensive, and high-throughput ways to assess hundreds of thousands of SNPs, and genomic sequence data available for increasing numbers of inbred strains.

Mouse inbred strains have been used with great success for the past 50 years to investigate genetic influences on behavior. Inbred strains are genetically homogeneous within a strain, but vary widely both genetically and phenotypically across strains. These reference populations represent a stable genetic resource that can be tested, analyzed, and compared across laboratories and across time. Inbred strain studies have provided a vast amount of information on anxiety and depression-related behaviors.

Two strains in particular, C57BL/6 (B6) and BALB/c (BALB), have repeatedly shown dramatically different behavioral profiles in anxiety and are commonly referred to as low (B6) and high (BALB) anxiety strains. The results of studies on anxiety-related behaviors, which generally have been shown to be somewhat labile (Crabbe et al., 1999), are surprisingly consistent in these two strains. BALB mice exhibit reduced locomotor activity and less time in unprotected and brightly lit areas in the open field (Carola et al., 2002; Tang et al., 2002; Francis et al., 2003; Priebe et al., 2005; Depino and Gross, 2007; Post et al., 2011) and light:dark assays (Crawley and Davis, 1982; Beuzen and Belzung, 1995; Griebel et al., 2000; Millstein and Holmes, 2007; O'Mahony et al., 2010b) in comparison to B6 mice with very few exceptions. Results from the elevated plus maze have been less consistent with at least one study showing no strain differences (Griebel et al., 2000) and some showing what appears to be less anxiety in the BALB strain (Trullas and Skolnick, 1993; Rogers et al., 1999; Post et al., 2011). These inconsistencies may be due to substrain differences (Trullas and Skolnick, 1993) or might reflect a strain-specific response to a particular apparatus that confounds interpretation of the results.

STRESS REACTIVITY IN B6 AND BALB MICE

Stressful life events have been shown to play an important role in the development and manifestation of psychiatric illnesses (Kendler et al., 1999; Charney and Manji, 2004; Anisman and Matheson, 2005). Interestingly, B6 and BALB mice also differ in response to stressful stimuli. BALB mice have consistently shown stressor-provoked hyperactivation of the HPA axis as reflected by stress-induced increases in corticosterone release (Shanks et al., 1994; Priebe et al., 2005; Prakash et al., 2006) and ACTH as well as basal differences in CRH (Anisman et al., 1998a). BALB mice have also been shown to exhibit stress-induced differences in CRH receptor immunoreactivity (Anisman et al., 2007) as well as basal and stress-induced differences in expression of $GABA_A$ receptor subunits (Poulter et al., 2010). Interestingly, $GABA_A$ receptor subunits have also been implicated in a mouse model of PPD (Maguire and Mody, 2008). O'Mahony et al. (2010b) have observed that

BALB mice show blunted stress-induced brain activation (as measured by c-Fos expression) in the prefrontal cortex in comparison to B6 mice, indicating that dysregulation in response to stress may be driving behavioral differences between these two strains.

Exposure to both acute and chronic stress differentially modulates depressive-like behavior in BALB mice as well. BALB mice showed significantly greater anhedonia (as measured by decreased sucrose consumption) following both acute and chronic stress in comparison to B6 mice (Poulter et al., 2010). BALB mice also show longer latencies to escape a shuttle box in which they have previously experienced an inescapable footshock (Shanks and Anisman, 1988) and exhibit decreased responding for reward after exposure to stress (Zacharko and Anisman, 1989).

MOTHERING BEHAVIOR IN ANIMAL MODELS

Behavioral differences among inbred strains of mice are frequently studied with regard to their genetic origins. However, environmental factors also play a significant role in the development of behavior in rodents. As has been demonstrated in humans, deficiencies in maternal care during the postpartum period have been shown to result in anxiety, stress, and depression-related behaviors in adult rodent offspring.

As discussed above, there is an extensive literature in humans demonstrating the link between maternal care and bonding and increased risk for development of mood disorders in offspring. This research extends to rat models where it has been shown that offspring of mothers that exhibit higher levels of arched back nursing (ABN) and licking and grooming (LG) exhibit reduced endocrine responses to stress as measured by adrenocorticotropic hormone and corticosterone and decreased anxiety behaviors (for a review see Francis and Meaney, 1999; Francis et al., 1999b; Champagne et al., 2003). Offspring of low LG mothers also exhibit decreased oxytocin receptor binding that is likely related to decreased levels of estrogen receptor alpha expression in the hypothalamus. Oxytocin is believed to promote mother–infant bonding in humans (Bartels and Zeki, 2004; Galbally et al., 2011). Interestingly, differences in maternal behavior have also been shown to be transmitted across generations (Francis et al., 1999a).

Daily removal of pups from the home cage for short periods of handling (3–15 min), results in decreases in anxiety-related behaviors. This observation seems counterintuitive but can be explained by the observation that dams of handled pups show increased ABN and LG when pups are returned to the cage (Liu et al., 1997). Pups exposed to maternal separation for longer periods (3–6 h daily) show increased endocrine responses to stress and increased behavioral reactivity to novelty (Champagne and Meaney, 2007; Curley et al., 2011). The effects of postnatal handling and maternal separation have been shown to change expression levels of genes involved in HPA reactivity including corticotropin releasing factor, glucocorticoid receptor, and subunits of the $GABA_A$ receptor (Francis and Meaney, 1999; Francis et al., 1999b; Curley et al., 2011).

Significant differences in mothering behavior have been observed in B6 and BALB strains of mice (Carlier et al., 1982; Anisman et al., 1998b; Priebe et al., 2005; Prakash et al., 2006) leading to the hypothesis that maternal care differences act separately from, or in conjunction with, genetic background to result in the observed behavioral differences between these strains. BALB mice have consistently been shown to perform less ABN, spend less time on the nest, exhibit less LG, and have longer latencies to retrieve pups that have been removed from the nest (**Table 1**). Very few studies have examined maternal separation or handling in mouse models. B6 mice have been exposed to both maternal separation and handling with mixed results. Male, but not female B6 mice show increased anxiety behaviors in both the EPM and OF after maternal separation from days 1 to 9 postpartum (Romeo et al., 2003) but showed no change in the defensive withdrawal test – an anxiety assay similar to the emergence test – after handling and under a similar schedule of maternal separation (Parfitt et al., 2004). A study by Millstein and Holmes

Table 1 | Maternal care differences in B6 and BALB mice.

Substrains	Maternal care observation	Mothering behavior (BALB relative to B6)	Reference
C57BL/6JOrl, BALB/cOrl	24 ± 10 h postpartum, between 10 AM and 4 PM	Increased latency of first contact with pup after removal from nest, longer latency to first retrieval, more time off nest	Carlier et al. (1982)
C57BL/6ByJ, BALB/cByJ	First 7 days postpartum, 1 h twice daily at 8 AM and 4 PM. 15 observations every hour at 4 min intervals	Less arched back nursing, less licking and grooming, less time spent on the nest	Anisman et al. (1998b)
C57BL/6J, BALB/cByJ	First 13 days postpartum, three 21 min observation periods per day	Poor nest building, less time spent on nest	Millstein and Holmes (2007)
C57BL/6ByJ, BALB/cByJ	2–6 ays postpartum, 1 h twice daily at 9 AM and 1 PM, 15 sec every 3 min	Less arched back nursing, less time on nest, longer latency to retrieve pups, poor nest building	Prakash et al. (2006)
C57BL/6J, BALB/cJ	1–14 days postpartum, 4 observations per day, once per minute in 30 min increments twice during lights on and twice during lights off	Less arched back nursing, less licking and grooming, less time spent on nest, nest building similar	Priebe et al. (2005)

(2007) examined strain differences in response to both handling and maternal separation and found that neither had an effect on B6 or BALB mice in multiple tests of anxiety and depression. These results indicate that the maternal separation and handling models of anxiety and depression may not be useful in mice, may be strain dependent or may be sensitive to procedural differences. However, too few studies in mice have been conducted to draw a conclusion (for a review see Millstein and Holmes, 2007).

The observation that B6 and BALB mice differ significantly for anxiety, stress, and mothering behaviors has led to research focused on the effects of both genetics and mothering on behavioral differences in these two strains.

NATURE OR NURTURE – IT'S LIKELY BOTH

The use of animal models to disentangle the roles of nature and nurture in the development of anxiety, stress and depression has advantages over human studies – in particular, the ability to control both environmental factors and genetics and perform experimental manipulations during pregnancy and the postpartum period as well as having access to brain tissue for analysis. However, this endeavor is not as straightforward as it may seem. Studies in humans have shown that mothers suffering from PPD demonstrate less attachment to their infants (Fleming and Corter, 1988), which can, in turn, lead to increased risk for psychiatric disorders in the offspring. However, genetic factors also play a role. Mothers contribute half of the genetic material to offspring, therefore, individuals with mothers who suffer from PPD already have an increased genetic risk making it difficult to separate genetic and environmental factors, both of which can act additively or interact to result in increased risk. Adoption studies in humans allow for partitioning of genetic and environmental influences on disease risk but these approaches often suffer from inadequate sample sizes (Merikangas and Low, 2004) along with other drawbacks common to human studies.

In rodents, cross fostering can be used to assess the role of genes and environment on the development of behavior. Cross-fostering involves removal of pups from their biological mother at birth and placing them with a foster mother. This manipulation can be used to study the effects of maternal care on behavior. In cross-fostering studies with rats, low LG offspring fostered to high LG dams exhibit decreased fear and stress behaviors similar to those observed in high LG offspring reared by their biological mothers. Conversely, high LG offspring fostered to low LG dams exhibited increases in fear and stress related behavior (Francis et al., 1999a). These data substantiate the role of early maternal care on subsequent behavior and, importantly, the non-genomic transmission of individual differences.

The cross-fostering approach has also been used with B6 and BALB mice in several studies with mixed results. Several studies have reported an increase in anxiety behaviors and corticosterone release in response to stress in B6 mice fostered by BALB mothers (Francis et al., 2003; Priebe et al., 2005) but other groups observed no change (Anisman et al., 1998b). BALB mice fostered to B6 mothers have been reported to show decreased anxiety in certain behavioral tests like the elevated plus maze (Priebe et al., 2005) and also improved performance in the Morris water maze (Anisman et al., 1998b), but no change in the open field (Priebe et al., 2005). These results indicate that the effects of maternal care are not sufficient to explain the behavioral differences between these strains, and variations in maternal care result in different outcomes depending upon which behavioral test is employed (even tests within the same domain).

It is likely that both genetics and environment interact to produce the behavioral differences observed in these inbred strains. The interaction of genes and the environment to produce phenotypic outcomes has been acknowledged and accepted for quite some time in the scientific community. However, the exact mechanism by which the environment can act on genetic material has only recently begun to be investigated in a more systematic manner.

A ROLE FOR EPIGENETICS IN THE LINK BETWEEN MATERNAL CARE AND BEHAVIORAL OUTCOMES IN ANIMAL MODELS

The observation that the behavioral effects of maternal care were associated with gene expression changes that persisted into adulthood and could be transmitted across generations suggested a potential role for epigenetic DNA modifications. The term "epigenetics" was coined in the 1940s to describe gene by environment interactions, but as the molecular mechanisms of those interactions have been better characterized, the term has evolved to be more specific. The modern definition of epigenetics is the study of DNA modification leading to changes in gene expression caused by a mechanism other than changes to the DNA sequence (Adrian, 2007). Epigenetic modifications can include DNA methylation, histone modification, and non-coding RNA as well as more recently identified mechanisms such as hydroxymethylcytosine residues in the brain (Kriaucionis and Heintz, 2009; Skinner et al., 2010). Of these, DNA methylation has been the most actively studied due to its role in developmental silencing of genes through imprinting or X-inactivation. DNA methylation refers to the process by which a methyl group attaches to DNA via cytosine at specific locations in the genome called CpG sites (Razin, 1998). The bond formed between the DNA cytosine and the methyl group is strong, causing a stable but potentially reversible change in gene expression (Jones and Taylor, 1980). At its most basic functional level, methylation results in the silencing of a gene, but recent evidence indicates that methylation may also be associated with gene activation (Metivier et al., 2008). It was commonly thought that DNA methylation changes that occurred during development were stable and unchangeable later in life. However, recent evidence suggests that DNA methylation is a dynamic process that allows the genome to adapt to alterations in the environment throughout life (Meaney and Szyf, 2005) providing a mechanism by which early life experiences can leave an indelible mark on the brain and influence behavior and health (Weaver et al., 2004).

Weaver et al. (2004) provided the first direct evidence of an epigenetic change in response to mothering behavior with the observation that rats exposed to poor maternal care exhibited increased methylation at a 5′ CpG site in the promoter region of the glucocorticoid receptor gene. The increase in methylation effectively reduced the number of receptors and resulted in heightened response to stress (Weaver et al., 2004). Champagne et al. (2006)

also reported increased methylation in response to maternal care in the signal transducer and activator of transcription 5 (*Stat5*) binding site in the estrogen receptor alpha (*Esr*) gene promoter region and cross-fostering reversed this effect. *Esr* is involved in the regulation of oxytocin receptor binding.

Franklin et al. (2010) have extended these studies to C57BL/6 mice and demonstrated that the stress of chronic and unpredictable early life maternal separation in male offspring alters the profile of DNA methylation in the promoter of several candidate genes including the *Mecp2* gene, a transcriptional regulator that binds methylated DNA, the cannabinoid receptor 1 (*Cb1*) that has been associated with emotionality in rodents and corticotropin releasing hormone receptor 2 (*Crhr2*), a stress hormone receptor (Franklin et al., 2010).

In sum, neurobehavioral epigenetics holds great promise for the future. The ability to conduct whole genome methylation analysis (Pokholok et al., 2005; Jeddeloh et al., 2008; Butcher and Beck, 2010; Li et al., 2010) along with the availability of novel resources in mouse systems genetics (Churchill et al., 2004) provides the starting point for further research into the complex genetic, environmental, and epigenetic mechanisms that mediate maternal mental illness during the perinatal period including the subsequent influence on maternal behavior and infant outcomes.

FUTURE DIRECTIONS: EXPANDING KNOWLEDGE OF GENE BY ENVIRONMENT INTERACTIONS IN B6 AND BALB MICE

Based on the behavioral and neuroendocrine data reviewed above, BALB and B6 mice may prove to be an excellent model for the effects of perinatal anxiety and depression on maternal care and bonding and subsequent behavior in offspring. Research in humans indicates that women who suffer from MDD and anxiety are more likely to develop PPD (Kammerer et al., 2006). It is clear that BALB mice display an increased basal level of anxiety. However, no studies have examined changes in anxiety- or depression-related behaviors in BALB mice during pregnancy or the postpartum period. In both humans and rodents, pregnancy is characterized as a period of high basal HPA activity (Brunton and Russell, 2008) – a phenomenon that has also not been characterized specifically in pregnant BALB mice who show significant basal differences in HPA reactivity.

Neuroendocrine changes during pregnancy and immediately postpartum have been shown to be important for the expression of maternal behavior in both human and rodent models. For example, oxytocin, which is essential for lactation, also plays a major role in facilitating maternal behavior and bonding (Neumann, 2008). Interestingly, oxytocin administered centrally or peripherally, has also been shown to have anxiolytic effects (Ring et al., 2006) and attenuate stress-induced activity of the HPA axis (Neumann, 2002). Prolactin, which also plays a role in milk production, has been shown to be involved in maternal behavior as indicated by the severe maternal behavior deficits observed in prolactin receptor knockout mice (Lucas et al., 1998). However, little or no published information exists regarding levels of oxytocin or prolactin during pregnancy and postpartum in either B6 or BALB mice specifically. Unpublished gene expression data from our own laboratory as well as publicly available data from multiple sources show decreased expression of oxytocin in BALB mice in comparison to B6 (**Figure 1**). Although these results have not yet been confirmed and gene expression differences by no means translate automatically to functional differences, these data offer tantalizing evidence regarding differences in the neuroendocrine systems of these two strains that may contribute to behavioral profiles.

Studies in rats have examined the development of mothering behavior in virgin females and suggest that animals that are stressed or anxious are less likely and take longer to display mothering behaviors (Bridges et al., 1972; Pereira et al., 2005; Mann and Gervais, 2011). These results are fairly intuitive based on the observation that oxytocin, which is known to induce mothering behavior, is also anxiolytic. Expanding upon these studies in mice may allow for more direct evidence in BALB for the role of innate anxiety and its effects on mothering behavior.

The environment in which an animal is raised can also have an effect on subsequent behaviors. Francis et al. (2002) have shown

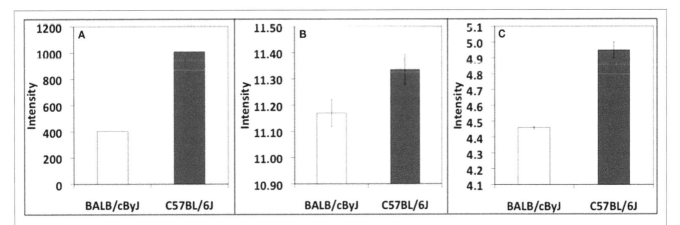

FIGURE 1 | Differential expression of *Oxt* in (A) hypothalamus, Wiltshire and Tarantino (unpublished), (B) whole brain, PhenoGen Informatics, University of Colorado at Denver Health Sciences Center (Bhave et al., 2007), and (C) hippocampus, Williams et al. (unpublished). Datasets (B,C) are available at http://webqtl.org, accessions GN123, GN273, respectively. The Wiltshire et al. data utilized the Affymetrix 430 v2 array. The Williams et al. data utilized the Affymetrix Mouse Exon 1.0 ST Array. The 3′ UTR probeset from the Exon 1.0 ST Array was utilized for comparison purposes.

that environmental enrichment from weaning until adulthood ameliorates HPA axis reactivity and stress behaviors in rats that have been exposed to maternal separation as pups. Environmental enrichment in BALB mice has been shown to decrease anxiety-related behaviors as well (Chapillon et al., 1999). Moreover, Curley et al. (2009) have also shown that social enrichment in BALB mice enhances maternal care and reduces anxiety behaviors and that these effects may be mediated by increased receptor densities of both oxytocin and vasopressin (V1a). These studies highlight the impact of early environment as a protective influence as well and present the potential for studying mechanisms that "rescue" phenotypes resulting from the detrimental environments early in life.

CONCLUSION

Postpartum depression is debilitating to women who experience it and potentially damaging to their offspring. Although the etiology of PPD remains unclear, headway is being made toward a better understanding of the complicated interplay of reproductive steroids with the HPA axis and other neuroregulatory systems implicated in depressive illness. Further study of alterations in the HPA axis during the transition from pregnancy to the postpartum period may provide new insights into the pathophysiology of PPD. Moreover, understanding the pathophysiology of PPD can potentially lead to the discovery of biomarkers specific for PPD so that prospective identification of those at risk may become feasible. This would have enormous implications for both the prevention and treatment of women at risk for PPD as well as the transmission of adverse sequelae to offspring exposed to mothers with PPD including adverse effects on neurobehavioral development and increased risk for psychiatric illness.

Although humans and mice evolved with very different sets of reproductive and selective pressures, complete genome sequencing has revealed that mouse and human genomes are highly conserved (Mouse Genome Sequencing Consortium et al., 2002), thereby substantiating the use of mouse models to study genetic aspects of human disease. Animal studies have been used successfully to model perinatal maternal behavior and to study the pathogenesis of perinatal anxiety, stress, and depression. Although animal models do not fully recapitulate human psychiatric syndromes and behaviors, many of the key characteristics observed in human disorders can be observed in mice and many of the same genetic and neuroendocrine factors are involved.

In particular, B6 and BALB mice exhibit divergent phenotypes for stress, anxiety, and mothering behaviors. Moreover, these phenotypic differences have been shown to be at least partially genetically determined, can be modulated by environmental manipulations and result in behavioral changes in adult offspring. The mechanism by which early environmental stress results in lasting changes in behavior and increased risk for psychiatric disorders has not yet been resolved. We believe that more detailed behavioral and neuroendocrine studies using genetic reference populations like B6 and BALB inbred mice will provide insight into the mechanisms by which early environment shapes later behavior and, more generally, into the etiology of anxiety and depression. Furthermore, the rapidly growing field of behavioral epigenetics offers an intriguing area of study that may provide new insights into the nature of gene–environment interactions during development. The dramatic expansion of genomic data and genetic resources in the mouse provides the perfect opportunity to expand on the building evidence for environmentally mediated epigenetic changes and their role, along with genetic predisposition, in increasing risk for psychiatric disorders.

REFERENCES

Adrian, B. (2007). Perceptions of epigenetics. *Nature* 447, 396–398.

Anisman, H., Lacosta, S., Kent, P., McIntyre, D. C., and Merali, Z. (1998a). Stressor-induced corticotropin-releasing hormone, bombesin, ACTH and corticosterone variations in strains of mice differentially responsive to stressors. *Stress* 2, 209–220.

Anisman, H., Zaharia, M. D., Meaney, M. J., and Merali, Z. (1998b). Do early-life events permanently alter behavioral and hormonal responses to stressors? *Int. J. Dev. Neurosci.* 16, 149–164.

Anisman, H., and Matheson, K. (2005). Stress, depression, and anhedonia: caveats concerning animal models. *Neurosci. Biobehav. Rev.* 29, 525–546.

Anisman, H., Prakash, P., Merali, Z., and Poulter, M. O. (2007). Corticotropin releasing hormone receptor alterations elicited by acute and chronic unpredictable stressor challenges in stressor-susceptible and resilient strains of mice. *Behav. Brain Res.* 181, 180–190.

Bartels, A., and Zeki, S. (2004). The neural correlates of maternal and romantic love. *Neuroimage* 21, 1155–1166.

Bennett, H. A., Einarson, A., Taddio, A., Koren, G., and Einarson, T. R. (2004). Prevalence of depression during pregnancy: systematic review. *Obstet. Gynecol.* 103, 698–709.

Beuzen, A., and Belzung, C. (1995). Link between emotional memory and anxiety states: a study by principal component analysis. *Physiol. Behav.* 58, 111–118.

Bhave, S. V., Hornbaker, C., Phang, T. L., Saba, L., Lapadat, R., Kechris, K., Gaydos, J., McGoldrick, D., Dolbey, A., Leach, S., Soriano, B., Ellington, A., Ellington, E., Jones, K., Mangion, J., Belknap, J. K., Williams, R. W., Hunter, L. E., Hoffman, P. L., and Tabakoff, B. (2007). The PhenoGen informatics website: tools for analyses of complex traits. *BMC Genet.* 8, 59. doi: 10.1186/1471-2156-8-59

Bloch, M., Daly, R. C., and Rubinow, D. R. (2003). Endocrine factors in the etiology of postpartum depression. *Compr. Psychiatry* 44, 234–246.

Bloch, M., Rubinow, D. R., Schmidt, P. J., Lotsikas, A., Chrousos, G. P., and Cizza, G. (2005). Cortisol response to ovine corticotropin-releasing hormone in a model of pregnancy and parturition in euthymic women with and without a history of postpartum depression. *J. Clin. Endocrinol. Metab.* 90, 695–699.

Bloch, M., Schmidt, P. J., Danaceau, M., Murphy, J., Nieman, L., and Rubinow, D. R. (2000). Effects of gonadal steroids in women with a history of postpartum depression. *Am. J. Psychiatry* 157, 924–930.

Bridges, R., Zarrow, M. X., Gandelman, R., and Denenberg, V. H. (1972). Differences in maternal responsiveness between lactating and sensitized rats. *Dev. Psychobiol.* 5, 123–127.

Brumariu, L. E., and Kerns, K. A. (2010a). Mother-child attachment patterns and different types of anxiety symptoms: is there specificity of relations? *Child Psychiatry Hum. Dev.* 41, 663–674.

Brumariu, L. E., and Kerns, K. A. (2010b). Parent-child attachment and internalizing symptoms in childhood and adolescence: a review of empirical findings and future directions. *Dev. Psychopathol.* 22, 177–203.

Brunton, P. J., and Russell, J. A. (2008). The expectant brain: adapting for motherhood. *Nat. Rev. Neurosci.* 9, 11–25.

Brunton, P. J., and Russell, J. A. (2010). Endocrine induced changes in brain function during pregnancy. *Brain Res.* 1364, 198–215.

Butcher, L. M., and Beck, S. (2010). AutoMeDIP-seq: a high-throughput, whole genome, DNA methylation assay. *Methods* 52, 223–231.

Campbell, S. B., Brownell, C. A., Hungerford, A., Spieker, S. I., Mohan, R., and Blessing, J. S. (2004). The course of maternal depressive symptoms and maternal sensitivity as predictors of attachment security at 36 months. *Dev. Psychopathol.* 16, 231–252.

Carlier, M., Roubertoux, P., and Cohen-Salmon, C. (1982). Differences in patterns of pup care in *Mus musculus* domesticus l-Comparisons between eleven inbred strains. *Behav. Neural Biol.* 35, 205–210.

Carola, V., D'Olimpio, F., Brunamonti, E., Mangia, F., and Renzi, P. (2002). Evaluation of the elevated plus-maze and open-field tests for the assessment of anxiety-related behaviour in inbred mice. *Behav. Brain Res.* 134, 49–57.

Champagne, F. A., Francis, D. D., Mar, A., and Meaney, M. J. (2003). Variations in maternal care in the rat as a mediating influence for the effects of environment on development. *Physiol. Behav.* 79, 359–371.

Champagne, F. A., and Meaney, M. J. (2007). Transgenerational effects of social environment on variations in maternal care and behavioral response to novelty. *Behav. Neurosci.* 121, 1353–1363.

Champagne, F. A., Weaver, I. C., Diorio, J., Dymov, S., Szyf, M., and Meaney, M. J. (2006). Maternal care associated with methylation of the estrogen receptor-alpha1b promoter and estrogen receptor-alpha expression in the medial preoptic area of female offspring. *Endocrinology* 147, 2909–2915.

Chapillon, P., Manneche, C., Belzung, C., and Caston, J. (1999). Rearing environmental enrichment in two inbred strains of mice: 1. Effects on emotional reactivity. *Behav. Genet.* 29, 41–46.

Charney, D. S., and Manji, H. K. (2004). Life stress, genes, and depression: multiple pathways lead to increased risk and new opportunities for intervention. *Sci. STKE* 2004, re5.

Churchill, G. A., Airey, D. C., Allayee, H., Angel, J. M., Attie, A. D., Beatty, J., Beavis, W. D., Belknap, J. K., Bennett, B., Berrettini, W., Bleich, A., Bogue, M., Broman, K. W., Buck, K. J., Buckler, E., Burmeister, M., Chesler, E. J., Cheverud, J. M., Clapcote, S., Cook, M. N., Cox, R. D., Crabbe, J. C., Crusio, W. E., Darvasi, A., Deschepper, C. F., Doerge, R. W., Farber, C. R., Forejt, J., Gaile, D., Garlow, S. J., Geiger, H., Gershenfeld, H., Gordon, T., Gu, J., Gu, W., de Haan, G., Hayes, N. L., Heller, C., Himmelbauer, H., Hitzemann, R., Hunter, K., Hsu, H. C., Iraqi, F. A., Ivandic, B., Jacob, H. J., Jansen, R. C., Jepsen, K. J., Johnson, D. K., Johnson, T. E., Kempermann, G., Kendziorski, C., Kotb, M., Kooy, R. F., Llamas, B., Lammert, F., Lassalle, J. M., Lowenstein, P. R., Lu, L., Lusis, A., Manly, K. F., Marcucio, R., Matthews, D., Medrano, J. F., Miller, D. R., Mittleman, G., Mock, B. A., Mogil, J. S., Montagutelli, X., Morahan, G., Morris, D. G., Mott, R., Nadeau, J. H., Nagase, H., Nowakowski, R. S., O'Hara, B. F., Osadchuk, A. V., Page, G. P., Paigen, B., Paigen, K., Palmer, A. A., Pan, H. J., Peltonen-Palotie, L., Peirce, J., Pomp, D., Pravenec, M., Prows, D. R., Qi, Z., Reeves, R. H., Roder, J., Rosen, G. D., Schadt, E. E., Schalkwyk, L. C., Seltzer, Z., Shimomura, K., Shou, S., Sillanpää, M. J., Siracusa, L. D., Snoeck, H. W., Spearow, J. L., Svenson, K., Tarantino, L. M., Threadgill, D., Toth, L. A., Valdar, W., de Villena, F. P., Warden, C., Whatley, S., Williams, R. W., Wiltshire, T., Yi, N., Zhang, D., Zhang, M, Zou, F., and Complex Trait Consortium. (2004). The collaborative cross, a community resource for the genetic analysis of complex traits. *Nat. Genet.* 36, 1133–1137.

Clancy, B., Darlington, R. B., and Finlay, B. L. (2001). Translating developmental time across mammalian species. *Neuroscience* 105, 7–17.

Crabbe, J. C., Wahlsten, D., and Dudek, B. C. (1999). Genetics of mouse behavior: interactions with laboratory environment. *Science* 284, 1670–1672.

Crawley, J. N., and Davis, L. G. (1982). Baseline exploratory activity predicts anxiolytic responsiveness to diazepam in five mouse strains. *Brain Res. Bull.* 8, 609–612.

Cryan, J. F., Mombereau, C., and Vassout, A. (2005). The tail suspension test as a model for assessing antidepressant activity: review of pharmacological and genetic studies in mice. *Neurosci. Biobehav. Rev.* 29, 571–625.

Curley, J. P., Davidson, S., Bateson, P., and Champagne, F. A. (2009). Social enrichment during postnatal development induces transgenerational effects on emotional and reproductive behavior in mice. *Front. Behav. Neurosci.* 3, 25. doi: 10.3389/neuro.08.025.2009

Curley, J. P., Jensen, C. L., Mashoodh, R., and Champagne, F. A. (2011). Social influences on neurobiology and behavior: epigenetic effects during development. *Psychoneuroendocrinology* 36, 352–371.

Cuthbert, B., and Insel, T. (2011). The data of diagnosis: new approaches to psychiatric classification. *Psychiatry* 73, 311–314.

Davis, E. P., Snidman, N., Wadhwa, P. D., Glynn, L. M., Schetter, C. D., and Sandman, C. A. (2004). Prenatal maternal anxiety and depression predict negative behavioral reactivity in infancy. *Infancy* 6, 319–331.

Depino, A. M., and Gross, C. (2007). Simultaneous assessment of autonomic function and anxiety-related behavior in BALB/c and C57BL/6 mice. *Behav. Brain Res.* 177, 254–260.

Feldman, R., Granat, A., Pariente, C., Kanety, H., Kuint, J., and Gilboa-Schechtman, E. (2009). Maternal depression and anxiety across the postpartum year and infant social engagement, fear regulation, and stress reactivity. *J. Am. Acad. Child Adolesc. Psychiatry* 48, 919–927.

Field, T. (2010). Postpartum depression effects on early interactions, parenting, and safety practices: a review. *Infant Behav. Dev.* 33, 1–6.

Fleming, A. S., and Corter, C. (1988). Factors influencing maternal responsiveness in humans: usefulness of an animal model. *Psychoneuroendocrinology* 13, 189–212.

Flynn, H. A., Davis, M., Marcus, S. M., Cunningham, R., and Blow, F. C. (2004). Rates of maternal depression in pediatric emergency department and relationship to child service utilization. *Gen. Hosp. Psychiatry* 26, 316–322.

Francis, D., Diorio, J., Liu, D., and Meaney, M. J. (1999a). Nongenomic transmission across generations of maternal behavior and stress responses in the rat. *Science* 286, 1155–1158.

Francis, D. D., Champagne, F. A., Liu, D., and Meaney, M. J. (1999b). Maternal care, gene expression, and the development of individual differences in stress reactivity. *Ann. N. Y. Acad. Sci.* 896, 66–84.

Francis, D. D., Diorio, J., Plotsky, P. M., and Meaney, M. J. (2002). Environmental enrichment reverses the effects of maternal separation on stress reactivity. *J. Neurosci.* 22, 7840–7843.

Francis, D. D., and Meaney, M. J. (1999). Maternal care and the development of stress responses. *Curr. Opin. Neurobiol.* 9, 128–134.

Francis, D. D., Szegda, K., Campbell, G., Martin, W. D., and Insel, T. R. (2003). Epigenetic sources of behavioral differences in mice. *Nat. Neurosci.* 6, 445–446.

Franklin, T. B., Russig, H., Weiss, I. C., Gräff, J., Linder, N., Michalon, A., Vizi, S., and Mansuy, I. M. (2010). Epigenetic transmission of the impact of early stress across generations. *Biol. Psychiatry* 68, 408–415.

Galbally, M., Lewis, A. J., Ijzendoorn, M., and Permezel, M. (2011). The role of oxytocin in mother-infant relations: a systematic review of human studies. *Harv. Rev. Psychiatry* 19, 1–14.

Gavin, N. I., Gaynes, B. N., Lohr, K. N., Meltzer-Brody, S., Gartlehner, G., and Swinson, T. (2005). Perinatal depression: a systematic review of prevalence and incidence. *Obstet. Gynecol.* 106(5 Pt 1), 1071–1083.

Gaynes, B. N., Gavin, N., Meltzer-Brody, S., Lohr, K. N., Swinson, T., Gartlehner, G., Brody, S., and Miller, W. C. (2005). Perinatal depression: prevalence, screening accuracy, and screening outcomes. *Evid. Rep. Technol. Assess. (Summ.)* 119, 1–8.

Gluckman, P. D., Hanson, M. A., Cooper, C., and Thornburg, K. L. (2008). Effect of in utero and early-life conditions on adult health and disease. *N. Engl. J. Med.* 359, 61–73.

Griebel, G., Belzung, C., Perrault, G., and Sanger, D. J. (2000). Differences in anxiety-related behaviours and in sensitivity to diazepam in inbred and outbred strains of mice. *Psychopharmacology (Berl.)* 148, 164–170.

Insel, T., Cuthbert, B., Garvey, M., Heinssen, R., Pine, D. S., Quinn, K., Sanislow, C., and Wang, P. (2010). Research domain criteria (RDoC): toward a new classification framework for research on mental disorders. *Am. J. Psychiatry* 167, 748–751.

Jeddeloh, J. A., Greally, J. M., and Rando, O. J. (2008). Reduced-representation methylation mapping. *Genome Biol.* 9, 231.

Jones, P. A., and Taylor, S. M. (1980). Cellular differentiation, cytidine analogs and DNA methylation. *Cell* 20, 85–93.

Kagan, J., Reznick, J. S., and Snidman, N. (1987). The physiology and psychology of behavioral inhibition in children. *Child Dev.* 58, 1459–1473.

Kammerer, M., Taylor, A., and Glover, V. (2006). The HPA axis and perinatal depression: a hypothesis. *Arch. Womens Ment. Health* 9, 187–196.

Kendler, K. S., Karkowski, L. M., and Prescott, C. A. (1999). Causal relationship between stressful life events and the onset of major depression. *Am. J. Psychiatry* 156, 837–841.

Kriaucionis, S., and Heintz, N. (2009). The nuclear DNA base 5-hydroxymethylcytosine is present in Purkinje neurons and the brain. *Science* 324, 929–930.

Krishnan, V., and Nestler, E. J. (2011). Animal models of depression: molecular perspectives. *Curr. Top. Behav. Neurosci.* 7, 121–147.

Li, N., Ye, M., Li, Y., Yan, Z., Butcher, L. M., Sun, J., Han, X., Chen, Q., Zhang, X., and Wang, J. (2010). Whole genome DNA methylation analysis based on high throughput sequencing technology. *Methods* 52, 203–212.

Lindahl, V., Pearson, J. L., and Colpe, L. (2005). Prevalence of suicidality during pregnancy and the postpartum. *Arch. Womens Ment. Health* 8, 77–87.

Liu, D., Diorio, J., Tannenbaum, B., Caldji, C., Francis, D., Freedman, A., Sharma, S., Pearson, D., Plotsky, P. M., and Meaney, M. J. (1997). Maternal care, hippocampal glucocorticoid receptors, and hypothalamic-pituitary-adrenal responses to stress. *Science* 277, 1659–1662.

Lucas, B. K., Ormandy, C. J., Binart, N., Bridges, R. S., and Kelly, P. A. (1998). Null mutation of the prolactin receptor gene produces a defect in maternal behavior. *Endocrinology* 139, 4102–4107.

Magiakou, M. A., Mastorakos, G., Rabin, D., Dubbert, B., Gold, P. W., and Chrousos, G. P. (1996). Hypothalamic corticotropin-releasing hormone suppression during the postpartum period: implications for the increase in psychiatric manifestations at this time. *J. Clin. Endocrinol. Metab.* 81, 1912–1917.

Maguire, J., and Mody, I. (2008). GABA(A)R plasticity during pregnancy: relevance to postpartum depression. *Neuron* 59, 207–213.

Mann, P. E., and Gervais, K. J. (2011). Environmental enrichment delays pup-induced maternal behavior in rats. *Dev. Psychobiol.* 53, 371–382.

Marmorstein, N. R., Malone, S. M., and Iacono, W. G. (2004). Psychiatric disorders among offspring of depressed mothers: associations with paternal psychopathology. *Am. J. Psychiatry* 161, 1588–1594.

Mastorakos, G., and Ilias, I. (2003). Maternal and fetal hypothalamic-pituitary-adrenal axes during pregnancy and postpartum. *Ann. N. Y. Acad. Sci.* 997, 136–149.

Meaney, M. J., and Szyf, M. (2005). Environmental programming of stress responses through DNA methylation: life at the interface between a dynamic environment and a fixed genome. *Dialogues Clin. Neurosci.* 7, 103–123.

Meltzer-Brody, S., Stuebe, A. M., Dole, N., Savitz, D., Rubinow, D., and Thorp, J. (2011). Elevated corticotropin releasing hormone (CRH) during pregnancy and risk of postpartum depression (PPD). *J. Clin. Endocrinol. Metab.* 96, E40–E47.

Merikangas, K. R., and Low, N. C. (2004). The epidemiology of mood disorders. *Curr Psychiatry Rep* 6, 411–421.

Metivier, R., Gallais, R., Tiffoche, C., Le Péron, C., Jurkowska, R. Z., Carmouche, R. P., Ibberson, D., Barath, P., Demay, F., Reid, G., Benes, V., Jeltsch, A., Gannon, F., and Salbert, G. (2008). Cyclical DNA methylation of a transcriptionally active promoter. *Nature* 452, 45–50.

Millstein, R. A., and Holmes, A. (2007). Effects of repeated maternal separation on anxiety- and depression-related phenotypes in different mouse strains. *Neurosci. Biobehav. Rev.* 31, 3–17.

Mitchell, B. F., and Taggart, M. J. (2009). Are animal models relevant to key aspects of human parturition? *Am. J. Physiol. Regul. Integr. Comp. Physiol.* 297, R525–R545.

Mouse Genome Sequencing Consortium, Waterston, R. H., Lindblad-Toh, K., Birney, E., Rogers, J., Abril, J. F., Agarwal, P., Agarwala, R., Ainscough, R., Alexandersson, M., An, P., Antonarakis, S. E., Attwood, J., Baertsch, R., Bailey, J., Barlow, K., Beck, S., Berry, E., Birren, B., Bloom, T., Bork, P., Botcherby, M., Bray, N., Brent, M. R., Brown, D. G., Brown, S. D., Bult, C., Burton, J., Butler, J., Campbell, R. D., Carninci, P., Cawley, S., Chiaromonte, F., Chinwalla, A. T., Church, D. M., Clamp, M., Clee, C., Collins, F. S., Cook, L. L., Copley, R. R., Coulson, A., Couronne, O., Cuff, J., Curwen, V., Cutts, T., Daly, M., David, R., Davies, J., Delehaunty, K. D., Deri, J., Dermitzakis, E. T., Dewey, C., Dickens, N. J., Diekhans, M., Dodge, S., Dubchak, I., Dunn, D. M., Eddy, S. R., Elnitski, L., Emes, R. D., Eswara, P., Eyras, E., Felsenfeld, A., Fewell, G. A., Flicek, P., Foley, K., Frankel, W. N., Fulton, L. A., Fulton, R. S., Furey, T. S., Gage, D., Gibbs, R. A., Glusman, G., Gnerre, S., Goldman, N., Goodstadt, L., Grafham, D., Graves, T. A., Green, E. D., Gregory, S., Guigó, R., Guyer, M., Hardison, R. C., Haussler, D., Hayashizaki, Y., Hillier, L. W., Hinrichs, A., Hlavina, W., Holzer, T., Hsu, F., Hua, A., Hubbard, T., Hunt, A., Jackson, I., Jaffe, D. B., Johnson, L. S., Jones, M., Jones, T. A., Joy, A., Kamal, M., Karlsson, E. K., Karolchik, D., Kasprzyk, A., Kawai, J., Keibler, E., Kells, C., Kent, W. J., Kirby, A., Kolbe, D. L., Korf, I., Kucherlapati, R. S., Kulbokas, E. J., Kulp, D., Landers, T., Leger, J. P., Leonard, S., Letunic, I., Levine, R., Li, J., Li, M., Lloyd, C., Lucas, S., Ma, B., Maglott, D. R., Mardis, E. R., Matthews, L., Mauceli, E., Mayer, J. H., McCarthy, M., McCombie, W. R., McLaren, S., McLay, K., McPherson, J. D., Meldrim, J., Meredith, B., Mesirov, J. P., Miller, W., Miner, T. L., Mongin, E., Montgomery, K. T., Morgan, M., Mott, R., Mullikin, J. C., Muzny, D. M., Nash, W. E., Nelson, J. O., Nhan, M. N., Nicol, R., Ning, Z., Nusbaum, C., O'Connor, M. J., Okazaki, Y., Oliver, K., Overton-Larty, E., Pachter, L., Parra, G., Pepin, K. H., Peterson, J., Pevzner, P., Plumb, R., Pohl, C. S., Poliakov, A., Ponce, T. C., Ponting, C. P., Potter, S., Quail, M., Reymond, A., Roe, B. A., Roskin, K. M., Rubin, E. M., Rust, A. G., Santos, R., Sapojnikov, V., Schultz, B., Schultz, J., Schwartz, M. S., Schwartz, S., Scott, C., Seaman, S., Searle, S., Sharpe, T., Sheridan, A., Shownkeen, R., Sims, S., Singer, J. B., Slater, G., Smit, A., Smith, D. R., Spencer, B., Stabenau, A., Stange-Thomann, N., Sugnet, C., Suyama, M., Tesler, G., Thompson, J., Torrents, D., Trevaskis, E., Tromp, J., Ucla, C., Ureta-Vidal, A., Vinson, J. P., Von Niederhausern, A. C., Wade, C. M., Wall, M., Weber, R. J., Weiss, R. B., Wendl, M. C., West, A. P., Wetterstrand, K., Wheeler, R., Whelan, S., Wierzbowski, J., Willey, D., Williams, S., Wilson, R. K., Winter, E., Worley, K. C., Wyman, D., Yang, S., Yang, S. P., Zdobnov, E. M., Zody, M. C., and Lander, E. S. (2002). Initial sequencing and comparative analysis of the mouse genome. *Nature* 420, 520–562.

NECCR, N. (1999). Chronicity of maternal depressive symptoms, maternal sensitivity, and child functioning at 36 months. NICHD Early Child Care Research Network. *Dev. Psychol.* 35, 1297–1310.

Nestler, E. J., and Hyman, S. E. (2010). Animal models of neuropsychiatric disorders. *Nat. Neurosci.* 13, 1161–1169.

Neumann, I. D. (2002). Involvement of the brain oxytocin system in stress coping: interactions with the hypothalamo-pituitary-adrenal axis. *Prog. Brain Res.* 139, 147–162.

Neumann, I. D. (2008). Brain oxytocin: a key regulator of emotional and social behaviours in both females and males. *J. Neuroendocrinol.* 20, 858–865.

Nolten, W. E., Lindheimer, M. D., Rueckert, P. A., Oparil, S., and Ehrlich, E. N. (1980). Diurnal patterns and regulation of cortisol secretion in pregnancy. *J. Clin. Endocrinol. Metab.* 51, 466–472.

O'Connor, T. G., Heron, J., Glover, V., and Alspac Study Team. (2002a). Antenatal anxiety predicts child behavioral/emotional problems independently of postnatal depression. *J. Am. Acad. Child Adolesc. Psychiatry* 41, 1470–1477.

O'Connor, T. G., Heron, J., Golding, J., Beveridge, M., and Glover, V. (2002b). Maternal antenatal anxiety and children's behavioural/emotional problems at 4 years. Report from the Avon longitudinal study of parents and children. *Br. J. Psychiatry* 180, 502–508.

O'Hara, M. W., and Swain, A. M. (1996). Rates and risk of postpartum depression-A meta-analysis. *Int. Rev. Psychiatry* 8, 37–54.

O'Mahony, C. M., Bravo, J. A., Dinan, T. G., and Cryan, J. F. (2010a). Comparison of hippocampal metabotropic glutamate receptor 7 (mGlu7) mRNA levels in two animal models of depression. *Neurosci. Lett.* 482, 137–141.

O'Mahony, C. M., Sweeney, F. F., Daly, E., Dinan, T. G., and Cryan, J. F. (2010b). Restraint stress-induced brain activation patterns in two strains of mice differing in their anxiety behaviour. *Behav. Brain Res.* 213, 148–154.

O'Mahony, C. M., Clarke, G., Gibney, S., Dinan, T. G., and Cryan, J. F. (2011). Strain differences in the neurochemical response to chronic restraint stress in the rat: relevance to depression. *Pharmacol. Biochem. Behav.* 97, 690–699.

Parfitt, D. B., Levin, J. K., Saltstein, K. P., Klayman, A. S., Greer, L. M., and Helmreich, D. L. (2004). Differential early rearing environments can accentuate or attenuate the responses to stress in male C57BL/6 mice. *Brain Res.* 1016, 111–118.

Paulson, J. F., Dauber, S., and Leiferman, J. A. (2006). Individual and combined effects of postpartum depression in mothers and fathers on parenting behavior. *Pediatrics* 118, 659–668.

Pereira, M., Uriarte, N., Agrati, D., Zuluaga, M. J., and Ferreira, A. (2005). Motivational aspects of maternal anxiolysis in lactating rats. *Psychopharmacology (Berl.)* 180, 241–248.

Pokholok, D. K., Harbison, C. T., Levine, S., Cole, M., Hannett, N. M., Lee, T. I., Bell, G. W., Walker, K., Rolfe, P. A., Herbolsheimer, E., Zeitlinger, J., Lewitter, F., Gifford, D. K., and Young, R. A. (2005). Genome-wide map of nucleosome acetylation and methylation in yeast. *Cell* 122, 517–527.

Post, A. M., Weyers, P., Holzer, P., Painsipp, E., Pauli, P., Wultsch, T., Reif, A., and Lesch, K. P. (2011). Gene-environment interaction influences anxiety-like behavior in ethologically based mouse models. *Behav. Brain Res.* 218, 99–105.

Poulter, M. O., Du, L., Zhurov, V., Merali, Z., and Anisman, H. (2010). Plasticity of the GABA(A) receptor subunit cassette in response to stressors in reactive versus resilient mice. *Neuroscience* 165, 1039–1051.

Prakash, P., Merali, Z., Kolajova, M., Tannenbaum, B. M., and Anisman, H. (2006). Maternal factors and monoamine changes in stress-resilient and susceptible mice: cross-fostering effects. *Brain Res.* 1111, 122–133.

Priebe, K., Romeo, R. D., Francis, D. D., Sisti, H. M., Mueller, A., McEwen, B. S., and Brake, W. G. (2005). Maternal influences on adult stress and anxiety-like behavior in C57BL/6J and BALB/cJ mice: a cross-fostering study. *Dev. Psychobiol.* 47, 398–407.

Rahman, A., Iqbal, Z., Bunn, J., Lovel, H., and Harrington, R. (2004). Impact of maternal depression on infant nutritional status and illness: a cohort study. *Arch. Gen. Psychiatry* 61, 946–952.

Razin, A. (1998). CpG methylation chromatin structure and gene silencing–a three-way connection. *EMBO J.* 17, 4905–4908.

Rich-Edwards, J. W., Mohllajee, A. P., Kleinman, K., Hacker, M. R., Majzoub, J., Wright, R. J., and Gillman, M. W. (2008). Elevated midpregnancy corticotropin-releasing hormone is associated with prenatal, but not postpartum, maternal depression. *J. Clin. Endocrinol. Metab.* 93, 1946–1951.

Ring, R. H., Malberg, J. E., Potestio, L., Ping, J., Boikess, S., Luo, B., Schechter, L. E., Rizzo, S., Rahman, Z., and Rosenzweig-Lipson, S. (2006). Anxiolytic-like activity of oxytocin in male mice: behavioral and autonomic evidence, therapeutic implications. *Psychopharmacology (Berl.)* 185, 218–225.

Rogers, D. C., Jones, D. N., Nelson, P. R., Jones, C. M., Quilter, C. A., Robinson, T. L., and Hagan, J. J. (1999). Use of SHIRPA and discriminant analysis to characterise marked differences in the behavioural pheno-

Romeo, R. D., Mueller, A., Sisti, H. M., Ogawa, S., McEwen, B. S., and Brake, W. G. (2003). Anxiety and fear behaviors in adult male and female C57BL/6 mice are modulated by maternal separation. *Horm. Behav.* 43, 561–567.

Ross, L. E., and Dennis, C. L. (2009). The prevalence of postpartum depression amongst women with substance use, an abuse history, or chronic illness: a systematic review. *J. Womens Health* 18, 475–486.

Shanks, N., and Anisman, H. (1988). Stressor-provoked behavioral changes in six strains of mice. *Behav. Neurosci.* 102, 894–905.

Shanks, N., Griffiths, J., and Anisman, H. (1994). Central catecholamine alterations induced by stressor exposure: analyses in recombinant inbred strains of mice. *Behav. Brain Res.* 63, 25–33.

Silverman, M. E., Loudon, H., Safier, M., Protopopescu, X., Leiter, G., Liu, X., and Goldstein, M. (2007). Neural dysfunction in postpartum depression: an fMRI pilot study. *CNS Spectr.* 12, 853–862.

Skinner, M. K., Manikkam, M., and Guerrero-Bosagna, C. (2010). Epigenetic transgenerational actions of environmental factors in disease etiology. *Trends Endocrinol. Metab.* 21, 214–222.

Smith, M. V., Shao, L., Howell, H., Lin, H., and Yonkers, K. A. (2011). Perinatal depression and birth outcomes in a Healthy Start project. *Matern Child Health J.* 15, 401–409.

Swain, J. E. (2008). Baby stimuli and the parent brain: functional neuroimaging of the neural substrates of parent-infant attachment. *Psychiatry (Edgmont)* 5, 28–36.

Swain, J. E., Lorberbaum, J. P., Kose, S., and Strathearn, L. (2007). Brain basis of early parent-infant interactions: psychology, physiology, and in vivo functional neuroimaging studies. *J. Child. Psychol. Psychiatry* 48, 262–287.

Talge, N. M., Neal, C., Glover, V., and Early Stress, Translational Research and Prevention Science Network: Fetal and Neonatal Experience on Child and Adolescent Mental Health. (2007). Antenatal maternal stress and long-term effects on child neurodevelopment: how and why? *J Child Psychol. Psychiatry* 48, 245–261.

Tang, X., Orchard, S. M., and Sanford, L. D. (2002). Home cage activity and behavioral performance in inbred and hybrid mice. *Behav. Brain Res.* 136, 555–569.

Tarantino, L. M., and Bucan, M. (2000). Dissection of behavior and psychiatric disorders using the mouse as a model. *Hum. Mol. Genet.* 9, 953–965.

Trullas, R., and Skolnick, P. (1993). Differences in fear motivated behaviors among inbred mouse strains. *Psychopharmacology (Berl.)* 111, 323–331.

Van den Bergh, B. R., and Marcoen, A. (2004). High antenatal maternal anxiety is related to ADHD symptoms, externalizing problems, and anxiety in 8- and 9-year-olds. *Child Dev.* 75, 1085–1097.

Van den Bergh, B. R., Mennes, M., Oosterlaan, J., Stevens, V., Stiers, P., Marcoen, A., and Lagae, L. (2005). High antenatal maternal anxiety is related to impulsivity during performance on cognitive tasks in 14- and 15-year-olds. *Neurosci. Biobehav. Rev.* 29, 259–269.

Wan, M. W., and Green, J. (2009). The impact of maternal psychopathology on child-mother attachment. *Arch. Womens Ment. Health* 12, 123–134.

Weaver, I. C., Cervoni, N., Champagne, F. A., D'Alessio, A. C., Sharma, S., Seckl, J. R., Dymov, S., Szyf, M., and Meaney, M. J. (2004). Epigenetic programming by maternal behavior. *Nat. Neurosci.* 7, 847–854.

Weinberg, M. K., and Tronick, E. Z. (1998). The impact of maternal psychiatric illness on infant development. *J. Clin. Psychiatry* 59(Suppl. 2), 53–61.

Yan, H. C., Cao, X., Das, M., Zhu, X. H., and Gao, T. M. (2010). Behavioral animal models of depression. *Neurosci. Bull.* 26, 327–337.

Zacharko, R. M., and Anisman, H. (1989). "Pharmacological, biochemical and behavioral analyses of depression: animal models," in *Animal Models of Depression*, eds G. F. Koob, C. L. Ehlers, and D. J. Kupfer (Boston: Birkhauser), 204–238.

Impaired neural synchrony in the theta frequency range in adolescents at familial risk for schizophrenia

Franc C. L. Donkers*, Shane R. Schwikert, Anna M. Evans, Katherine M. Cleary, Diana O. Perkins and Aysenil Belger

Department of Psychiatry, University of North Carolina at Chapel Hill, Chapel Hill, NC, USA

*Correspondence:
Franc C. L. Donkers, Department of Psychiatry, University of North Carolina at Chapel Hill, Campus Box 7160, 367 Medical School Wing C, Chapel Hill, NC 27599, USA.
e-mail: franc_donkers@med.unc.edu

Puberty is a critical period for the maturation of the fronto-limbic and fronto-striate brain circuits responsible for executive function and affective processing. Puberty also coincides with the emergence of the prodromal signs of schizophrenia, which may indicate an association between these two processes. Time-domain analysis and wavelet based time–frequency analysis was performed on electroencephalographic (EEG) data of 30 healthy control (HC) subjects and 24 individuals at familial risk (FR) for schizophrenia. All participants were between the ages of 13 and 18 years and were carefully matched for age, gender, ethnicity, education, and Tanner Stage. Electrophysiological recordings were obtained from 32 EEG channels while participants performed a visual oddball task, where they identified rare visual targets among standard "scrambled" images and rare aversive and neutral distracter pictures. The time-domain analysis showed that during target processing the FR group showed smaller event-related potentials in the P2 and P3 range as compared to the HC group. In addition, EEG activity in the theta (4–8 Hz) frequency range was significantly reduced during target processing in the FR group. Inefficient cortical information processing during puberty may be an early indicator of altered brain function in adolescents at FR for schizophrenia and may represent a vulnerability marker for illness onset. Longitudinal assessments will have to determine their predictive value for illness onset in populations at FR for psychotic illness.

Keywords: schizophrenia, familial risk, P300, ERP, wavelet analysis, time–frequency decomposition, theta frequency, phase-locking factor

INTRODUCTION

Little is known about how or why psychotic disorders like schizophrenia develop. Although structural brain abnormalities occurring early in life may be necessary for the future emergence of psychotic symptoms, the notion that psychotic symptoms do not typically manifest until after puberty has led researchers to believe that neurodevelopmental processes active during this period may also play a role in the pathogenesis of schizophrenia (Feinberg, 1982; Weinberger, 1987). Adolescence represents a period of active brain development, during which increases in neuronal efficiency are accompanied by a reduction (i.e., pruning) of excess synapses and by myelination of axonal connections in regions critical for higher order cognition, particularly the prefrontal cortex (Huttenlocher, 1979; Keshavan et al., 1994; Woods, 1998). The behavioral expression of schizophrenia-related neural disturbances also seems to vary with maturation, and becomes more "psychosis-like" the closer to the onset of a psychotic episode (Cannon, 2005). The fact that schizophrenia is increasingly viewed as a neurodevelopmental disorder suggests that potential precursors to psychotic illness may be detectable in individuals at familial risk (FR) for developing schizophrenia. Although, the idea of examining individuals at FR for developing schizophrenia is not new (e.g., Fish et al., 1992; Marcus et al., 1993; McNeil et al., 1993) to date there has been relatively little study into the neurodevelopmental changes occurring around puberty, and comparing those to the changes occurring in subjects at FR for developing schizophrenia. Focusing attention on young at-risk individuals provides a unique window on the unfolding pathophysiology of the illness, and does not suffer from the clouding effects of disease chronicity or long-term treatment that plague studies of patients with established illness. Longitudinal assessments of young at-risk relatives also provides an opportunity to determine whether biological or biobehavioral differences are present prior to typical onset of schizophrenia in those individuals who progress. These differences hold the potential to serve as vulnerability markers or predictors of illness, and may inform targets for prevention.

Electroencephalography (EEG) has long been used in search for biomarkers of schizophrenia through the analysis of event-related potentials (ERPs). ERPs can provide detailed information about neuronal events underlying sensory, cognitive, or motor functions. One of the most reliably demonstrated ERP abnormalities in schizophrenia is the amplitude reduction of the P3 (e.g., Ford, 1999; Jeon and Polich, 2003). The P3 is a late scalp-positive ERP component usually recorded in an auditory or visual "oddball" experimental paradigm in which a subject detects an infrequent deviant or task-relevant "target" stimulus randomly presented within a series of frequent non-target or "standard" stimuli. The P3 in oddball task paradigms has been associated with attention and memory processes (e.g., Donchin and Coles, 1998; Polich and Herbst, 2000). Evidence for the idea that the P3 indexes a genetic and biological vulnerability to schizophrenia has come from family based high-risk studies showing that this ERP component is also impaired in clinically unaffected family members who, by reason of their family history, are at high-risk for developing schizophrenia (see Bramon et al., 2005 for a meta-analysis). Few studies have examined the P3 in adolescents at FR for schizophrenia and the results of these studies have been mixed (e.g., Friedman et al., 1988; Schreiber et al., 1992). However, recent advances in neurophysiological techniques provide new opportunities to measure abnormal brain function in adolescents at FR for schizophrenia. Traditional ERP analysis assumes that the EEG response to relevant task processing is contained within a background of irrelevant neuroelectric noise. By averaging a large number of EEG trials, the background neuroelectric noise is minimized allowing only the "relevant" neural signal to remain. However, a growing body of evidence suggests that the activity removed in the ERP averaging process is not random or irrelevant, and that event-related changes in the magnitude and phase of the EEG signal across all frequencies may be relevant to information processing (e.g. Kolev and Yordanova, 1997; Demiralp et al., 1999; Makeig et al., 2004). A more thorough understanding of neuronal events can be gained through time–frequency decomposition of (single-trial) EEG data.

Time–frequency decomposition comprises many methods and can reveal the time evolution of the magnitude and phase of the EEG signals in different frequency bands in response to particular events. When the magnitude values of each time–frequency point are squared and then averaged over trials, all the signal change in the post-event period is captured irrespective of their phase angles. This measure quantifies the total activity [or total power (TP)] after event onset and is comprised of both phase-locked and non-phase-locked event-related EEG activity. Computing the time–frequency transform of the trial-averaged ERP and then squaring the magnitude values associated with each time–frequency point captures activity that is phase-locked to the event only since averaging across trials tends to cancel out the non-phase-locked activity [also known as evoked power (EP)]. When the magnitude values of each time–frequency point are unit normalized and then averaged across trials, a measure of cross-trial phase synchrony [or phase-locking factor (PLF)] is obtained. This measure describes the consistency of phase angles with respect to an event's onset. Time–frequency decomposition of the ERP to target trials in oddball task paradigms has shown that the late scalp-positive P3 ERP occupies the delta (1–4 Hz) and theta (4–8 Hz) frequency range (e.g. Kolev et al., 1997; Spencer and Polich, 1999; Demiralp and Ademoglu, 2001) and abnormal activity in these low-frequency ranges has been observed during oddball task paradigms in patients with schizophrenia (e.g., Roschke and Fell, 1997; Ergen et al., 2008; Ford et al., 2008; Doege et al., 2009). Slow frequency EEG activity has been associated with long range interactions in larger scale brain networks (von Stein et al., 2000). Since the core cognitive domains affected in schizophrenia are the attention and memory systems that involve the activation of larger scale brain networks, it has been hypothesized that the cognitive deficits observed in schizophrenia can be attributed to abnormalities in the synchronization and efficiency of neural processes that integrate information from different brain regions. Time–frequency decomposition of (single-trial) EEG data could provide additional insight into whether abnormalities in the synchronization and efficiency of neural processes are compromised in schizophrenia.

In the current study we employed a visual oddball task in conjunction with EEG measurements to assess brain function associated with executive processing in a group of adolescents at FR for schizophrenia and a group of adolescents without such risk. We applied traditional time-domain analysis and wavelet based time–frequency analysis to the EEG data obtained from target response trials in order to assess potential group differences in ERPs and time–frequency decomposition measures between both groups. We hypothesized that compared to the HC group the FR group would show a reduction of the P3 amplitude accompanied by a reduction of low-frequency EEG activity in response to the target stimuli. We further aimed to establish whether these reductions are produced by deficits in (a) synchronization mechanisms, which would be reflected by a decrease in the EP and PLF measures, (b) by a decrease in the power of signals generated by underlying neural mechanisms, which would be reflected in a decrease in the TP measure, or (c) by a combination of both.

MATERIALS AND METHODS
PARTICIPANTS

Subjects consisted of 24 adolescents at FR for schizophrenia and 30 HC subjects. All subjects were between the ages of 13–18 years and in Tanner Stage 3 or higher according to the Tanner Stage growth chart (Marshall and Tanner, 1969, 1970). Participants with FR were recruited from a referral network including community-based health providers and the UNC PRIME (Prevention through Risk Identification, Management and Education) research clinic. No participants with FR were seeking treatment. Controls were recruited from local schools and the general community. The groups did not significantly differ according to age, gender, race, education, handedness, and Tanner Stage (see Table 1). FR was defined as having a first-degree family member (sibling or parent) with a diagnosis of schizophrenia or schizoaffective disorder, as determined by the Family Interview for Genetics conducted with the participant's parent (Maxwell, 1992). Diagnosis of the affected relative was confirmed by the Structured Interview for DSM-IV Disorders for adults and the Washington University Kiddie Schedule for Affective Disorders and Schizophrenia for children (Orvaschel et al., 1982). Of the 24 subjects with FR, six had an affected parent and 18 had an affected sibling. Race was classified by participant self-report at the time of screening by options defined by the investigators in order to match between groups. Tanner Stages were determined by a physical exam performed by a licensed medical physician, a questionnaire answered by a parent, or a cartoon illustration depicting the stages completed by the participant.

Table 1 | Demographic and clinical characteristics of study groups.

Characteristic	Familial risk subjects (N = 24)	Healthy control subjects (N = 30)	One-way ANOVA or Chi-square test		
			F or χ^2	df	p
Age	16.29 ± 1.45	15.64 ± 1.35	2.85	1, 52	0.097
Gender (m/f)	10/14	11/19	0.140	1	0.708
Handedness (r/l)	19/5	26/4	0.540	1	0.462
Education (years)	9.46 ± 1.84	8.87 ± 1.36	1.85	1, 52	0.180
Tanner stage	3.88 ± 0.711	3.67 ± 0.711	1.145	1, 52	0.290
SCALE OF PRODROMAL SYMPTOMS					
Positive subscale	2.42 ± 2.45	1 ± 1.66	6.39	1, 52	0.015
Negative subscale	3.42 ± 3.36	0.7 ± 1.37	16.29	1, 52	<0.001
Disorganization subscale	1.38 ± 1.79	0.38 ± 0.85	7.45	1, 52	0.009
General subscale	2.04 ± 2.42	0.6 ± 1.13	8.37	1, 52	0.006

Exclusion criteria for the FR group included presence of a past or current DSM-IV Axis I psychotic or bipolar affective disorder. Because FR for schizophrenia is associated with a high likelihood of premorbid disorders (Keshavan et al., 2008), we chose not to exclude high-risk individuals with other Axis I disorders. In our sample, 14 participants with FR had other diagnoses including attention-deficit hyperactivity disorder, learning disorder, conduct disorder, adjustment disorder, specific phobia, depressive disorder – not otherwise specified, and anxiety disorder. Other exclusion criteria for the FR group included central nervous system disorder (e.g., seizure disorder) or mental retardation (IQ less than 65), current treatment with an antipsychotic medication, and past history of over 12 weeks lifetime cumulative treatment with an antipsychotic. Exclusion criteria for the control group included history of a DSM-IV Axis I psychiatric disorder, any psychiatric disorder in a first-degree relative, neurological disorder, and substance abuse disorder. After complete description of the study to the subjects, written informed assent (or consent, if age 18) was obtained, with parents providing written consent as approved by the University of North Carolina at Chapel Hill Institutional Review Board.

The presence of positive, negative, disorganization, and general symptoms was assessed for all participants using the schedule of prodromal symptoms (SOPS; Miller et al., 1999). The FR group showed significantly more symptoms than the control group in positive, negative, disorganization, and general symptoms (Table 1).

EXPERIMENTAL PROCEDURE

Participants were seated in a dimly illuminated and sound attenuated room 80 cm in front of a computer monitor. Electrophysiological data were collected while subjects performed a visual oddball task with novel distracters. Subjects attended to a series of four types of visual stimuli and where required to press a button to the infrequently occurring target stimulus only. The four stimulus types consisted of frequent "standard" scrambled images (N = 1040, 87.4%), aversive novel images (N = 50, 4.2%), neutral novel images (N = 50, 4.2%), and simple colored "target" circles (N = 50, 4.2%). The aversive and neutral novel stimuli were chosen from the International Affective Picture System database, which consists of complex pictures with standardized ratings from adults for arousal (calm to exiting) and valence (unpleasant to pleasant; Lang et al., 2005). The aversive IAPS pictures were selected to be age-appropriate for the children and adolescents in the study. The average valence and arousal ratings for the aversive stimuli were 3.38 (SD = 1.78) and 6.14 (SD = 2.08), respectively. Average valence and arousal ratings for the neutral stimuli were 6.21 (SD = 0.26) and 3.72 (SD = 2.15). All images were pseudo-randomized, with target or novel stimuli never occurring twice in a row. All stimuli were presented centrally for 500 ms on a black background, with a white fixation cross appearing during inter-stimulus intervals. The stimuli were presented on an Intel Core2 Quad computer, using Presentation software (Neurobehavioral Systems, Inc., Albany, CA, USA). The images occupied a maximum of 11.4° of visual angle vertically and 16.2° of visual angle horizontally. The inter-stimulus interval varied from 1050 to 1450 ms, with an average of 1200 ms. The task consisted of 40 unique aversive images (with 10 images being repeated twice, resulting in a total of 50 aversive images), 50 unique neutral images, 50 unique targets, and 140 unique "standard" images which repeated throughout the experiment. Total task time was 25 min, divided up into 10 time blocks of approximately two and a half minutes each. Here we report on the results obtained from the target trials only. Results for the novel stimuli will be presented elsewhere.

ELECTROPHYSIOLOGICAL RECORDING

The EEG was recorded from 30 electrode positions (Fp1, Fp2, F7, F3, Fz, F4, F8, FT7, FC3, FCz, FC4, FT8, T7, C3, Cz, C4, T8, TP7, CP3, CPz, CP4, TP8, P7, P3, Pz, P4, P8, O1, Oz, and O2) using an elastic cap (Electro-Cap International Inc.). The right mastoid served as the reference electrode and AFz as the ground. Bipolar recordings of the vertical and horizontal electro-oculogram were obtained by electrodes placed above and below the right eye and on the outer canthus of each eye, respectively. The EEG and electro-oculogram were amplified, bandpass filtered between

0.15 and 70 Hz (notch filter at 60 Hz), and digitized at 500 Hz. The EEG was acquired with a Neuroscan 4.3 (Neurosoft, Inc., Sterling, VA, USA) system and analyzed with Neuroscan Edit 4.4 and custom MATLAB scripts built on the open source EEGLAB (Delorme and Makeig, 2004) and FieldTrip (Oostenveld et al., 2011) toolboxes.

BEHAVIORAL DATA ANALYSIS

Behavioral performance measures consisted of the percentage of correctly detected targets (hit rate) and the time needed to respond correctly to targets (reaction time). Only button-press responses occurring between 200 and 1000 ms after target onset were considered correct responses.

EEG DATA ANALYSIS

Electroencephalography data sets from each participant were corrected for eye-movements using regression analysis as implemented in Neuroscan Edit 4.4 (Semlitsch et al., 1986) Continuous EEG data from all channels were subsequently segmented into epochs ranging from 4 s before target stimulus onset to 4 s after onset. The extended length of the epochs was necessary in order to perform the time–frequency analyses. EEG epochs associated with incorrect behavioral responses and responses occurring faster than 200 ms or slower than 1000 ms after target onset and containing amplitudes exceeding ±100 μV at any scalp electrode were excluded. Finally, epochs containing abnormally distributed data (i.e., joint probability or kurtosis >5 SD from expected mean values) were rejected. Extended infomax independent component analysis (ICA) using a weight change <10-7 as stop criterion was applied to the continuous data of one subject to remove heart rate artifact (Jung et al., 2000). Independent components representing heart rate were removed from the EEG data by back-projecting all but these components. Channel F7 was interpolated on two subjects and channel FP1 was interpolated on another subject to remove artifact caused by faulty electrodes. After data pre-processing, an average of 41 trials for the FR group and 45 trials for the control group remained for final analysis [$F(1,52) = 4.57$, $p = 0.037$].

Time-domain computations

Baseline correction was implemented by subtracting the average amplitude computed from the 200 ms interval immediately preceding the stimulus onset from each epoch. ERPs were obtained by averaging the baseline corrected EEG epochs for targets of each participant. After filtering the data with a low-pass 15 Hz filter an automatic peak detection procedure identified the most positive peak ranging from 300 to 700 ms to quantify the P3 amplitudes. A second time window identified the most positive peak ranging from 150 to 300 ms to quantify the P2 amplitudes[1]. Both peaks were identified on electrode channels F3, Fz, F4, C3, Cz, C4, P3, Pz, and P4 and were then manually checked to ensure correct selection.

Time–frequency computations

Time–frequency analysis was performed using a complex Morlet wavelet transform as implemented by the FieldTrip toolbox for MATLAB. Conceptually, a Morlet wavelet transformation is related to a windowed short-term Fourier transformation. By applying the wavelet transform to successive intervals of EEG data, both temporal and spectral information can be extracted from the signal. The Morlet wavelet $f(t)$ is obtained by multiplying a complex sinusoidal waveform with a Gaussian envelope. The Morlet wavelet is characterized by a center frequency f_0, a temporal SD σ_t, a center position t_c and a width W: $f(t|t_c,f_0,W) = e^{i2\pi f_0 t}e^{-(t-t_c)^2/2\sigma_t^2}$ $|t-t_c| < W$, and f is zero otherwise. The Morlet wavelet is simultaneously localized in time (σ_t) and frequency (σ_f). These quantities are related as $\sigma_t = 1/(2\pi\sigma_f)$, therefore an increased temporal specificity of the transform compromises spectral specificity, and *vice versa*. In the time–frequency literature (see Roach and Mathalon, 2008, for an overview), the parameters σ_t and the width W of the wavelet are commonly expressed in terms of two parameters: $c = f_0/\sigma_f = 2\pi(\sigma_t/T_0)$ (or 2π multiplied by the number of cycles that fit in the Gaussian envelope) and $m = W/\sigma_t$, which is the width of the wavelet in terms of the width of the Gaussian envelope. In this analysis we used $c = 7$ (more than one cycle in the Gaussian envelope) and $m = 3$ (a wavelet width that is three times the length of the Gaussian envelope). These values represent an appropriate trade-off between frequency and time resolution (Roach and Mathalon, 2008).

The Morlet wavelet was convolved with the EEG data at specified time (t_c) and frequency (f_0) center points, yielding for each trial n a wavelet spectrogram $WS_n(t_c, f_0)$; a two dimensional matrix of complex values. The measure of TP, as a function of frequency and time relative to stimulus onset, was derived by taking the squared absolute value of each point in the wavelet spectrogram and subsequently averaging across trials. We also estimated the PLF, which quantifies phase consistency across trials in response to the event (Tallon-Baudry et al., 1996). To calculate PLF, for each trial the complex value of the wavelet spectrogram is normalized to unit length and averaged across trials, taking the absolute value of the product. In mathematical terms: $\text{PLF}(t_c,f_0) = |\sum_{n=1}^{N_t} e^{i\varphi_n(t_c,f_0)}|/\sum_{n=1}^{N_t} |e^{i\varphi_n(t_c,f_0)}|$, here N_t is the number of trials and |.| denotes the absolute value. A PLF of 1 represents complete phase coherence, whereas a value of 0 reflects a completely random distribution of phases across trials. The measure of EP was obtained by applying the Morlet wavelet transformation to the averaged ERP calculated using epochs aligned to the onset of the visual targets.

The time–frequency analysis procedure was applied using a 1300-ms (ranging from −500 ms before to 800 ms after) window within each epoch, whose location was shifted in steps of 10 ms. The wavelet's central frequencies f_0 ranged from 1.5 to 60 Hz in 0.5 Hz steps. In order to highlight changes in TP, it was divided by the mean baseline $\text{TP}_{\text{baseline}}$ (the power in the 500-ms preceding stimulus onset, averaged across trials) and expressed in decibels, specifically $10 \log_{10}(\text{TP}/\text{TP}_{\text{baseline}})$. Therefore, the color scale in the TP figures reflects the deviation of the power from the baseline in decibels at each frequency and time point from

---

[1] Based on previous research in adults with schizophrenia our main ERP of interest was the P3 ERP. Since our data also seemed to show a group difference around the time of the P2 peak we also quantified group differences in this earlier time window.

the stimulus. For each subject, the maximum value of TP, PLF, and EP was identified during an early (150–300 ms) and a later (300–700 ms) time window after target onset at electrode locations F3, Fz, F4, C3, Cz, C4, P3, Pz, and P4. These two analyses windows were centered on the maxima of the P2 and the P3 peak respectively. Five frequency bands were analyzed: 1.5–3.5 Hz (delta), 4–8 Hz (theta), 8–16 Hz (alpha), 16–30 Hz (beta), and 30–50 Hz (gamma). These frequency windows were selected *a priori* based on the well know "natural frequencies" that occur in the brain in response to various cognitive functions (Basar et al., 2001). For each subject the TP, PLF, and EP mean values were quantified as the mean value in a window surrounding the TP, PLF, and EP peak. The window width was specifically tailored to each frequency band with slower oscillating bands having a larger window width than faster oscillating ones (i.e., ±95 ms for delta, ±75 ms for theta, ±50 ms for alpha, ±30 ms for beta, and ±20 ms for gamma).

STATISTICAL ANALYSIS

All statistical analyses were performed using SPSS (SPSS Inc., Chicago, IL, USA). In order to cope with the different correlations between electrode sites (Vasey and Thayer, 1987) individual means and latencies of EP, PLF, and TP for each frequency band of interest were subjected to a repeated measure multivariate analyses of variance (MANOVA) with Region (Frontal, Central, Parietal) and Laterality (Left, Middle, Right) as the within-subjects factors and Group as the between subjects factor. Follow-up separate ANOVAs were conducted for each electrode position to examine further the main effect of group for that electrode position. ERP amplitude and latency measures were subjected to the same analysis. Cohen's d was computed to determine effect sizes if results on individual electrodes were significant.

RESULTS
PERFORMANCE DATA

Table 2 shows behavioral performance data for both subject groups. Reaction times to target stimuli did not differ between groups $[F(1,52) = 0.87, p = 0.356]$ but subjects with a FR for schizophrenia had a significant lower hit rate to target stimuli $[F(1,52) = 8.90, p = 0.004]$ than the HC group.

TIME-DOMAIN DATA

Figure 1 depicts the ERPs to target stimuli at electrodes F3, Fz, F4, C3, Cz, C4, P3, Pz, and P4 for both groups.

Table 2 | Means and SD (in parentheses) of behavioral performance data.

Group	Reaction time	Hit rate
HC	521 (81)	**97(4)***
FR	543 (99)	**91(10)**

HC, healthy control; FR, familial risk. Reaction time is given in milliseconds after stimulus presentation. Hit rate is given in percent correct.
*Bold numberings denote significant group difference with p < 0.05.

P2

P2 peak amplitude was larger at the central and parietal electrode locations than at the frontal electrode locations $[F(2,51) = 10.81, p < 0.001]$, and was larger at the midline electrode locations than at the lateral electrode locations $[F(2,51) = 7.68, p = 0.001]$ for both groups. *Post hoc* analyses revealed that P2 amplitude was significantly smaller in the FR group than in the HC group on electrode locations: F3 $[F(1,52) = 5.42, p = 0.024; d = 0.65]$, Fz $[F(1,52) = 4.67, p = 0.035; d = 0.60]$, F4 $[F(1,52) = 5.83, p = 0.020; d = 0.67]$, C3 $[F(1,52) = 5.89, p = 0.019; d = 0.68]$, C4 $[F(1,52) = 4.73, p = 0.034; d = 0.61]$, Cz $[F(1,52) = 4.58, p = 0.037; d = 0.60]$, P3 $[F(1,52) = 5.59, p = 0.022; d = 0.66]$, and Pz $[F(1,52) = 5.65, p = 0.021; d = 0.66]$. There were no group effects observed for P2 latency at these electrode locations.

P3

The P3 amplitude showed the characteristic scalp distribution with a parietal maximum $[F(2,51) = 86.04, p < 0.001]$ and midline amplitudes being larger than lateral amplitudes $[F(2,51) = 12.40, p < 0.001]$ for both groups (e.g., Duncan-Johnson and Donchin, 1977). *Post hoc* analyses showed that the P3 amplitude was larger in the HC group than in the FR group for the parietal electrode locations only: P3 $[F(1,52) = 4.68, p < 0.035; d = 0.60]$, Pz $[F(1,52) = 4.40, p < 0.041; d = 0.59]$, P4 $[F(1,52) = 5.32, p = 0.025; d = 0.64]$. No differences in P3 latency were observed. Means and SD of the P2 and the P3 amplitude and latency for nine electrode channels are listed in **Table A1** in Appendix.

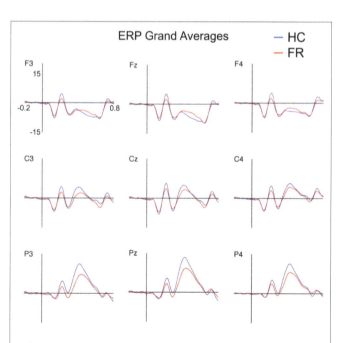

FIGURE 1 | Grand-average event-related potentials to targets (15 Hz low-pass filtered) for the healthy control (HC) and familial risk (FR) groups for electrodes F3, Fz, F4, C3, Cz, C4, P3, Pz, and P4. Amplitude is indicated on the y-axis and ranges from +20 to −10 μV (positive plotted upward). Time is indicated on the x-axis and ranges from −0.2 to 0.8 s. Target onset is at time = 0 s.

TIME–FREQUENCY DATA

Figures 2–4 depict group comparisons of EP, PLF, and TP for both groups. Since group differences in EP, PLF, and TP were most prominent in the lower frequency ranges we restricted our statistical analyses to the delta, theta and alpha frequency ranges. Means and latencies for the EP, PLF, and TP peaks for the early (150–300 ms) and late (300–700 ms) time windows were assessed across delta, theta, and alpha frequency bands at nine electrode positions are listed in **Tables A2** and **A3** in Appendix.

Evoked Power

Figure 2 shows EP plots for nine electrode locations for both groups. Group differences in EP values were observed in the theta frequency range only. For both groups EP_{theta} in the early time window was largest at the central electrode locations $[F(2,51) = 10.50, p < 0.001]$ and was larger at the midline electrode positions compared to the lateral electrode positions $[F(2,51) = 90.57, p < 0.001]$. Post hoc analyses showed that compared to the HC group EP_{theta} was significantly reduced in the FR group on electrode position Pz only $[F(1,52) = 5.27, p = 0.026; d = 0.64]$. EP_{theta} in the later time window was also largest at the central electrode locations $[F(2,51) = 11.98, p < 0.001]$ and was larger at the midline electrode position compared to the lateral electrode locations $[F(2,51) = 95.10, p < 0.001]$. Post hoc analyses showed that compared to the HC group EP_{theta} was significantly reduced in the FR group on electrode position Pz only $[F(1,52) = 4.98, p = 0.030; d = 0.62]$. There were no group differences in EP_{theta} peak latency during the early time window but during the later time window EP_{theta} peaked slightly earlier in the HC group than in the FR group on electrode positions Cz $[F(1,52) = 4.43, p = 0.040; d = -0.57]$ and Pz $[F(1,52) = 4.20, p = 0.045; d = -0.58]$.

Phase-Locking Factor

Figure 3 shows PLF plots for nine electrode locations for both groups. Group differences in PLF values were also confined to the theta frequency range. For both groups PLF_{theta} during the earlier time window was largest across the central electrode locations $[F(2,51) = 35.02, p < 0.001]$ and was smaller at the left electrode locations compared to the central and right electrode locations $[F(2,51) = 21.95, p < 0.001]$. Post hoc analyses showed that PLF_{theta} during the early time window was significantly smaller in the FR group than in the HC group on electrode locations F3 $[F(1,52) = 4.47, p = 0.039; d = 0.59]$, Fz $[F(1,52) = 4.58, p = 0.037; d = 0.60]$, F4 $[F(1,52) = 5.38, p = 0.024; d = 0.65]$, C3 $[F(1,52) = 4.72, p = 0.034; d = 0.61]$, Cz $[F(1,52) = 6.27, p = 0.015; d = 0.70]$, and C4 $[F(1,52) = 4.67, p = 0.035; d = 0.60]$. PLF_{theta} during the later time window was also largest at the central electrode locations $[F(2,51) = 23.89, p < 0.001]$ and was smaller at the left electrode locations compared to the central and right electrode locations $[F(2,51) = 9.58, p < 0.001]$ for both groups. Post hoc analyses showed that PLF_{theta} during the later time window was significantly smaller in the FR group than in the HC group on electrode locations F3 $[F(1,52) = 4.16, p = 0.046; d = 0.57]$, Fz $[F(1,52) = 5.29, p = 0.025; d = 0.64]$, F4 $[F(1,52) = 7.04, p = 0.011; d = 0.74]$, C3 $[F(1,52) = 4.03, p = 0.050; d = 0.56]$, and Cz $[F(1,52) = 5.55, p = 0.022; d = 0.66]$. There were no group effects observed for PLF_{theta} latency at these electrode locations during either the early or the later time window.

Total Power

Figure 4 shows TP plots for nine electrode locations for both groups. Group differences in TP values were observed in the alpha frequency range only. For both groups TP_{alpha} during the early time window was most negative (i.e., reduced compared to baseline activity) at the parietal electrode locations $[F(2,51) = 22.76, p < 0.001]$ and was more negative at the left and right electrode positions compared to the midline electrode positions $[F(2,51) = 9.59, p < 0.001]$. Post hoc analyses showed that TP_{alpha} in the earlier time window was significantly less negative in the FR group than in the HC group on electrode positions P3 $[F(1,52) = 7.08, p = 0.010; d = -0.74]$, Pz $[F(1,52) = 7.01, p = 0.11; d = -0.74]$, and P4 $[F(1,52) = 5.59, p = 0.022; d = -0.66]$. TP_{alpha} during the later time window was also most negative (i.e., reduced compared to baseline activity) at the parietal electrode locations $[F(2,51) = 90.91, p < 0.001]$ and more negative at the left and right electrode positions than at the midline electrode positions $[F(2,51) = 3.99, p = 0.021]$ for both groups. Post hoc analyses showed that TP_{alpha} in the later time window was significantly less negative in the FR group than in the HC group on electrode position Pz only $[F(1,52) = 5.07, p = 0.029; d = -63]$. There were no group effects observed for TP_{alpha} peak latency at these electrode locations during either the early or the later time window.

ADDITIONAL ANALYSES

In order to determine if there was a relationship between clinical variables and the electrophysiological measures, we computed correlations between the SOPS scores (positive, negative, organizational, and general scales) and the P2, P3, EP, PLF, and TP peaks for the delta, theta and alpha frequency bands for both groups. However, none of these correlations were significant below a p-level of 0.01.

To differentiate the effects of comorbidity in the FR group, all analyses were also conducted on a subgroup that had no other psychopathologies. In spite of the fact that the remaining FR group was small ($N = 10$) our most important result remained stable. That is, PLF in the theta frequency range was still significantly smaller across the majority of the frontal and central electrode positions during both the early time window: F3 $[F(1,38) = 3.22, p = 0.080]$, Fz $[F(1,38) = 4.13, p = 0.049]$, F4 $[F(1,38) = 4.78, p = 0.035]$, C3 $[F(1,38) = 4.58, p = 0.039]$, Cz $[F(1,38) = 4.85, p = 0.034]$ and C4 $[F(1,38) = 4.43, p = 0.042]$ and the later time window: F3 $[F(1,38) = 2.97, p = 0.093]$, Fz $[F(1,38) = 4.00, p = 0.053]$, F4 $[F(1,38) = 6.30, p = 0.016]$, C3 $[F(1,38) = 4.30, p = 0.045]$, Cz $[F(1,38) = 4.21, p = 0.047]$ and C4 $[F(1,38) = 4.71, p = 0.036]$.

DISCUSSION

The aim of this study was to examine whether neurophysiological response patterns associated with executive processing in a

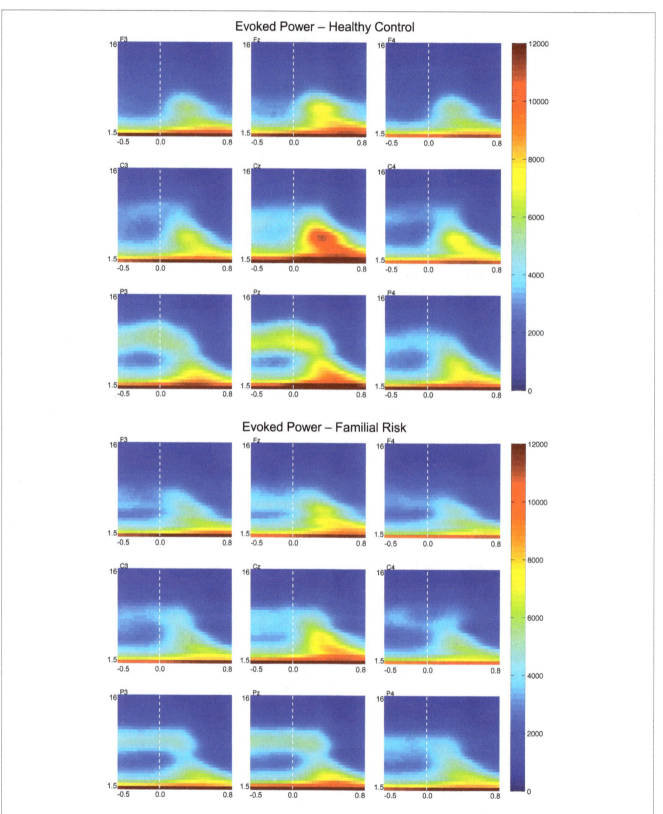

FIGURE 2 | Grand-average evoked power (EP) time–frequency transformations for healthy control (HC) and familial risk (FR) groups at electrodes F3, Fz, F4, C3, Cz, C4, P3, Pz, and P4. EEG frequency is indicated on the y-axis for all panels ranging from 1.5 Hz to 16 Hz. Time is indicated on the x-axis and ranges from −0.5 to 0.8 s. Target onset is at time = 0.0 s. EP value is indicated on the far right and ranges from 0 to 12000. Greater EP values with respect to target onset are shown in warm colors.

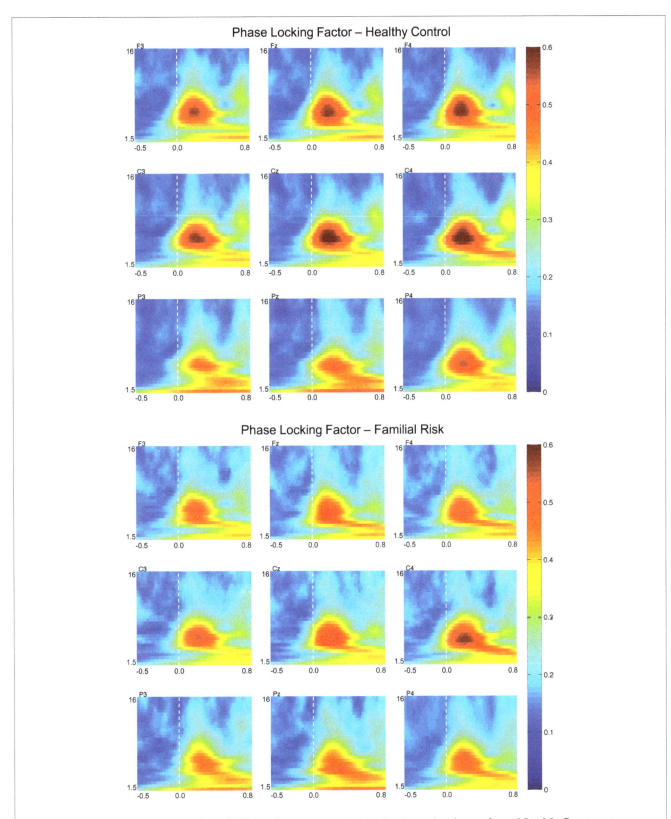

FIGURE 3 | Grand-average phase-locking factor (PLF) time–frequency transformations for healthy control (HC) and familial risk (FR) groups at electrodes F3, Fz, F4, C3, Cz, C4, P3, Pz, and P4. EEG frequency is indicated on the y-axis for all panels ranging from 1.5 Hz to 16 Hz. Time is indicated on the x-axis and ranges from −0.5 to 0.8 s. Target onset is at time = 0.0 s. PLF value is indicated on the far right and ranges from 0 to 0.6. Greater PLF values with respect to target onset are shown in warm colors.

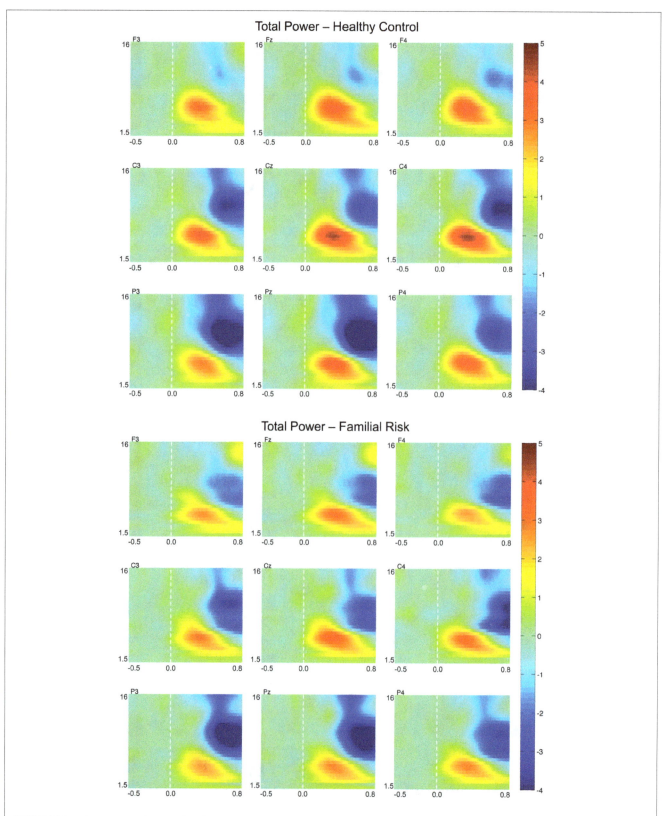

FIGURE 4 | Grand-average total power time–frequency transformations for healthy control (HC) and familial risk (FR) groups at electrodes F3, Fz, F4, C3, Cz, C4, P3, Pz, and P4. EEG frequency is indicated on the y-axis for all panels ranging from 1.5 Hz to 16 Hz. Time is indicated on the x-axis and ranges from −0.5 to 0.8 s. Target onset is at time = 0.0 s. TP value is indicated on the far right and ranges from −4 to 5. Greater TP values with respect to target onset are shown in warm colors.

group of adolescents at FR for schizophrenia would differ from a group of adolescents without such risk. We examined traditional time-domain measures and wavelet based time–frequency domain measures of EEG data obtained during target trials in a visual oddball task. The results demonstrated that adolescents at FR for schizophrenia process target stimuli in an oddball task differently from healthy control subjects. The ERP results showed that the FR group had diminished P2 amplitudes across the frontal and central electrode locations as well as diminished P3 amplitudes across the parietal electrode locations compared to the healthy control (HC) group. Wavelet transformation of the averaged ERP to target trials showed that EP in the theta frequency range (4–8 Hz) was significantly reduced in the FR group at the midline parietal electrode location. Wavelet transformation of the single-trial target data showed that PLF in the theta frequency range was significantly smaller in the FR group than in the HC group across central and frontal electrode locations. The single-trial based TP computations did not show differences between groups in the theta frequency range but showed differences in the alpha frequency range instead. The FR group exhibited less of a reduction in alpha TP after target stimulus occurrence at parietal electrode locations than the HC group.

Significant group effects were observed in the P2 and P3 ERPs amplitude measures and in theta range EP and theta range PLF, but not in theta range TP. This finding suggests that weaker theta synchronization across target trials in the FR group is driving the observed differences as opposed to a decrease in the strength of the theta signal. Scalp topography of theta EP had a more posterior maximum whereas theta PLF had a more anterior maximum, suggesting that these measures are not reflecting identical processes. In spite of the fact that both measures are biased toward phase-locked EEG activity they could be reflective of a different cognitive and/or different neuroelectric process. On the other hand, a difference in scalp topography alone is not sufficient to assume a different neuroelectric source is driving them. Activity generated by the same neuroelectrical source could manifest itself on the scalp surface as being different by means of volume conduction effects. The functional meaning of the P2 ERP in visual task paradigms is ill-described but has been related to stimulus categorization processes (e.g., Pernet et al., 2003), while the P3 ERP has been associated with attention and memory processes (Donchin and Coles, 1998; Polich and Herbst, 2000). Both theta PLF and theta EP were reduced in the FR group in the absence of a reduction in theta TP, suggesting that cortical theta band timing with respect to stimulus presentation may be impaired and not the production of theta band activity. Theta band activity after target detection has been related to processes associated with focused attention and signal detection (e.g., Basar-Eroglu et al., 1992). Yordanova et al. (2000) have proposed that theta activity is related to cortico-hippocampal feedback loops related to the evaluation of stimuli that become activated in case of physical context deviations, which may lead to a subsequent controlled processing in the frontal cortex. Abnormal neural synchrony has been associated with aberrant neurodevelopmental changes that alter myelination and affect synchronous brain function. Accordingly, multiple genetic and environmental factors may interfere with the neurodevelopmental processes, resulting in a dysregulation of the complementary changes occurring in gray and white matter. These changes result in insufficient capacity to maintain temporal synchrony of widely distributed neural networks (Bartzokis, 2002). More recent studies have further demonstrated that a core deficit in fronto-temporal connectivity may indeed be associated with abnormal theta band synchronization in schizophrenia (Sigurdsson et al., 2010). Hence the smaller P2 and P3 amplitude and reduced theta activity observed in the FR group may be indicative of impaired stimulus categorization and/or attention allocation processes in this group and may reflect neurodevelopmental abnormalities in fronto-temporal connectivity.

It remains to be determined if abnormalities in fronto-temporal connectivity is really the cause of our observed findings, but our results are not in disagreement with such an account. If there is a malfunction in the feedback loop between frontal and hippocampal brain areas, a reduction in theta band inter-trial phase synchrony such as we reported here may be expected. The observation that alpha TP after target onset was reduced *less* in the FR group than in the HC group is not necessarily inconsistent with the observation of reduced theta findings. A reduction in alpha TP might actually be indicative of an *increase* in activation of the underlying neural sources. Since our task required visual attention to target stimuli it can be expected that cortical areas involved in the processing of visual stimuli should become more active after a visual stimulus is being presented. TP reductions in the alpha frequency range were progressively larger at electrode positions close to the visual cortex than at electrodes farther removed from it. The HC group might be better able to allocate their attention to the visual target stimulus and hence alpha activity was more suppressed in the short period that follows stimulus presentation in this group than it was in the FR group. This effect was primarily observed for the alpha TP measure and not for the alpha EP or PLF measures suggesting that it is the strength of the alpha activity, not its timing that is diminished in response to the occurrence of a visual stimulus.

The present results are in line with previous findings demonstrating that patients with full blown schizophrenia show reduced P3 amplitudes as well as reduced low-frequency EEG activity during target processing in oddball tasks compared to healthy control groups (e.g., Roschke and Fell, 1997; Ergen et al., 2008; Ford et al., 2008; Doege et al., 2009). Our findings extend these observations to adolescents at FR for schizophrenia and therefore hold promise to unfold the pathophysiology of the illness. It is important to acknowledge some limitations to the present study. First, group sizes were relatively small, and the findings require replication in larger subject samples before firm conclusions can be drawn. Second, the results might be compromised by confounding comorbid disorders. Finally, this cross-sectional study does not address the predictive value of the observed findings for illness onset in populations at FR for psychotic illness. Longitudinal follow-up will determine the true predictive value of our findings.

ACKNOWLEDGMENTS

We thank Erin Douglas, M.S., Kathleen Monforton, B.S., and Carolyn Bellion, M.A. for their contributions to participant recruitment and clinical assessment. Nicholas Musisca, M.A., Nathaniel Lucena, M.A., and Josh Bizzell, M.S. contributed to data collection and/or analysis. We thank Zoë Englander, B.S. and Paul Tiesinga, Ph.D for their contribution to the development of the time-frequency analysis pipeline. Hongbin Gu, Ph.D. provided consultation on statistical analysis. We thank the two reviewers for their valuable comments on an earlier version of the manuscript. Finally, we would like to thank the children and their families for participating in this study. This study was supported by Conte center grant P50 MH064065 from the National Institute of Mental Health.

REFERENCES

Bartzokis, G. (2002). Schizophrenia: breakdown in the well-regulated lifelong process of brain development and maturation. Neuropsychopharmacology 27, 672–683.

Basar, E., Schurmann, M., Demiralp, T., Basar-Eroglu, C., and Ademoglu, A. (2001). Event-related oscillations are "real brain responses"-wavelet analysis and new strategies. Int. J. Psychophysiol. 39, 91–127.

Basar-Eroglu, C., Basar, E., Demiralp, T., and Schurmann, M. (1992). P300-response: possible psychophysiological correlates in delta and theta frequency channels. A review. Int. J. Psychophysiol. 13, 161–179.

Bramon, E., Mcdonald, C., Croft, R. J., Landau, S., Filbey, F., Gruzelier, J. H., Sham, P. C., Frangou, S., and Murray, R. M. (2005). Is the P300 wave an endophenotype for schizophrenia? A meta-analysis and a family study. Neuroimage 27, 960–968.

Cannon, T. D. (2005). Clinical and genetic high-risk strategies in understanding vulnerability to psychosis. Schizophr. Res. 79, 35–44.

Delorme, A., and Makeig, S. (2004). EEGLAB: an open source toolbox for analysis of single-trial EEG dynamics including independent component analysis. J. Neurosci. Methods 134, 9–21.

Demiralp, T., and Ademoglu, A. (2001). Decomposition of event-related brain potentials into multiple functional components using wavelet transform. Clin. Electroencephalogr. 32, 122–138.

Demiralp, T., Yordanova, J., Kolev, V., Ademoglu, A., Devrim, M., and Samar, V. J. (1999). Time-frequency analysis of single-sweep event-related potentials by means of fast wavelet transform. Brain Lang. 66, 129–145.

Doege, K., Bates, A. T., White, T. P., Das, D., Boks, M. P., and Liddle, P. F. (2009). Reduced event-related low frequency EEG activity in schizophrenia during an auditory oddball task. Psychophysiology 46, 566–577.

Donchin, E., and Coles, M. G. H. (1998). Context updating and the P300. Behav. Brain Sci. 21, 149–168.

Duncan-Johnson, C. C., and Donchin, E. (1977). On quantifying surprise: the variation of event-related potentials with subjective probability. Psychophysiology 14, 456–467.

Ergen, M., Marbach, S., Brand, A., Basar-Eroglu, C., and Demiralp, T. (2008). P3 and delta band responses in visual oddball paradigm in schizophrenia. Neurosci. Lett. 440, 304–308.

Feinberg, I. (1982). Schizophrenia: caused by a fault in programmed synaptic elimination during adolescence? J. Psychiatr. Res. 17, 319–334.

Fish, B., Marcus, J., Hans, S. L., Auerbach, J. G., and Perdue, S. (1992). Infants at risk for schizophrenia: sequelae of a genetic neurointegrative defect. A review and replication analysis of pandysmaturation in the Jerusalem Infant Development Study. Arch. Gen. Psychiatry 49, 221–235.

Ford, J. M. (1999). Schizophrenia: the broken P300 and beyond. Psychophysiology 36, 667–682.

Ford, J. M., Roach, B. J., Hoffman, R. S., and Mathalon, D. H. (2008). The dependence of P300 amplitude on gamma synchrony breaks down in schizophrenia. Brain Res. 1235, 133–142.

Friedman, D., Cornblatt, B., Vaughan, H. Jr., and Erlenmeyer-Kimling, L. (1988). Auditory event-related potentials in children at risk for schizophrenia: the complete initial sample. Psychiatry Res 26, 203–221.

Huttenlocher, P. R. (1979). Synaptic density in human frontal cortex – developmental changes and effects of aging. Brain Res. 163, 195–205.

Jeon, Y. W., and Polich, J. (2003). Meta-analysis of P300 and schizophrenia: patients, paradigms, and practical implications. Psychophysiology 40, 684–701.

Jung, T. P., Makeig, S., Humphries, C., Lee, T. W., Mckeown, M. J., Iragui, V., and Sejnowski, T. J. (2000). Removing electroencephalographic artifacts by blind source separation. Psychophysiology 37, 163–178.

Keshavan, M., Montrose, D. M., Rajarethinam, R., Diwadkar, V., Prasad, K., and Sweeney, J. A. (2008). Psychopathology among offspring of parents with schizophrenia: relationship to premorbid impairments. Schizophr. Res. 103, 114–120.

Keshavan, M. S., Anderson, S., and Pettegrew, J. W. (1994). Is schizophrenia due to excessive synaptic pruning in the prefrontal cortex? The Feinberg hypothesis revisited. J. Psychiatr. Res. 28, 239–265.

Kolev, V., Demiralp, T., Yordanova, J., Ademoglu, A., and Isoglu-Alkac, U. (1997). Time-frequency analysis reveals multiple functional components during oddball P300. Neuroreport 8, 2061–2065.

Kolev, V., and Yordanova, J. (1997). Analysis of phase-locking is informative for studying event-related EEG activity. Biol. Cybern. 76, 229–235.

Lang, P. J., Bradely, M. M., and Cuthbert, B. N. (2005). International Affective Picture System (IAPS): Digitized Photographs, Instruction Manual and Affective Ratings. Technical Report A-6. Gainesville, FL: The Center for Research in Psychophysiology, University of Florida.

Makeig, S., Debener, S., Onton, J., and Delorme, A. (2004). Mining event-related brain dynamics. Trends Cogn. Sci. 8, 204–210.

Marcus, J., Hans, S. L., Auerbach, J. G., and Auerbach, A. G. (1993). Children at risk for schizophrenia: the Jerusalem Infant Development Study. II. Neurobehavioral deficits at school age. Arch. Gen. Psychiatry 50, 797–809.

Marshall, W. A., and Tanner, J. M. (1969). Variations in pattern of pubertal changes in girls. Arch. Dis. Child. 44, 291–303.

Marshall, W. A., and Tanner, J. M. (1970). Variations in the pattern of pubertal changes in boys. Arch. Dis. Child. 45, 13–23.

Maxwell, M. E. (1992). Manual for the FIGS (Family Interview for Genetic Studies). Bethesda, MD: Clinical Neurogenetics Branch, Intramural Research Program, National Institute of Mental Health.

McNeil, T. F., Cantor-Graae, E., and Cardenal, S. (1993). Prenatal cerebral development in individuals at genetic risk for psychosis: head size at birth in offspring of women with schizophrenia. Schizophr. Res. 10, 1–5.

Miller, T. J., Mcglashan, T. H., Woods, S. W., Stein, K., Driesen, N., Corcoran, C. M., Hoffman, R., and Davidson, L. (1999). Symptom assessment in schizophrenic prodromal states. Psychiatr. Q. 70, 273–287.

Oostenveld, R., Fries, P., Maris, E., and Schoffelen, J. M. (2011). FieldTrip: open source software for advanced analysis of MEG, EEG, and invasive electrophysiological data. Comput. Intell. Neurosci. 2011, 156869.

Orvaschel, H., Puig-Antich, J., Chambers, W., Tabrizi, M. A., and Johnson, R. (1982). Retrospective assessment of prepubertal major depression with the Kiddie-SADS-e. J. Am. Acad. Child Psychiatry 21, 392–397.

Pernet, C., Basan, S., Doyon, B., Cardebat, D., Demonet, J. F., and Celsis, P. (2003). Neural timing of visual implicit categorization. Brain Res. Cogn. Brain Res. 17, 327–338.

Polich, J., and Herbst, K. L. (2000). P300 as a clinical assay: rationale, evaluation, and findings. Int. J. Psychophysiol. 38, 3–19.

Roach, B. J., and Mathalon, D. H. (2008). Event-related EEG time-frequency analysis: an overview of measures and an analysis of early gamma band phase locking in schizophrenia. Schizophr. Bull. 34, 907–926.

Roschke, J., and Fell, J. (1997). Spectral analysis of P300 generation in depression and schizophrenia. Neuropsychobiology 35, 108–114.

Schreiber, H., Stolz-Born, G., Kornhuber, H. H., and Born, J. (1992). Event-related potential correlates of impaired selective attention in children at high risk for schizophrenia. Biol. Psychiatry 32, 634–651.

Semlitsch, H. V., Anderer, P., Schuster, P., and Presslich, O. (1986). A solution for reliable and valid reduction of ocular artifacts, applied to the P300 ERP. Psychophysiology 23, 695–703.

Sigurdsson, T., Stark, K. L., Karayiorgou, M., Gogos, J. A., and Gordon, J. A. (2010). Impaired hippocampal-prefrontal synchrony in a genetic mouse model of schizophrenia. Nature 464, 763–767.

Spencer, K. M., and Polich, J. (1999). Poststimulus EEG spectral analysis and P300: attention, task, and probability. Psychophysiology 36, 220–232.

Tallon-Baudry, C., Bertrand, O., Delpuech, C., and Pernier, J. (1996). Stimulus specificity of phase-locked and non-phase-locked 40 Hz visual responses in human. *J. Neurosci.* 16, 4240–4249.

Vasey, M. W., and Thayer, J. F. (1987). The continuing problem of false positives in repeated measures ANOVA in psychophysiology: a multivariate solution. *Psychophysiology* 24, 479–486.

von Stein, A., Chiang, C., and Konig, P. (2000). Top-down processing mediated by interareal synchronization *Proc. Natl. Acad. Sci. U.S.A.* 97, 14748–14753.

Weinberger, D. R. (1987). Implications of normal brain development for the pathogenesis of schizophrenia. *Arch. Gen. Psychiatry* 44, 660–669.

Woods, B. T. (1998). Is schizophrenia a progressive neurodevelopmental disorder? Toward a unitary pathogenetic mechanism. *Am. J. Psychiatry* 155, 1661–1670.

Yordanova, J., Devrim, M., Kolev, V., Ademoglu, A., and Demiralp, T. (2000). Multiple time-frequency components account for the complex functional reactivity of P300. *Neuroreport* 11, 1097–1103.

APPENDIX

Table A1 | Means and SD (in parentheses) for ERP measures at nine electrode locations.

Electrode position	Group	P2 amplitude	P2 latency	P3 amplitude	P3 latency
F3	HC	**5.15(4.40)***	218(11)	2.61(4.68)	575(163)
	FR	**2.73(2.86)**	217(17)	2.22(4.54)	546(154)
Fz	HC	**5.64(4.99)**	216(11)	1.95(5.14)	564(156)
	FR	**3.07(3.32)**	216(13)	1.97(4.80)	526(152)
F4	HC	**5.59(4.66)**	217(11)	3.12(4.70)	565(155)
	FR	**2.88(3.28)**	215(13)	2.63(4.08)	543(142)
C3	HC	**6.29(4.04)**	218(10)	8.34(5.91)	480(130)
	FR	**3.76(3.50)**	219(16)	6.21(5.14)	495(117)
Cz	HC	**8.25(4.98)**	216(10)	10.42(6.98)	487(126)
	FR	**5.51(4.28)**	218(13)	8.46(5.49)	489(118)
C4	HC	**6.83(4.01)**	217(10)	10.27(5.98)	482(112)
	FR	**4.67(3.09)**	220(13)	8.32(4.92)	489(123)
P3	HC	**7.43(4.94)**	237(23)	**16.45(7.42)**	437(47)
	FR	**4.40(4.35)**	235(25)	**12.24(6.71)**	451(67)
Pz	HC	**8.15(5.06)**	231(17)	**19.39(8.73)**	429(35)
	FR	**5.04(4.39)**	225(13)	**14.70(7.40)**	444(64)
P4	HC	7.74(4.80)	236(22)	**16.71(7.29)**	430(32)
	FR	5.85(3.80)	237(25)	**12.51(5.72)**	451(64)

HC, healthy control; FR, familial risk.
*Bold numberings denote significant group difference with $p < 0.05$.

Table A2 | Means and SD (in parentheses) for time–frequency decomposition measures. Time range 150–300 ms.

TF	Pos	Grp	Delta Value	Delta Latency	Theta Value	Theta Latency	Alpha Value	Alpha Latency
EP	F3	HC	8301(3434)	282(48)	4862(2039)	263(37)	1658(823)	203(62)
		FR	7775(3257)	297(14)	4601(3190)	268(50)	1572(1884)	219(61)
	Fz	HC	8958(3341)	294(28)	6193(2593)	269(37)	1780(818)	216(66)
		FR	8160(3673)	300(0)	5750(3983)	267(52)	1695(1917)	217(61)
	F4	HC	7164(2762)	292(31)	4611(1870)	260(39)	1465(676)	218(66)
		FR	6721(3300)	294(31)	4180(2833)	259(53)	1395(1453)	216(59)
	C3	HC	8132(3176)	295(27)	5654(2481)	267(40)	2234(1381)	198(62)
		FR	7502(3459)	295(20)	4691(3136)	259(53)	2124(2333)	225(57)
	Cz	HC	11000(4237)	295(27)	8604(3674)	266(42)	2542(1380)	211(63)
		FR	9751(4383)	299(6)	6580(4123)	269(48)	2256(2251)	232(59)
	C4	HC	7560(3173)	295(27)	5593(2731)	263(41)	2152(1717)	215(62)
		FR	6857(3338)	296(18)	4502(2865)	264(42)	1867(1838)	243(48)
	P3	HC	10226(4459)	286(40)	5518(3219)	268(44)	2789(1978)	169(42)
		FR	8396(4332)	294(31)	4114(2804)	283(27)	2444(2478)	207(53)
	Pz	HC	11952(5111)	289(35)	**6885(3935)***	266(47)	3305(2477)	183(51)
		FR	9917(5196)	288(42)	**4665(2939)**	281(35)	2538(2417)	214(55)
	P4	HC	8662(3687)	286(41)	4918(3361)	269(46)	2426(2124)	185(53)
		FR	7823(4346)	280(48)	3830(2589)	278(40)	2066(1888)	215(58)

(Continued)

Table A2 | Continued

TF	Pos	Grp	Frequency band					
			Delta		Theta		Alpha	
			Value	Latency	Value	Latency	Value	Latency
PLF	F3	HC	0.3416(0.099)	249(66)	**0.5152(0.110)**	184(40)	0.2842(0.083)	207(58)
		FR	0.3388(0.068)	280(48)	**0.4531(0.103)**	171(24)	0.2565(0.098)	215(65)
	Fz	HC	0.3506(0.089)	248(63)	**0.5312(0.111)**	182(38)	0.2888(0.088)	212(58)
		FR	0.3546(0.065)	288(35)	**0.4675(0.105)**	168(22)	0.2644(0.096)	200(54)
	F4	HC	0.3635(0.106)	262(56)	**0.5479(0.115)**	182(35)	0.2883(0.089)	197(52)
		FR	0.3493(0.082)	280(41)	**0.4768(0.107)**	167(21)	0.2697(0.099)	207(55)
	C3	HC	0.3411(0.111)	294(23)	**0.5243(0.093)**	207(45)	0.2655(0.075)	208(57)
		FR	0.3302(0.098)	289(27)	**0.4611(0.119)**	209(44)	0.2574(0.096)	208(60)
	Cz	HC	0.3403(0.113)	275(51)	**0.5503(0.093)**	192(32)	0.2700(0.080)	213(59)
		FR	0.3419(0.091)	289(29)	**0.4818(0.107)**	180(36)	0.2698(0.077)	195(50)
	C4	HC	0.3461(0.117)	287(40)	**0.5641(0.090)**	201(38)	0.2775(0.072)	217(55)
		FR	0.3511(0.101)	295(24)	**0.5050(0.110)**	193(31)	0.2717(0.091)	200(55)
	P3	HC	0.4097(0.116)	294(24)	0.4304(0.098)	238(53)	0.2535(0.079)	216(49)
		FR	0.3874(0.116)	285(42)	0.4287(0.105)	230(39)	0.2565(0.094)	199(51)
	Pz	HC	0.4265(0.129)	293(29)	0.4542(0.105)	241(49)	0.2484(0.068)	219(55)
		FR	0.4134(0.105)	298(6)	0.4516(0.111)	211(38)	0.2703(0.104)	212(58)
	P4	HC	0.4217(0.108)	292(31)	0.4511(0.112)	239(48)	0.2717(0.074)	222(58)
		FR	0.3915(0.107)	290(29)	0.4461(0.109)	237(40)	0.2735(0.117)	220(59)
TP	F3	HC	0.89(0.70)	295(27)	2.52(1.28)	262(36)	0.34(1.13)	232(61)
		FR	1.01(0.78)	279(51)	2.24(1.51)	268(50)	0.42(1.26)	225(61)
	Fz	HC	1.10(0.65)	299(5)	2.98(1.28)	269(37)	0.54(1.25)	236(67)
		FR	1.19(0.71)	294(3)	2.68(1.71)	274(45)	0.67(1.44)	213(60)
	F4	HC	1.01(0.65)	297(18)	2.93(1.26)	259(39)	0.51(1.33)	241(64)
		FR	1.01(0.75)	283(46)	2.41(1.63)	266(47)	0.56(1.27)	233(60)
	C3	HC	0.89(0.75)	295(27)	2.74(1.37)	267(40)	0.16(1.15)	239(64)
		FR	0.97(0.79)	283(44)	2.40(1.36)	259(53)	0.39(1.10)	248(62)
	Cz	HC	1.13(0.74)	300(0)	3.37(1.45)	266(42)	0.56(1.40)	235(65)
		FR	1.16(0.86)	286(42)	2.95(1.52)	274(41)	0.80(1.43)	243(53)
	C4	HC	1.08(0.73)	297(16)	3.21(1.42)	263(41)	0.39(1.33)	233(66)
		FR	1.07(0.73)	283(46)	2.87(1.55)	259(44)	0.58(1.09)	235(41)
	P3	HC	1.14(0.77)	291(31)	2.09(1.20)	273(38)	**−1.18(1.61)**	272(56)
		FR	1.07(0.81)	294(31)	1.96(1.30)	281(36)	**−0.15(1.14)**	259(51)
	Pz	HC	1.35(0.83)	295(22)	2.42(1.38)	266(47)	**−0.87(1.68)**	267(51)
		FR	1.23(0.94)	294(29)	2.45(1.53)	283(29)	**0.22(1.26)**	237(58)
	P4	HC	1.19(0.71)	291(32)	2.33(1.38)	269(47)	**−1.15(1.66)**	273(43)
		FR	0.96(0.91)	292(32)	2.28(1.61)	273(48)	**−0.11(1.54)**	249(54)

TF, time–frequency measure; Pos, electrode position; Grp, group; EP, evoked power; PLF, phase-locking factor; TP, total power; HC, healthy control; FR, familial risk.
Bold numberings denote significant group difference with p < 0.05.

Table A3 | Means and SD (in parentheses) for time–frequency decomposition measures. Time range 300–700 ms.

TF	Pos	Grp	Frequency band					
			Delta		Theta		Alpha	
			Value	Latency	Value	Latency	Value	Latency
EP	F3	HC	8859(3898)	493(126)	4798(2035)	313(42)	1636(1083)	439(187)
		FR	8543(3617)	558(110)	4485(2796)	353(100)	1437(1385)	404(155)
	Fz	HC	9657(3781)	510(111)	6195(2703)	333(85)	1812(1209)	393(159)
		FR	8960(3981)	545(93)	5662(3613)	357(89)	1588(1560)	413(153)
	F4	HC	7516(2844)	471(111)	4526(1849)	310(40)	1393(734)	366(133)
		FR	7341(4105)	523(113)	4032(2518)	343(80)	1283(1225)	398(137)
	C3	HC	8522(3386)	477(109)	5510(2362)	310(25)	1942(1177)	328(99)
		FR	8075(3716)	502(110)	4548(2910)	331(63)	1844(1793)	358(126)
	Cz	HC	11573(4657)	460(84)	8413(3585)	**308(14)**	2304(1211)	344(121)
		FR	10415(4614)	493(95)	6429(3782)	**328(50)**	1987(1725)	314(40)
	C4	HC	7927(3358)	447(85)	5460(2609)	305(9)	1925(1447)	350(121)
		FR	7195(3459)	474(98)	4370(2636)	312(25)	1833(1860)	317(35)
	P3	HC	10466(4551)	409(91)	5338(2898)	316(28)	2233(1633)	352(136)
		FR	8735(4462)	453(100)	4104(2707)	344(75)	2130(2258)	302(6)
	Pz	HC	12286(5272)	413(82)	**6592(3454)***	**313(22)**	2664(1978)	328(101)
		FR	10328(5461)	438(87)	**4649(2797)**	**335(53)**	2293(2292)	301(4)
	P4	HC	8919(3776)	412(98)	4713(2803)	315(25)	1906(1527)	347(122)
		FR	8040(4397)	414(99)	3772(2407)	334(45)	1876(1748)	306(18)
PLF	F3	HC	0.3754(0.086)	546(164)	**0.4486(0.102)**	355(138)	0.2688(0.057)	519(183)
		FR	0.3914(0.080)	612(130)	**0.3935(0.093)**	331(104)	0.2608(0.067)	524(174)
	Fz	HC	0.3895(0.080)	588(139)	**0.4620(0.104)**	338(115)	0.2734(0.056)	489(178)
		FR	0.4175(0.069)	626(92)	**0.3990(0.095)**	373(148)	0.2558(0.078)	556(152)
	F4	HC	0.4013(0.094)	536(168)	**0.4803(0.103)**	341(122)	0.2802(0.053)	517(181)
		FR	0.4160(0.080)	628(76)	**0.4076(0.096)**	317(82)	0.2610(0.079)	523(167)
	C3	HC	0.3949(0.106)	616(101)	**0.4808(0.082)**	320(74)	0.2666(0.073)	511(172)
		FR	0.3888(0.104)	604(101)	**0.4285(0.110)**	364(130)	0.2685(0.071)	530(167)
	Cz	HC	0.3897(0.109)	583(143)	**0.4965(0.091)**	316(74)	0.2752(0.076)	543(166)
		FR	0.3936(0.100)	583(111)	**0.4340(0.103)**	331(102)	0.2644(0.067)	540(160)
	C4	HC	0.4008(0.112)	611(108)	0.5153(0.084)	318(76)	0.2936(0.081)	512(182)
		FR	0.4075(0.101)	589(107)	0.4640(0.106)	318(74)	0.2751(0.084)	533(179)
	P3	HC	0.4399(0.112)	504(105)	0.4202(0.088)	354(113)	0.2659(0.064)	496(183)
		FR	0.4188(0.119)	530(98)	0.4192(0.100)	359(115)	0.2485(0.086)	530(162)
	Pz	HC	0.4599(0.122)	540(97)	0.4409(0.095)	336(103)	0.2640(0.067)	531(173)
		FR	0.4380(0.107)	538(80)	0.4363(0.108)	355(112)	0.2582(0.067)	519(182)
	P4	HC	0.4511(0.106)	503(97)	0.4434(0.099)	341(101)	0.2840(0.055)	534(181)
		FR	0.4194(0.1059)	514(115)	0.4291(0.105)	350(109)	0.2644(0.077)	545(165)
TP	F3	HC	1.05(1.03)	555(119)	2.13(1.93)	366(140)	−0.95(2.16)	553(136)
		FR	1.46(0.89)	557(107)	1.98(2.03)	393(139)	−0.56(1.88)	533(160)
	Fz	HC	1.33(0.99)	549(101)	2.83(1.65)	346(108)	−0.92(2.28)	564(150)
		FR	1.61(0.91)	544(90)	2.51(2.26)	390(129)	−0.27(2.09)	525(171)
	F4	HC	1.18(0.87)	486(114)	2.59(1.88)	346(108)	−0.85(2.31)	518(160)
		FR	1.33(0.99)	521(113)	1.74(2.67)	409(153)	−0.87(1.84)	572(150)
	C3	HC	1.03(0.98)	504(112)	2.15(2.31)	362(133)	−2.77(2.29)	593(122)
		FR	1.26(0.96)	530(112)	1.57(2.51)	414(162)	−2.25(2.38)	572(137)
	Cz	HC	1.29(0.99)	473(87)	3.02(2.14)	335(101)	−1.85(2.71)	542(149)
		FR	1.47(0.95)	491(94)	2.15(2.78)	394(148)	−1.25(2.44)	526(166)

(Continued)

Table A3 | Continued

TF	Pos	Grp	Frequency band					
			Delta		Theta		Alpha	
			Value	Latency	Value	Latency	Value	Latency
	C4	HC	1.21(1.01)	485(103)	2.61(2.56)	358(137)	−2.75(2.62)	589(135)
		FR	1.24(0.93)	510(116)	2.15(2.78)	377(149)	−2.44(2.17)	597(135)
	P3	HC	1.10(1.08)	475(127)	0.80(2.79)	444(179)	−4.18(1.99)	607(80)
		FR	1.18(1.01)	506(126)	0.78(2.77)	488(182)	−3.56(1.87)	604(80)
	Pz	HC	1.34(1.14)	474(124)	1.05(3.19)	439(175)	**−4.58(2.06)**	614(71)
		FR	1.32(1.19)	494(120)	1.75(2.72)	413(157)	**−3.37(1.82)**	608(95)
	P4	HC	1.21(1.02)	463(128)	1.30(2.98)	432(175)	−3.94(2.19)	594(101)
		FR	1.01(1.17)	482(130)	1.23(2.98)	444(168)	−3.06(2.45)	612(117)

TF, time–frequency measure; Pos, electrode position; Grp, group; EP, evoked power; PLF, phase-locking factor; TP, total power; HC, healthy control; FR, familial risk.
*Bold numberings denote significant group difference with $p < 0.05$.

Adolescent opiate exposure in the female rat induces subtle alterations in maternal care and transgenerational effects on play behavior

Nicole L. Johnson, Lindsay Carini, Marian E. Schenk, Michelle Stewart and Elizabeth M. Byrnes*

Department of Biomedical Science, Cummings School of Veterinary Medicine, Tufts University, North Grafton, MA, USA

*Correspondence:
Elizabeth M. Byrnes, Section of Neuroscience and Reproductive Biology, Department of Biomedical Science, Cummings School of Veterinary Medicine, Tufts University, 200 Westboro Road, North Grafton, MA 01536, USA.
e-mail: elizabeth.byrnes@tufts.edu

The non-medical use of prescription opiates, such as Vicodin® and MSContin®, has increased dramatically over the past decade. Of particular concern is the rising popularity of these drugs in adolescent female populations. Use during this critical developmental period could have significant long-term consequences for both the female user as well as potential effects on her future offspring. To address this issue, we have begun modeling adolescent opiate exposure in female rats and have observed significant transgenerational effects despite the fact that all drugs are withdrawn several weeks prior to pregnancy. The purpose of the current set of studies was to determine whether adolescent morphine exposure modifies postpartum care. In addition, we also examined juvenile play behavior in both male and female offspring. The choice of the social play paradigm was based on previous findings demonstrating effects of both postpartum care and opioid activity on play behavior. The findings revealed subtle modifications in the maternal behavior of adolescent morphine-exposed females, primarily related to the amount of time females' spend nursing and in non-nursing contact with their young. In addition, male offspring of adolescent morphine-exposed mothers (MOR-F1) demonstrate decreased rough and tumble play behaviors, with no significant differences in general social behaviors (i.e., social grooming and social exploration). Moreover, there was a tendency toward increased rough and tumble play in MOR-F1 females, demonstrating the sex-specific nature of these effects. Given the importance of the postpartum environment on neurodevelopment, it is possible that modifications in maternal–offspring interactions, related to a history of adolescent opiate exposure, plays a role in the observed transgenerational effects. Overall, these studies indicate that the long-term consequences of adolescent opiate exposure can impact both the female and her future offspring.

Keywords: morphine, offspring, rough and tumble play, nursing, maternal attachment

INTRODUCTION

Since the early 1990s there has been a steady increase in prescription rates for opiates (Substance Abuse and Mental Health Services Administration [SAMHSA], 2009), including prescribing for conditions ranging from routine dental procedures to menstrual cramps. This escalation in prescribing, coupled with increased availability of these substances online (Forman et al., 2006), and the advent of long-acting forms of opiate analgesics such as OxyContin®, have combined to create a dangerous upsurge in both the medical and non-medical use of prescription pain medications (Paulozzi et al., 2006; Cai et al., 2010). Of great concern is the increased use of these potent opiates in adolescent populations (Sung et al., 2005), with 60.6% of respondents in a recent survey reporting initiation of use before the age of 15 (Wu et al., 2008). Misuse in younger populations is likely due to the decreased risk perception associated with prescription opiates (e.g., as compared to heroin), in conjunction with their increased availability. Indeed, overall, prescription drugs are reported as the "drug of choice" in 12- and 13-year-old populations (SAMHSA, 2007) and unlike other drugs of abuse, they are used at higher rates in young female populations (Sung et al., 2005; Alemagno et al., 2009). Currently, the long-term impact of this increased use of opiates in adolescent female populations remains unknown.

Given that adolescence represents a period of significant brain maturation, perturbation of the endogenous opioid system during this period may induce significant long-term effects. Endogenous opioids (beta-endorphin, dynorphin, and enkephalin) and their receptor targets (mu, kappa, and delta) are ubiquitous, serving as critical modulators of neural, endocrine, and immune function. For example, during adolescence, endogenous opioids modulate the timing of sexual maturation (Cicero et al., 1986; Reiter, 1987; Sizonenko, 1987). Opioids also regulate stress responsiveness as well as modulating numerous cognitive and reward-related processes (Zager and Black, 1985; McCubbin, 1993; Van Ree et al., 2000; Drolet et al., 2001; Kreek, 2007). Thus, adaptations in response to high levels of opioids during adolescent development could impact a wide-range of opioid-mediated functions.

A significant body of literature indicates that endogenous opioids play a role in maternal behavior. Initial studies conducted with morphine, showed a disruption of postpartum maternal behavior (Bridges and Grimm, 1982; Rubin and Bridges, 1984;

Kinsley and Bridges, 1986, 1990; Mann et al., 1990; Kinsley et al., 1995; Sukikara et al., 2007). These disruptive effects were even more pronounced when the female was pre-exposed to morphine during pregnancy (Bridges and Grimm, 1982; Miranda-Paiva et al., 2001; Slamberova et al., 2001). In a number of species, including humans and non-human primates, endogenous opioids modulate affiliative behaviors, including mother–infant attachment (Panksepp et al., 1994; Kalin et al., 1995; Nelson and Panksepp, 1998; Saltzman and Maestripieri, 2010). Indeed, there is evidence in women, that opioid use (e.g., methadone) can induce subtle alterations in mother–infant contact and attachment (Goodman et al., 1999). Moreover, studies indicate that endogenous opioids in both the mother, and the infant, are important for infant emotional regulation and attachment (Schino and Troisi, 1992; Weller and Feldman, 2003; Barr et al., 2008). If this system is altered by prior exposure to opiates, then postpartum maternal–offspring interactions could be affected.

We have previously documented significant effects of adolescent morphine exposure on the expression of opioid-related genes, including increased expression of mu- and kappa-opioid receptor genes and decreased expression of the proopiomelanocortin gene in the mediobasal hypothalamus (Byrnes, 2008). In addition, we observed attenuated suckling-stimulated prolactin secretion during early lactation in these females (Byrnes, 2005b, 2008). These findings demonstrate long-term changes in the endogenous opioid system of adolescent-exposed females, as well as alterations in physiological parameters that can influence maternal care. One additional component of these studies was an examination of rudimentary aspects of maternal behavior, such as the latency to retrieve and crouch over pups following a brief separation. No differences in maternal behavior latencies were observed, however, such measures do not assess quantitative or qualitative aspects of maternal care.

In addition to observing direct effects of adolescent morphine exposure on the female rat, we have also demonstrated transgenerational effects in both male and female offspring. These offspring effects include differences in anxiety-like behavior, shifts in morphine sensitization and alterations in morphine analgesia (Byrnes, 2005a; Byrnes et al., 2011). It is important to note that all adolescent-exposed females in our studies are drug-free for several weeks prior to mating. Thus, the developing embryo/fetus is never directly exposed to morphine. These findings indicate that even when morphine exposure is confined to the adolescent period, there can be significant effects on future offspring. Moreover, the nature of these transgenerational effects suggests an alteration in the endogenous opioid system of the offspring. Variations in maternal care can significantly impact offspring neurodevelopment, including the development of the endogenous opioid system (Weaver et al., 2007; Gustafsson et al., 2008; Michaels and Holtzman, 2008). Thus, one potential mechanism underlying transgenerational effects of adolescent morphine exposure may be altered maternal–offspring interactions.

The current study was designed to examine maternal behavior in females exposed to morphine during adolescent development. In addition, we also investigated social play behavior in their male and female offspring. The choice of social play behavior was based upon studies indicating that play behavior is modulated by opioids (Niesink and Van Ree, 1989; Vanderschuren et al., 1995; Van den Berg et al., 2000) and can be altered by changes in the postnatal environment (Janus, 1987; Veenema and Neumann, 2009). Our working hypothesis is that adolescent morphine exposure induces significant changes in the endogenous opioid system of both the female and her offspring.

MATERIALS AND METHODS
EXPERIMENTAL ANIMALS
Sixty female Sprague-Dawley rats (22 days of age) were purchased from Charles River Breeding Laboratories [Crl:CD(SD)BR; Kingston, NY, USA]. All animals were group-housed in light- (on 0700–1900 hours) and temperature- (21–24°C) controlled rooms and provided with food and water *ad libitum*. All animals were maintained in accordance with the National Research Council (NRC) Guide for the Care and Use of Laboratory Animals and all procedures were approved by the Institutional Animals Care and Use Committee of Tufts University.

ADOLESCENT MORPHINE EXPOSURE
Beginning at 30 days of age, females were treated with morphine (morphine sulfate; Butler-Schein, Dublin, OH, USA) for a total of 10 days using an increasing dose regimen. The doses used in the current study were based on allometric scaling to approximate human use (Chiou et al., 1998). Moreover, the use of increasing doses is more compatible with human use patterns, allowing for rising and falling levels of opiates. On day 1 of exposure, 30 animals received 5 mg/kg morphine sulfate (s.c.) once daily (between 0900 and 1100 hours). Every other day, the dose of morphine was increased by 5 mg/kg such that by the final day of treatment subjects received 25 mg/kg. Thirty, age-matched control animals received the saline vehicle (0.9% NaCl, s.c.) with volumes adjusted to match those of drug-treated females. Bodyweights were recorded daily throughout the treatment. Bodyweight gain during drug exposure was calculated by subtracting each animal's bodyweight on exposure day 1 from their bodyweight on exposure day 10. Bodyweight gain was also measured at additional time points post-withdrawal (1, 2, 12, and 19 days after withdrawal). Again, bodyweight gain was calculated relative to exposure day 1 (i.e., prior to their first injection). Adolescent-exposed females will subsequently be referred to as SAL-F0 and MOR-F0 females.

MATING AND MATERNAL BEHAVIOR OBSERVATIONS – F0 FEMALES
At 60 days of age (i.e., 3 weeks after their final injection), SAL-F0 and MOR-F0 females were mated with colony males. A total of 27 SAL-F0 and 28 MOR-F0 became pregnant. The day of parturition was designated as postnatal day 0 (PND0). On PND1 all litters were weighed and culled to 10 pups (five males: five females). In a subset of these females, home-cage maternal behavior was observed at multiple time points throughout PND4, PND10, and PND16. A behavioral checklist was used to monitor maternal behavior with frequencies recorded every 60 s during a 30-min observation period. A total of five observation periods per day were included; three during the light phase (0900, 1200, and 1500 hours), and two during the dark phase (0500 and 2000 hours). Behaviors monitored included nesting (in nest with pups regardless of nursing status), nursing (actively nursing at least one pup), pup grooming, and self-directed behaviors (eating, drinking, self-grooming). In addition,

on PND5 and PPD12 maternal behavior was digitally recorded for 30 min during the light phase (0800 hours; 1 h after lights on) or the dark phase (2000 hour; 1 h after lights off). Maternal behavior durations were then scored. The behaviors included the following: nursing (arched back, side, or low posture), hovering (female is in the nest but no pups are nursing), pup grooming, and self-directed behavior. Care was taken to minimize any disturbance to mothers and litters during these home-cage observations. Sample sizes for frequency data were 15 SAL-F0 and 18 MOR-F0 mothers, sizes for the video analysis were 12 SAL-F0 and 10 MOR-F0 mothers.

SOCIAL PLAY TESTING – F1 MALES AND FEMALES

On PND21 all litters from F0 mothers were weighed and weaned. F1 male and female offspring were then group-housed with same sex siblings. Between PND24 and 26, SAL-F1 and MOR-F1 males and females were tested for social play behavior in a novel environment. Only one male and one female per litter were used in social play testing to eliminate potential litter effects. On the day of testing, animals were socially isolated in a holding cage for 3.5 h. Following isolation, unfamiliar subject pairs of the same sex and maternal adolescent exposure condition (i.e., SAL-F1 or MOR-F1) were placed in a novel test chamber (40 cm × 30 cm × 60 cm) under dim lighting conditions. Behavior was then digitally recorded for 15 min. Sample size was based on pairs, with each pair scored for the frequency and duration of select play behaviors using ODlog software. The scored behaviors included the following: boxing/wrestling, pinning, chasing/following, crawling over/under, social exploration (sniffing any part of the conspecific), and social grooming. Sample sizes were 10 SAL-F1 male and 10 SAL-F1 female pairs; 12 MOR-F1 male and 12 MOR-F1 female pairs. These subjects represent data from $N = 20$ SAL-F0 litters and $N = 24$ MOR-F0 litters.

STATISTICAL ANALYSES

Differences in bodyweight gain during the morphine exposure regimen were analyzed using a Student's t-test. Post-withdrawal bodyweight gain was analyzed using a two-way repeated-measures ANOVA with day as the within subject factor and drug exposure (SAL or MOR) as the between-subject factor. Maternal behavior frequency data were analyzed using a two-way repeated-measures ANOVA with phase of the light cycle as the within subject factor and adolescent maternal exposure as the between-subject factor. Each postnatal day was analyzed separately. Social play behavior data was analyzed using a two-way ANOVA with sex and adolescent maternal exposure (SAL-F1 versus MOR-F1) as factors. All significant effects were followed by post hoc analyses using the Tukey's test. For all data, significance was designated as $p < 0.05$.

RESULTS
EFFECTS OF ADOLESCENT MORPHINE EXPOSURE ON BODYWEIGHT

All females continued to gain weight during the 10-day injection regimen (SAL-F0 = 51.8 ± 1.2 g; MOR-F0 = 43.8 ± 0.89 g), however, MOR-F0 females gained significantly less than SAL-F0 controls [$t_{(58)} = -5.43, p < 0.001$]. Attenuated bodyweight gain continued to be observed when measured soon after drug-withdrawal, but these differences did not persist at later time points [day × drug interaction; $F_{(3,179)} = 4.5, p < 0.01$]. As shown in **Figure 1**, MOR-F0 females had reduced weight gain on the first 2 days following withdrawal,

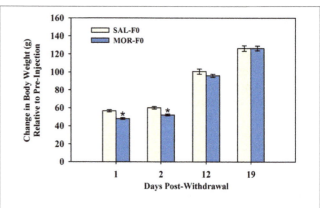

FIGURE 1 | Mean (±SEM) body weight gain (gram) following cessation of daily injections. *$p < 0.001$ as compared to SAL-F0 within day. $N = 27$ SAL-F0; $N = 28$ MOR-F0.

however, by the 12th day post-withdrawal these differences were no longer observed. Prior to mating (i.e., 20 days post-withdrawal), all females were of similar weights.

Data recorded on PND1 did not reveal any significant differences in litter size, gender ratio, or total litter weight (all $ps > 0.2$). At weaning (PND21) there was a significant difference between the groups, with MOR-F1 subjects weighing more than SAL-F1 controls [$t_{(53)} = 2.17, p < 0.05$]. These data are reported in **Table 1**. As post-culling bodyweights were not taken on PND1, we were unable to determine whether MOR-F1 pups that remained post-culling were heavier. Thus, whether these differences reflect increased bodyweight gain in MOR-F1 pups during the postnatal period remains to be determined.

MATERNAL BEHAVIOR IN ADOLESCENT MORPHINE-EXPOSED FEMALES – FREQUENCIES

All maternal behavior frequency data are presented in **Figure 2**. On PND4, there was a main effect of light phase [$F_{(1,31)} = 55.4, p < 0.001$], adolescent exposure [$F_{(1,31)} = 6.9, p < 0.02$], as well as a significant interaction [$F_{(1,31)} = 4.3, p < 0.05$] on the frequency of nursing behavior. Specifically, all females showed reduced nursing during the dark phase, however, MOR-F0 mothers nursed less frequently during the dark phase ($p < 0.01$). On PND10 there was a main effect of light phase [$F_{(1,31)} = 11.0, p < 0.001$], with no other significant effects. Finally, on PND16 there was both a main effect of light phase [$F_{(1,31)} = 9.4, p < 0.01$] and a significant interaction [$F_{(1,31)} = 5.2, p < 0.05$]. Post hoc analyses indicate that SAL-F0 mothers nursed less frequently during the dark phase, while MOR-F0 mothers did not reduce nursing frequency during the dark phase.

The decreased frequency of nursing observed in MOR-F0 was related to an increase in their frequency away from the nest. As shown in **Figure 2**, MOR-F0 mothers tended to be away from their nests more frequently than SAL-F0 mothers during the dark phase. On PND4, there was a main effect of light phase [$F_{(1,31)} = 71.2, p < 0.001$] as well as a significant interaction [$F_{(1,31)} = 6.9, p < 0.02$]. All females were off the nest more frequently during the dark, however, this effect was significantly greater in MOR-F0 mothers ($p < 0.01$). On PND10 there was a main effect of both light phase [$F_{(1,31)} = 119.9, p < 0.001$] and adolescent exposure [$F_{(1,31)} = 4.3$,

Table 1 | The effects of adolescent morphine exposure on postnatal parameters.

	Litter size (no. of pups)	No. of females	No. of males	Bodyweight (g, PND1)	Bodyweight (g, PND21)
SAL-F0	14.1 ± 0.5	6.7 ± 0.4	7.4 ± 0.4	91.2 ± 2.7	550.9 ± 8.8
MOR-F0	14.2 ± 0.4	7.5 ± 0.3	6.6 ± 0.5	96.5 ± 2.3	582.1 ± 11.0*

*$p < 0.05$ as compared to SAL-F0 on PND21.

$p < 0.05$], with MOR-F0 off the nest more frequently than SAL-F0 mothers. Finally, on PND16 there was a main effect of light phase [$F_{(1,31)} = 30.86, p < 0.001$] and a significant interaction [$F_{(1,31)} = 7.16$, $p < 0.02$]. *Post hoc* analyses indicate an increased frequency for MOR-F0 mothers to be away from the nest when compared to SAL-F0 mothers during the light phase only.

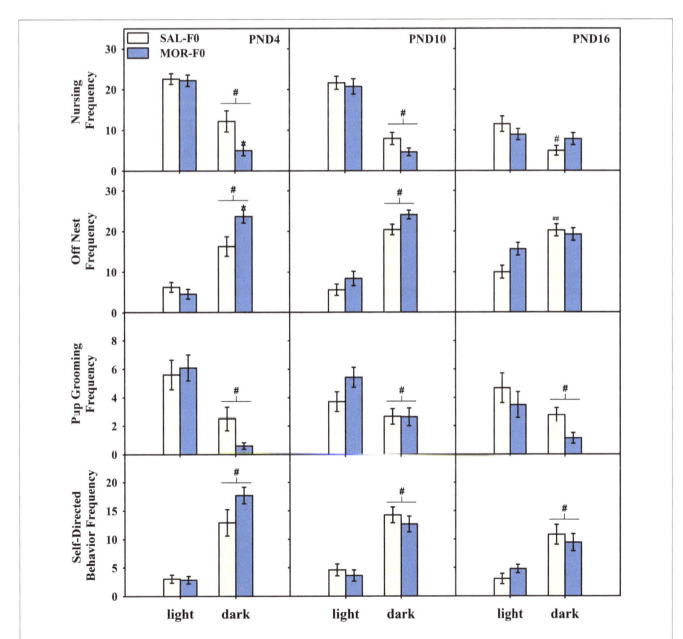

FIGURE 2 | Mean (±SEM) frequency nursing, off nest, pup grooming, or engaged in self-directed behaviors on PND4, 10, and 16. Data collected during the light phase was averaged across three observation periods (0900, 1200, and 1500 hours). Data collected during the dark phase was averaged across two observation periods (0500 and 2000 hours). #$p < 0.01$ compared to light phase collapsed across maternal adolescent exposure condition. ##$p < 0.05$ compared to light phase within SAL-F0. *$p < 0.02$ compared to SAL-F0 females within day. N = 15 SAL-F0; N = 18 MOR-F0.

As expected, the frequency of pup grooming decreased while self-directed behaviors increased in the dark phase when compared to the light phase. These effects were similar across all postnatal days examined (see **Figure 2**; main effect of light phase, all $ps < 0.05$). No significant effects of adolescent morphine exposure were observed on frequency of pup grooming or self-directed behaviors, nor were there any significant interactions (all $ps > 0.1$).

MATERNAL BEHAVIOR IN ADOLESCENT MORPHINE-EXPOSED FEMALES – DURATION

As illustrated in **Figure 3** (left panels), significant effects of both the light phase and maternal adolescent exposure were observed on PND5. All females nursed more during the light phase [$F_{(1,19)} = 8.21$, $p < 0.05$], with no significant differences between MOR-F0 and SAL-F0 mothers ($ps > 0.6$). However, when we examined the amount of time female's spent hovering over their litter (i.e., contacting but not actively nursing pups), there was a significant main effect of light phase [$F_{(1,19)} = 9.13$, $p < 0.01$] and maternal adolescent exposure [$F_{(1,19)} = 8.93$, $p < 0.01$]. Overall, MOR-F0 mothers spent more time hovering then SAL-F0 mothers. Finally, no significant effects on pup grooming were observed, while all females spent more time engaged in self-directed behaviors during the dark phase [main effect of light phase; $F_{(1,19)} = 17.4$, $p < 0.01$].

Few statistically significant effects were observed on PND12, however, some interesting trends were observed (see **Figure 3**, right panels). For example, while no significant effects of light phase or maternal adolescent exposure on nursing behavior were observed (both $ps > 0.3$), there was a trend [$F_{(1,19)} = 3.78$, $p = 0.067$] toward a light phase by maternal adolescent exposure interaction. This trend appears to be due to a tendency toward increased time spent nursing during the dark phase by MOR-F0 mothers. No significant effects on either hovering or pup grooming were observed. Finally, similar to the effects observed in PND5, all females engaged in more self-directed behaviors during the dark phase [main effect of light phase; $F_{(1,19)} = 5.12$, $p < 0.05$].

SOCIAL PLAY BEHAVIOR IN THE OFFSPRING OF ADOLESCENT MORPHINE-EXPOSED MOTHERS

Frequency and duration data were combined from separate measures to form two categories of social play behavior. These categories were (1) general social behavior, which included both social exploration and social grooming, and (2) rough and tumble play, which included pinning, boxing, wrestling, chasing, following, crawling over/under, and tail pulling. These data are shown in **Figure 4**. There was no significant effect of either sex or maternal adolescent exposure on either the frequency or duration of general social behaviors, although there was a modest trend toward a main effect of sex on durations ($p = 0.07$). Maternal adolescent exposure did, however, significantly affect both the frequency and duration of rough and tumble play. Moreover, these effects were sex-specific with a significant sex by maternal adolescent exposure interaction [frequency– $F_{(1,43)} = 4.89$, $p < 0.05$; duration– $F_{(1,43)} = 5.2$, $p < 0.03$]. Post hoc analyses indicate that these effects were largely due to the decreased expression of rough and tumble play by MOR-F1 males ($p < 0.05$). In addition to decreased play in MOR-F1 males, there was also a trend ($p = 0.07$) toward increased rough and tumble play in MOR-F1 females. Thus, significant sex differences were observed in MOR-F1 subjects (both $ps < 0.03$), but not in SAL-F1 (both

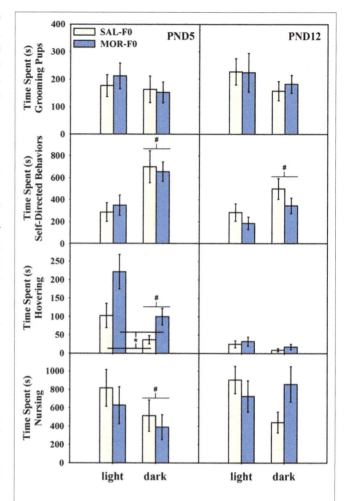

FIGURE 3 | Mean (±SEM) time (seconds) engaged in pup-directed and non-pup-directed activities on PND5 (left panels) and PND12 (right panels). Behavior was recorded at 0800 hours (light phase) and 2000 hours (dark phase). #$p < 0.01$ as compared to light phase collapsed across adolescent exposure groups. *$p < 0.01$ MOR-F0 compared to SAL-F0 collapsed across light cycle phase. $N = 11$ SAL-F0; $N = 10$ MOR-F0.

$ps > 0.3$). Overall, these findings demonstrate a sex-specific shift in rough and tumble play in MOR-F1 subjects, which is not associated with alterations in other aspects of social behavior at this age.

DISCUSSION

The current findings demonstrate that exposure to escalating doses of morphine, confined to the adolescent period, can induce subtle modifications in subsequent maternal care and can alter the behavioral phenotype of subsequent offspring. These effects were largely expressed as differences in frequency of nursing and contact time during early lactation. In addition, the offspring of MOR-F0 mothers showed sex-specific differences in rough and tumble play. These results indicate that even when opiates are withdrawn several weeks prior to mating, a history of opiate exposure can influence both maternal care and offspring development.

A number of animal models have documented the effects of changes in maternal care on developing offspring. For example, the amount of licking and grooming that a female exhibits in

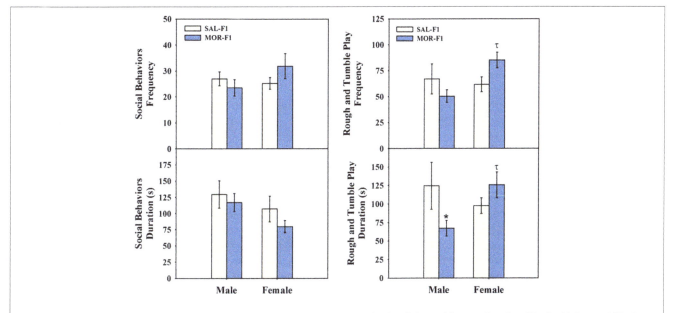

FIGURE 4 | Mean (±SEM) frequency and duration (seconds) of either general social behaviors (left panels) or rough and tumble play (right panels) in the offspring of females exposed to either morphine (MOR-F1) or saline (SAL-F1) during adolescence. *$p < 0.05$ as compared SAL-F1 males, τ$p < 0.05$ as compared to MOR-F1 males. $N = 10$ SAL-F1 male; $N = 10$ SAL-F1 female pairs and $N = 12$ MOR-F1 male; $N = 12$ MOR-F1 female pairs.

the first week postpartum, can modify the behavioral phenotype of her offspring (Caldji et al., 1998). These offspring effects include shifts in the maternal behavior of adult female offspring (Champagne et al., 2003; Kikusui et al., 2005), as well as changes in stress responsiveness (Fish et al., 2004), play behavior (Moore and Power, 1992), and cognition (Liu et al., 2000; Champagne et al., 2008). Other models, focusing on the effects of either brief or prolonged maternal separation, have also illustrated the importance of mother–offspring interactions (D'Amato et al., 1998), with significant effects on the regulation of fear and anxiety, stress responsiveness, and motivated behaviors observed in adult offspring (Romeo et al., 2003; Lee et al., 2007; Michaels et al., 2007; George et al., 2010; Skripuletz et al., 2010; Macri et al., 2011). Often, these effects are sex-specific (Slotten et al., 2006). It is not clear whether all of these alterations in offspring development are directly related to maternal behavior. It is certainly possible that a number of these effects are mediated by factors present in the milk (e.g., corticosterone or prolactin) or represent some interplay between maternal care, maternal endocrine milieu, and the offspring's own physiology. When considering how these findings might translate to human mothers and their infants, it is important to remember that there are significant developmental differences between rodents and humans. Indeed, neurodevelopment in the postnatal rat is comparable to that observed in second and third trimester infants (Bayer et al., 1993). By determining what mechanisms underlie changes in adult phenotype that are induced by alterations in maternal care, we may gain significant insight into how early life experience, both *in utero* and during the early postpartum period, may alter neurodevelopment. Overall, these findings on maternal care in rodents clearly indicate that even ostensibly modest changes in the postpartum environment can significantly impact offspring development.

How then might adolescent morphine exposure induce alterations in maternal care? One possible mechanism may be a shift in the endogenous opioid system. Indeed, we previously observed significant shifts in the regulation hypothalamic, opioid-related gene transcription following adolescent opioid exposure (Byrnes, 2008). These effects on gene transcription persisted for at least 10 weeks following cessation of morphine administration. Thus, a shift in endogenous opioid-mediated regulation of maternal behavior may be one consequence of adolescent morphine exposure.

The importance of endogenous opioids in both the pre- and postnatal period has been well documented. Opioids directly regulate numerous aspects of embryonic and fetal development (Kar and Quirion, 1995; Leslie et al., 1998; Zagon et al., 1999; Kivell et al., 2004; Cooney et al., 2009). Moreover, during pregnancy and parturition, endogenous opioids modulate both the maternal and fetal hypothalamic–pituitary–adrenal axis (Taylor et al., 1997; Douglas et al., 1998), and regulate maternal central oxytocin activity (Douglas et al., 1995; Douglas and Russell, 2001; Kutlu et al., 2004). The role of endogenous opioids in the regulation of specific aspects of maternal care in the rat is not well-defined. There is evidence, however, that the administration of an opioid antagonist increases the duration of nursing bouts and mother–offspring contact time during early lactation (Byrnes et al., 2000). These data fit well with the hypothesis that opioids regulate maternal–offspring attachment processes (Nelson and Panksepp, 1998; Weller and Feldman, 2003). Thus, in the face of opioid receptor blockade, the female may prolong contact and/or nursing bouts to achieve a similar level of reward associated with pup contact. In this context, one would postulate that MOR-F0 females may have more sensitive opioid receptors and therefore may terminate their nursing bouts sooner. While we observed significantly increased mu- and kappa-opioid receptor mRNA in non-lactating MOR-F0 females, no differences in the expression of these receptor subtypes were observed during lactation (Byrnes, 2008). Of course, protein expression and/or postsynaptic response of these receptors could be modified in MOR-F0 females. Moreover, our previous studies only examined changes in the mediobasal hypothalamus. Certainly, significant differences in opioid receptor number and/or function in any number of brain regions could underlie changes in nursing behavior during early lactation. This would not, however, explain the increased contact time (i.e., hovering) observed in MOR-F0 mother. Perhaps then, some other change in the female's behavior might underlie the observed effects on nursing frequency.

Examination of the differences in nursing behavior and contact time reveal a significant influence of both the time of day and the testing method. MOR-F0 females only spent more time away from the nest during the dark and these differences were only significant when tested using frequency data. Similarly, when recorded continuously, no decrease in the duration of nursing was observed during early lactation. One obvious difference between our frequency and duration data was the presence of an observer during frequency data collection. We have noticed that qualitatively, MOR-F0 females appear to be more sensitive to any disturbance in their environment. Thus, while all of our observations were conducted in the home cage, and care was taken not to disturb the female and her litter, MOR-F0 females would often come off the nest and rear up toward the front of the cage during the 30-min observation session. In addition, this behavioral pattern appeared more robust during the dark phase. Thus, the simple act of observing MOR-F0 females may have altered their nursing frequency. These effects would be more robust during early lactation when immature pups are unable to maintain nipple contact when the dam rears or changes positions. If a more general, non-specific, increase in "distractibility" underlies these changes in maternal care, this would suggest that MOR-F0 mothers may be more likely to decrease the care of their offspring in the presence of substantial environmental distracters.

The data on the duration of nursing suggests that during later postnatal time points, MOR-F0 mothers have more prolonged nursing bouts. As mentioned previously, during these later time points pups are more able to maintain nursing contact even when the female moves either within or even off of the nest. Thus, rearing up in the presence of any distracter would not be as detrimental to nursing when pups are older. However, this would not explain why the female nurses for longer periods when compared to SAL-F0 females. One possibility is that the female and/or offspring are compensating for decreased nutrition during early lactation with more sustained lactation during later development. Indeed, the bodyweight data demonstrate that MOR-F1 weanlings are heavier than their SAL-F1 counterparts. To what extent maternal nursing behavior, as opposed to some other metabolic factor, induces this difference in body weight is unknown. However, we have previous data suggesting differences in the lactogenic hormone prolactin in MOR-F1 mothers, with lower levels observed during early lactation and higher levels observed during late lactation (Byrnes, 2005b). Thus, MOR-F0 females may not necessarily be deficient in their nursing behavior, but rather may demonstrate a shift in the developmental profile of this behavior over the course of lactation. Overall, these data suggest that subtle modifications in maternal care, especially relating to nursing and non-nursing contact, are a consequence of adolescent morphine exposure. To what extent these differences play a role in the behavioral phenotype of their offspring remains to be determined.

In addition to modifying maternal care, adolescent morphine exposure induced transgenerational effects on juvenile play behavior. MOR-F1 males demonstrated a significant reduction in rough and tumble play, with no change in other aspects of social behavior (social grooming or exploration). In addition, there was a trend toward increased rough and tumble play behavior in MOR-F1 females, although these effects did not achieve significance. Rough and tumble play is displayed by a wide-range of species and is an important developmental marker (Auger and Olesen, 2009; Auger et al., 2011). It has been suggested that low levels of rough and tumble play may indicate vulnerability toward reduced motivated behavior in adulthood (Trezza et al., 2010). For example, animal models have demonstrated a relationship between rough and tumble play and future sexual and aggressive behaviors (van den Berg et al., 1999a; Cervantes et al., 2007; Wommack and Delville, 2007). Thus, decreased rough and tumble play in MOR-F1 males may suggest an increased risk for deficits in other motivated behavior in adulthood.

The neural systems underlying rough and tumble play have been fairly well elucidated (Gordon et al., 2002), with opioids playing a significant role in the regulation of this behavioral repertoire. Specifically, administration of morphine enhances play behavior, while administration of the mu-opiate receptor antagonist naloxone, reduces rough and tumble play (Panksepp et al., 1985; Vanderschuren et al., 1995; Guard et al., 2002; Trezza and Vanderschuren, 2008). Moreover, when juveniles are socially isolated, thereby eliminating all experiences of play, both mu and kappa receptors are significantly up-regulation in several nuclei related to emotional regulation (Van den Berg et al., 1999b). Thus, the reduction in rough and tumble play behavior could be a symptom of a down-regulation of functional mu-opiate receptors in MOR-F1 males or conversely, their low levels of play could induce alterations in opiate receptors. In line with these data, previous findings in adult MOR-F1 males, demonstrate significant alterations in their response to opiates (Byrnes, 2005a; Byrnes et al., 2011). Thus, one intriguing possibility is that MOR-F0 females transfer modifications in neural opioid systems to their offspring. The mechanism underlying this type of epigenetic effect is unknown, but could certainly involve alterations in maternal care or maternal endocrine milieu.

Finally, consideration of the current findings in the context of effects following prenatal morphine administration is warranted. Certainly, morphine exposure during the prenatal period has been shown to significantly impact offspring development (Sobrian, 1977; Vathy and Katay, 1992; Lesage et al., 1996; Vathy et al., 2000; Slamberova et al., 2005), with many of these effects involving changes in opioidergic function (O'Callaghan and Holtzman, 1976; Ramsey et al., 1993; Gagin et al., 1997; Chiou et al., 2003; Villarreal et al., 2008). Interestingly, the effects we observed in MOR-F1 animals are in the opposite direction of those observed in the offspring of females exposed to morphine *in utero*, with rough and tumble play behavior found to be increased in the offspring of females exposed to morphine during gestation (Hol et al., 1996; Niesink et al., 1996). In fact, our effects are more similar to those observed following administration of opioid antagonists during fetal development (Shepanek et al., 1995; Medina Jimenez et al., 1997). Thus, the transgenerational effects observed in the offspring of adolescent morphine-exposed females may be indicative of a down-regulation of the endogenous opioid system in their mothers, perhaps both pre- and postnatally, which is then transmitted to their offspring via currently unidentified, epigenetic processes. Such processes could include modifications in maternal–offspring interactions.

CONCLUSION

Adolescent use of prescription pain relievers has increased dramatically in the past decade, especially in young females. Beyond the risks of overdose or addiction, the long-term effects of exposure to such powerful opiates during a critical period of neurodevelopment are unknown. As endogenous opioids play such a significant role in reproductive function, prior opiate use could influence pre- and/or postnatal factors. Given the importance of opioids in maternal–offspring interactions, and the critical role that mothers play in the healthy development of their children, it is possible that opiate use in adolescent girls could have repercussions for future generations. To begin to elucidate the possible long-term effects of adolescent opiate use, animal models examining the impact of adolescent opiate exposure on both the female and her future offspring are required. The current findings demonstrate that exposure to increasing doses of morphine during adolescent development can induce subtle changes in maternal care and offspring development. While the neural and/or endocrine mechanisms underlying these effects remain to be determined, a shift in the endogenous opioid system of both mother and offspring seems likely. These findings strongly suggest that adolescent female opiate use, occurring prior to mating, and in the absence of any further use pre- or postnatally, can impact maternal–offspring interactions and the behavioral phenotype of their offspring. Thus, concerns about the impact of maternal drug use on children's health, should not only include consideration of *in utero* exposure, but prior drug history as well.

ACKNOWLEDGMENT

This work was supported by a grant from the National Institute on Drug Abuse R01 DA025674 (EMB).

REFERENCES

Alemagno, S. A., Stephens, P., Shaffer-King, P., and Teasdale, B. (2009). Prescription drug abuse among adolescent arrestees: correlates and implications. *J. Correct. Health Care* 15, 35–46.

Auger, A. P., Jessen, H. M., and Edelmann, M. N. (2011). Epigenetic organization of brain sex differences and juvenile social play behavior. *Horm. Behav.* 59, 358–363.

Auger, A. P., and Olesen, K. M. (2009). Brain sex differences and the organisation of juvenile social play behaviour. *J. Neuroendocrinol.* 21, 519–525.

Barr, C. S., Schwandt, M. L., Lindell, S. G., Higley, J. D., Maestripieri, D., Goldman, D., Suomi, S. J., and Heilig, M. (2008). Variation at the mu-opioid receptor gene (OPRM1) influences attachment behavior in infant primates. *Proc. Natl. Acad. Sci. U.S.A.* 105, 5277–5281.

Bayer, S. A., Altman J., Russo, R. J., and Zhang, X. (1993). Timetables of neurogenesis in the human brain based on experimentally determined patterns in the rat. *Neurotoxicology* 14, 83–144.

Bridges, R. S., and Grimm, C. T. (1982). Reversal of morphine disruption of maternal behavior by concurrent treatment with the opiate antagonist naloxone. *Science* 218, 166–168.

Byrnes, E. M. (2005a). Transgenerational consequences of adolescent morphine exposure in female rats: effects on anxiety-like behaviors and morphine sensitization in adult offspring. *Psychopharmacology (Berl.)* 182, 537–544.

Byrnes, E. M. (2005b). Chronic morphine exposure during puberty decreases postpartum prolactin secretion in adult female rats. *Pharmacol. Biochem. Behav.* 80, 445–451.

Byrnes, E. M. (2008). Chronic morphine exposure during puberty induces long-lasting changes in opioid-related mRNA expression in the mediobasal hypothalamus. *Brain Res.* 1190, 186–192.

Byrnes, E. M., Rigero, B. A., and Bridges, R. S. (2000). Opioid receptor antagonism during early lactation results in the increased duration of nursing bouts. *Physiol. Behav.* 70, 211–216.

Byrnes, J. J., Babb, J. A., Scanlan, V. F., and Byrnes, E. M. (2011). Adolescent opioid exposure in female rats: transgenerational effects on morphine analgesia and anxiety-like behavior in adult offspring. *Behav. Brain Res.* 218, 200–205.

Cai, R., Crane, E., Poneleit, K., and Paulozzi, L. (2010). Emergency department visits involving nonmedical use of selected prescription drugs in the United States, 2004–2008. *J. Pain Palliat. Care Pharmacother.* 24, 293–297.

Caldji, C., Tannenbaum, B., Sharma, S., Francis, D., Plotsky, P. M., and Meaney, M. J. (1998). Maternal care during infancy regulates the development of neural systems mediating the expression of fearfulness in the rat. *Proc. Natl. Acad. Sci. U.S.A.* 95, 5335–5340.

Cervantes, M. C., Taravosh-Lahn, K., Wommack, J. C., and Delville, Y. (2007). Characterization of offensive responses during the maturation of play-fighting into aggression in male golden hamsters. *Dev. Psychobiol.* 49, 87–97.

Champagne, D. L., Bagot, R. C., van Hasselt, F., Ramakers, G., Meaney, M. J., de Kloet, E. R., Joels, M., and Krugers, H. (2008). Maternal care and hippocampal plasticity: evidence for experience-dependent structural plasticity, altered synaptic functioning, and differential responsiveness to glucocorticoids and stress. *J. Neurosci.* 28, 6037–6045.

Champagne, F. A., Francis, D. D., Mar, A., and Meaney, M. J. (2003). Variations in maternal care in the rat as a mediating influence for the effects of environment on development. *Physiol. Behav.* 79, 359–371.

Chiou, L. C., Yeh, G. C., Fan, S. H., How, C. H., Chuang, K. C., and Tao, P. L. (2003). Prenatal morphine exposure decreases analgesia but not K+ channel activation. *Neuroreport* 14, 239–242.

Chiou, W. L., Robbie, G., Chung, S. M., Wu, T., and Ma, C. (1998). Correlation of plasma clearance of 54 extensively metabolized drugs between humans and rats: mean allometric coefficient of 0.66. *Pharm. Res.* 15, 1474–1479.

Cicero, T. J., Schmoeker, P. F., Meyer, E. R., Miller, B. T., Bell, R. D., Cytron, S. M., and Brown, C. C. (1986). Ontogeny of the opioid-mediated control of reproductive endocrinology in the male and female rat. *J. Pharmacol. Exp. Ther.* 236, 627–633.

Cooney, T. E., Konieczko, E. M., Roach, L., and Poole, B. (2009). Fate of mu receptors during rat skeletogenesis. *Orthopedics* 32, 95.

D'Amato, F. R., Cabib, S., Ventura, R., and Orsini, C. (1998). Long-term effects of postnatal manipulation on emotionality are prevented by maternal anxiolytic treatment in mice. *Dev. Psychobiol.* 32, 225–234.

Douglas, A. J., Bicknell, R. J., and Russell, J. A. (1995). Pathways to parturition. *Adv. Exp. Med. Biol.* 395, 381–394.

Douglas, A. J., Johnstone, H. A., Wigger, A., Landgraf, R., Russell, J. A., and Neumann, I. D. (1998). The role of endogenous opioids in neurohypophysial and hypothalamo-pituitary-adrenal axis hormone secretory responses to stress in pregnant rats. *J. Endocrinol.* 158, 285–293.

Douglas, A. J., and Russell, J. A. (2001). Endogenous opioid regulation of oxytocin and ACTH secretion during pregnancy and parturition. *Prog. Brain Res.* 133, 67–82.

Drolet, G., Dumont, E. C., Gosselin, I., Kinkead, R., Laforest, S., and Trottier, J. F. (2001). Role of endogenous opioid system in the regulation of the stress response. *Prog. Neuropsychopharmacol. Biol. Psychiatry* 25, 729–741.

Fish, E. W., Shahrokh, D., Bagot, R., Caldji, C., Bredy, T., Szyf, M., and Meaney, M. J. (2004). Epigenetic programming of stress responses through variations in maternal care. *Ann. N. Y. Acad. Sci.* 1036, 167–180.

Forman, R. F., Woody, G. E., McLellan, T., and Lynch, K. G. (2006). The availability of web sites offering to sell opioid medications without prescriptions. *Am. J. Psychiatry* 163, 1233–1238.

Gagin, R., Kook, N., Cohen, E., and Shavit, Y. (1997). Prenatal morphine enhances morphine-conditioned place preference in adult rats. *Pharmacol. Biochem. Behav.* 58, 525–528.

George, E. D., Bordner, K. A., Elwafi, H. M., and Simen, A. A. (2010). Maternal separation with early weaning: a novel mouse model of early life neglect. *BMC Neurosci.* 11, 123. doi: 10.1186/1471-2202-11-123

Goodman, G., Hans, S. L., and Cox, S. M. (1999). Attachment behavior and its antecedents in offspring born to methadone-maintained women. *J. Clin. Child Psychol.* 28, 58–69.

Gordon, N. S., Kollack-Walker, S., Akil, H., and Panksepp, J. (2002). Expression of c-fos gene activation during rough and tumble play in juvenile rats. *Brain Res. Bull.* 57, 651–659.

Guard, H. J., Newman, J. D., and Roberts, R. L. (2002). Morphine administration selectively facilitates social play in common marmosets. *Dev. Psychobiol.* 41, 37–49.

Gustafsson, L., Oreland, S., Hoffmann, P., and Nylander, I. (2008). The impact of postnatal environment on opioid peptides in young and adult male Wistar rats. *Neuropeptides* 42, 177–191.

Hol, T., Niesink, M., van Ree, J. M., and Spruijt, B. M. (1996). Prenatal exposure to morphine affects juvenile play behavior and adult social behavior in rats. *Pharmacol. Biochem. Behav.* 55, 615–618.

Janus, K. (1987). Early separation of young rats from the mother and the development of play fighting. *Physiol. Behav.* 39, 471–476.

Kalin, N. H., Shelton, S. E., and Lynn, D. E. (1995). Opiate systems in mother and infant primates coordinate intimate contact during reunion. *Psychoneuroendocrinology* 20, 735–742.

Kar, S., and Quirion, R. (1995). Neuropeptide receptors in developing and adult rat spinal cord: an in vitro quantitative autoradiography study of calcitonin gene-related peptide, neurokinins, mu-opioid, galanin, somatostatin, neurotensin and vasoactive intestinal polypeptide receptors. *J. Comp. Neurol.* 354, 253–281.

Kikusui, T., Isaka, Y., and Mori, Y. (2005). Early weaning deprives mouse pups of maternal care and decreases their maternal behavior in adulthood. *Behav. Brain Res.* 162, 200–206.

Kinsley, C. H., and Bridges, R. S. (1986). Opiate involvement in postpartum aggression in rats. *Pharmacol. Biochem. Behav.* 25, 1007–1011.

Kinsley, C. H., and Bridges, R. S. (1990). Morphine treatment and reproductive condition alter olfactory preferences for pup and adult male odors in female rats. *Dev. Psychobiol.* 23, 331–347.

Kinsley, C. H., Morse, A. C., Zoumas, C., Corl, S., and Billack, B. (1995). Intracerebroventricular infusions of morphine, and blockade with naloxone, modify the olfactory preferences for pup odors in lactating rats. *Brain Res. Bull.* 37, 103–107.

Kivell, B. M., Day, D. J., McDonald, F. J., and Miller, J. H. (2004). Developmental expression of mu and delta opioid receptors in the rat brainstem: evidence for a postnatal switch in mu isoform expression. *Brain Res. Dev. Brain Res.* 148, 185–196.

Kreek, M. J. (2007). Opioids, dopamine, stress, and the addictions. *Dialogues Clin. Neurosci.* 9, 363–378.

Kutlu, S., Yilmaz, B., Canpolat, S., Sandal, S., Ozcan, M., Kumru, S., and Kelestimur, H. (2004). Mu opioid modulation of oxytocin secretion in late pregnant and parturient rats. Involvement of noradrenergic neurotransmission. *Neuroendocrinology* 79, 197–203.

Lee, J. H., Kim, H. J., Kim, J. G., Ryu, V., Kim, B. T., Kang, D. W., and Jahng, J. W. (2007). Depressive behaviors and decreased expression of serotonin reuptake transporter in rats that experienced neonatal maternal separation. *Neurosci. Res.* 58, 32–39.

Lesage, J., Bernet, F., Montel, V., and Dupouy, J. P. (1996). Effects of prenatal morphine on hypothalamic metabolism of neurotransmitters and gonadal and adrenal activities, during the early postnatal period in the rat. *Neurochem. Res.* 21, 723–732.

Leslie, F. M., Chen, Y., and Winzer-Serhan, U. H. (1998). Opioid receptor and peptide mRNA expression in proliferative zones of fetal rat central nervous system. *Can. J. Physiol. Pharmacol.* 76, 284–293.

Liu, D., Diorio, J., Day, J. C., Francis, D. D., and Meaney, M. J. (2000). Maternal care, hippocampal synaptogenesis and cognitive development in rats. *Nat. Neurosci.* 3, 799–806.

Macri, S., Zoratto, F., and Laviola, G. (2011). Early-stress regulates resilience, vulnerability and experimental validity in laboratory rodents through mother–offspring hormonal transfer. *Neurosci. Biobehav. Rev.* doi: 10.1016/j.neubiorev.2010.12.014 [Epub ahead of print].

Mann, P. E., Pasternak, G. W., and Bridges, R. S. (1990). Mu 1 opioid receptor involvement in maternal behavior. *Physiol. Behav.* 47, 133–138.

McCubbin, J. A. (1993). Stress and endogenous opioids: behavioral and circulatory interactions. *Biol. Psychol.* 35, 91–122.

Medina Jimenez, M., Lujan Estrada, M., and Rodriguez, R. (1997). Influence of chronic prenatal and postnatal administration of naltrexone in locomotor activity induced by morphine in mice. *Arch. Med. Res.* 28, 61–65.

Michaels, C. C., Easterling, K. W., and Holtzman, S. G. (2007). Maternal separation alters ICSS responding in adult male and female rats, but morphine and naltrexone have little affect on that behavior. *Brain Res. Bull.* 73, 310–318.

Michaels, C. C., and Holtzman, S. G. (2008). Early postnatal stress alters place conditioning to both mu- and kappa-opioid agonists. *J. Pharmacol. Exp. Ther.* 325, 313–318.

Miranda-Paiva, C. M., Nasello, A. G., Yin, A. J., and Felicio, L. F. (2001). Morphine pretreatment increases opioid inhibitory effects on maternal behavior. *Brain Res. Bull.* 55, 501–505.

Moore, C. L., and Power, K. L. (1992). Variation in maternal care and individual differences in play, exploration, and grooming of juvenile Norway rat offspring. *Dev. Psychobiol.* 25, 165–182.

Nelson, E. E., and Panksepp, J. (1998). Brain substrates of infant–mother attachment: contributions of opioids, oxytocin, and norepinephrine. *Neurosci. Biobehav. Rev.* 22, 437–452.

Niesink, R. J., Vanderschuren, L. J., and van Ree, J. M. (1996). Social play in juvenile rats after in utero exposure to morphine. *Neurotoxicology* 17, 905–912.

Niesink, R. J., and Van Ree, J. M. (1989). Involvement of opioid and dopaminergic systems in isolation-induced pinning and social grooming of young rats. *Neuropharmacology* 28, 411–418.

O'Callaghan, J. P., and Holtzman, S. G. (1976). Prenatal administration of morphine to the rat: tolerance to the analgesic effect of morphine in the offspring. *J. Pharmacol. Exp. Ther.* 197, 533–544.

Panksepp, J., Jalowiec, J., DeEskinazi, F. G., and Bishop, P. (1985). Opiates and play dominance in juvenile rats. *Behav. Neurosci.* 99, 441–453.

Panksepp, J., Nelson, E., and Siviy, S. (1994). Brain opioids and mother–infant social motivation. *Acta Paediatr. Suppl.* 397, 40–46.

Paulozzi, L. J., Budnitz, D. S., and Xi, Y. (2006). Increasing deaths from opioid analgesics in the United States. *Pharmacoepidemiol. Drug. Saf.* 15, 618–627.

Ramsey, N. F., Niesink, R. J., and Van Ree, J. M. (1993). Prenatal exposure to morphine enhances cocaine and heroin self-administration in drug-naive rats. *Drug Alcohol Depend.* 33, 41–51.

Reiter, E. O. (1987). Neuroendocrine control processes. Pubertal onset and progression. *J. Adolesc. Health Care* 8, 479–491.

Romeo, R. D., Mueller, A., Sisti, H. M., Ogawa, S., McEwen, B. S., and Brake, W. G. (2003). Anxiety and fear behaviors in adult male and female C57BL/6 mice are modulated by maternal separation. *Horm. Behav.* 43, 561–567.

Rubin, B. S., and Bridges, R. S. (1984). Disruption of ongoing maternal responsiveness in rats by central administration of morphine sulfate. *Brain Res.* 307, 91–97.

Saltzman, W., and Maestripieri, D. (2010). The neuroendocrinology of primate maternal behavior. *Prog. Neuropsychopharmacol. Biol. Psychiatry*, doi:10.1016/j.pnpbp.2010.09.017

Schino, G., and Troisi, A. (1992). Opiate receptor blockade in juvenile macaques: effect on affiliative interactions with their mothers and group companions. *Brain Res.* 576, 125–130.

Shepanek, N. A., Smith, R. F., Anderson, L. A., and Medici, C. N. (1995). Behavioral and developmental changes associated with prenatal opiate receptor blockade. *Pharmacol. Biochem. Behav.* 50, 313–319.

Sizonenko, P. C. (1987). Normal sexual maturation. *Pediatrician* 14, 191–201.

Skripuletz, T., Kruschinski, C., Pabst, R., von Horsten, S., and Stephan, M. (2010). Postnatal experiences influence the behavior in adult male and female Fischer and Lewis rats. *Int. J. Dev. Neurosci.* 28, 561–571.

Slamberova, R., Riley, M. A., and Vathy, I. (2005). Cross-generational effect of prenatal morphine exposure on neurobehavioral development of rat pups. *Physiol. Res* 54, 655–660.

Slamberova, R., Szilagyi, B., and Vathy, I. (2001). Repeated morphine administration during pregnancy attenuates maternal behavior. *Psychoneuroendocrinology* 26, 565–576.

Slotten, H. A., Kalinichev, M., Hagan, J. J., Marsden, C. A., and Fone, K. C. (2006). Long-lasting changes in behavioural and neuroendocrine indices in the rat following neonatal maternal separation: gender-dependent effects. *Brain Res.* 1097, 123–132.

Sobrian, S. K. (1977). Prenatal morphine administration alters behavioral development in the rat. *Pharmacol. Biochem. Behav.* 7, 285–288.

Substance Abuse and Mental Health Services Administration (SAMHSA). (2007). *Results from the 2006 National Survey on Drug Use and Health: National Findings*. NSDUH Series H-32, DHHS Publication No. SMA 07-4293. Rockville, MD: Office of Applied Studies.

Substance Abuse and Mental Health Services Administration (SAMHSA). (2009). *Results from the 2008 National Survey on Drug Use and Health: National Findings*. NSDUH Series H-36, HHS Publication No. SMA 09-4434. Rockville, MD: Office of Applied Studies.

Sukikara, M. H., Platero, M. D., Canteras, N. S., and Felicio, L. F. (2007). Opiate regulation of behavioral selection during lactation. *Pharmacol. Biochem. Behav.* 87, 315–320.

Sung, H. E., Richter, L., Vaughan, R., Johnson, P. B., and Thom, B. (2005). Nonmedical use of prescription opioids among teenagers in the United States: trends and correlates. *J. Adolesc. Health* 37, 44–51.

Taylor, C. C., Wu, D., Soong, Y., Yee, J. S., and Szeto, H. H. (1997). Opioid modulation of the fetal hypothalamic–pituitary–adrenal axis: the role of receptor subtypes and route of administration. *J. Pharmacol. Exp. Ther.* 281, 129–135.

Trezza, V., Baarendse, P. J., and Vanderschuren, L. J. (2010). The pleasures of play: pharmacological insights into social reward mechanisms. *Trends Pharmacol. Sci.* 31, 463–469.

Trezza, V., and Vanderschuren, L. J. (2008). Cannabinoid and opioid modulation of social play behavior in adolescent rats: differential behavioral mechanisms. *Eur. Neuropsychopharmacol.* 18, 519–530.

van den Berg, C. L., Hol, T., Van Ree, J. M., Spruijt, B. M., Everts, H., and Koolhaas, J. M. (1999a). Play is indispensable for an adequate development of coping with social challenges in the rat. *Dev. Psychobiol.* 34, 129–138.

Van den Berg, C. L., Van Ree, J. M., Spruijt, B. M., and Kitchen, I. (1999b). Effects of juvenile isolation and morphine treatment on social interactions and opioid receptors in adult rats: behavioural and autoradiographic studies. *Eur. J. Neurosci.* 11, 3023–3032.

Van den Berg, C. L., Van Ree, J. M., and Spruijt, B. M. (2000). Morphine attenuates the effects of juvenile isolation in rats. *Neuropharmacology* 39, 969–976.

Vanderschuren, L. J., Niesink, R. J., Spruijt, B. M., and Van Ree, J. M. (1995). Effects of morphine on different aspects of social play in juvenile rats. *Psychopharmacology (Berl.)* 117, 225–231.

Van Ree, J. M., Niesink, R. J., Van Wolfswinkel, L., Ramsey, N. F., Kornet, M. M., Van Furth, W. R., Vanderschuren, L. J., Gerrits, M. A., and Van den Berg, C. L. (2000). Endogenous opioids and reward. *Eur. J. Pharmacol.* 405, 89–101.

Vathy, I., He, H. J., Iodice, M., Hnatczuk, O. C., and Rimanoczy, A. (2000). Prenatal morphine exposure differentially alters TH-immunoreactivity in the stress-sensitive brain circuitry of adult male and female rats. *Brain Res. Bull.* 51, 267–273.

Vathy, I., and Katay, L. (1992). Effects of prenatal morphine on adult sexual behavior and brain catecholamines in rats. *Brain Res. Dev. Brain Res.* 68, 125–131.

Veenema, A. H., and Neumann, I. D. (2009). Maternal separation enhances offensive play-fighting, basal corticosterone and hypothalamic vasopressin mRNA expression in juvenile male rats. *Psychoneuroendocrinology* 34, 463–467.

Villarreal, D. M., Derrick, B., and Vathy, I. (2008). Prenatal morphine exposure attenuates the maintenance of late LTP in lateral perforant path projections to the dentate gyrus and the CA3 region in vivo. *J. Neurophysiol.* 99, 1235–1242.

Weaver, S. A., Diorio, J., and Meaney, M. J. (2007). Maternal separation leads to persistent reductions in pain sensitivity in female rats. *J. Pain.* 8, 962–969.

Weller, A., and Feldman, R. (2003). Emotion regulation and touch in infants: the role of cholecystokinin and opioids. *Peptides* 24, 779–788.

Wommack, J. C., and Delville, Y. (2007). Stress, aggression, and puberty: neuroendocrine correlates of the development of agonistic behavior in golden hamsters. *Brain Behav. Evol.* 70, 267–273.

Wu, L. T., Pilowsky, D. J., and Patkar, A. A. (2008). Non-prescribed use of pain relievers among adolescents in the United States. *Drug Alcohol Depend.* 94, 1–11.

Zager, E. L., and Black, P. M. (1985). Neuropeptides in human memory and learning processes. *Neurosurgery* 17, 355–369.

Zagon, I. S., Wu, Y., and McLaughlin, P. J. (1999). Opioid growth factor and organ development in rat and human embryos. *Brain Res.* 839, 313–322.

Mesolimbic dopamine transients in motivated behaviors: Focus on maternal behavior

Donita L. Robinson[1,2,3]*, Dawnya L. Zitzman[1] and Sarah K. Williams[2,3]

[1] Bowles Center for Alcohol Studies, University of North Carolina, Chapel Hill, NC, USA
[2] Department of Psychiatry, University of North Carolina, Chapel Hill, NC, USA
[3] Curriculum in Neurobiology, University of North Carolina, Chapel Hill, NC, USA

*Correspondence:
Donita L. Robinson, Center for Alcohol Studies, University of North Carolina, CB #7178, Chapel Hill, NC 27599-7178, USA.
e-mail: dlr@unc.edu

Phasic activity of the mesolimbic dopamine pathway – burst-firing of dopamine neurons and the resulting dopamine release events at striatal targets – have been associated with a variety of motivational events, such as novelty, salient stimuli, social interaction, and reward prediction. Over the past decade, advances in electrochemical techniques have allowed measurement of naturally occurring dopamine release events, or dopamine transients, in awake animals during ongoing behavior. Thus, a growing body of studies has revealed dynamic dopamine input to ventral striatum during motivated behavior in a variety of experimental paradigms. We propose that dopamine transients may be important neural signals in pup-directed aspects of maternal behavior, as preliminary data suggest that dopamine transients in dams are associated with pup cues. Measurements of dopamine transients may be useful to investigate not only typical maternal behavior but also maternal inattention induced by drug exposure or stress.

Keywords: dopamine, phasic, voltammetry, *in vivo*, maternal, social, reward

Dopamine exerts considerable influence on animal behavior. In addition to the control of voluntary movement (e.g., Parkinson's disease), dopamine plays an important role in reward and motivation (preliminary data: Ikemoto and Panksepp, 1999; Salamone et al., 2005, 2007; Alcaro et al., 2007). Thus, it is central not only to many natural behaviors, such as reproduction and ingestion, but also to pathologic ones, like addiction and other compulsive disorders. Telencephalic dopamine projections arise from the ventral tegmental area (VTA) and the substantia nigra in the midbrain and ascend to multiple forebrain structures, most notably the caudate, putamen, and nucleus accumbens (NAc; collectively called the striatum). All of these projections have been implicated in various aspects of motivated behavior. For example, nigral dopaminergic afferents to the dorsolateral striatum participate in habit-learning and automatic responses to cues, while those to the dorsomedial striatum have been implicated in goal-directed behaviors and action selection (Yin and Knowlton, 2006; Wickens et al., 2007; Lovinger, 2010; de Wit et al., 2011). Furthermore, the dopaminergic system most closely associated with cue-reward associations is the mesolimbic pathway, projecting from the VTA in the midbrain to anterior targets that include the NAc, olfactory tubercle, and prefrontal cortex. This review will focus on the mesolimbic dopamine system as it is the dopamine projection most studied in the context of maternal behavior. Nevertheless, dopaminergic input to each striatal region is likely to play important roles in maternal behavior.

By using *in vivo* neurochemical methods, many studies have demonstrated that extracellular dopamine concentrations in the NAc increase in the minutes to hours during natural reward such as sex and food, during stress, or following administration of addictive drugs (for review, see Westerink, 1995; Phillips et al., 2008; Willuhn et al., 2010). More recent research suggests that one aspect of dopamine release – fast fluctuations in dopamine called *dopamine transients* – is a neural correlate of reward salience, approach initiation, and learning (for review, see Robinson et al., 2008; Willuhn et al., 2010). As such, mesolimbic dopamine transients may be a useful window on reward processing in maternal behavior. The goal of this review is to describe the expression of dopamine transients during behavior in studies to date and consider how these fast dopamine events can instruct us on the dopaminergic contribution to both normal and disrupted maternal behavior.

DOPAMINE TRANSIENTS AS A WINDOW INTO REWARD AND REINFORCEMENT PROCESSING

Much of what we have learned of extracellular dopamine dynamics has been dependent on the neurochemical methods to measure them *in vivo*. Microdialysis (Westerink, 1995; Watson et al., 2006) has been used to successfully measure dopamine in various terminal regions. Because the diffusion-based technique has limited ability to track dynamic concentration changes, it is best suited for monitoring slow (over minutes) changes in dopamine concentrations over broad (mm) areas of tissue. Microdialysis research has yielded a wealth of information about dopamine levels during a range of motivated behaviors, including maternal behavior. For example, dopamine levels rise in the NAc during active maternal behaviors, such as nursing and licking pups (Hansen et al., 1993). However, microdialysis lacks the resolution to observe brief changes in dopamine that result from burst-firing of dopamine neurons and are time-locked to specific behavioral events or environmental stimuli (Borland et al., 2005; Yang and Michael, 2007). In contrast, fast scan cyclic voltammetry (FSCV, **Box 1**) is used to measure

---

Abbreviations: FSCV, fast scan cyclic voltammetry; MPOA, medial preoptic area; NAc, nucleus accumbens; VTA, ventral tegmental area.

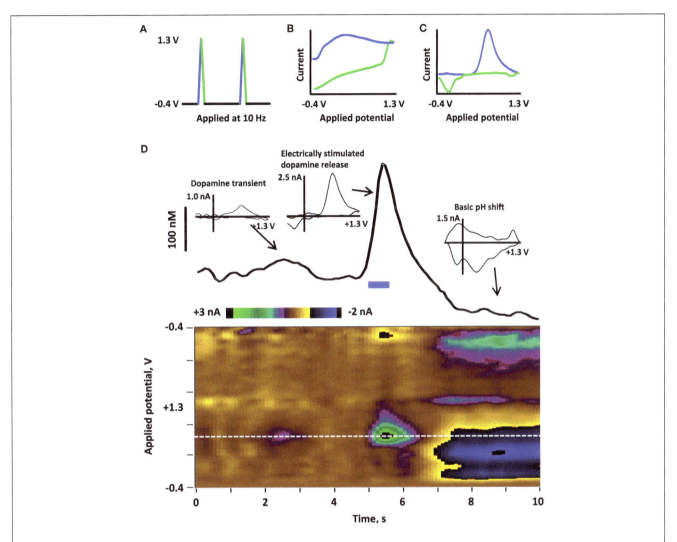

BOX 1 | Fast scan cyclic voltammetry (FSCV) to detect dopamine release

FSCV is a method used to electrochemically detect dopamine *in situ* at the surface of a carbon-fiber microelectrode (Robinson et al., 2008). First, a potential is applied to the electrode; the triangle waveform shown in **(A)** is typically used for electrochemical detection of extracellular dopamine in freely moving rats. This waveform ramps from −0.4 to +1.3 V and back, applied at 400 V/s and repeated at 10 Hz. The precise parameters of the applied waveform (such as the range of potentials, the shape of the waveform, and the speed and frequency at which it is applied) will vary depending on the analyte. Next, current is detected at the electrode due to redox reactions on the electrode surface as well as charging of the double layer around the electrode. This current is depicted in the cyclic voltammogram in **(B)** current associated with the positive, oxidative sweep of the applied waveform is in blue, while current at the negative, reductive sweep is in green. The charging current is large but stable over short time frames (~60 s); thus, the charging current can be subtracted to reveal smaller currents associated with fast changes, such as the oxidation and reduction of dopamine release depicted in **(C)** (background-subtracted cyclic voltammogram of dopamine; oxidation in blue, reduction in green). Importantly, analyte selectivity is obtained by choosing waveform parameters that yield distinguishing background-subtracted cyclic voltammograms for the analyte versus other biological compounds (Robinson and Wightman, 2007). **(D)** Illustrates electrically evoked dopamine release in an awake rat recorded by using FSCV. Current detected at the electrode across time is depicted in a color plot to visualize changes in current at the range of applied potentials (Michael et al., 1998); potential is on the y-axis, time is on the x-axis and current is in color). To better illustrate changes in dopamine, the current at the oxidation potential of dopamine (white dotted line, approximately +0.6 V versus an Ag/AgCl reference electrode) is shown in the trace above the color plot. Dopamine neurons in the midbrain were stimulated with a bipolar electrode (indicated by the blue bar at 5 s; 40 Hz, 16 p, biphasic, 2 ms/phase, 120 μA) and the resulting dopamine release in the nucleus accumbens is observed by increased oxidative current. By calibrating the electrode after the experiment (Logman et al., 2000), current can be converted to dopamine concentration to estimate the amount of dopamine release (~250 nM). This change in current can be confirmed as dopaminergic by evaluation of the cyclic voltammogram (inset). Such electrical stimulation is often followed by basic changes in pH (Kawagoe et al., 1992; Venton et al., 2003; Takmakov et al., 2010), as is observed by the negative current at the oxidative sweep and positive current at the reductive sweep in 7–10 s; the cyclic voltammogram (inset) associated with this change in pH is clearly distinguished from dopamine. FSCV can also be used to detect spontaneous dopamine release events, or dopamine transients. A small transient is observed between 2 and 3 s, identified by the cyclic voltammogram (inset).

these fast and often sub-second, dopamine fluctuations due to the temporal (100 ms) and spatial (typically 100 μm) resolution of the method.

Extracellular dopamine concentrations can be considered within the framework of tonic and phasic release. Tonic dopamine concentrations arise from the population activity of dopamine neurons innervating a target region. While estimates of basal, tonic dopamine levels in striatum range from 5 to 100 nM (Ross, 1991; Kawagoe et al., 1992; Suaud-Chagny et al., 1992; Justice, 1993), these concentrations are likely sufficient to occupy dopamine autoreceptors and high-affinity postsynaptic receptors (Richfield et al., 1989). This "tone" at the dopamine receptors is thought to be important to facilitate movement and gate a variety of dopamine-dependent behaviors (Berke and Hyman, 2000). Furthermore, mesolimbic dopamine tone is an important regulator of effort that an animal will expend to obtain a reward (Salamone et al., 2005). Phasic, burst-firing of dopamine neurons, on the other hand, produces dopamine transients (Kawagoe et al., 1992; Suaud-Chagny et al., 1995; Garris and Rebec, 2002; Sombers et al., 2009): brief, higher concentrations of dopamine that may activate low-affinity dopamine receptors. These phasic dopamine signals are important, for example, for cue-associated learning about reward and salient stimuli (Schultz, 1998; Tsai et al., 2009; Zweifel et al., 2009). Moreover, these brief bursts of firing and the resulting dopamine transients are thought to be important in behavioral switching (Redgrave et al., 1999). Interestingly, dopamine terminals in the ventral striatum appear to corelease glutamate upon phasic firing, which adds another dimension to the function of dopamine transients (Sulzer and Rayport, 2000; Lapish et al., 2006; Hnasko et al., 2010; Stuber et al., 2010a; Tecuapetla et al., 2010). Specifically, the addition of a time-locked glutamatergic signal may provide a transient the true ability to time-lock to stimuli and reward because glutamate activates fast ligand-coupled ion channels. In contrast, postsynaptic dopamine actions via G-protein coupled receptors are slower and may modulate postsynaptic responses to converging inputs (Lapish et al., 2006). Nevertheless, although the complex molecular signaling interactions are still under investigation, it is clear that dopamine transients play a critical contributory role in learning about and appropriate responding to the environment.

Thus, tonic and phasic dopamine firing and release are thought to have distinct receptor targets and different functions in the behaving animal (Garris and Rebec, 2002; Schultz, 2007; Hauber, 2010). In light of this duality, it is important to note that microdialysis and FSCV provide complementary measurements of dopamine dynamics; for example, increases in the number of dopamine neurons that are spontaneously active influence the tonic dopamine concentrations measured with microdialysis (Floresco et al., 2003), whereas increases in dopamine burst-firing do not necessarily affect measurements of dopamine tone (Lu et al., 1998; Floresco et al., 2003; Borland et al., 2005). In contrast, FSCV detects variation in dopamine transient rates that reflect burst rates of dopamine neurons (Sombers et al., 2009), but the method has limited utility to detect slower changes in extracellular dopamine concentrations (Robinson et al., 2008). It is interesting that while the general role of dopamine in maternal behavior is well established

and associated with a rise in tonic dopamine levels (Numan, 2007; Stolzenberg and Numan, 2011), little is known of phasic dopamine activity during maternal behavior.

Transient increases in firing rate, or burst-firing, of dopamine neurons have been recorded in many animal models at numerous events, such as salient environmental stimuli (experimenter hand approach, whisker touch) and reward delivery (for review, see Overton and Clark, 1997). Perhaps the most iconic illustration of phasic dopamine activity during reward processing comes from experiments by Wolfram Schultz and colleagues (Schultz et al., 1997; Schultz, 1998). Recording from midbrain dopamine neurons in primates during a simple Pavlovian task, they found that dopaminergic neurons briefly increased firing rate in response to an unexpected squirt of juice (reward). However, when the animal learned that a cue predicted the reward, the phasic dopamine activity shifted from the reward delivery to the presentation of the conditioned cue. Since FSCV instrumentation and techniques advanced to the point that they could be used in freely moving rats, dopamine transients have been measured at these same events: salient environmental stimuli, reward delivery, and conditioned cues (for review, see Robinson et al., 2008). One advantage of measuring dopamine release as opposed to neuronal firing rate is that while electrophysiology reveals firing patterns of individual neurons, FSCV reveals the extracellular dopamine concentrations available to activate target receptors. This distinction can be important, as recent studies suggest that dopamine transients can arise from influences, perhaps inputs onto dopaminergic axon terminals, other than NMDA receptor activation at the dopamine cell bodies (Sombers et al., 2009; Parker et al., 2010). Related to this, electrophysiology yields firing patterns of individual neurons but cannot confirm their neurochemical identity (e.g., dopaminergic versus GABAergic neuron). In contrast, dopamine fluctuations measured with FSCV are positively identified as dopamine. In addition, regional variation in dopamine release is more easily determined by measuring dopamine release than dopamine neuronal firing (Garris and Rebec, 2002), as there is heterogeneity in the projection targets of various cell groups within the midbrain and especially the VTA (Ikemoto, 2007). While the majority of reports of dopamine transient activity to date have focused on the NAc core and shell, spontaneous transients have also been characterized in dorsomedial striatum (Robinson et al., 2002) and olfactory tubercle (Robinson et al., 2002; Robinson and Wightman, 2004).

The first reports of dopamine transients were in the NAc in response to a novel environment (Rebec et al., 1997) and to the presentation of a sexually receptive rat (Robinson et al., 2001) both arguably important stimuli to a rat. Additional studies demonstrated that dopamine transients were not associated with any particular movement or behavior; instead, they were followed by approach and appetitive behaviors toward the stimulus rat (Robinson et al., 2002), consistent with theories of dopamine function in behavioral switching and reward-seeking. Some studies, including these initial reports, monitored dopamine release across time and at individual experimental events, such as a stimulus presentation or a drug injection. However, other studies have explored dopamine release during multiple-trial sessions, such as Pavlovian conditioning (e.g., Day et al., 2007) and operant self-administration of a reinforcer (e.g., Phillips et al., 2003; Roitman et al., 2004). These multi-trial paradigms allow more sensitive dopamine measurements due to signal-averaging to enhance the signal-to-noise of dopamine release that is consistently expressed at a repeated event such as an operant response or cue presentation. As more and more studies employ FSCV to monitor dopamine transients, some common findings have emerged.

(1) *Dopamine transients occur across the striatum at a basal rate that varies across recording sites and can be pharmacologically manipulated.* Just as individual dopamine neurons burst at a basal frequency (Freeman and Bunney, 1987; Overton and Clark, 1997; Hyland et al., 2002), dopamine transients are expressed at a basal rate in target areas. Generally, transients are more frequent in ventral striatum than dorsal striatum (Robinson et al., 2002), and few basal differences have been detected among the NAc core, shell, and olfactory tubercle (Robinson and Wightman, 2004; Aragona et al., 2008; Robinson et al., 2009). However, within a target nucleus, one may observe dramatic variability in transient expression from one recording site to another as the 100-μm carbon-fiber microelectrode is lowered through the tissue (Wightman et al., 2007). This heterogeneity has resulted in the observation of "hot" and "cold" sites of dopamine transients that is independent of dopamine innervation, as dopamine release can be evoked with electrical stimulation even in the "cold" sites that do not readily support spontaneous dopamine transients (Robinson and Wightman, 2007; Wightman et al., 2007; Robinson et al., 2009). Moreover, these basal rates of dopamine transients can be increased by administration of dopamine transporter blockers, autoreceptor antagonists, and addictive drugs (Robinson and Wightman, 2004; Stuber et al., 2005; Cheer et al., 2007; Aragona et al., 2008). Thus, basal frequencies of dopamine transients are thought to reflect both the burst-firing characteristics of the dopaminergic neurons that innervate the recording site as well as the complement of transporter and receptors on those neurons. As dopaminergic tone is lower in the postpartum period (Afonso et al., 2009), understanding changes in basal rates of transients could be very informative.

(2) *Dopamine transients are often coincident with the presentation of unexpected, salient stimuli.* Just as burst-firing of dopamine neurons in awake animals were initially recorded during unexpected sensory stimulation such as experimenter approach, whisker stimulation, and novelty (for review, see Overton and Clark, 1997), dopamine transients have been reported to occur at the presentation of experimenter approach, novelty, sounds, and unfamiliar rats (for review, see Robinson and Wightman, 2007). Indeed, the unexpected nature of a stimulus appears to be an important factor in whether it evokes dopaminergic burst-firing (Mirenowicz and Schultz, 1994) and dopamine transients, as repeated presentation of a novel stimulus reduced the phasic dopaminergic response to that stimulus (Ljungberg et al., 1992; Rebec et al., 1997; Robinson et al., 2002). Thus, phasic dopamine signals to unexpected events may facilitate behavioral responses and learning about potentially important environmental stimuli (Redgrave et al., 1999, 2008; Alcaro et al., 2007; Schultz, 2007), and thus could play very important roles in the response to newly born pups and the various stimuli (olfactory, auditory, sensory) they create. Additionally, dopamine transients may contribute to the recognition of the subtly altered pup-produced stimuli as they change over pup development.

(3) *Dopamine transients reflect learned cue-reward associations.* The expression of both burst-firing of dopamine neurons and dopamine transients has been explicitly tied to reward and learning. Not only do unexpected rewards reliably induce phasic dopamine release, but cues that predict reward can do the same. In fact, phasic dopamine is hypothesized to act as an error predictor of reward (Schultz, 1998): when a reward is better than expected, phasic dopamine is increased, and when it is worse than expected, it is decreased. In this way, unexpected presentations of reward or reward-predictive cues are "better than expected" and trigger dopamine release. Furthermore, the phasic dopamine signal emerges over time as the relationship between the conditioned cue and the reward is learned (Schultz, 1998; Day et al., 2007; Owesson-White et al., 2008). Dopamine transients associated with cue-reward associations have been demonstrated both in Pavlovian and operant settings, with dopamine release time-locked to the presentation of cues predicting cocaine, sucrose, food, and intracranial stimulation. **Figure 1** shows examples of dopamine release to the cue and a reward in the NAc of a rat after several days of Pavlovian conditioning. As previously reported (Day et al., 2007; Stuber et al., 2008), dopamine release is more robust to the cue than to the reward delivery after Pavlovian conditioning. Recently, optogenetics has been combined with FSCV to experimentally induce firing in dopaminergic neurons expressing the light-activated cation channel channelrhodopsin-2 (Tsai et al., 2009; Vickrey et al., 2009; Bass et al., 2010; Tecuapetla et al., 2010). Using light to stimulate these neurons, Tsai et al. (2009) demonstrated that phasic dopamine was sufficient to induce a conditioned place preference, providing an elegant confirmation that phasic dopamine release (and potentially glutamate corelease) regulates cue-reward learning. In the context of maternal behavior, this technique holds promise to also determine how phasic dopamine might regulate learning of pup stimuli.

(4) *Dopamine transients appear to facilitate reward-seeking behavior.* It has long been known that electrical stimulation of the mesolimbic dopamine pathway is reinforcing and can induce context-dependent motivated behavior (Valenstein et al., 1968), such as approaching and gnawing on a woodchip when it is available, or approaching a bottle and drinking when water is available. Indeed, a unifying theory of dopamine function is that it serves as a seeking system in the brain that is vital to the recognition of and approach toward rewarding stimuli that are necessary to survival, such as food, sex, and safety (Ikemoto and Panksepp, 1999; Alcaro et al., 2007). Thus, it is not surprising that dopamine transients have also been associated with appetitive and approach behaviors. In the first report of dopamine transients during operant self-administration of a reward, electrical stimulation of dopamine was followed by approach to the lever (Phillips et al.,

2003). However, electrical stimulation of dopamine fibers inevitably includes stimulation of other neurons as well, so the effects are non-specific. Thus, an important finding was that spontaneous transients were observed at the initiation of approach to a lever in rats trained to self-administer sucrose (Roitman et al., 2004). In the future, we expect that more selective techniques such as optogenetic control of dopamine release can be used to confirm whether transients are necessary and sufficient to elicit approach behavior to obtain a reward.

DOPAMINE TRANSIENTS DURING SOCIAL BEHAVIOR

While several studies have now reported dopamine transients at the presentation of unexpected stimuli, social stimuli appear to be particularly effective. For example, in one recent study the frequency of dopamine transients in adult male rats increased 2-fold from basal rates at the most effective non-social stimulus (a combination of a novel odor and experimenter approach), while it increased 3.6-fold at the presentation and brief interaction with another male rat (Robinson et al., 2011). **Figure 2** shows examples of dopamine transients in the NAc of a male rat during interaction with another male. Dopamine release is evident at initial whisker contact and sniffing (left), as well as during anogenital sniffing (right). There are several interesting aspects of phasic dopamine release in this paradigm. First, the dopamine transients often occur at initial contact with the partner rat and are followed by appetitive behaviors such as orientation, approach, and sniffing (Robinson et al., 2002). Second, the number and amplitude of the dopamine transients to social stimuli appear to reflect motivation toward the partner rat. When dopamine release in adult male rats was monitored during brief interaction with sexually receptive females, non-receptive females or males, dopamine transients were most frequent with sexually receptive females and least frequent with males (Robinson et al., 2002). Third, the phasic dopamine response appears to habituate with repeated presentation of the same partner rat; that is, fewer dopamine transients are observed at a second presentation of a particular rat, despite the observation that behavior directed at the partner rat is not diminished (Robinson et al., 2002, 2011).

These findings suggest that the phasic dopamine release helps to shift the rat's behavior toward an unexpected partner rat, especially when the partner rat is motivationally significant, consistent with the role of phasic dopamine in behavioral switching (Redgrave et al., 1999), reward-seeking (Alcaro et al., 2007) and reward prediction (Schultz, 1998). Theories of dopamine function would suggest that dopamine transients at the presentation of social stimuli and initial interaction would reflect both the salience of the social stimulus and the unexpected nature. For example, while a sexually receptive female may be effective to trigger transients in a male rat when she unexpectedly appears, she does not necessarily continue to evoke transients when his behavior is already directed toward her. This may explain the habituation of dopamine transients to repeated presentations of stimulus rats, although recognition of the partner rat (lack of novelty) or simply an expectation that the rat will reappear (lack of surprise) may contribute as well. Interestingly, we recently monitored dopamine transients in socially deprived adolescent rats and found that dopamine transients during brief social interaction in adolescent rats did not habituate to a repeat presentation as occurs in socially deprived adults (Robinson et al., 2011). As previous studies have shown that social interaction is particularly rewarding in adolescent rats (Douglas et al., 2004), it is possible that the persistence of dopamine transients also reflects increased reward.

Our studies support the hypothesis that dopamine transients reflect appetitive aspects of social behavior rather than consummatory aspects. This was most clearly shown when, after measuring dopamine release to several brief interaction episodes, the male rat was allowed to copulate with the receptive female (Robinson et al., 2002). Fewer dopamine transients were observed during copulation as opposed to brief interactions, but most of these transients were followed within 5 s by sexual behaviors such as mounting, intromission, and ejaculation. Thus, even within copulatory episodes, the timing of transients is consistent with appetitive rather than consummatory aspects of sexual behavior.

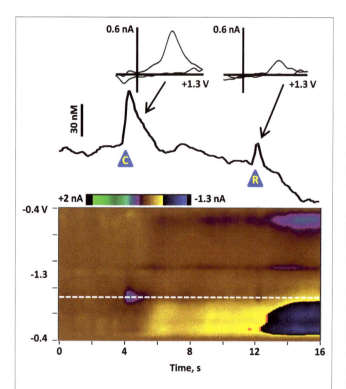

FIGURE 1 | Average dopamine release in the NAc core of a rat at the presentation of a cue and reward after Pavlovian conditioning. The rat was trained for 7 days on a Pavlovian conditioning paradigm: each day it received 25 pairings of a cue (8-s lever extension and cue light illumination) and a reward (0.1 ml of Ensure® chocolate drink). On the eighth day, dopamine was recorded in the NAc core during an identical Pavlovian session. The figure illustrates the dopamine release associated with cue and reward presentation, signal-averaged across the 25 trials. The color plot shows the changes in current at each applied potential over a 16-s window; cue presentation ("C") is at 4 s and reward delivery ("R") is at 12 s. Current at the oxidation potential of dopamine (white dotted line) is depicted in the line trace above the color plot. The transients are confirmed to be dopaminergic by evaluation of the cyclic voltammograms (inset above). As previously reported (Day et al., 2007; Stuber et al., 2008), dopamine release is more robust to the cue than to the reward delivery after Pavlovian conditioning.

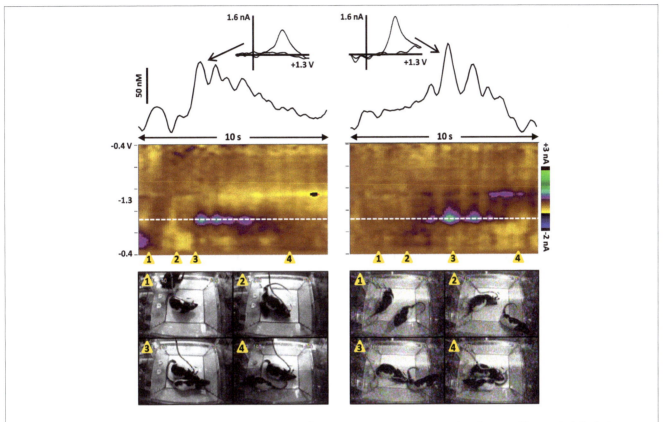

FIGURE 2 | Dopamine transients in the NAc core of male rats during brief interaction with another male. Left: Dopamine release is associated with initial whisker contact and sniffing of the peer. Right: Dopamine transients in a different rat occur during anogenital sniffing. The color plot shows the changes in current at each applied potential over a 10-s window, and current at the oxidation potential of dopamine (white dotted line) is depicted in the line trace above the color plot. The transients are confirmed to be dopaminergic by evaluation of the cyclic voltammograms (inset above). Snapshots from the video record of the interactions are shown below the color plot and illustrate the behavioral events that co-occur with dopamine release; the timing of each snapshot is indicated by the orange triangles. Note that the test rats had been in the recording chamber for over 30 min prior to presentation of the peer rats. Left: 1, the peer rat is placed in the test chamber; 2, The peer rat begins to walk around the test rat; 3, the test rat sniffs the peer rat; 4, the peer rat moves away from the test rat. Right: 1, the test rat is facing away from the peer rat; 2, the test rat orients toward the peer rat; 3, the test rat sniffs the peer rat; 4, the peer rat moves away from the test rat.

DOPAMINE TRANSIENTS DURING MATERNAL BEHAVIOR

In light of this research, it seems reasonable to speculate that dopamine transients are also important neural signals in maternal behavior, another stimulus-driven, motivated behavior. Maternal behavior represents a critical survival behavior, and one that is induced by both the unique postpartum hormonal state and by the sensory stimuli of the pups. Interestingly, male rats or virgin females actively avoid pups, but the incentive value of pups to postpartum dams overcomes any tendency to avoid or reject them; instead, a postpartum dam will approach and exhibit maternal behaviors toward pups immediately after delivery, even pups from another dam (Rosenblatt, 1994). These maternal-specific behaviors include nest building, pup retrieval, pup grooming (body and anogenital licking), and crouching to nurse the pups. Furthermore, these activities can be divided into appetitive (goal-directed behaviors, such as pup retrieval) and consummatory (behaviors once the goal has been obtained, such as nursing). Bouts of licking and grooming, another pup-directed behavior, may have both appetitive (approaching and handling the pup) and consummatory (licking and grooming sequences) aspects. The medial preoptic area (MPOA) of the hypothalamus coordinates all of these events, as its various projections can suppress avoidance and rejection of the pups, activate approach and appetitive behaviors toward the pups, and modulate consummatory aspects such as nursing posture (for review, see Numan and Woodside, 2010; Stolzenberg and Numan, 2011).

Thus, the MPOA and other hypothalamic nuclei, primed by the hormonal milieu of parturition, enhance the incentive salience of pups to a parturient dam to trigger appetitive, approach behavior. Mechanisms by which this influence can occur are the direct projections from the MPOA and from the adjacent ventral bed nucleus of the stria terminalis to the VTA (Numan and Smith, 1984; Numan and Numan, 1997), where they presumably affect dopamine neurons; the input from the MPOA includes oxytocin-expressing neurons (Shahrokh et al., 2010). Oxytocin is a neuropeptide that plays an important role in modulating appetitive aspects of maternal behavior (Pedersen and Boccia, 2002; Numan and Stolzenberg, 2009; Numan and Woodside, 2010). Notably, oxytocin likely arising from the parvocellular neurons of the paraventricular nucleus is released into both the MPOA and the VTA, where it modulates maternal behavior (Pedersen et al., 1994). Moreover, microinfusion of oxytocin into the VTA can trigger dopamine release into the NAc (Melis et al., 2007).

When tonic dopamine concentrations in the NAc are compared between early postpartum dams and cycling virgin females, levels are lower in the dams at baseline (Afonso et al., 2009) despite having similar tissue concentrations of dopamine (Olazabal et al., 2004). However, extracellular dopamine concentrations rise in dams when pups are returned after a brief separation, and they rise even higher during vigorous maternal behaviors such as grooming dirt off of pups (Hansen et al., 1993; Lavi-Avnon et al., 2008). This tonic dopamine response to pup presentation is dependent on parturient hormones early postpartum (Afonso et al., 2009), but it is also experience-dependent, as tonic dopamine release can be induced by foster pups in dams that previously had litters (Afonso et al., 2008). The magnitude of dopamine release appears to vary with individual differences in maternal behavior: when dams were separated into high-licking and low-licking groups based on their pup-directed licking and grooming behavior, the high-licking dams exhibited larger dopamine-like signals in the NAc during a pup-directed licking and grooming bout than low-licking dams (Champagne et al., 2004). Interestingly, mere presentation of pup cues in the absence of maternal behavior can also induce tonic dopamine increases in postpartum dams but not in virgin rats (Afonso et al., 2009). Supporting these findings, EEG recordings in the VTA show distinct electrophysiological profiles in lactating dams versus cycling females in response to pup odors (Hernandez-Gonzalez et al., 2005). Together, these studies clearly indicate that tonic mesolimbic dopamine release increases during maternal interaction with pups and pup-associated cues, but the role of phasic dopamine transients has not been determined.

Based on observations of dopamine transients in other behaviors, we can make specific predictions regarding the potential role of dopamine transients in maternal behavior and when dopamine transients might occur. Consistent with its role to signal unexpected reward, dopamine transients would be expected to occur at pup presentation in parturient dams more frequently than in virgin female or male rats; this prediction is consistent with the ability of pups to act as reward (Wansaw et al., 2008) and reinforcers (Lee et al., 2000) in dams. While dopamine transients may also occur in virgin female or male rats in response to the novel and perhaps aversive salience of pups (Fleming and Luebke, 1981), we expect that this dopaminergic response would be less consistent or persistent than the response in postpartum dams, reflecting the different motivational value the pups hold for the various adult rats. Similarly, pup-predictive cues, such as ultrasonic pup vocalizations, would also be expected to trigger dopamine transients in dams. These transients would likely be followed by approach and retrieval, similar to the approach and appetitive behaviors we observed following dopamine transients in male sexual behavior (Robinson et al., 2002) and the approach to the lever observed rats trained to self-administer cocaine and sucrose (Phillips et al., 2003; Roitman et al., 2004). Thus, the function of dopamine transients in these instances would be to facilitate initiation and maintenance of seeking and appetitive aspects of maternal behavior. It would follow that disruption of this signal would block appetitive maternal behaviors. While local infusion of GABA agonists into the VTA (Numan et al., 2009) and dopamine D1 receptor antagonists in the NAc (Keer and Stern, 1999; Numan et al., 2005) block pup retrieval, these manipulations are not specific for phasic dopamine responses. A more explicit test of phasic dopamine would be to use optogenetics to selectively excite or inhibit dopaminergic inputs to the NAc at discrete times and observe the effect on appetitive behaviors such as pup retrieval.

What is less straightforward is whether dopamine transients might occur during consummatory aspects of maternal behavior, such as nursing and pup-directed licking and grooming. While these behaviors can be considered consummatory – behaviors that emerge once the desired object has been obtained – they also involve sensory stimuli to maintain the behavior, and those stimuli may trigger dopamine transients when they are salient. Of particular importance may be the pulsatile release of oxytocin during nursing bouts (Armstrong and Hatton, 2006), which can increase tonic DA release in the NAc (Melis et al., 2007). In addition, a bout of licking and grooming involves approaching, selecting, and picking up the pup – these may be mini-episodes of appetitive behaviors, in contrast to the more consummatory behavior of licking once the pup is obtained. Due to its time resolution, FSCV is an ideal method to investigate these different aspects of a licking and grooming bout as individual dopamine transients can be time-locked to specific events in the sequence.

We have recently recorded dopamine transients in the NAc core of a dam at postpartum day 4 to demonstrate the feasibility of recording during maternal behaviors and to begin to test our hypotheses of when dopamine transients will occur. While the data are preliminary, they suggest that dopamine transients do occur during maternal behavior, especially at pup cues and appetitive behaviors. Pups were removed from the dam and placed in a holding cage for 30 min. Next, we monitored dopamine transients during the process of pup return and found that transients occur in a manner that is consistent with phasic dopamine triggered by unexpected, salient stimuli. Dopamine transients were detected and analyzed as previously described (Robinson et al., 2011). **Movie S1** in Supplementary Material and **Figure 3** show the neurochemical recording during a 15-s period while the external chamber door is open and the investigator is gathering pups from the holding cage to return to the dam. During this time, the dam is oriented toward the investigator and the pups and actively sniffing and whisking. It is unknown whether sensory stimuli are associated with the exact timing of the transients, but we predict that pup-associated stimuli such as vocalizations and odors could trigger transients. Consistent with this idea, the largest dopamine transient occurred as the investigator began to gather pups (**Figure 3**, snapshot 2), which may have induced pup vocalizations heard by the dam. Such a finding would be consistent with measurements of tonic dopamine levels (Afonso et al., 2009) and reports of phasic dopamine signals to reward-predictive cues (Schultz, 1998; Robinson et al., 2008).

Next, we recorded dopamine immediately following pup return as the dam initiated pup retrieval, as shown in **Movie S2** in Supplementary Material and **Figure 4**. In the seconds following pup return, the dam initially scanned and sniffed several pups as well as the test chamber. However, a large dopamine transient occurred while the rat was facing away from the pups and apparently sniffing the test cage (snapshots 5 and 6). As with the dopamine transients observed in **Figure 3**, is it possible that ultrasonic pup vocalizations triggered the dopamine release, as pup vocalizations can act as auditory cues

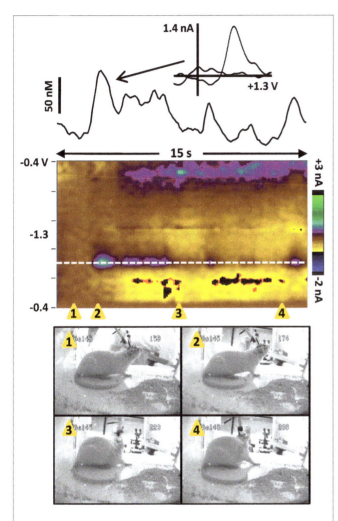

FIGURE 3 | Dopamine transients in the NAc core of a dam in the seconds before pup return (data also shown in Movie S1 in Supplementary Material). The color plot shows the changes in current at each applied potential over a 15-s window, and current at the oxidation potential of dopamine (white dotted line) is depicted in the line trace above the color plot. The timing of the snapshots is indicated by the orange triangles. In this sequence, the investigator has opened the door of the test chamber (snapshot 1) and is gathering pups to return to the dam (snapshots 2–4). The dam is positioned by the plexiglass front of the chamber, actively sniffing/whisking and leaning in the direction of the investigator and the pups. Several dopamine transients occur while the dam is oriented toward the investigator and the pups. The transients are confirmed to be dopaminergic by evaluation of the cyclic voltammograms (inset above).

1) 0.5 s – **touch/sniff pup while experimenter closes cage door**
2) 1.3 s – **turn toward door and investigator's hand, sniff**
3) 3.4 s – touch/sniff pup
4) 5 s – **touch/sniff different pup**
5) 6 s – **turn away from pups, sniffing cage**
6) 7 s – **sniffing cage**
7) 7.8 s – **turn back toward pups**
8) 8.3 s – **touch/sniff pup**
9) 9 s – touch/sniff pup
10) 9.5 s – touch/sniff different pup
11) 10 s – touch/sniff different pup
12) 10.4 s – **grasp pup with mouth**
13) 10.8 s – **pull pup back toward nest**
14) 11.4 s – touch/sniff pup
15) 11.8 s – move forward, touch/sniff pup
16) 12.6 s – touch/sniff different pup
17) 12.9 s – grasp pup with mouth
18) 13.8 s – pull pup back to nest

Thus, these preliminary data indicate that dopamine transients can occur as predicted during maternal behavior: at salient stimuli, during pup investigation, and immediately before and during pup retrieval. Future studies will need to delineate the contribution of pup-associated cues such as vocalizations by concurrently monitoring ultrasonic frequencies. In addition, the potential role of phasic dopamine during lactation should be explored, as the connection between oxytocin and dopamine transmission is evident but not fully understood. It is interesting to note that the second act of pup retrieval was neither preceded nor followed by a large dopamine transient, suggesting that transients may be especially important for the initiation of such behavior, but that once the behavior is initiated it continues via other mechanisms. This interpretation is consistent with dopamine transients' role in behavioral switching. Further investigation is clearly needed to understand this phenomenon more clearly.

There are experimental considerations that may guide future studies of phasic dopamine release during maternal behavior. One important focus of research would be to monitor dopamine release during ongoing maternal behavior in as naturalistic a situation as possible, such as shown in **Figure 4**. The advantage of this type of "free behavior" measurement is that we can determine when dopamine transients occur and associate them with stimuli and behaviors that precede or follow them. This is the approach we have successfully used for dopamine release during brief social interaction and male sexual behavior (Robinson et al., 2001, 2002, 2011), and differences in the frequency of dopamine transients during multiple behavioral epochs can be detected (e.g., solitude versus social interaction; interaction with a male versus a receptive female). Using this approach, we expect that dopamine transients would be higher during epochs of appetitive maternal behaviors as compared to solitude or lactation, and that the frequency of dopamine transients would be proportional to the amount of maternal behavior exhibited, similar to the tonic measurements previously described (Hansen et al., 1993; Champagne et al., 2004; Lavi-Avnon et al., 2008). In addition to a video record of the test session that is time-stamped to

to direct maternal behavior (Brunelli et al., 1994; Zimmerberg et al., 2003). Alternatively, the dam may have been scanning the chamber to see where pups were scattered before initiating retrieval. Notably, immediately after the peak of that transient, the rat turned toward the pups (snapshot 7) and began to touch and sniff them (snapshot 8), inducing further dopamine release. Finally a smaller dopamine transient occurred as the dam retrieved the first pup (snapshots 12 and 13). The following is a detailed description of the dam's behavior at each snapshot in the sequence of **Figure 4**, and those events concurrent with confirmed dopamine release (meeting criteria described in Robinson et al., 2011) are depicted in bold type:

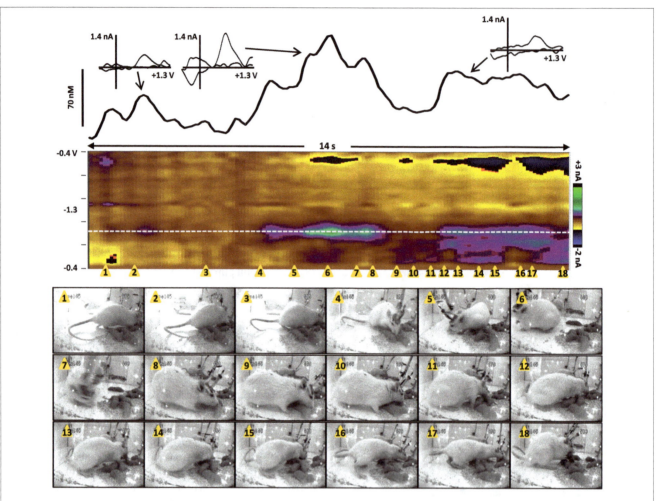

FIGURE 4 | Dopamine transients in the NAc core of a dam at the onset of retrieval after pups are returned (data also shown in Movie S2 in Supplementary Material). The color plot shows the changes in current at each applied potential over a 14-s window, and current at the oxidation potential of dopamine (white dotted line) is depicted in the line trace above the color plot. The timing of the snapshots is indicated by the orange triangles. This sequence begins 4 s after the pups were returned; for full description of the dam's behavior, see the text. Dopamine transients are associated with closing the test chamber door, investigating the pups and test chamber, and pup retrieval. The largest dopamine release at 6.3–8.3 s (near snapshots 5–8) preceded a series of pup retrievals that started at 10.4 s (snapshot 12) and continued for two more minutes until the dam crouched for nursing. The transients are confirmed to be dopaminergic by evaluation of the cyclic voltammograms (inset above).

the neurochemical measurement, the ideal experiment will include a time-stamped recording of ultrasonic vocalizations, as these may be important auditory cues to the dam (Brunelli et al., 1994; Zimmerberg et al., 2003).

However, a major limitation to dopamine measurement during free behavior is the fact that it yields correlational rather than causal relationships. Thus, follow-up studies can employ experimental paradigms that allow more precise determination of antecedents of dopamine release as well as comparison among experimental groups. For example, various pup cues (odors, vocalizations, movements) can be separately presented to dams or to virgin rats to compare their relative efficacy to trigger dopamine release. This design can include time-locked and repeated cue presentations, which has the advantage of allowing signal-averaging of the dopamine signal. Moreover, non-pup cues can be presented as positive controls. Similarly, retrieval of pups can be constrained such that only one pup is retrieved at a time from a particular spot, such that more consistent approach, lifting, and delivery of pup retrieval can be elicited and associated with dopamine release. Interestingly, dams can be trained to perform an operant behavior for access to pups (Lee et al., 2000), allowing measurements of pup-seeking behavior and the associated dopamine release, similar to self-administration of drugs and consumed reward (e.g., Phillips et al., 2003; Roitman et al., 2004). Another level of investigation would be to examine the effectiveness of various pup cues to elicit dopamine release and maternal behavior in dams. For example, ultrasonic vocalizations of pups are more effective to elicit maternal response when pup odors are also present (Rohitsingh et al., 2011), and preliminary data suggest that the quality (e.g., frequency, harmonics, rate) of pup vocalizations can be influenced by genetic manipulation (Scattoni et al., 2009) or prenatal events such as cocaine exposure (preliminary data: Cox et al., 2010) and may, thus, contribute to changes in maternal behavioral and neurochemical responses.

SUMMARY AND FUTURE DIRECTIONS

Phasic dopamine release has a special function in motivated behaviors that is still being elucidated, but appears to be focused on predictive and appetitive aspects of reward-seeking. Dopamine transients are qualitatively different than tonic dopamine levels, both due to the time frames in which they occur, their potential receptor targets, and corelease of glutamate. When examined during social behavior and reward conditioning, transients tend to occur during unexpected salient stimuli and appetitive and approach behaviors. Therefore, we expect that they also play an important role in maternal behavior: particularly in the expression of incentive value of pup cues that lead to retrieval and appetitive aspects of licking and grooming. Systematic studies during maternal behavior are needed to first describe the occurrence of dopamine transients at various events, then to manipulate the expression of transients and observe effects on behavior, or vice versa. For example, predictions can be made based on the hormonal state of the female: pup-associated cues would be expected to trigger more dopamine transients in dams early versus late postpartum, and more in maternally experienced rats than in virgins. Furthermore, blocking dopamine transients pharmacologically or with optogenetic manipulation would be predicted to substantially reduce or delay appetitive maternal behaviors. Finally, dopamine transients in regions beyond the NAc can be investigated to explore their potential role in pup-directed action selection or the development of habitual responses driven by pup-associated cues.

Once the role of dopamine transients in normal maternal behavior is better understood, that knowledge can be used as the foundation to study animal models of disrupted maternal behavior, such as inattention and neglect due to stress or drug exposure. For example, chronic and acute cocaine exposures cause deficits in retrieval, crouching, and licking behaviors in postpartum rats (Johns et al., 1994, 1998, 2005). These drug treatments also decrease oxytocin in the VTA (Johns et al., 1997), which could affect VTA neuronal firing and, thus, dopamine release (Melis et al., 2007). As exposure to drugs of abuse can alter dopamine neuronal plasticity (Stuber et al., 2010b) and phasic release (Stuber et al., 2005), it is possible that the neuroadaptations induced by pregnancy and lactation are prevented or delayed in the drug-exposed dam. Similarly, maternal behaviors can be disrupted by exposure to stressful environments during pregnancy or lactation as well as by increased circulating stress hormones (Bosch et al., 2007; Brummelte and Galea, 2010). Stress response signaling systems, including corticotrophin releasing factor and corticosterone acting respectively through CRF1 and glucocorticoid receptors, can influence dopaminergic neuronal firing in the VTA, dopamine release in the NAc and synaptic plasticity in NAc neurons (Lodge and Grace, 2005; Campioni et al., 2009). Thus, it is possible that disruptions of phasic dopamine transmission could be one neurobiological mechanism underlying deficits in maternal behavior following drug use or stress, and that further study of this aspect of dopamine transmission may open avenues for intervention and restoration of maternal function.

ACKNOWLEDGMENTS

The authors gratefully acknowledge the lab of Dr. Josephine M. Johns for supply of rats for dopamine measurements in maternal behavior and technical support from Abigail Jamieson-Drake. We thank the NIH-National Institute of Alcoholism and Alcohol Abuse (NADIA Project 1-U01-AA019972 and 1-U24-AA020024, R01 AA018008, and 5-P60-AA011605-11-14), the NIH-National Institute of Drug Abuse (P01 DA022446 to JMJ), the Foundation of Hope and the Bowles Center for Alcohol Studies at the University of North Carolina for support. We also thank Dr. Tatiana Shnitko and Dr. Katherine Smith for critical reading of the manuscript. The content is solely the responsibility of the authors and does not necessarily represent the official views of the National Institute of Alcoholism and Alcohol Abuse, the National Institute on Drug Abuse, or the National Institutes of Health.

REFERENCES

Afonso, V. M., Grella, S. L., Chatterjee, D., and Fleming, A. S. (2008). Previous maternal experience affects accumbal dopaminergic responses to pup-stimuli. Brain Res. 1198, 115–123.

Afonso, V. M., King, S., Chatterjee, D., and Fleming, A. S. (2009). Hormones that increase maternal responsiveness affect accumbal dopaminergic responses to pup- and food-stimuli in the female rat. Horm. Behav. 56, 11–23.

Alcaro, A., Huber, R., and Panksepp, J. (2007). Behavioral functions of the mesolimbic dopaminergic system: an affective neuroethological perspective. Brain Res. Rev. 56, 283–321.

Aragona, B. J., Cleaveland, N. A., Stuber, G. D., Day, J. J., Carelli, R. M., and Wightman, R. M. (2008). Preferential enhancement of dopamine transmission within the nucleus accumbens shell by cocaine is attributable to a direct increase in phasic dopamine release events. J. Neurosci. 28, 8821–8831.

Armstrong, W. E., and Hatton, G. I. (2006). The puzzle of pulsatile oxytocin secretion during lactation: some new pieces. Am. J. Physiol. Regul. Integr. Comp Physiol. 291, R26–R28.

Bass, C. E., Grinevich, V. P., Vance, Z. B., Sullivan, R. P., Bonin, K. D., and Budygin, E. A. (2010). Optogenetic control of striatal dopamine release in rats. J. Neurochem. 114, 1344–1352.

Berke, J. D., and Hyman, S. E. (2000). Addiction, dopamine, and the molecular mechanisms of memory. Neuron 25, 515–532.

Borland, L. M., Shi, G., Yang, H., and Michael, A. C. (2005). Voltammetric study of extracellular dopamine near microdialysis probes acutely implanted in the striatum of the anesthetized rat. J. Neurosci. Methods 146, 149–158.

Bosch, O. J., Musch, W., Bredewold, R., Slattery, D. A., and Neumann, I. D. (2007). Prenatal stress increases HPA axis activity and impairs maternal care in lactating female offspring: implications for postpartum mood disorder. Psychoneuroendocrinology 32, 267–278.

Brummelte, S., and Galea, L. A. (2010). Chronic corticosterone during pregnancy and postpartum affects maternal care, cell proliferation and depressive-like behavior in the dam. *Horm. Behav.* 58, 769–779.

Brunelli, S. A., Shair, H. N., and Hofer, M. A. (1994). Hypothermic vocalizations of rat pups (*Rattus norvegicus*) elicit and direct maternal search behavior. *J. Comp. Psychol.* 108, 298–303.

Campioni, M. R., Xu, M., and McGehee, D. S. (2009). Stress-induced changes in nucleus accumbens glutamate synaptic plasticity. *J. Neurophysiol.* 101, 3192–3198.

Champagne, F. A., Chretien, P., Stevenson, C. W., Zhang, T. Y., Gratton, A., and Meaney, M. J. (2004). Variations in nucleus accumbens dopamine associated with individual differences in maternal behavior in the rat. *J. Neurosci.* 24, 4113–4123.

Cheer, J. F., Wassum, K. M., Sombers, L. A., Heien, M. L., Ariansen, J. L., Aragona, B. J., Phillips, P. E., and Wightman, R. M. (2007). Phasic dopamine release evoked by abused substances requires cannabinoid receptor activation. *J. Neurosci.* 27, 791–795.

Cox, E., Jones, G., Williams, S., McMurray, M., Jamieson-Drake, A., Zeskind, P., Hodge, C., Grewen, K., and Johns, J. M. (2010). "Prenatal cocaine exposure alters human and rodent infant vocalizations: implications for maternal care and neural integrity," in *Abstracts of the International Behavioral Neuroscience Society, Villasimius, Italy,* 19, #136.

Day, J. J., Roitman, M. F., Wightman, R. M., and Carelli, R. M. (2007). Associative learning mediates dynamic shifts in dopamine signaling in the nucleus accumbens. *Nat. Neurosci.* 10, 1020–1028.

de Wit, S., Barker, R. A., Dickinson, A. D., and Cools, R. (2011). Habitual versus goal-directed action control in Parkinson disease. *J. Cogn. Neurosci.* 23, 1218–1229.

Douglas, L. A., Varlinskaya, E. I., and Spear, L. P. (2004). Rewarding properties of social interactions in adolescent and adult male and female rats: impact of social versus isolate housing of subjects and partners. *Dev. Psychobiol.* 45, 153–162.

Fleming, A. S., and Luebke, C. (1981). Timidity prevents the virgin female rat from being a good mother: emotionality differences between nulliparous and parturient females. *Physiol. Behav.* 27, 863–868.

Floresco, S. B., West, A. R., Ash, B., Moore, H., and Grace, A. A. (2003). Afferent modulation of dopamine neuron firing differentially regulates tonic and phasic dopamine transmission. *Nat. Neurosci.* 6, 968–973.

Freeman, A. S., and Bunney, B. S. (1987). Activity of A9 and A10 dopaminergic neurons in unrestrained rats: further characterization and effects of apomorphine and cholecystokinin. *Brain Res.* 405, 46–55.

Garris, P. A., and Rebec, G. V. (2002). Modeling fast dopamine neurotransmission in the nucleus accumbens during behavior. *Behav. Brain Res.* 137, 47–63.

Hansen, S., Bergvall, A. H., and Nyiredi, S. (1993). Interaction with pups enhances dopamine release in the ventral striatum of maternal rats: a microdialysis study. *Pharmacol. Biochem. Behav.* 45, 673–676.

Hauber, W. (2010). Dopamine release in the prefrontal cortex and striatum: temporal and behavioural aspects. *Pharmacopsychiatry* 43(Suppl. 1), S32–S41.

Hernandez-Gonzalez, M., Prieto-Beracoechea, C., Navarro-Meza, M., Ramos-Guevara, J. P., Reyes-Cortes, R., and Guevara, M. A. (2005). Prefrontal and tegmental electrical activity during olfactory stimulation in virgin and lactating rats. *Physiol. Behav.* 83, 749–758.

Hnasko, T. S., Chuhma, N., Zhang, H., Goh, G. Y., Sulzer, D., Palmiter, R. D., Rayport, S., and Edwards, R. H. (2010). Vesicular glutamate transport promotes dopamine storage and glutamate corelease in vivo. *Neuron* 65, 643–656.

Hyland, B. I., Reynolds, J. N., Hay, J., Perk, C. G., and Miller, R. (2002). Firing modes of midbrain dopamine cells in the freely moving rat. *Neuroscience* 114, 475–492.

Ikemoto, S. (2007). Dopamine reward circuitry: two projection systems from the ventral midbrain to the nucleus accumbens-olfactory tubercle complex. *Brain Res. Rev.* 56, 27–78.

Ikemoto, S., and Panksepp, J. (1999). The role of nucleus accumbens dopamine in motivated behavior: a unifying interpretation with special reference to reward-seeking. *Brain Res. Brain Res. Rev.* 31, 6–41.

Johns, J. M., Elliott, D. L., Hofler, V. E., Joyner, P. W., McMurray, M. S., Jarrett, T. M., Haslup, A. M., Middleton, C. L., Elliott, J. C., and Walker, C. H. (2005). Cocaine treatment and prenatal environment interact to disrupt intergenerational maternal behavior in rats. *Behav. Neurosci.* 119, 1605–1618.

Johns, J. M., Lubin, D. A., Walker, C. H., Meter, K. E., and Mason, G. A. (1997). Chronic gestational cocaine treatment decreases oxytocin levels in the medial preoptic area, ventral tegmental area and hippocampus in Sprague-Dawley rats. *Neuropeptides* 31, 439–443.

Johns, J. M., Nelson, C. J., Meter, K. E., Lubin, D. A., Couch, C. D., Ayers, A., and Walker, C. H. (1998). Dose-dependent effects of multiple acute cocaine injections on maternal behavior and aggression in Sprague-Dawley rats. *Dev. Neurosci.* 20, 525–532.

Johns, J. M., Noonan, L. R., Zimmerman, L. I., Li, L., and Pedersen, C. A. (1994). Effects of chronic and acute cocaine treatment on the onset of maternal behavior and aggression in Sprague-Dawley rats. *Behav. Neurosci.* 108, 107–112.

Justice, J. B. Jr. (1993). Quantitative microdialysis of neurotransmitters. *J. Neurosci. Methods* 48, 263–276.

Kawagoe, K. T., Garris, P. A., Wiedemann, D. J., and Wightman, R. M. (1992). Regulation of transient dopamine concentration gradients in the microenvironment surrounding nerve terminals in the rat striatum. *Neuroscience* 51, 55–64.

Keer, S. E., and Stern, J. M. (1999). Dopamine receptor blockade in the nucleus accumbens inhibits maternal retrieval and licking, but enhances nursing behavior in lactating rats. *Physiol. Behav.* 67, 659–669.

Lapish, C. C., Seamans, J. K., and Chandler, L. J. (2006). Glutamate-dopamine cotransmission and reward processing in addiction. *Alcohol. Clin. Exp. Res.* 30, 1451–1465.

Lavi-Avnon, Y., Weller, A., Finberg, J. P., Gispan-Herman, I., Kinor, N., Stern, Y., Schroeder, M., Gelber, V., Bergman, S. Y., Overstreet, D. H., and Yadid, G. (2008). The reward system and maternal behavior in an animal model of depression: a microdialysis study. *Psychopharmacology (Berl.)* 196, 281–291.

Lee, A., Clancy, S., and Fleming, A. S. (2000). Mother rats bar-press for pups: effects of lesions of the mpoa and limbic sites on maternal behavior and operant responding for pup-reinforcement. *Behav. Brain Res.* 108, 215–231.

Ljungberg, T., Apicella, P., and Schultz, W. (1992). Responses of monkey dopamine neurons during learning of behavioral reactions. *J. Neurophysiol.* 67, 145–163.

Lodge, D. J., and Grace, A. A. (2005). Acute and chronic corticotropin-releasing factor 1 receptor blockade inhibits cocaine-induced dopamine release: correlation with dopamine neuron activity. *J. Pharmacol. Exp. Ther.* 314, 201–206.

Logman, M. J., Budygin, E. A., Gainetdinov, R. R., and Wightman, R. M. (2000). Quantitation of in vivo measurements with carbon fiber microelectrodes. *J. Neurosci. Methods* 95, 95–102.

Lovinger, D. M. (2010). Neurotransmitter roles in synaptic modulation, plasticity and learning in the dorsal striatum. *Neuropharmacology* 58, 951–961.

Lu, Y., Peters, J. L., and Michael, A. C. (1998). Direct comparison of the response of voltammetry and microdialysis to electrically evoked release of striatal dopamine. *J. Neurochem.* 70, 584–593.

Melis, M. R., Melis, T., Cocco, C., Succu, S., Sanna, F., Pillolla, G., Boi, A., Ferri, G. L., and Argiolas, A. (2007). Oxytocin injected into the ventral tegmental area induces penile erection and increases extracellular dopamine in the nucleus accumbens and paraventricular nucleus of the hypothalamus of male rats. *Eur. J. Neurosci.* 26, 1026–1035.

Michael, D., Travis, E. R., and Wightman, R. M. (1998). Color images for fast-scan CV measurements in biological systems. *Anal. Chem.* 70, 586A–592A.

Mirenowicz, J., and Schultz, W. (1994). Importance of unpredictability for reward responses in primate dopamine neurons. *J. Neurophysiol.* 72, 1024–1027.

Numan, M. (2007). Motivational systems and the neural circuitry of maternal behavior in the rat. *Dev. Psychobiol.* 49, 12–21.

Numan, M., and Numan, M. J. (1997). Projection sites of medial preoptic area and ventral bed nucleus of the stria terminalis neurons that express Fos during maternal behavior in female rats. *J. Neuroendocrinol.* 9, 369–384.

Numan, M., Numan, M. J., Pliakou, N., Stolzenberg, D. S., Mullins, O. J., Murphy, J. M., and Smith, C. D. (2005). The effects of D1 or D2 dopamine receptor antagonism in the medial preoptic area, ventral pallidum, or nucleus accumbens on the maternal retrieval response and other aspects of maternal behavior in rats. *Behav. Neurosci.* 119, 1588–1604.

Numan, M., and Smith, H. G. (1984). Maternal behavior in rats: evidence for the involvement of preoptic projections to the ventral tegmental area. *Behav. Neurosci.* 98, 712–727.

Numan, M., and Stolzenberg, D. S. (2009). Medial preoptic area interactions with dopamine neural systems in the control of the onset and maintenance of maternal behavior in rats. *Front. Neuroendocrinol.* 30:1. doi: 10.1016/j.yfrne.2008.10.002

Numan, M., Stolzenberg, D. S., Dellevigne, A. A., Correnti, C. M., and Numan, M. J. (2009). Temporary inactivation of ventral tegmental area neurons with either muscimol or baclofen reversibly disrupts maternal behavior in rats through different underlying mechanisms. *Behav. Neurosci.* 123, 740–751.

Numan, M., and Woodside, B. (2010). Maternity: neural mechanisms, motivational processes, and physiological adaptations. *Behav. Neurosci.* 124, 715–741.

Olazabal, D. E., Abercrombie, E., Rosenblatt, J. S., and Morrell, J. I. (2004). The content of dopamine, serotonin, and their metabolites in the neural circuit that mediates maternal behavior in juvenile and adult rats. *Brain Res. Bull.* 63, 259–268.

Overton, P. G., and Clark, D. (1997). Burst firing in midbrain dopaminergic neurons. *Brain Res. Rev.* 25, 312–334.

Owesson-White, C. A., Cheer, J. F., Beyene, M., Carelli, R. M., and Wightman, R. M. (2008). Dynamic changes in accumbens dopamine correlate with learning during intracranial self-stimulation. *Proc. Natl. Acad. Sci. U.S.A.* 105, 11957–11962.

Parker, J. G., Zweifel, L. S., Clark, J. J., Evans, S. B., Phillips, P. E., and Palmiter, R. D. (2010). Absence of NMDA receptors in dopamine neurons attenuates dopamine release but not conditioned approach during Pavlovian conditioning. *Proc. Natl. Acad. Sci. U.S.A.* 107, 13491–13496.

Pedersen, C. A., and Boccia, M. L. (2002). Oxytocin links mothering received, mothering bestowed and adult stress responses. *Stress* 5, 259–267.

Pedersen, C. A., Caldwell, J. D., Walker, C., Ayers, G., and Mason, G. A. (1994). Oxytocin activates the postpartum onset of rat maternal behavior in the ventral tegmental and medial preoptic areas. *Behav. Neurosci.* 108, 1163–1171.

Phillips, A. G., Vacca, G., and Ahn, S. (2008). A top-down perspective on dopamine, motivation and memory. *Pharmacol. Biochem. Behav.* 90, 236–249.

Phillips, P. E., Stuber, G. D., Heien, M. L., Wightman, R. M., and Carelli, R. M. (2003). Subsecond dopamine release promotes cocaine seeking. *Nature* 422, 614–618.

Rebec, G. V., Christensen, J. R., Guerra, C., and Bardo, M. T. (1997). Regional and temporal differences in real-time dopamine efflux in the nucleus accumbens during free-choice novelty. *Brain Res.* 776, 61–67.

Redgrave, P., Gurney, K., and Reynolds, J. (2008). What is reinforced by phasic dopamine signals? *Brain Res. Rev.* 58, 322–339.

Redgrave, P., Prescott, T. J., and Gurney, K. (1999). Is the short-latency dopamine response too short to signal reward error? *Trends Neurosci.* 22, 146–151.

Richfield, E. K., Penney, J. B., and Young, A. B. (1989). Anatomical and affinity state comparisons between dopamine D1 and D2 receptors in the rat central nervous system. *Neuroscience* 30, 767–777.

Robinson, D. L., Heien, M. L., and Wightman, R. M. (2002). Frequency of dopamine concentration transients increases in dorsal and ventral striatum of male rats during introduction of conspecifics. *J. Neurosci.* 22, 10477–10486.

Robinson, D. L., Hermans, A., Seipel, A. T., and Wightman, R. M. (2008). Monitoring rapid chemical communication in the brain. *Chem. Rev.* 108, 2554–2584.

Robinson, D. L., Howard, E. C., McConnell, S., Gonzales, R. A., and Wightman, R. M. (2009). Disparity between tonic and phasic ethanol-induced dopamine increases in the nucleus accumbens of rats. *Alcohol. Clin. Exp. Res.* 33, 1187–1196.

Robinson, D. L., Phillips, P. E., Budygin, E. A., Trafton, B. J., Garris, P. A., and Wightman, R. M. (2001). Sub-second changes in accumbal dopamine during sexual behavior in male rats. *Neuroreport* 12, 2549–2552.

Robinson, D. L., and Wightman, R. M. (2004). Nomifensine amplifies subsecond dopamine signals in the ventral striatum of freely-moving rats. *J. Neurochem.* 90, 894–903.

Robinson, D. L., and Wightman, R. M. (2007). "Rapid dopamine release in freely moving rats," in *Electrochemical Methods for Neuroscience*, eds A. C. Michael and L. M. Borland (Boca Raton: CRC Press), 17–34.

Robinson, D. L., Zitzman, D. L., Smith, K. J., and Spear, L. P. (2011). Fast dopamine release events in the nucleus accumbens of early adolescent rats. *Neuroscience* 176, 296–307.

Rohitsingh, S. A., Smith, J. A., and Shair, H. N. (2011). Sex and experience influence behavioral responses of adult rats to potentiated and nonpotentiated ultrasonic vocalizations of pups. *Dev. Psychobiol.* PMID: 21432845. [Epub ahead of print].

Roitman, M. F., Stuber, G. D., Phillips, P. E., Wightman, R. M., and Carelli, R. M. (2004). Dopamine operates as a subsecond modulator of food seeking. *J. Neurosci.* 24, 1265–1271.

Rosenblatt, J. S. (1994). Psychobiology of maternal behavior: contribution to the clinical understanding of maternal behavior among humans. *Acta Paediatr. Suppl.* 397, 3–8.

Ross, S. B. (1991). Synaptic concentration of dopamine in the mouse striatum in relationship to the kinetic properties of the dopamine receptors and uptake mechanism. *J. Neurochem.* 56, 22–29.

Salamone, J. D., Correa, M., Farrar, A., and Mingote, S. M. (2007). Effort-related functions of nucleus accumbens dopamine and associated forebrain circuits. *Psychopharmacology (Berl.)* 191, 461–482.

Salamone, J. D., Correa, M., Mingote, S. M., and Weber, S. M. (2005). Beyond the reward hypothesis: alternative functions of nucleus accumbens dopamine. *Curr. Opin. Pharmacol.* 5, 34–41.

Scattoni, M. L., Crawley, J., and Ricceri, L. (2009). Ultrasonic vocalizations: a tool for behavioural phenotyping of mouse models of neurodevelopmental disorders. *Neurosci. Biobehav. Rev.* 33, 508–515.

Schultz, W. (1998). Predictive reward signal of dopamine neurons. *J. Neurophysiol.* 80, 1–27.

Schultz, W. (2007). Multiple dopamine functions at different time courses. *Annu. Rev. Neurosci.* 30, 259–288.

Schultz, W., Dayan, P., and Montague, P. R. (1997). A neural substrate of prediction and reward. *Science* 275, 1593–1599.

Shahrokh, D. K., Zhang, T. Y., Diorio, J., Gratton, A., and Meaney, M. J. (2010). Oxytocin-dopamine interactions mediate variations in maternal behavior in the rat. *Endocrinology* 151, 2276–2286.

Sombers, L. A., Beyene, M., Carelli, R. M., and Wightman, R. M. (2009). Synaptic overflow of dopamine in the nucleus accumbens arises from neuronal activity in the ventral tegmental area. *J. Neurosci.* 29, 1735–1742.

Stolzenberg, D. S., and Numan, M. (2011). Hypothalamic interaction with the mesolimbic DA system in the control of the maternal and sexual behaviors in rats. *Neurosci. Biobehav. Rev.* 35, 826–847.

Stuber, G. D., Hnasko, T. S., Britt, J. P., Edwards, R. H., and Bonci, A. (2010a). Dopaminergic terminals in the nucleus accumbens but not the dorsal striatum corelease glutamate. *J. Neurosci.* 30, 8229–8233.

Stuber, G. D., Hopf, F. W., Tye, K. M., Chen, B. T., and Bonci, A. (2010b). Neuroplastic alterations in the limbic system following cocaine or alcohol exposure. *Curr. Top. Behav. Neurosci.* 3, 3–27.

Stuber, G. D., Klanker, M., de Ridder, B., Bowers, M. S., Joosten, R. N., Feenstra, M. G., and Bonci, A. (2008). Reward-predictive cues enhance excitatory synaptic strength onto midbrain dopamine neurons. *Science* 321, 1690–1692.

Stuber, G. D., Roitman, M. F., Phillips, P. E., Carelli, R. M., and Wightman, R. M. (2005). Rapid dopamine signaling in the nucleus accumbens during contingent and noncontingent cocaine administration. *Neuropsychopharmacology* 30, 853–863.

Suaud-Chagny, M. F., Chergui, K., Chouvet, G., and Gonon, F. (1992). Relationship between dopamine release in the rat nucleus accumbens and the discharge activity of dopaminergic neurons during local in vivo application of amino acids in the ventral tegmental area. *Neuroscience* 49, 63–72.

Suaud-Chagny, M. F., Dugast, C., Chergui, K., Msghina, M., and Gonon, F. (1995). Uptake of dopamine released by impulse flow in the rat mesolimbic and striatal systems in vivo. *J. Neurochem.* 65, 2603–2611.

Sulzer, D., and Rayport, S. (2000). Dale's principle and glutamate corelease from ventral midbrain dopamine neurons. *Amino Acids* 19, 45–52.

Takmakov, P., Zachek, M. K., Keithley, R. B., Bucher, E. S., McCarty, G. S., and Wightman, R. M. (2010). Characterization of local pH changes in brain using fast-scan cyclic voltammetry with carbon microelectrodes. *Anal. Chem.* 82, 9892–9900.

Tecuapetla, F., Patel, J. C., Xenias, H., English, D., Tadros, I., Shah, F., Berlin, J., Deisseroth, K., Rice, M. E., Tepper, J. M., and Koos, T. (2010). Glutamatergic signaling by mesolimbic dopamine neurons in the nucleus accumbens. *J. Neurosci.* 30, 7105–7110.

Tsai, H. C., Zhang, F., Adamantidis, A., Stuber, G. D., Bonci, A., de Lecea, L., and Deisseroth, K. (2009). Phasic firing in dopaminergic neurons is sufficient for behavioral conditioning. *Science* 324, 1080–1084.

Valenstein, E. S., Cox, V. C., and Kakolewski, J. W. (1968). Modification of motivated behavior elicited by electrical stimulation of the hypothalamus. *Science* 159, 1119–1121.

Venton, B. J., Michael, D. J., and Wightman, R. M. (2003). Correlation of local changes in extracellular oxygen and pH that accompany dopaminergic terminal activity in the rat caudate-putamen. *J. Neurochem.* 84, 373–381.

Vickrey, T. L., Condron, B., and Venton, B. J. (2009). Detection of endogenous dopamine changes in *Drosophila melanogaster* using fast-scan cyclic voltammetry. *Anal. Chem.* 81, 9306–9313.

Wansaw, M. P., Pereira, M., and Morrell, J. I. (2008). Characterization of maternal motivation in the lactating rat: contrasts between early and late postpartum responses. *Horm. Behav.* 54, 294–301.

Watson, C. J., Venton, B. J., and Kennedy, R. T. (2006). In vivo measurements of neurotransmitters by microdialysis sampling. *Anal. Chem.* 78, 1391–1399.

Westerink, B. H. (1995). Brain microdialysis and its application for the study of animal behaviour. *Behav. Brain Res.* 70, 103–124.

Wickens, J. R., Horvitz, J. C., Costa, R. M., and Killcross, S. (2007). Dopaminergic mechanisms in actions and habits. *J. Neurosci.* 27, 8181–8183.

Wightman, R. M., Heien, M. L., Wassum, K. M., Sombers, L. A., Aragona, B. J., Khan, A. S., Ariansen, J. L., Cheer, J. F., Phillips, P. E., and Carelli, R. M. (2007). Dopamine release is heterogeneous within microenvironments of the rat nucleus accumbens. *Eur. J. Neurosci.* 26, 2046–2054.

Willuhn, I., Wanat, M. J., Clark, J. J., and Phillips, P. E. (2010). Dopamine signaling in the nucleus accumbens of animals self-administering drugs of abuse. *Curr. Top. Behav. Neurosci.* 3, 29–71.

Yang, H., and Michael, A. C. (2007). "In vivo fast-scan cyclic voltammetry of dopamine near microdialysis probes," in *Electrochemical Methods for Neuroscience*, eds A. C. Michael and L. M. Borland (Boca Raton: CRC Press), 489–501.

Yin, H. H., and Knowlton, B. J. (2006). The role of the basal ganglia in habit formation. *Nat. Rev. Neurosci.* 7, 464–476.

Zimmerberg, B., Kim, J. H., Davidson, A. N., and Rosenthal, A. J. (2003). Early deprivation alters the vocalization behavior of neonates directing maternal attention in a rat model of child neglect. *Ann. N. Y. Acad. Sci.* 1008, 308–313.

Zweifel, L. S., Parker, J. G., Lobb, C. J., Rainwater, A., Wall, V. Z., Fadok, J. P., Darvas, M., Kim, M. J., Mizumori, S. J., Paladini, C. A., Phillips, P. E., and Palmiter, R. D. (2009). Disruption of NMDAR-dependent burst firing by dopamine neurons provides selective assessment of phasic dopamine-dependent behavior. *Proc. Natl. Acad. Sci. U.S.A.* 106, 7281–7288.

# Synergy of image analysis for animal and human neuroimaging supports translational research on drug abuse

Guido Gerig[1], Ipek Oguz[2], Sylvain Gouttard[1], Joohwi Lee[3], Hongyu An[4], Weili Lin[4], Matthew McMurray[5], Karen Grewen[2], Josephine Johns[2] and Martin Andreas Styner[2,3]*

[1] Scientific Computing and Imaging Institute, University of Utah, Salt Lake City, UT, USA
[2] Department of Psychiatry, University of North Carolina, Chapel Hill, NC, USA
[3] Department of Computer Science, University of North Carolina, Chapel Hill, NC, USA
[4] Biomedical Research Imaging Center, University of North Carolina, Chapel Hill, NC, USA
[5] Department of Psychology, University of North Carolina, Chapel Hill, NC, USA

*Correspondence:
Martin Andreas Styner, Neuro Image Research and Analysis Laboratory, Department of Psychiatry, University of North Carolina, Chapel Hill, NC 27599-7160, USA.
e-mail: styner@cs.unc.edu

The use of structural magnetic resonance imaging (sMRI) and diffusion tensor imaging (DTI) in animal models of neuropathology is of increasing interest to the neuroscience community. In this work, we present our approach to create optimal translational studies that include both animal and human neuroimaging data within the frameworks of a study of post-natal neuro-development in intra-uterine cocaine-exposure. We propose the use of non-invasive neuroimaging to study developmental brain structural and white matter pathway abnormalities via sMRI and DTI, as advanced MR imaging technology is readily available and automated image analysis methodology have recently been transferred from the human to animal imaging setting. For this purpose, we developed a synergistic, parallel approach to imaging and image analysis for the human and the rodent branch of our study. We propose an equivalent design in both the selection of the developmental assessment stage and the neuroimaging setup. This approach brings significant advantages to study neurobiological features of early brain development that are common to animals and humans but also preserve analysis capabilities only possible in animal research. This paper presents the main framework and individual methods for the proposed cross-species study design, as well as preliminary DTI cross-species comparative results in the intra-uterine cocaine-exposure study.

Keywords: small animal imaging, neonatal neuroimaging, drug abuse, brain segmentation, white matter pathways, magnetic resonance imaging, diffusion tensor imaging

INTRODUCTION

In the last decade, research in many psychiatric disorders has focused on a potential onset very early in life (Bale et al., 2010), perhaps even *in utero* (Brown and Derkits, 2010), before any onset of clinical symptoms (NIMII, 2008). While many neuroimaging research projects have provided novel insights (Kennedy et al., 2003; Shaw et al., 2008; Hazlett et al., 2009; Mosconi et al., 2009; Gilmore et al., 2010), overall progress into the neurobiological etiology of mental illness can be considered slow, as no major breakthrough toward a more complete understanding of a major psychiatric disorder has yet been reported. Main reasons include the necessary time scale to study a neuro-developmental disorder into adolescence, the correspondingly large monetary requirements, the difficulty of rigorously controlling the developmental environment and the need for handling ethical limitations on the collection of human developmental neurobiological data. In contrary to human clinical studies, animal models have several advantages, such as a well controlled environment and access to genetic modifications that allow for the creation of knock-out models (Nieman et al., 2005; Bugos et al., 2009), as well as the typically shorter lifespan of small animals, which provides ample time to study the disease from conception to adulthood. With respect to neuroimaging, rodent imaging has the advantage that scan time is commonly only limited by access to the imaging facility availability; another advantage is the availability of contrast enhancers that can be used in rodents that are not fit for use in human studies (Nieman et al., 2005). These enhancements result in higher resolution scans as well as increased signal to noise ratio (SNR) as compared human neuroimaging. Finally, there are inherent benefits to using rodent MRI models, such as the capability to augment and validate the neuroimaging results with traditional histology (Nieman et al., 2005).

While few experimental tools have shown themselves to be of use for the in-vivo study of neurobiological mechanisms in clinical human neuro-development, magnetic resonance imaging (MRI) has proven itself an invaluable tool for such research. MRI provides a non-invasive tool to probe brain anatomy and function. As it has no known, detectable influence on neuro-development, it allows for repeated longitudinal assessments (Paus et al., 1999; Gilmore et al., 2007; NIMH, 2008). Furthermore, MRI can be applied both in the clinical settings for humans and in animal research, as the MR data can be acquired and processed using similar methodology in both humans and animals as illustrated in this paper. Thus, findings have the potential to directly translate from basic science to clinical science, within reason. Rodent imaging is commonly acquired with specialized coils and high-field scanners (up to 17.4 T), although commercial-grade clinical scanners can be used for studies with less stringent requirements on spatial resolution and SNR (Pfefferbaum et al., 2004; Lee et al., 2006; Mayer et al., 2007; Pillai et al., 2011). The higher field strength and the smaller bore size of such high-field magnet not only allow for sub-millimeter resolution at appropriate SNR, but also provide a more homogeneous static magnetic field (Nieman et al., 2005). Nevertheless, the basic science community has been rather cautious to embrace MRI, as small animal researchers have a number of non-MRI tools at their disposal such as microscopy and electrophysiology that allow for dramatically enhanced neurochemical and anatomical assessment at considerably higher spatial resolution. On the other hand, MRI offers the advantage of assessing undistorted, three-dimensional structural changes (Nieman et al., 2005). Consequently, the use of rodent MRI has increased significantly in the last few years in order to study small animal models of human neuropathology via knock-outs (Badea et al., 2007; Lerch et al., 2008), lesion models (VanCamp et al., 2009; Zhang et al., 2009), as well as exposure models (Fatemi et al., 2009; Fernandes de Abreu et al., 2010; O'Leary-Moore et al., 2010). *However, to our knowledge, none have attempted to do both human and rodent imaging in a parallel fashion and compare results across-species directly.* Comparisons are usually *ad hoc* and compare a mouse model against human literature, or human neuroimaging results against mouse model literature. Here, we describe our approach to simultaneously study both aspects. This allows for the analysis to be as comparable as possible between human and rodent study settings. The standard comparison across existing studies usually entails mismatched study paradigms and measurements related to the drug exposure, assessment time points, assessed structures, and tracts, as well as MR protocols. Our proposed approach is designed to maximize the ability to infer findings from the rodent setting to the human one.

The overall focus of our research project is the elucidation of neurobiological and behavioral characteristics and responses of mothers that have used primarily cocaine during pregnancy, and of offspring prenatally exposed to cocaine, that could impact negatively on normal mother–infant interactions. Assessment of neurobiological changes includes structural imaging as a measure in human and animal infants and mothers to assess differences in brain structure and maturation.

In this paper, we present our proposed approach toward a cross-species neuroimaging with synchronized, comparative assessments of rodent pups and human neonates. In the next sections, we will first discuss the general concept of our parallel assessment approach. This approach demands comparative settings with respect to assessment age, MR imaging acquisition sequences as well as the MR image analysis methodology. These aspects are all discussed by presenting data from our ongoing study on intra-uterine cocaine-exposure and its effect on early post-natal brain development. It is also important to note that while this paper focuses on the neuroimaging aspects, our ongoing project devotes similar attention toward physiological, behavioral, and biosample measurements.

MATERIALS AND METHODS
STUDY ON POST-NATAL BRAIN DEVELOPMENT FOLLOWING INTRA-UTERINE COCAINE-EXPOSURE

We are illustrating our parallel assessment approach for cross-species neuroimaging studies employing an ongoing multidisciplinary, translational research project that focuses on the elucidation of neurobiological, and behavioral characteristics of offspring prenatally exposed to cocaine. While maternal cocaine use is known to be highly correlated with maternal neglect and poorer mother–infant interactions in both human and animal models, there is little known about the potentially pathologic brain development and the ensuing abnormal physiological/behavioral responses in infants prenatally exposed to cocaine that may in turn impact parenting behaviors of both drug using and non-using mothers.

The project assesses both intra-uterine cocaine-exposure in humans as well as a small animal model using Sprague-Dawley rats. The human part of our study was approved by the institutional review board of the University of North Carolina School of Medicine. All rodent procedures were approved by the institutional animal care and use committee of the University of North Carolina. While characterizing the influence of prenatal cocaine-exposure on post-natal development directly in human infants is the main goal of the project, such a study is nearly impossible within controlled settings. Cocaine abusing mothers often also abuse other drugs such as alcohol and nicotine during pregnancy. Also social environment in both pre and post-natally settings is commonly non-conventional. These factors are all potential confounders for an appropriate analysis. In contrast, prenatal cocaine-exposure in rodent models can be tightly controlled such that effects on the rodent brain can be clearly described.

We focus here on the neuroimaging aspects of this project, where brain structural abnormalities are hypothesized in regions important for the production of relevant sensory stimuli and integration of complex signals. Cocaine-exposed individuals are hypothesized to exhibit increased ventricular size, reduced hypothalamic, limbic, auditory, and olfactory regions, as well as delayed myelination of tracts. Deficits in myelination following long term cocaine-exposure in humans has been a consistent finding, as well as enlarged ventricles and localized white matter (WM) reduction (Moeller et al., 2005; Schlaepfer et al., 2005). Moeller et al. (2005) correlated reduced myelination in the genu and rostral body of the corpus callosum in cocaine-abusers to behavioral scores of impulsivity. This translational, interdisciplinary project aims to better understand how drug abuse affects brain development in the intra-uterine exposed offspring, as well as how the resulting behavioral characteristics may influence neglect. This could result in early and continuing intervention strategies to offset some of the negative consequences of cocaine abuse during and post pregnancy.

GENERAL CONCEPT

Magnetic resonance imaging follows a parallel design (see **Figure 1**) where human subjects are imaged on high-field human scanners (3 T Siemens Trio for adults, 3 T Siemens Allegra for neonates), whereas rodent imaging is using a dedicated high-field

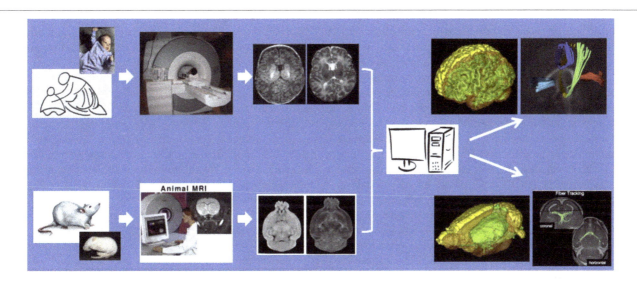

FIGURE 1 | Mother and infant neuroimaging of humans and animals using dedicated scanners, and comparable imaging sequences and image processing methods for inter-species studies.

animal scanner (9.4 T Bruker). With primary interest in anatomical and WM diffusion imaging, we selected optimal imaging sequences on all scanners in regard to maximum contrast for brain tissue types, fluid, and WM diffusivity. Image processing and analysis methodologies and tools developed by our group are generic with respect to the type of species imaged, and we apply the same processing tools to characterize tissue types, to extract anatomical structures, and to quantify WM integrity properties at each voxel and also for selected fiber tracts of interest. In processing steps that require subject-specific anatomical templates, often in the form of probabilistic, normative brain atlases (Cocosco et al., 1997; Prastawa et al., 2005), we use existing atlases for human brain analysis and generate new atlases for rodent adult and pup analysis. Anatomical structures and WM tracts hypothesized to show changes due to drug abuse or drug exposure can then be compared at the subsequent stage of biostatistical analysis.

SUBJECT AGE

Assessment of both behavioral and neuroimaging measurements at comparative ages for humans and rodents is quite difficult to establish, as not all brain development processes happen along parallel trajectories. For example, rodent pups are born with their eyes closed and remain so until post-natal day 5–6, resulting in a comparatively slower visual system development. Similar disparate relationships between the two species exist in social systems, learning and memory, stress, and numerous other brain systems. This inconsistency in developmental trajectories a cross-species means that it is important to define *a priori* the measurements of interest and choose the assessment age in the studied species according to a similar stage in development. In addition to the consideration of developmental stage, we also need to take into account that neuroimaging of human infants in their first year of life is usually restricted to annual or biannual measurements by local institutional review boards (IRB). No such considerations are in place for small animal imaging, which offers thus a chance to capture a

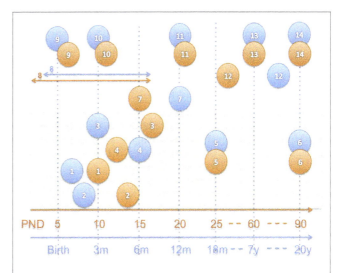

FIGURE 2 | Approximate neuro-development comparison in humans (blue) and rats (orange; Watson et al., 2006). 1–6 = myelination, 1 = myelination onset internal capsule, 2 = onset olfactory tract, 3 = onset anterior commissure, 4 = onset fornix, 5 = 50% myelination of corpus callosum, 6 = mature myelination, 7 = 50% cerebellum size, 8 = peak synaptogenesis period, 9 = maximum brain growth velocity (peak), 10 = cortical dominance established, 11 = mature cerebral metabolism, 12 = adult pattern of slow wave and REM sleep, 13 = adult brain weight, 14 = mature prefrontal cortex.

more detailed characterization of the neuro-development process with respect to the developmental time scale than is possible in human clinical research studies. In **Figure 2** several milestones of post-natal brain development are compared between humans and rats (data from Watson et al., 2006). While several neuro-developmental milestones are mapped across-species well in **Figure 2**, others clearly are mismatched such as cerebellar growth or olfactory tract myelination.

For our cocaine-exposure study we chose to study auditory, emotional, and olfactory aspects. Consequently, hippocampus, amygdala, and olfactory bulb are some of the main target measures. The human neonate imaging time point was preset at 1–6 weeks of age (median at 3 weeks) by the availability of prior control data from a large study of normal development (Gilmore et al., 2007; Marc et al., 2010). We selected two pup imaging time points, one early time point at post-natal day (PND) five where pups are at a similar neuro-developmental stage for the selected measures to human 1-week-old neonates, as well as a second later time point at PND 14 with myelination stages in the olfactory bulb comparable to human infants at about 8 weeks of age, as well as established cortical dominance comparable to human development at about 12 weeks of age (Bayer et al., 1993; Watson et al., 2006). All image assessments occur during peak synaptogenesis, which ends at PND 16 in rats and 8 months in humans, as well as prior to mature cerebral metabolism, adult sleep patterns, and 50% cerebral myelination. The use of two separate time points as compared to the single human time point also allows us to better characterize the developmental impact of intra-uterine cocaine-exposure in the rat model.

MR IMAGING

We chose anatomical and structural imaging protocols on the various high-field MRI scanners which provided optimal contrast for tissue type and fluid, and adequate WM diffusion information This includes high-resolution sequences for T1- and T2-weighted scans, which are mainly used for structural volumetry analysis, as well as for diffusion tensor imaging (DTI) scans, which are used for brain WM connectivity information. Derived DTI property maps focus on the local fiber integrity [fractional anisotropy (FA) and axonal diffusivity (AD)], the local degree of myelination [Zhang et al., 2009; radial diffusivity (RD)] as well as the level of micro-organization [mean diffusivity (MD)].

Animal imaging

Animal imaging is performed on a Bruker 9.4 T horizontal 30 cm MR scanner with a 800 mT/m gradient coil. The system has a 35 mm quad volume coil for transmit and receive. In addition to allowing acquisition of high-resolution images, the available high gradient coil greatly facilitates the proposed DTI. A small animal heating system is integrated with the animal bed. Finally, a MR compatible small animal monitoring system is available to provide the physiological monitoring, including respiration, ECG and body temperature, while animals are being scanned. Several imaging sequences are used to provide high-resolution anatomical as well as DTI images. A high-resolution (minimally $150\,\mu m \times 150\,\mu m \times 110\,\mu m$) 3D RARE DTI sequence with diffusion gradients applied in six non-collinear directions is used to acquire DTI imagery (Cai et al., 2009). Two navigator-echoes are utilized in this sequence to correct for motion artifacts. The total data acquisition time is within 3–4 h. Animals are maintained under ad lib conditions for 24 h prior to imaging. General anesthesia is induced via gas isoflurane (1–2% for induction and 0.75–1% for maintaining anesthesia). The study design includes a total of 165 rat and pup MRI and DTI scans.

Human infant imaging

The high-field 3 T scanning (Siemens 3 T Allegra head-only) of newborns uses parallel imaging (eight-channel receiver array head coil) to provide optimal contrast-to-noise ratio and optimal success rate for motion-free scans of non-sedated newborns. Structural imaging sequences include a turboflash, rapid gradient echo (MP-RAGE) T1-weighted and a turbo spin echo, dual-echo (proton density and T2-weighted). Spatial resolution is $1\,mm \times 1\,mm \times 1\,mm$ voxel for T1-weighted images and $1.25\,mm \times 1.25\,mm \times 1.5\,mm$ voxel for proton density/T2-weighted images. For diffusion weighted imaging, a single shot echo planar SE DTI imaging sequence is used. Forty-two unique gradient direction images at $b = 1000\,s/mm^2$ are acquired and seven images without diffusion gradient ($b = 0$; Gilmore et al., 2007). The total scan time is about 20 min. At the final stage of the project, 120 children are planned to be enrolled in this study, 60 with prenatal exposure to cocaine and 60 normal controls.

IMAGE ANALYSIS

In this section we will focus on the methods and design of the brain MR image analysis pipelines. As was the case for our selection of the MR imaging sequences, while these pipelines have been developed for our cocaine-exposure projects, they are generally applicable to any human or rodent MR neuroimaging projects. Regional selections for the structural analysis as well as the fiber selection for the DTI analysis are synchronized, such that the findings can be compared between the human and rodent arms of our project.

Structural MRI analysis workflow

Atlas space. A general necessity in neuroimaging is the ability to compare findings across different studies, and for that purpose MR datasets are commonly reoriented to a standard, prior atlas space, usually a variant of the MNI (Mazziotta et al., 2001) atlas space in human neuroimaging and the Paxinos (Paxinos and Franklin, 2001; MacKenzie-Graham et al., 2004) or Waxholm (Johnson et al., 2010) atlas space in rodents. While such atlas spaces are commonly well defined and publicly available for the adult brain, this is not the case for developing subjects. As part of our neuro-developmental projects we generated atlas images that represent an average brain anatomy at every developmental stage of study. In this study, we employed a prior human neonate T1-weighted atlas image (Prastawa et al., 2005; Gilmore et al., 2010), and we computed novel average DTI atlas images for Sprague-Dawley rats at PND five and 14 from 10 post-mortem subject each (see also **Figure 3**). All these atlases were built using a joint deformable registration of all training datasets into a single, iteratively improving the unbiased average image that has a minimal deformation to all training images, as described in (Joshi et al., 2004; Styner et al., 2009; AtlasWerks[1]). Prior to the deformable atlas building, one selected training image was rigidly aligned to a prior atlas space (such as the adult MNI space) and then all other training images were affinely registered to it. Furthermore, skull stripping, initialized via

---

[1] http://www.sci.utah.edu/software/13/370-atlaswerks.html

the automatic BET2 (Jenkinson et al., 2005) method followed by manual post-processing using ITKSnap[2] (Yushkevich et al., 2006), and intensity calibration using pairwise histogram quantile matching via AutoSeg[3] (Gouttard et al., 2007) was performed prior to atlas building.

Atlas priors. On the above mentioned atlas image space, we further define additional prior information that is employed in the subsequent image analysis steps. Such spatial prior information can be encoding both voxel-wise attributes, such as spatial tissue probability maps, and geometric attributes, such as surfaces or WM fiber tracts. In our structural MRI atlases, we define the following voxel-wise attribute maps: (a) probabilistic tissue maps for WM, gray matter (GM), and cerebrospinal fluid (CSF) in humans (Prastawa et al., 2005), for WM and two separate classes of GM (Lee et al., 2009) in rodents; (b) probabilistic or hard label maps for brain structures (hippocampus, amygdala, caudate/putamen/striatum, globus pallidus, and lateral ventricles in both human and rodent atlas); and (c) hard label maps for cortical lobe parcellations (hemispheric definitions of occipital, temporal, parietal, frontal, and prefrontal lobes in both human and rodent atlas). All label definitions (b, c) were established by experts via manual outlining with ITKSnap.

Brain tissue segmentation. Following rigid registration into the atlas space, all MR images are automatically segmented into the major brain tissue regions using an atlas-based expectation maximization (EM) scheme (Van Leemput et al., 1999; Prastawa et al., 2005; see also brain renderings in **Figure 1**). Human neonate data employed an adapted EM version that allows the separation WM into unmyelinated an myelinated regions (Prastawa et al., 2005). Rodent brain segmentations use the same parameter settings but separate atlases and tissue priors (via ABC[4]). It is noteworthy that the relative sizes of GM and WM regions is vastly different in the human and rodent brain, e.g., the hippocampus is an order of magnitude larger, measured relative to the overall brain size (Lee et al., 2009). Thus, whole brain tissue measurements are difficult to compare between species and thus are of limited use in cross-species studies. Nevertheless, our brain tissue segmentation step provides an overall segmentation of the brain without the need for skull stripping. In fact, the computed tissue segmentation serves as a mean to strip the skull from the images, a necessary processing step before the regional segmentation step can be computed (Oguz et al., 2011). Manual post-processing is employed if necessary. It further noteworthy that our EM based segmentation method provides an intensity inhomogeneity correction that ensures that the different tissue classes appear homogeneously with similar intensities across the image.

Regional segmentation. In this step, we subdivide the brain into several regions via a deformable fluid registration (Joshi et al., 2004; AtlasWerks/AutoSeg) of the prior atlas (Gouttard et al., 2007; Lee et al., 2009; see **Figure 4** for an example). Since the registration method is matching directly the intensities of the atlas image with the intensities in the subject MR images, intensity calibration using pairwise histogram quantile matching (Gouttard et al., 2007) is applied before registration. Using the computed deformable transform, prior regional atlas maps are propagated to the individual image (a) to directly define the subcortical structure measurements and (b) to be combined with the tissue segmentations for cortical, lobar parcellation measurement.

While the same registration method should be employed in human and rodent MRI data, the registration parameters have to be optimized separately for each setting. In general, human brain anatomy exhibits much higher inter-subject variability than small animal models due to the fact that such small animal models do not have any complex cortical folds which are the main contributors to the inter-subject variability in humans; the variability is further reduced due to the fact that the animals are commonly only investigated within a genetically similar population, such as only Sprague-Dawley rats in our study. In order to match major cortical folds in the human settings, registration parameters are chosen to provide a considerably more relaxed deformation model than in the small animal settings. The parameters used in our human study are the default parameters in the AutoSeg package.

---

[2] http://www.itksnap.org
[3] http://www.nitrc.org/projects/autoseg
[4] http://www.nitrc.org/projects/abc/

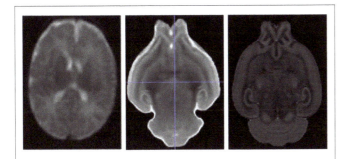

FIGURE 3 | Human neonate T2-weighted atlas (left) and rodent MD atlas at PND 5 (middle) and PND 14 (right).

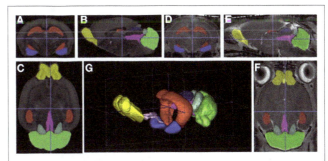

FIGURE 4 | Visualization of the atlas registration based regional segmentation for PND14: (A–C) Orthogonal slice views of the atlas; (D–F) views on an example dataset; (G) 3D-rendering of example segmentation. Red: hippocampus, green: cerebellum, blue: amygdala, yellow: olfactory bulb.

Cortical thickness analysis. As a final step in the structural analysis workflow, we compute local cortical thickness measurements using the cortical GM segmentation in humans (Vachet et al., 2011; via GAMBIT[5]) and the regional neocortex segmentation in rodents (via ShapeWorks[6]; Lee et al., 2011; **Figure 5**). While the cortical thickness is estimated from the segmentations in a voxel-wise fashion, it is analyzed on the cortical surface in a surface location wise fashion. For this purpose, a group-wise correspondence is established on the cortical surface (Oguz et al., 2008) using a particle-based entropy optimization over surface location, as well as sulcal depth measurements in human data due to the folded nature of the human cortex (GAMBIT). Cortical thickness measurements at corresponding surface locations are then extracted and statistically analyzed using the statistical analysis toolbox SurfStat[7].

DTI analysis workflow

Prior to any processing, a strict diffusion weighted images (DWI)/DTI quality control (QC), eddy current and motion correction was performed for all DWI scans via DWI/DTI data suffers from inherent low SNR, motion, and eddy current artifacts. These artifacts can be too severe for a correct and stable estimation of the diffusion tensor without strict QC and correction methods. Thus, all datasets are subjected to a strict QC using DTIPrep[8] (Liu et al., 2010), which identifies signal corruption artifacts in the DWI, as well as corrects for motion and eddy current artifacts.

---

[5] http://www.nitrc.org/projects/gambit/
[6] http://www.nitrc.org/projects/shapeworks/
[7] http://www.nitrc.org/projects/surfstat/
[8] http://www.nitrc.org/projects/dtiprep

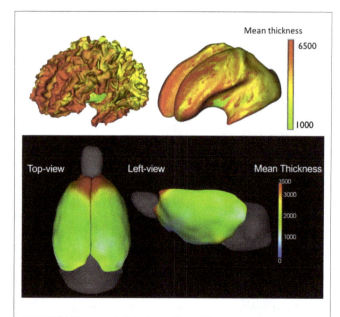

FIGURE 5 | Mean cortical thickness (in μm) in a human 2 year old population (top, seen on the original white matter surface and the corresponding inflated brain surface; Vachet et al., 2011) and an adolescent rat population (bottom, seen from two viewpoints; Lee et al., 2011).

Skull stripping is performed automatically via tissue segmentation masks from co-registered structural MRI data. Diffusion tensor images are computed by standard weighted least-square estimation.

Regional analysis using structural segmentations. White matter integrity is assessed in our DTI analysis at three levels of scale. The first step analyzes WM properties within larger regions using the previously computed regional segmentation of the structural MRI data. For human DTI datasets, the corresponding T2-weighted structural image is registered with the baseline ($b=0$) scan and the regional segmentations are propagated accordingly. We employ affine registration within 3D Slicer[9] due to the presence of DTI distortion artifacts. As we compute the regional segmentations directly on the DTI property maps for the rat MRI datasets, no registration is required for this data. Within each region, including both the cortical parcellations as well as the subcortical structures, we compute the mean and median DTI FA, MD, AD, and RD measures for further statistical analysis. While region analysis usually provides stable measurements of both white and GM regions, WM regions are not well represented, as different fiber tracts with likely different developmental maturation trajectories are lumped together. For example, the frontal lobe WM region contains information from fiber tracts such as the cerebrospinal tract, which myelinates early in development mainly during the first year of life (Goodlett et al., 2009), as well as the arcuate fasciculus, which myelinates later.

Voxel-wise analysis via atlas mapping. The second DTI analysis step provides a highly localized voxel-wise analysis (Liu et al., 2009), in contrast to the regional step that lumps together rather large regions. For this voxel-wise analysis, all datasets are mapped into a common reference space using the fluid diffeomorphic registration based atlas building (Joshi et al., 2004) also employed in the structural analysis (via AtlasWerks). This creates an unbiased analysis space, which allows the examination of the whole WM. The discovered findings are often considered for hypothesis generation or as preliminary findings that have to be confirmed in the third DTI analysis step.

Tract-based DTI analysis via atlas mapping. In the third DTI analysis step, we measure WM diffusion properties along selected tracts of interest (see **Figure 6**). This step thus provides a curvi-linear regional analysis at an intermediate scale between the first two analysis steps. Using the atlas space generated in the previous step, Goodlett et al. (2009) developed a population-based analysis scheme that uses fiber tractography in the common atlas space to generate statistics of tract-based diffusion properties across all images in the population. DTI fibers on the DTI atlas are computed with standard streamline tractography in 3D Slicer. Measurements of FA mean diffusivity (MD), and axial and radial diffusivity (AD, RD) are extracted at well defined locations along each tract (Fillard et al., 2003; Corouge et al., 2005; Goodlett et al., 2005; via DTI-TractStat[10]) to do group comparisons. In our cocaine study, the

---

[9] http://www.slicer.org
[10] http://www.nitrc.org/projects/dti_tract_stat/

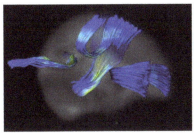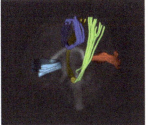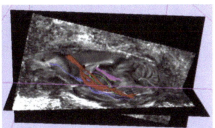

FIGURE 6 | Left/middle: white matter fiber tracts (splenium/red, genu/cyan, mid-corpus callosum/blue and motor tracts/green) obtained from population-based analysis of neonatal DTI with color coding of fractional anisotropy (left) and as multi-colored fiber tracts (middle). Right: genu fiber tract (red) in a rodent DTI scan (anterior commissure = blue, hippocampal commissure = pink).

selected tracts of interest include major tracts such as the motor tract, sensory tract, uncinate fasciculus, fornix, arcuate fasciculus, splenium tract, genu tract, and the inferior longitudinal fasciculus. This fiber based DTI analysis method has previously been used in large clinical studies, such as our ongoing large neonatal MRI study (Gilmore et al., 2007). **Figure 6** demonstrates tract-based visualizations of WM diffusion properties based on 67 neonatal subjects in our cocaine study (31 controls, 13 cocaine, and 23 nicotine only subjects (Gerig et al., 2010; Gouttard et al., 2010).

PRELIMINARY COMPARATIVE DTI ANALYSIS

Our proposed cross-species analysis framework is currently being applied to the previously described study on intra-uterine cocaine-exposure and brain development. To highlight the proposed framework, we present preliminary results that focus on the fiber tract-based DTI analysis of the inter-hemispheric genu tract, which connect the left and right hemispheric prefrontal cortices through the corpus callosum. In **Figure 6**/middle, the human genu tract is highlight in light blue, whereas in **Figure 6**/right, the rodent genu tract is shown in red including also non-prefrontal projections, which were excluded in the preliminary results presented in **Figure 7**. The human results were computed from scans of 10 neonates exposed to cocaine intra-uterinely as well as 22 age matched controls. Rodent results were computed from scans of 20 cocaine-exposed Wistar rats at PND 14 and 20 ages matched untreated controls. **Figure 7** shows the surprising, though non-significant (trends at $p = 0.08$ to 0.10) results of heightened FA measures in the corpus callosum region (center section of the profile) of the genu fiber tract in both human and rodent analyses. The similarities of group differences between the human and rodent results are also quite evident.

DISCUSSION

This report describes the study design of the neuroimaging and image processing setup for a translational animal–human translational project to study effects of drug-abuse in mothers and drug-exposure of infants. It is discussed that the choice of scanners and imaging protocols for 3D anatomical and diffusion imaging is carefully optimized with respect to the type of species and age of subjects. Human adult imaging uses a full-body 3 T scanner, whereas neonatal imaging makes use of a head-only 3 T device which facilitates subject management. Animal imaging requires much higher field strength due to much smaller structures, and

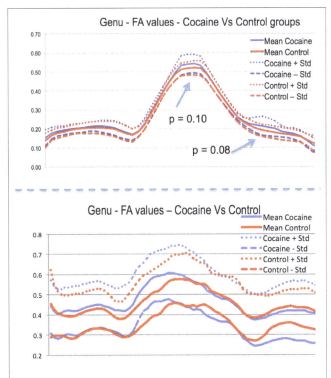

FIGURE 7 | Preliminary DTI–FA profile results of the genu fiber tract in the intra-uterine cocaine-exposure study (plot shows left hemisphere to right hemisphere). Top: human subjects, bottom: rodent subjects. Few locations show statistical trends with surprising similarities across-species in group differences along most of the tract.

this study therefore make use of a 9.4 T special animal research scanner. It is discussed that pulse sequences are optimized on each device to achieve maximum soft tissue contrast and also WM diffusion information. Image processing, on the other hand, uses exactly the same underlying methodological and computational concepts, and can make use of the same toolboxes originally developed for human imaging. We can thus measure brain WM, GM, cortical thickness, size, and shapes of subcortical structures, volume of lobar regions, and WM diffusion in regions and along fiber tracts in animals and humans and in infants and adults. This allows us to capture relevant anatomical and WM property changes from normal due to drug exposure across-species. Comparison across-species is not done at the imaging level, but at the level of statistical analysis of image-derived assessments of brain changes. Information obtained from animal models can thus help us to generate possible hypothesis for human brain maturation and changes as observed in non-invasive MRI and DTI imaging.

It is noteworthy to keep in mind that despite all the efforts toward a cross-species analysis framework, no rodent model of neuro-development will sufficiently characterize the human teratologic impact of drug abuse. Nevertheless, such rodent models provide highly valuable information highlighted as evidenced by the vast literature on this topic. With respect to the framework presented here, we cannot compare the brain morphology between humans and rodents directly, e.g., by combining human and rodent atlases based results in a voxel-wise fashion. Rather we can compare findings indirectly, e.g., reproducible findings of delayed maturation in WM fibers within the genu region of the corpus callosum both in humans and rodents would be a strong indication that such a finding in infants would be due to the cocaine-exposure and not one of the many possible confounding factors. Our framework aims to enhance the confidence in such inferred cross-species findings.

Animal and human capabilities for imaging carry significant differences that make such a parallel approach very attractive and potentially a powerful way to get better insight in brain changes due to drug abuse or exposure but also in other scenarios. Human brains show large individual variability within a population, which presents significant challenges for measurements of comparable regional and functional properties. Rat brains, on the other hand, show very small anatomical variability due to the fact that they can be genetically controlled. Further, human *in vivo* imaging inherently is limited by safety and patient comfort constraints that affect scan times and repetition of scanning for longitudinal assessment. Choices of spatial resolution and of multi-modal imaging sequences are therefore always limited by the total scan time but also maximum time per image sequence to avoid artifacts due to patient motion. These limitations are even more pronounced in imaging infants since sedation is limited to subjects with indication of pathology, which permits clinical scanning. Animal imaging brings much more flexibility concerning scanning types and times since subjects are imaged under general anesthesia.

ACKNOWLEDGMENTS

We would like to acknowledge the following funding sources UNC IDDRC HD 03110, NINDS R42 NS059095, NIDA P01 DA022446-01, RC1AA019211. Furthermore, we would like to thanks Fulton Crews, Allan Johnson and Sheryl Moy for their insightful discussion on the topic of cross-species studies and small animal imaging. NICHD P30 HD03110 awarded to J. Piven.

REFERENCES

Badea, A., Nicholls, P., Johnson, G., and Wetsel, W. (2007). Neuroanatomical phenotypes in the reeler mouse. *Neuroimage* 34, 1363–1374.

Bale, T. J., Baram, T. Z., Brown, A. S., Goldstein, J. M., Insel, T. M., McCarthy, M. M., Nemeroff, C. B., Reyes, T. M., Simerly, R. B., Susser, E. S., and and Nestler, E. J. (2010). Early life programming and neuro-developmental disorders. *Biol. Psychiatry* 68, 314–319.

Bayer, S. A., Altman, J., Russo, R. J., and, Zhang X. (1993). Time-tables of neurogenesis in the human brain based on experimentally determined patterns in the rat. *Neurotoxicology* 14, 83–144.

Brown, A. S., and Derkits, E. J. (2010). Prenatal infection and schizophrenia: a review of epidemiologic and translational studies. *Am. J. Psychiatry* 167, 261–280.

Bugos, O., Bhide, M., and Zilka, N. (2009). Beyond the rat models of human neurodegenerative disorders. *Cell. Mol. Neurobiol.* 29, 859–869.

Cai, Y., Hong, Y. L., McMurray, M. S., Johns, J. M., Lin, W., and An, H. (2009). "High-field diffusion tensor magnetic resonance histology using rapid acquisition with relaxation enhancement (DTI RARE)," in *Annual Meeting of the Society for Neuroscience*, Chicago.

Cocosco, C. A., Kollokian, V., Kwan, R. S., and Evans, A. C. (1997). BrainWeb: online interface to a 3D MRI simulated brain database. *Neuroimage* 5, S425.

Corouge, I., Fletcher, T., Joshi, S., Gilmore, J. H., and Gerig, G. (2005). "Fiber tract-oriented statistics for quantitative diffusion tensor MRI analysis," in *Lecture Notes in Computer Science LNCS*, Vol. 3749, eds J. S. Duncan and G. Gerig (Palm Springs, CA: Springer Verlag), 131–138.

Fatemi, S. H., Folsom, T., Reutiman, T., Abu-Odeh, D., Mori, S., Huang, H., and Oishi, K. (2009). Abnormal expression of myelination genes and alterations in white matter fractional anisotropy following prenatal viral influenza infection at E16 in mice. *Schizophr. Res.* 112, 46–53.

Fernandes de Abreu, D., Nivet, E., Baril, N., Khrestchatisky, M., Roman, F., and Féron, F. (2010). Developmental vitamin D deficiency alters learning in C57Bl/6J mice. *Behav. Brain Res.* 208, 603–608.

Fillard, P., Gilmore, J., Lin, W., and Gerig, G. (2003). "Quantitative analysis of white matter fiber properties along geodesic paths," in *Lecture Notes in Computer Science LNCS #2879*, eds R. E. Ellis and T. M. Peters (Montreal, CA: Springer), 16–23.

Gerig, G., Grewen, K., Gouttard, S., Gilmore, J., Bitaud, E., and Johns, J. (2010). "Prenatal cocaine effects on neonatal white matter development," in *Annual Meeting of the Society for Neuroscience*, San Diego, CA.

Gilmore, J., Kang, C., Evans, D., Wolfe, H., Smith, J. K., Lieberman, J. A., Lin, W., Hamer, R., Styner, M., and Gerig, G. (2010). Prenatal and neonatal brain structure and white matter maturation in children at high risk for schizophrenia. *Am. J. Psychiatry* 167, 1083–1091.

Gilmore, J. H., Lin, W., Corouge, I., Vetsa, Y. S. K., Smith, J. K., Kang, C., Gu, H., Hamer, R. M., Lieberman, J. A., and Gerig, G. (2007). Early postnatal development of corpus callosum and corticospinal white matter assessed with quantitative tractography. *AJNR Am. J. Neuroradiol.* 28, 1789–1795.

Goodlett, C., Corouge, I., Jomier, M., and Gerig, G. (2005). "A Quantitative DTI Fiber Tract Analysis Suite," *The Insight Journal*, Vol. ISC/NAMIC/MICCAI Workshop on Open-Source Software, Palm Springs, CA.

Goodlett, C. B., Thomas, Fletcher, P. T., Gilmore, J. H., and Gerig, G. (2009). Group analysis of DTI fiber tract statistics with application to neurodevelopment. *Neuroimage* 45(Supp. 1), S133–S142.

Gouttard, S., Grewen, K., Gerig, G., Gilmore, J., Bitaud, E., and Johns, J. (2010). "Prenatal cocaine effects on infant brain development," in *Annual Meeting of the Society for Neuroscience*, San Diego.

Gouttard, S., Styner, M., Joshi, S., Smith, R. G., Cody, H., and Gerig, G. (2007). "Subcortical structure segmentation using probabilistic atlas priors," in *Proceedings in SPIE Medical Imaging*, San Diego, CA.

Hazlett, H., Poe, M., Lightbody, A., Gerig, G., Macfall, J. R., Ross, A. K., Provenzale, J., Martin, A., Reiss, A., and Piven, J. (2009). Teasing apart the heterogeneity of autism: same behavior, different brains in toddlers with fragile X syndrome and autism. *J. Neurodev. Disord.* 1, 81–90.

Jenkinson, M., Pechaud, M., and Smith, S. (2005). "BET2: MR-based estimation of brain, skull and scalp surfaces," in *Eleventh Annual Meeting of the Organization for Human Brain Mapping*, Toronto, CA.

Johnson, G. A., Badea, A., Brandenburg, J., Cofer, G., Fubara, B., Liu, S., and Nissanov, J. (2010). Waxholm space: an image-based reference for coordinating mouse brain research. *Neuroimage* 53, 365–372.

Joshi, S., Davis, B., Jomier, M., and Gerig, G. (2004). Unbiased diffeomorphic atlas construction for computational anatomy. *Neuroimage* 23, S151–S160.

Kennedy, D., Haselgrove, C., and McInerney, S. (2003). MRI-based morphometric of typical and atypical brain development. *Ment. Retard. Dev. Disabil. Res. Rev.* 9, 155–160.

Lee, F. K. H., Fang, M., Antonio, G. E., Yeung, D. K. W., Chan, E. T. Y., Zhang, L., Yew, D. T., and Ahuja, A. T. (2006). Dti of rodent brains in vivo using a 1.5t clinical MR scanner. *J. Magn. Reson. Imaging* 23, 747–751.

Lee, J., Jomier, J., Aylward, S., Tyszka, M., Moy, S., Lauder, J., and Styner, M. (2009). Evaluation of atlas based mouse brain segmentation. *Proc. SPIE* 7259, 137–148.

Lee, J., Ehlers, C., Crews, F., Niethammer, M., Budin, F., Paniagua, B., Sulik, K., Johns, J., Styner, M., and Oguz, I. (2011). "Automatic cortical thickness analysis on rodent brain," in *SPIE Medical Imaging: Image Processing*, Orlando, FL, 7962, 7962481–79624811.

Lerch, J., Carroll, J., Dorr, A., Spring, S., Evans, A., Hayden, M., Sled, J., and Henkelman, R. (2008). Cortical thickness measured from MRI in the YAC128 mouse model of Huntington's disease. *Neuroimage* 41, 243–251.

Liu, Z., Wang, Y., Gerig, G., Gouttard, S., and Styner, M. (2010). "Quality control of diffusion weighted images. Medical imaging 2010: advanced PACS-based imaging informatics and therapeutic applications," in *Proceedings of SPIE*, San Diego, CA.

Liu, Z., Zhu, H., Marks, B., Katz, L., Goodlett, C. B., Gerig, G., and Styner, M. (2009). "Voxel-wise group analysis of DTI," in *IEEE International Symposium on Biomedical Imaging*, Orlando, FL.

MacKenzie-Graham, A., Lee, E., Dinov, I. D., Bota, M., Shattuck, D., Ruffins, S., Yuan, H., Konstantinidis, F., Pitiot, A., Ding, Y., Hu, G., Jacobs, R., and Toga, A. (2004). A multimodal, multidimensional atlas of the C57BL/6J mouse brain. *J. Anat.* 204, 93–102.

Marc, C., Vachet, C., Gerig, G., Blocher, J., Gilmore, J., and Styner, M. (2010). "Changes of MR and DTI appearance in early human brain development," in *SPIE Medical Imaging: Image Processing*, San Diego, CA.

Mayer, D., Zahr, N. M., Adal-steinsson, E., Rutt, B., Sullivan, E. V., and Pfefferbaum, A. (2007). In vivo fiber tracking in the rat brain on a clinical 3t MRI system using a high strength insert gradient coil. *Neuroimage* 35, 1077–1085.

Mazziotta, J., Toga, A., Evans, A., Fox, P., Lancaster, J., Zilles, K., Woods, R., Paus, T., Simpson, G., Pike, B., Holmes, C., Collins, L., Thompson, P., MacDonald, D., Iacoboni, M., Schormann, T., Amunts, K., Palomero-Gallagher, N., Geyer, S., Parsons, L., Narr, K., Kabani, N., Le Goualher, G., Boomsma, D., Cannon, T., Kawashima, R., and Mazoyer, B. (2001). A probabilistic atlas and reference system for the human brain: International Consortium for Brain Mapping (ICBM). *Philos. Trans. R. Soc. Lond. B Biol. Sci.* 356, 1293–1322.

Moeller, F. G., Hasan, K. M., Steinberg, J. L., Kramer, L. A., Dougherty, D. M., Santos, R. M., Valdes, I., Swann, A. C., Barratt, E. S., and Narayana, P. A. (2005). Reduced anterior corpus callosum white matter integrity is related to increased impulsivity and reduced discriminability in cocaine-dependent subjects: diffusion tensor imaging. *Neuropsychopharmacology* 30, 610–617.

Mosconi, M. W., Hazlett, H., Poe, M. D., Gerig, G., Smith, R., and Piven, J. (2009). Longitudinal study of amygdala volume and joint attention in 2- to 4-year-old children with autism. *Arch. Gen. Psychiatry* 66, 509–516.

Nieman, B. J., Bock, N. A., Bishop, J., Chen, X. J., Sled, J. G., Rossant, J., and Henkelman, R. M. (2005). Magnetic resonance imaging for detection and analysis of mouse phenotypes. *NMR Biomed.* 18, 447–468.

NIMH. (2008). "Transformative neurodevelopmental research in mental illness," in *National Advisory Mental Health Council Workgroup*, Bethesda, MD.

Oguz, I., Cates, J., Fletcher, T., Whitaker, R., Cool, D., Aylward, S., and Styner, M. (2008). "Cortical correspondence using entropy-based particle systems and local features," in *IEEE International Symposium on Biomedical Imaging*, Paris.

Oguz, I., Lee, J., Budin, F., Rumple, A., McMurray, M., Ehlers, C., Crews, F., Johns, J., and Styner, M. (2011). "Automatic skull-stripping of rat MRI/DTI scans and atlas building," in *SPIE Medical Imaging: Image Processing*, Orlando, FL, 7962, 7962251–7962257.

O'Leary-Moore, S. K., Parnell, S. E., Godin, E., Dehart, D., Ament, J., Khan, A., Johnson, G. A., Styner, M. A., and Sulik, K. (2010). Magnetic resonance microscopy-based analyses of the brains of normal and ethanol-exposed fetal mice. *Birth Defects Res. A Clin. Mol. Teratol.* 88, 953–964.

Paus, T., Zijdenbos, A., Worsley, K., Collins, D. L., Blumenthal, J., Giedd, J. N., Rapoport, J. L., and Evans, A. C. (1999). Structural maturation of neural pathways in children and adolescents: in vivo study. *Science* 283, 1908–1911.

Paxinos, G., and Franklin, K. B. J. (2001). *The Mouse Brain in Stereotaxic Coordinates*, 2nd Edn, San Diego: Academic Press.

Pfefferbaum, A., Adal-steinsson, E., and Sullivan, E. V. (2004). In vivo structural imaging of the rat brain with a 3-t clinical human scanner. *J. Magn. Reson. Imaging* 20, 779–785.

Pillai, D., Heidemann, R., Kumar, P., Shanbhag, N., Lanz, T., Dittmar, M., Sandner, B., Beier, C., Weidner, N., Greenlee, M., Schuierer, G., Bogdahn, U., and Schlachetzki, F. (2011). Comprehensive small animal imaging strategies on a clinical 3 T dedicated head MR-scanner; adapted methods and sequence protocols in cns pathologies. *PLoS ONE* 6, e16091. doi:10.1371/journal.pone.0016091

Prastawa, M., Gilmore, J. H., Lin, W., and Gerig, G. (2005). Automatic segmentation of MR images of the developing newborn brain. *Med. Image Anal.* 9, 457–466.

Schlaepfer, T. E., Lancaster, E., Heidbreder, R., Strain, E. C., Kosel, M., Fisch, H. U., and Pearlson, G. D. (2005). Decreased frontal white-matter volume in chronic substance abuse. *J. Neuropsychopharmacol.* 9, 1–7.

Shaw, P., Kabani, N., Lerch, J. P., Eckstrand, K., Lenroot, R., Gogtay, N., Greenstein, D., Clasen, L., Evans, A., Rapoport, J. L., Giedd, J., and Wise, S. (2008). Neurodevelopmental trajectories of the human cerebral cortex. *J. Neurosci.* 28, 3586–3594.

Styner, M. A., Joshi, S., Overstreet, D. H., Mc Murray, M. S., and Johns, J. M. (2009). "Unbiased population atlas building of early postnatal rat development at PND 5 and 14 for atlas based analysis," in *Annual Meeting of the Society for Neuroscience*, Chicago.

Vachet, C., Hazlett, H. C., Niethammer, M., Oguz, I., Cates, J., Whitaker, R., Piven, J., and Styner, M. (2011). "Group-wise automatic mesh-based analysis of cortical thickness," in *Medical Imaging 2011: Image Processing*, 796227.

Van Leemput, K., Maes, F., Vandermeulen, D., and Suetens, P. (1999). Automated model-based tissue classification of MR images of the brain. *IEEE Trans. Med. Imaging* 18, 897–908.

VanCamp, N., Blockx, I., Verhoye, M., Casteels, C., Coun, F., Leemans, A., Sijbers, J., Baekelandt, V., Van Laere, K., and Van der Linden, A. (2009). Dti in a rat model of Parkinson's disease after lesioning of the nigrostriatal tract. *NMR Biomed.* 22, 697–706.

Watson, R. E., DeSesso, J. M., Hurtt, M. E., and Cappon, G. D. (2006). Postnatal growth and morphological development of the brain: a species comparison. *Birth Defects Res. B Dev. Reprod. Toxicol.* 77, 471–484.

Yushkevich, P. A., Piven, J., Hazlett, H. C., Smith, R. G., Ho, S., Gee, J. C., and Gerig, G. (2006). User-guided 3D active contour segmentation of anatomical structures: significantly im-proved efficiency and reliability. *Neuroimage* 31, 1116–1128.

Zhang, J., Jones, M., DeBoy, C., Reich, D., Farrell, J., Hoffman, P., Griffin, J., Sheikh, K., Miller, M., Mori, S., and Calabresi, P. (2009). Diffusion tensor magnetic resonance imaging of Wallerian degeneration in rat spinal cord after dorsal root axotomy. *J. Neurosci.* 29, 3160–3171.

Addiction, adolescence, and innate immune gene induction

Fulton T. Crews[1,2]* and Ryan Peter Vetreno[1,2]

[1] Department of Pharmacology, Bowles Center for Alcohol Studies, The University of North Carolina at Chapel Hill, Chapel Hill, NC, USA
[2] Department of Psychiatry, Bowles Center for Alcohol Studies, The University of North Carolina at Chapel Hill, Chapel Hill, NC, USA

*Correspondence:
Fulton T. Crews, Bowles Center for Alcohol Studies, The School of Medicine, The University of North Carolina at Chapel Hill, CB #7178, 1021 Thurston-Bowles Building, Chapel Hill, NC 27599-71780, USA.
e-mail: fulton_crews@med.unc.edu

Repeated drug use/abuse amplifies psychopathology, progressively reducing frontal lobe behavioral control, and cognitive flexibility while simultaneously increasing limbic temporal lobe negative emotionality. The period of adolescence is a neurodevelopmental stage characterized by poor behavioral control as well as strong limbic reward and thrill seeking. Repeated drug abuse and/or stress during this stage increase the risk of addiction and elevate activator innate immune signaling in the brain. Nuclear factor kappa-light-chain-enhancer of activated B cells (NF-κB) is a key glial transcription factor that regulates proinflammatory chemokines, cytokines, oxidases, proteases, and other innate immune genes. Induction of innate brain immune gene expression (e.g., NF-κB) facilitates negative affect, depression-like behaviors, and inhibits hippocampal neurogenesis. In addition, innate immune gene induction alters cortical neurotransmission consistent with loss of behavioral control. Studies with anti-oxidant, anti-inflammatory, and anti-depressant drugs as well as opiate antagonists link persistent innate immune gene expression to key behavioral components of addiction, e.g., negative affect-anxiety and loss of frontal–cortical behavioral control. This review suggests that persistent and progressive changes in innate immune gene expression contribute to the development of addiction. Innate immune genes may represent a novel new target for addiction therapy.

Keywords: addiction, alcoholism, chemokines, microglia, neurogenesis

INTRODUCTION

Chronic use of alcohol, stimulants, and/or opiates leads to progressive changes in brain and behavior. Addiction is the continued use of a drug despite harm, e.g., a loss of behavioral control over drug use. The frontal cortex regulates decision making and other executive functions, such as motivation, planning, goal setting, and inhibition of impulses. In contrast, the amygdala, hippocampus, and other limbic structures contribute to emotion, emotional learning, and mood. Persistent use of alcohol and other drugs of abuse result in changes to neurobiology that culminate in a loss of attention, poor decision making, increased impulsivity, and anxious urgency that promotes the progressive loss of behavioral control over drug use. Although it is well accepted that drug intoxication changes neurochemistry ultimately leading to altered behavior, the importance of persistent drug-induced changes in the brain that underlie persistent harmful behaviors has only recently been appreciated. Indeed, drug dependence and addiction involves a disruption of the normal balance between self-control mechanisms and emotional needs. Across drugs of addiction, the progression from abuse to addiction involves increased drug wanting, negative emotional urgency, and diminished behavioral control (Jentsch and Taylor, 1999; Robinson and Berridge, 2003). Frontal lobe executive function involves the ability to recognize future consequences, choose between good and bad actions (or better and best), override and suppress unacceptable social responses, and determine similarities and differences between things or events. This cortical region also plays an important role in retaining long-term memories associated with emotions derived from the brain's limbic system. These emotions are then modified via the frontal cortex to generally fit societal norms important for individual integration into society. In addition, the frontal lobes also inhibit impulsivity, making predictions that adjust behavior to current rewards when environment changes (Schoenbaum and Shaham, 2008). Thus, a key element of the behavioral pathology of addiction and substance dependence centers on the loss of frontal–cortical executive behavioral control, increased impulsivity, reduced behavioral flexibility, and a mounting limbic anxiety and urgency.

ADOLESCENT BRAIN DEVELOPMENT AND ADDICTION
ADOLESCENCE: A UNIQUE PERIOD OF DEVELOPMENT

Adolescence is a critical developmental period that encompasses the transition from childhood to adulthood. It is best defined by characteristic behaviors that include high levels of risk-taking, increased exploration, novelty and sensation seeking, social interaction, high activity, and play behaviors that likely promote the acquisition of skills necessary for maturation and independence (Spear, 2000; Ernst et al., 2009). These behaviors are suggested to facilitate the adolescents' development of social skills necessary to gain independence from their family or become senior adults in their group. In rodents, increased social interactions help guide their food choices (Galef, 1977) and other adult actions, such as sexual and aggressive behaviors (see e.g., Fagen, 1976; Smith, 1982). Unfortunately, the increased incidence of novelty/sensation-seeking behaviors during adolescence are also strong predictors of drug and alcohol use (Baumrind, 1987; Andrucci et al., 1989; Wills et al., 1994; Faden, 2006). Indeed, the adolescent brain is in a unique state of transition as it undergoes both progressive and regressive changes providing a biological basis for unique adolescent behaviors and the associated changes in these behaviors during maturation to adulthood. Human magnetic resonance imaging (MRI) studies have demonstrated an inverted U-shape change in gray matter volume during the adolescent period, with pre-adolescent increases followed by post-adolescent reductions (Giedd et al., 1999; Giedd, 2004). At the cellular level, these changes correspond with a marked overproduction of axons and synapses during early puberty, but rapid pruning in later adolescence (Giedd et al., 1999; Andersen et al., 2000; Andersen and Teicher, 2004). Although the exact mechanisms underlying such synaptic changes are not well understood, it is speculated that such remodeling is the biological basis of developmental plasticity wherein the neurological circuits are effectively shaped to adapt to environmental needs leading to mature adult behavior. Such a period of remodeling could also make the adolescent brain more vulnerable to external insults and other psychiatric disorders.

The prefrontal cortex (PFC) and the limbic system, which includes the hippocampus, amygdala, nucleus accumbens (NAcc), and the hypothalamus, undergo prominent reorganization during adolescence. Indeed, absolute PFC gray matter volumes decline in humans (Sowell et al., 1999, 2001) as well as in rats (van Eden et al., 1990) during adolescence. Similarly, a substantial loss of synapses, especially excitatory glutamatergic inputs to the PFC, occur during the adolescent period in humans and non-human primates (Huttenlocher, 1984; Zecevic et al., 1989). In contrast to such adolescent-associated pruning, dopaminergic, and serotonergic inputs to the PFC increase to peak levels well above those observed earlier or later in life (Kalsbeek et al., 1988; Rosenberg and Lewis, 1994). In a similar fashion, cholinergic innervation of the PFC also increases at this time point, ultimately reaching mature levels in rats (Gould et al., 1991) and humans (Kostovic, 1990). Within the hippocampus, the exuberant outgrowth of excitatory axon collaterals and synapses during youth are morphologically remodeled, and branches within dendritic arbors are pruned during this period of maturation (Swann et al., 1999 #3027). Similarly, significant dendritic pruning and synaptic regression also occurs in the medial amygdala (Zehr et al., 2006), NAcc (Teicher et al., 1995; Tarazi et al., 1998b), and hypothalamus (Choi and Kellogg, 1992; Choi et al., 1997). Although most synaptic pruning is likely glutamatergic, dopaminergic receptor expression peaks in early adolescence at postnatal day (P) 28 followed by a one-third reduction of receptors between P35 and P60 (Tarazi et al., 1998a). In terms of hypothalamic function, adolescent rats often exhibit more prolonged stress-induced increases in cortisol than adults (Walker et al., 2001). In addition, rats at P28 evidence less stress-induced Fos-like immunoreactivity in cortical and amygdaloid nuclei than adult rats (Kellogg et al., 1998), but higher novelty-induced Fos activation in the hippocampus during this period (Waters et al., 1997). Thus, significant maturation of the cortical and limbic systems characterizes the adolescent period of development.

Behavioral studies have demonstrated that performance on tasks involving inhibitory control, decision making, and processing speed continues to develop during adolescence. During this developmental stage, selective attention, working memory, and problem solving skills consistently improve as frontal–cortical synaptic pruning and myelination progress (Blakemore and Choudhury, 2006). Similarly, executive inhibitory control improves from adolescence through to adulthood. Studies measuring behavioral inhibition on a Go–No-Go task and functional MRI data reveal greater activation of dorsolateral frontal and orbitofrontal cortices in children than adolescence, and greater activation during adolescence than adults with the adults showing the lowest dorsolateral, but equal orbitofrontal activation and greater inhibitory control performance (Casey et al., 1997; Tamm et al., 2002). These studies support the concept that the immature brain, with excess synapses, possesses more extensive, and less efficient frontal activation and lower performance than adults that have a more efficient frontal cortex that results in more focused, lower overall activation and faster reaction times and better performance (Blakemore and Choudhury, 2006). Taken together, these studies suggest that remodeling of the cortex during the developmental transition from youth to adolescence to adulthood has functional implications for the adult stages of life.

NEUROGENIC PROCESSES IN THE ADOLESCENT BRAIN

Although neurogenesis is primarily an early developmental process with most neurons generated during the prenatal and early postnatal periods, it continues throughout adulthood in discrete brain regions, including the forebrain subventricular zone and subgranular zone of the hippocampal dentate gyrus. The generation and functional integration of nascent neurons into preexisting adult neural circuits is believed to enable the hippocampus to adapt to novel and more complex situations (Kempermann, 2002). Indeed, the contribution of hippocampal neurogenesis to learning and memory (Shors et al., 2001) as well as mood and affective state (Malberg et al., 2000) is supported by many studies. Adolescent neurogenesis, and its role in brain remodeling and unique adolescent behaviors, has to date not been investigated. Studies indicate that adolescent animals have higher levels of hippocampal neurogenesis (He and Crews, 2007), but that neurogenesis in the adolescent brain is very sensitive to alcohol-induced degeneration (Crews et al., 2006a). Thus, disruption of the neurogenic process by drugs and alcohol use during adolescence might produce long-lasting changes that persist into adulthood.

BINGE DRINKING DURING CRITICAL PERIODS IN CORTICAL DEVELOPMENT MIGHT LEAD TO LIFELONG CHANGES IN EXECUTIVE FUNCTION

The effect of alcohol on the adolescent brain is different from those observed in adulthood. Adolescents are less sensitive to the sedative effects of alcohol (Silveri and Spear, 1998), which allows them to binge drink. However, they are more vulnerable to alcohol-induced neurotoxicity (Monti et al., 2005; Crews et al., 2007). The increased sensitivity of the adolescent brain to alcohol-induced toxicity (Peleg-Oren et al., 2009), coupled with the dynamic synaptic remodeling that characterizes this stage, might strengthen the learning components of heavy drinking behaviors and perpetuate the loss of important self-control and goal setting components of the maturing brain's executive centers. Indeed, studies of adolescent individuals with alcohol use disorder have demonstrated smaller prefrontal gray and white matter volumes than age-matched controls. These lower PFC volumes, in turn, correlate with a higher maximum number of drinks per drinking episode (De Bellis et al., 2005). Furthermore, binge ethanol exposure during adolescence reduces D1 and D2 receptors in the frontal cortex while simultaneously increased histone acetylation in the frontal cortex and limbic system (Pascual et al., 2009). Thus, it is likely that both genetics and environment (heavy drinking) contribute to the development of an alcohol use disorder and lower PFC volumes in adolescents. Studies of social drinkers have found that the heaviest binge drinkers have more negative moods and performed worse on executive function tasks (Townshend and Duka, 2003; Weissenborn and Duka, 2003). Furthermore, alcoholics report more fear in facial expressions and animal studies have suggested these alterations in fear response are the result of alcohol-induced deficits in associative learning (Duka et al., 2004). Additional studies have demonstrated perseverative relearning deficits following a rat model of binge drinking that relates to damage of the association cortex (Obernier et al., 2002). However, none of these studies directly reveal a critical period during adolescence when executive function is liable to disruption by ethanol. In contrast, other work on the deleterious effects of ethanol on critical periods involving of visual cortical development, coupled with ethanol-induced cortical neurotoxicity and ethanol-induced alterations in executive function, support the theory that disruption of frontal–cortical development and executive function maturation occurs in adolescent alcohol abusers. It is plausible that adolescent alcohol abuse might disrupt impulse inhibition, attention, and motivation thereby promoting adult alcohol dependence and underlie the high risk of lifetime alcohol dependence found among those who begin drinking as adolescents. In total, the evidence does support a link between adolescent alcohol abuse during a critical period of executive function maturation and an increased risk of lifetime alcohol dependence and perhaps other psychopathologies.

DRUGS AND STRESS INDUCE INNATE IMMUNE GENES THROUGH ACTIVATION OF NF-κB TRANSCRIPTION

Neuroimmune signaling contributes to enteric, sensory, and endocrine hypothalamic–pituitary–adrenal (HPA) responses to external and internal environmental factors. Monocytes and tissue specific monocytes, such as brain microglia, are key cells involved in neuroimmune signaling. These cells are regularly generated from bone marrow stem cells where they migrate to blood, and under normal states, replenish tissue resident macrophages and dendritic cells, including brain microglia. Monocytes have multiple stages of activation that represent a progressive cascade of innate immune gene activation (Graeber, 2010). Monocyte responses regulate cellular movement to sites of tissue damage, secretion of chemokine signals to other cells, secretion of proinflammatory cytokines, proteases, and "danger" signaling molecules, and increased expression of Toll-like receptors (TLRs), oxidases [nicotinamide adenine dinucleotide phosphate (NADPH) oxidase, cyclooxygenase (COX), and inducible nitric oxide synthases (iNOS)], and other innate immune molecules that increase across a spectrum of activation states that range from proinflammatory to trophic. Microglia have a low threshold of activation with initial states of activation secreting signaling molecules, slight morphological changes, upregulation of major histocompatibility complex (MHC) and TLR proteins, and activation of synaptic stripping. In contrast, highly activated microglia progress to mitosis, proliferation, and phagocytic oxidative bursts that oxidize and engulf waste (Graeber, 2010). Under healthy conditions, microglia as well as monocytes in the peripheral sensory nerves and endocrine organs contributes to the integration of sensory systems aimed at maintaining health. However, stress, alcohol, and other addictive drugs as well

as sensory and hormonal signals activate the oxidation sensitive transcription factor NF-κB that is highly expressed in microglia (see **Figure 1**).

The transcription factor NF-κB is involved in the induction of innate immune genes in microglia and other monocyte-like cells in the periphery. Stimuli such as stress, cytokines, oxidative free radicals, ultraviolet irradiation, bacterial or viral antigens, and many other signaling molecules increase NF-κB–DNA binding and transcription of many genes, particularly chemokines, cytokines, oxidases, and proteases. Our laboratory has previously demonstrated that ethanol increases NF-κB–DNA binding in the brain *in vivo* (Crews et al., 2006b) and *in vitro* in hippocampal–entorhinal cortex slice cultures (Zou and Crews, 2006). Furthermore, work from our laboratory and others indicate that ethanol also increases the transcription of NF-κB target

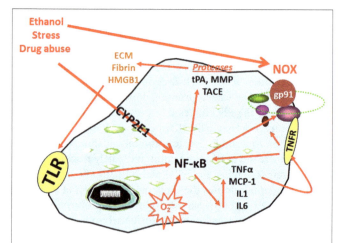

FIGURE 1 | Nuclear factor kappa-light-chain-enhancer of activated B cells transcription increases the expression of chemokines, cytokines, oxidases, and proteases. The transcription factor NF-κB is involved in the induction of innate immune genes (Ghosh and Hayden, 2008). Stimuli such as stress, drugs of abuse, peptides, chemokines, cytokines, reactive oxygen species (ROS), ultraviolet irradiation, bacteria, viruses, trauma, and other factors all increase NF-κB-DNA binding and transcription. Reactive oxygen species resulting from oxidases such as NADPH-oxidase or ethanol metabolism by CYP2E1 increase NF-κB transcription of $NOX2^{phox}$, a key NOX catalytic subunit (Cao et al., 2005) that produces ROS (Qin et al., 2008). Loops of activation also occur through induction of genes that stimulate further NF-κB activation leading to autocrine and paracrine amplification and persistent signals. Cytokines and chemokines, such as TNFα, IL1β, IL6, and MCP-1 as well as their receptors (TNFR in figure), are also induced resulting in amplification loops. Toll-like receptors are increased by ethanol (Dolganiuc et al., 2006; Alfonso-Loeches et al., 2010) as are other damage-associated molecular pattern receptors and there agonists resulting in the formation of positive activation loops (Garg et al., 2010). Toll-like receptors and HMGB1 interact to create another activation-amplification loop. Persistent and repeated activation occurs through positive cycles of activation. These loops spread innate immune signaling across the brain causing altered neurocircuitry and neurobiology. Figure abbreviations: CYP2E1, cytochrome P450 2E1; ECM, extracellular matrix; EtOH, ethanol; gp91, NADPH-oxidase flavocytochrome *b* components; HMGB1, high-mobility group box 1; IL-1β, interleukin 1 beta; IL1, interleukin-1; LPS, lipopolysaccharide; MMP, matrix metalloproteinase; MCP-1, monocyte chemoattractant protein-1; NOX, nicotinamide adenine dinucleotide phosphate (NADPH) oxidases; NF-κB, nuclear factor kappa-light-chain-enhancer of activated B cells; TACE, TNFα converting enzyme; TLR, toll-like receptor; TNFα, tissue necrosis factor-alpha; tPA, tissue plasminogen activator.

genes, including chemokine monocyte chemoattractant protein-1 (MCP-1, CCL2; He and Crews, 2008), proinflammatory cytokines [tumor necrosis factor-α (TNFα), Interleukin (IL)-1β, and IL-6], proinflammatory oxidases [iNOS (Zou and Crews, 2010), cyclooxygenase (COX; Knapp and Crews, 1999), and NOX (Qin et al., 2008)], and proteases (TACE and tPA; Zou and Crews, 2010). Similarly, stress increases the expression of NF-κB (Madrigal et al., 2001), cytokines, prostaglandin E2, and COX-2 levels (Madrigal et al., 2003) in the brain. In addition, chronic stress causes the reversal of acute glucocorticoid anti-inflammatory responses to proinflammatory NF-κB activation in the cortex (Munhoz et al., 2010). Similarly, all addictive drugs cause chronic elevations of basal glucocorticoids (Armario, 2010) that likely contribute to activation of brain NF-κB. Thus, activation of NF-κB by stress and drugs of abuse is a common molecular mechanism involving innate immune gene induction that is consistent with a stress-drug synergy culminating in progressive increases in loss of behavioral control and addiction.

Astrocytes and microglia show morphological changes in response to exposure to drugs of abuse. Using both *in vitro* and *in vivo* models through a series of elegant studies, Guerri and colleagues have established that chronic ethanol treatment induces astroglial activation and astrogliosis in the brain as indicated by marked upregulation of glial fibrillary acidic protein immunoreactivity along with hypertrophic astrocytes (Alfonso-Loeches et al., 2010). In addition to the altered astrocyte morphology, microglia also evidence increased expression of TLRs, which are both NF-κB target genes and activators of NF-κB transcription. Recently, TLR4 was discovered to contribute to persistent innate immune gene induction following ethanol exposure. Indeed, chronic ethanol exposure produces upregulation and activation of TLR4-glial NF-κB signaling that contributes to alcohol-induced neurodegeneration (Alfonso-Loeches et al., 2010). Similarly, acute ethanol exposure disrupts membrane lipid rafts thereby activating TLR4 signaling to NF-κB as well as increased expression of TLR4 (Blanco et al., 2008). Indomethacin, an anti-inflammatory drug, reduces chronic intermittent ethanol induction of brain innate immune genes (iNOS and COX-2) in astrocytes and reduces markers of cell death and behavioral dysfunction (Pascual et al., 2007). Innate immune activation resulting from oxidized phospholipids (Yang et al., 2010), and/or release of damage-associated molecular pattern danger sensing molecules such as high-mobility group box 1 (Garg et al., 2010), activate TLR and other signals that contribute to innate immune gene induction (Huang et al., 2010). Loops of NF-κB activation likely vary across individuals and exposure to specific addictive drugs. However, all addictive drugs activate NF-κB transcription across the development of addiction (Russo et al., 2009; Loftis et al., 2010). In an extensive series of studies, repeated bouts of moderate ethanol consumption and/or stress or innate immune activator exposure increased negative affect and anxiety in rats. The finding that the effects of ethanol and stress on brain function can be mimicked by injection of the chemokine MCP-1, the cytokine TNFα, or lipopolysaccharide (LPS), is consistent with the notion that stress and ethanol act through induction of innate immune genes to progressively increase negative affect (Breese et al., 2008). Thus, NF-κB transcription of innate immune genes in the brain occurs during exposure to ethanol and other addictive drugs as well as stress promoting vicious cycles of NF-κB induction of innate immune genes that culminate in changes to neurocircuitry and neurobiology.

In addition to alcohol, opiates are known to be addicting drugs, and endogenous opioid receptors and agonists clearly contribute to the neurobiology of addiction (Koob and Volkow, 2010). In contrast, opiate antagonists are used to treat both alcohol and opiate addiction. Interestingly, a potential mechanism of opiate antagonists appears to involve blockade of innate immune gene activation. Indeed, studies have found that opiate antagonists blunt LPS inherent immune responses (Liu et al., 2000b) and protect dopaminergic neurons via inhibition of microglial activation and reduced NOX formation of reactive oxygen species (Liu et al., 2000a; Qin et al., 2005). Other studies have demonstrated that opiate antagonists block TLR4 activation of innate immune transcription, which is a site of action in innate immune loops (Hutchinson et al., 2008, 2010). Thus, opiate antagonist therapy might exert some of its beneficial effects through blockade of innate immune gene induction. However, the progressive nature of innate immune gene induction and addictive behaviors suggest that therapeutic treatments aimed at reducing the induction of these genes would be more advantageous at preventing than reversing addiction.

INNATE IMMUNE ACTIVATION IS INVOLVED IN ETHANOL DRINKING, DEPRESSION-LIKE BEHAVIOR, AND ADDICTION

Numerous studies have investigated the neurobiological consequences of addiction. Our laboratory demonstrated that MCP-1 (CCL2), a key chemokine induced by chronic ethanol treatment in mice known to regulate ethanol consumptive behavior, is upregulated in post-mortem human alcoholic brains (see **Figure 2**). Neuroanatomical assessment of MCP-1 protein levels as well as

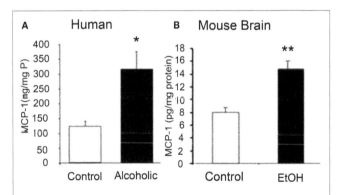

FIGURE 2 | Comparisons of increased levels of CCL2 in post-mortem human alcoholic brain and mouse brain following chronic ethanol treatment. Shown is data from different studies within our laboratory illustrating increased levels of the chemokine MCP-1 (CCL2) in humans and mice following ethanol exposure. **(A)** MCP-1 protein levels from human hippocampal homogenate measured using ELISA. Increased MCP-1 levels were also found in ventral tegmental area, substantia nigra, and amygdala (see He and Crews, 2008). **(B)** Levels of MCP-1 in mouse brain increased following chronic ethanol treatment. Mice (C57Bl/6) treated with 10 daily doses of ethanol (5.0 g/kg. i.g.) and brain MCP-1 levels were determined 24 h after the last ethanol administration (see Qin et al., 2008 for details). These studies indicate that ethanol upregulates the innate immune chemokine MCP-1 in post-mortem human alcoholic and mouse brain samples, which is consistent with ethanol activation of innate immune genes.

histological assessment of microglia from alcoholic human brains indicate increased levels in the ventral tegmental area, substantia nigra, hippocampus, and amygdala relative to healthy control subjects (He and Crews, 2008). In another post-mortem human alcoholic brain study, Okvist et al. (2007) reported increased NF-κB nuclear binding of p50 subunits with 479 NF-κB driven genes being generally upregulated in the frontal cortex, but not motor cortex. In addition, a human gene expression analysis conducted on post-mortem tissue (Liu et al., 2006) revealed altered expression of a group of cell adhesion genes that is consistent with altered extracellular membrane components and innate immune activation. Thus, studies of human alcoholic brain are consistent with the hypothesis that drug addiction activates brain innate immune gene expression.

The induction of innate immune gene expression is known to alter behavior. Perhaps the most serious consequence of cancer treatment with proinflammatory interferon and interleukin is the development of severe depression that requires treatment with anti-depressant medication (O'Connor et al., 2007). Several other studies have linked negative affect and depression to innate immune activation (see e.g., Kelley and Dantzer, 2011). For instance, bacterial endotoxin induces sickness behavior and negative affect across multiple species. Indeed, Eisenberger et al. (2010) recently demonstrated that infusions of LPS into healthy humans reduced reward responses and increased depressed mood. Similarly, cycles of drug abuse, stress, and other environmental changes amplify anxiety and negative affect. Interestingly, animal studies determining the genetic basis of behavior find that innate immune genes increase alcohol drinking behavior. For example, gene expression studies of genetically paired rats and mice that differ primarily in their preference for ethanol consumption find that NF-κB, its regulatory proteins, and many innate immune genes are central to high ethanol drinking behaviors (Mulligan et al., 2006). Furthermore, beta-2 microglobulin (β2M), which is a NF-κB target gene involved in MHC immune signaling (Pahl, 1999) evidenced the largest increase in high ethanol preferring brain transcriptomes (Mulligan et al., 2006). In addition, work from Blednov et al. (2005, 2011b) have provided interesting and novel data supporting the hypothesis that innate immune genes regulate ethanol drinking behavior. Across multiple strains of transgenic mice with innate immune gene deletion, these animals universally drink significantly less ethanol than matched controls across multiple ethanol drinking paradigms. Recently, Blednov et al. (2011a) discovered that innate immune activation through LPS can cause long-lasting increases in ethanol drinking. Indeed, strains of mice show varied innate immune responses to LPS that correspond to increases in the consumption of ethanol. Furthermore, a single injection of LPS is capable of producing a delayed, but long-lasting increase in ethanol consumption even in strains of high drinking mice. Similarly, a single LPS treatment induces persistent increases in brain innate immune gene expression (Qin et al., 2007). Taken together, these findings are consistent with genetic regulation of brain innate immune gene expression contributing to risk for alcoholism, alcohol drinking (both preference and quantity), and behavioral sensitivity to alcohol across multiple species.

A significant body of evidence supports the hypothesis that innate immune gene induction in the brain results in negative affect and depression-like behavior (Raison et al., 2009). Patients with major depressive disorder evidence increased blood inflammatory markers, and anti-depressant therapy is associated with a reduction of these markers. In addition to increased innate immune gene expression, human depression involves structural changes in the hippocampus as multiple studies have demonstrated decreased hippocampal volume in patients with depression (see e.g., Videbech and Ravnkilde, 2004). These findings are consistent with depression-associated diminution of hippocampal neurogenesis and anti-depressant-induced increases in neurogenesis, hippocampal volume in humans, and reversal of depressive symptomology (Dranovsky and Hen, 2006). The reductions of adult hippocampal neurogenesis may underlie depression and provide an index of mood and negative affect that allow for molecular studies. Indeed, both alcoholism and depression may be mediated by changes in adult hippocampal neurogenesis (Crews and Nixon, 2003; Koo et al., 2011). Similarly, stress, multiple addictive drugs, and other factors that precipitate depression also reduce neurogenesis (Tanapat et al., 2001; Malberg and Duman, 2003; Gregus et al., 2005). Many of the factors that reduce neurogenesis also increase depression-like behaviors (Johnson et al., 2006; see **Figure 3**). Recent research has revealed that activation of NF-κB is necessary for stress-induced inhibition of neurogenesis and induction of depression-like behaviors (Koo and Duman, 2008), such as the social defeat model of depression (Christoffel et al., 2011). In addition, anti-depressant efficacy in rodent behavioral models is dependent upon hippocampal neurogenesis (Santarelli et al., 2003). In animal studies, endotoxin-induced increases in innate immune genes reduce neurogenesis and increase depression-like behavior (Kelley and Dantzer, 2011). Immune activation includes induction of microglial tryptophan metabolism that could reduce serotonin thereby contributing to depression (Kelley and Dantzer, 2011). TLRs are necessary components of both ethanol neurotoxicity (Alfonso-Loeches et al., 2010) and innate immune-induced depressive behavior and reduction of neurogenesis (Kelley and Dantzer, 2011). We have found that chronic ethanol increases brain innate immune genes, reduces brain neurogenesis, and increases depression-like behavior. In addition, mice self-administering ethanol in a chronic heavy drinking model evidenced depression-like behavior during abstinence that was associated with reduced neurogenesis (Stevenson et al., 2009). Ethanol-induced loss of neurogenesis parallels the onset of depression-like behavior, which is reversed via anti-depressant treatment. Similarly, stress-induced IL-1β reduces neurogenesis causing depression-like behaviors (Koo and Duman, 2008). Inhibition of neurogenesis is also associated with negative affect and depression, which are key elements in the neurobiology of addiction. Thus, neurogenesis reflects mood, with reduced neurogenesis associated with innate immune gene induction, drug-induced negative affect, and depression-like behavior.

Innate immune gene activation in the brain persists for long periods (Qin et al., 2007, 2008), consistent with the persistence of addiction. This persistent nature is likely amplified in the adolescent brain (Spear, 2000) because of their increased ethanol consumption (Silveri and Spear, 1998) and greater vulnerability to the neurotoxic effects of alcohol (Monti et al., 2005; Crews et al., 2007). As such, chronic intermittent ethanol exposure during adolescence increases COX-2 and iNOS expression as well as apoptotic cell death in the neocortex and hippocampus (see **Figure 4**). Importantly, and relevant to the potential involvement of innate immune

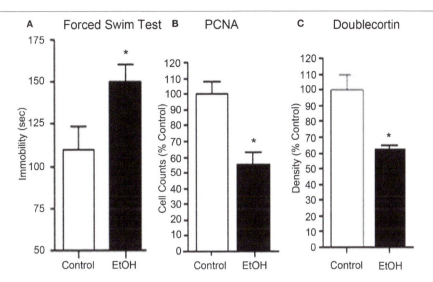

FIGURE 3 | Chronic ethanol self-administration induces depression-like behavior and inhibits hippocampal neurogenesis. C57BL/6J mice self-administered either ethanol (10% v/v) or water for 28 days. **(A)** Abstinence-induced increase in immobility (seconds) on the forced swim test provides an index of depression-like behavior. Abstinence from chronic ethanol consumption resulted in increased negative affect. **(B)** Ethanol self-administration decreased PCNA, a marker of cell proliferation, in the neurogenic region of the hippocampal dentate gyrus. **(C)** Ethanol self-administration decreased doublecortin expression, a marker of neurogenesis, in the dentate gyrus. Reduced progenitor cell proliferation and neurogenesis is associated with increased depression-like behavior. Furthermore, these studies are consistent with the research suggesting that decreased hippocampal neurogenesis is linked to depression. Finally, desipramine treatment, an anti-depressant, reversed both the reduced hippocampal neurogenesis and the depression-like behavior in abstinent mice (see Stevenson et al., 2009).

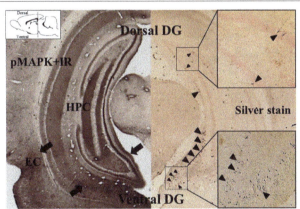

pMAPK+IR and Silver stain following 4 day EtOH binge

FIGURE 4 | Ventral hippocampus shows greater activation (pMAPK + IR) and neurotoxicity (Silver stain) following binge ethanol treatment. Coronal sections of rats exposed to a 4-day binge ethanol model are shown [approximately −5.80 mm from bregma, adapted from Crews et. al. (2006a; The position of the coronal histological sections are depicted in the sagittal diagram in the upper left corner. The histological coronal sections show both dorsal (upper) and ventral (lower) dentate gyrus of hippocampus)]. Left: Mitogen-activated protein kinase (MAPK) is a family of kinases activated by phosphorylation. Phosphorylated MAPK (pMAPK) provides an index of kinase activation. Note the lower-ventral dentate gyrus, hippocampus, and entorhinal cortex (indicated by black arrows) contains more pMAPK + IR than the upper-dorsal sections consistent with greater activation of ventral hippocampus. Right: Silver stain identifies dying neurons (see Crews et. al., 2006a). Note that the ventral hippocampus contains many more silver stained neurons (black arrowheads) compared to the ventral hippocampus. Boxes on the right show higher magnification of silver stained dorsal and ventral hippocampus. These findings are consistent with ethanol causing greater emotional ventral hippocampus activation (pMAPK + IR) and cell death (silver stain).

gene induction in adolescent binge drinking, administration of indomethacin attenuates the behavioral dysfunction associated with adolescent intermittent ethanol in early adulthood (Pascual et al., 2007).

Maturation of the frontal cortex during adolescence is paralleled by the development of behavioral control (Ernst et al., 2009). Adolescence is a recognized risk period for the initiation of drug experimentation and addiction due to the vulnerability of the developing frontal cortex (Crews et al., 2007). Other studies have suggested that genetic factors linked to a hyperglutamatergic state might contribute to alcoholism (Spanagel et al., 2005) and ethanol-induced NF-κB activation to increased extracellular glutamate (Ward et al., 2009). Innate immune gene induction results in hyperexcitability in the spinal cord related to neuropathic pain (Graeber, 2010) and in the hippocampus related to seizures (Maroso et al., 2010). Similarly, hyperexcitability in the frontal cortex results in loss of cognitive flexibility creating addiction-like behavior (Gruber et al., 2010). In elegant studies by Kaliva and colleagues have established that cocaine and stimulant addiction are related to a hyperglutamatergic states due to alterations of the cortical glutamate transporters (Reissner and Kalivas, 2010). Studies of both human cocaine and alcohol addicts have revealed dysfunctional decision making on tasks involving delayed reward for more value and reversal learning tasks that probe cognitive flexibility and frontal lobe function (Bechara et al., 2002). Thus, frontal–cortical hyperexcitability due to innate immune gene induction likely contributes to the neurobiology of addiction.

Frontal–cortical dysfunction is often investigated using reversal learning tasks. During reversal learning, expected outcomes are incorrect requiring flexible behavior in response to outcomes that do not match those predicted by the preceding cues (Stalnaker

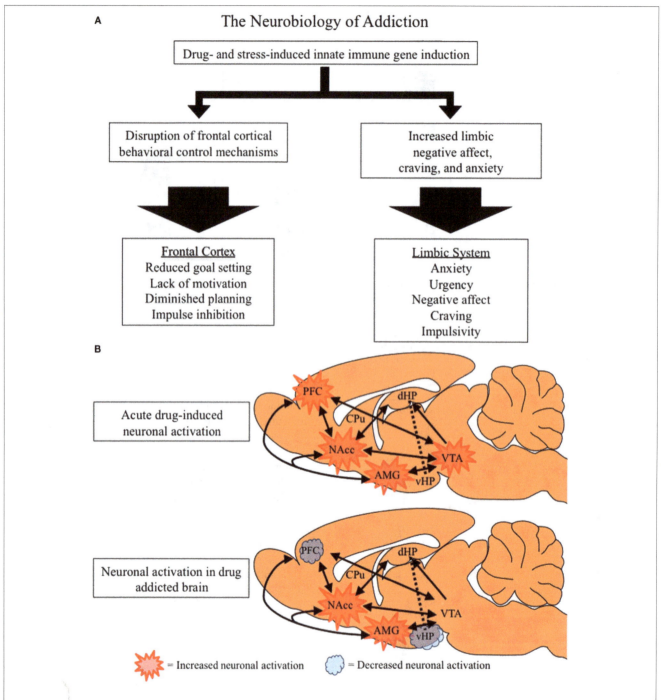

FIGURE 5 | The neurobiology of addiction. (A) Flow chart distinguishing the frontal–cortical and limbic changes associated with drug addiction. Both stress and drug abuse activate innate immune gene expression, which increases limbic activation and disrupts frontal–cortical function. **(B)** A simplified schematic of the frontal–cortical and limbic circuitry that contributes to addictive behavior. Depicted is a rat brain with internal structures highlighted and accompanying projections (as indicated by black arrows). The frontal–cortical areas include the medial prefrontal, anterior cingulate, and orbitofrontal cortices, and are involved in attention, goal setting, planning, and impulse control (Schoenbaum et al., 2006; Schoenbaum and Shaham, 2008). The limbic circuitry, comprising the nucleus accumbens (NAcc), amygdala (AMG), hippocampus (HPC), and ventral tegmental area (VTA), is involved in emotion, learning, and memory. Acute drug abuse activates frontal–cortical attention mechanisms, prompting limbic learning. Similarly, innate immune gene induction in the brain leads to PFC hyperexcitability (Zou and Crews 2005; Crews et al., 2006a) that inactivates frontal–cortical regulation of limbic structures (Gruber et al., 2010). Innate immune gene induction in limbic regions increases negative affect and depression-like behaviors prompting further drug abuse and self-medication. The harmful consequences of prolonged alcohol, opiate and stimulant drug dependence result in diminished activation of frontal–cortical circuits leading to a loss of attention and poor decision combined with increasing urgency and negative affect motivating persistent drug taking behaviors. Decreased ventral hippocampal activation likely contributes to frontal hyperexcitability and loss of cognitive flexibility (Gruber et al., 2010). Thus, an inactivated PFC, loss of behavioral flexibility, and increasing limbic negative emotion characterizes the drug-addicted brain.

et al., 2009). In behavioral studies, this learning paradigm mimics the inability of drug addicted individuals to learn new healthy behaviors. Thus, proper frontal cortex function is needed to weigh the value of decisions and is important when new learning and/or behavior is necessary. Our laboratory found that models of binge ethanol drinking induces persistent deficits in reversal learning in rats (Obernier et al., 2002) and in adult mice following a model of adolescent binge drinking (Coleman et al., 2011). Other studies have demonstrated that rats with previous experience, either with self-administration of cocaine or with passive cocaine injections, are abnormally slow to learn reversals even though they learn initial contingencies at a normal rate (Schoenbaum et al., 2004; Calu et al., 2007). Furthermore, lesion of the frontal cortex produce reversal learning deficits similar in nature to chronic drug abuse-induced deficits (Schoenbaum et al., 2006). In addition, frontal cortex dysfunction results in perseveration and repetition of previously learned behaviors due to failure to associate new information (e.g., negative consequences) into decision making. Thus, innate immune gene induction disrupts frontal–cortical functions leading to loss of behavioral control. Similarly, limbic negative affect is promoted by innate immune gene induction. Together, the loss of behavioral control and increased limbic drive due to innate immune gene induction is consistent with innate immune gene induction culminating in the neurobiology of addiction.

CONCLUSION

The neurobiology of addiction is complex (see **Figure 5**) and high rates of co-morbid depression psychopathology suggest common overlapping molecular changes in the brain (Grant and Dawson, 1998). Drug-induced induction of brain innate immune genes was initially thought to reflect drug-induced neurodegeneration. However, more recent studies suggest that increased glutamate hyperexcitability in the frontal cortex occurs as well as increased sensitivity to excitotoxicity. Recent research supports a role for innate immune gene induction in altered neurotransmission and neurocircuitry that contribute to the dysfunctional behaviors associated with addiction. Indeed, increased innate immune gene expression in increasingly associated with the molecular mechanisms underlying negative affect, anxiety, and depression that are known to increase in the addicted brain. The recent discovery that chronic glucocorticoids, elevated by stress and/or drug abuse, promote NF-κB proinflammatory transcription in the frontal cortex support a common molecular mechanism of drug abuse and stress promoting common changes in neurobiology that parallel the progressive and persistent psychopathology of addiction. Increased innate immune gene expression in post-mortem brain tissue of addicted individuals' mimic findings in pre-clinical studies of drug- and stress-induced activation of brain NF-κB transcription and the prolonged psychopathology of chronic addiction. Stimuli that activate brain innate immune gene expression independent of any addictive drug experience promote addiction-like behaviors and increase drug consumption. Human genetic studies on alcohol dependence have also found innate immune gene polymorphisms that are associated with risk for alcoholism. A promising recent discovery that anti-opiate drugs used to treat addiction also disrupt innate immune gene induction suggests new and unanticipated mechanisms of action. Taken together, these findings support innate immune gene induction as a key mechanism causing addiction. This new mechanism includes many new and novel targets for addiction, depression, and other psychopathology. It is hoped that the discoveries of the role of innate immune genes in addiction will lead to improved prevention and/or therapy for addiction.

ACKNOWLEDGMENTS

The Authors wish to acknowledge support from the Bowles Center for Alcohol Studies, School of Medicine, University of North Carolina and the National Institutes of Health, National Institute on Alcoholism and Alcohol Abuse, AA020023, AA020024, AA020022, AA019767, AA11605, and AA007573.

REFERENCES

Alfonso-Loeches, S., Pascual-Lucas, M., Blanco, A. M., Sanchez-Vera, I., and Guerri, C. (2010). Pivotal role of TLR4 receptors in alcohol-induced neuroinflammation and brain damage. *J. Neurosci.* 30, 8285–8295.

Andersen, S. L., and Teicher, M. H. (2004). Delayed effects of early stress on hippocampal development. *Neuropsychopharmacology* 29, 1988–1993.

Andersen, S. L., Thompson, A. T., Rutstein, M., Hostetter, J. C., and Teicher, M. H. (2000). Dopamine receptor pruning in prefrontal cortex during the periadolescent period in rats. *Synapse* 37, 167–169.

Andrucci, G. L., Archer, R. P., Pancoast, D. L., and Gordon, R. A. (1989). The relationship of MMPI and sensation seeking scales to adolescent drug use. *J. Pers. Assess.* 53, 253–266.

Armario, A. (2010). Activation of the hypothalamic–pituitary–adrenal axis by addictive drugs: different pathways, common outcome. *Trends Pharmacol. Sci.* 31, 318–325.

Baumrind, D. (1987). "A developmental perspective on adolescent risk taking in contemporary America," in *Adolescent Social Behavior and Health*, ed. C. E. Irwin Jr. (San Francisco, CA: Jossey-Bass), 93–125.

Bechara, A., Dolan, S., and Hindes, A. (2002). Decision-making and addiction (part II): myopia for the future or hypersensitivity to reward? *Neuropsychologia* 40, 1690–1705.

Blakemore, S. J., and Choudhury, S. (2006). Development of the adolescent brain: implications for executive function and social cognition. *J. Child Psychol. Psychiatry* 47, 296–312.

Blanco, A. M., Perez-Arago, A., Fernandez-Lizarbe, S., and Guerri, C. (2008). Ethanol mimics ligand-mediated activation and endocytosis of IL-1RI/TLR4 receptors via lipid rafts caveolae in astroglial cells. *J. Neurochem.* 106, 625–639.

Blednov, Y. A., Benavidez, J. M., Geil, C., Perra, S., Morikawa, H., and Harris, R. A. (2011a). Activation of neuroinflammatory signaling by lipopolysaccharide produces a prolonged increase of voluntary alcohol intake in mice. *Brain Behav. Immun.* doi: 10.1016/j.bbi.2011.01.008. [Epub ahead of print].

Blednov, Y. A., Ponomarev, I., Geil, C., Bergeson, S., Koob, G. F., and Harris, R. A. (2011b). Neuroimmune regulation of alcohol consumption: behavioral validation of genes obtained from genomic studies. *Addict. Biol.* doi: 10.1111/j.1369-1600.2010.00284.x. [Epub ahead of print].

Blednov, Y. A., Bergeson, S. E., Walker, D., Ferreira, V. M., Kuziel, W. A., and Harris, R. A. (2005). Perturbation of chemokine networks by gene deletion alters the reinforcing actions of ethanol. *Behav. Brain Res.* 165, 110–125.

Breese, G. R., Knapp, D. J., Overstreet, D. H., Navarro, M., Wills, T. A., and Angel, R. A. (2008). Repeated lipopolysaccharide (LPS) or cytokine treatments sensitize ethanol withdrawal-induced anxiety-like behavior. *Neuropsychopharmacology* 33, 867–876.

Calu, D. J., Roesch, M. R., Stalnaker, T. A., and, Schoenbaum, G. (2007). Associative encoding in posterior piriform cortex during odor discrimination and reversal learning. *Cereb. Cortex* 17, 1342–1349.

Cao, Q., Mak, K. M., and Lieber, C. S. (2005). Cytochrome P4502E1 primes macrophages to increase TNF-alpha production in response to lipopolysaccharide.

Am. J. Physiol. Gastrointest. Liver Physiol. 289, G95–G107.

Casey, B. J., Trainor, R. J., Orendi, J. L., Schubert, A. B., Nystrom, L. E., Giedd, J. N., Castellanos, F. X., Haxby, J. V., Noll, D. C., Cohen, J. D., Forman, S. D., Dahl, R. E., and Rapoport, J. L. (1997). A developmental functional MRI study of prefrontal activation during performance of a go–no-go task. J. Cogn. Neurosci. 9, 835–847.

Choi, S., and Kellogg, C. K. (1992). Norepinephrine utilization in the hypothalamus of the male rat during adolescent development. Dev. Neurosci. 14, 369–376.

Choi, S., Weisberg, S. N., and Kellogg, C. K. (1997). Control of endogenous norepinephrine release in the hypothalamus of male rats changes over adolescent development. Brain Res. Dev. Brain Res. 98, 134–141.

Christoffel, D. J., Golden, S. A., Dumitriu, D., Robinson, A. J., Janssen, W. G., Ahn, H. F., Krishnan, V., Reyes, C. M., Han, M. H., Ables, J. L., Eisch, A. J., Dietz, D. M., Ferguson, D., Neve, R. L., Greengard, P., Kim, Y., Morrison, J. H., and Russo, S. J. (2011). IkB kinase regulates social defeat stress-induced synaptic and behavioral plasticity. J. Neurosci. 31, 314–321.

Coleman, L., Jun, H., Joohwi, L., Styner, M., and Crews, F. T. (2011). Adolescent binge drinking alters adult brain neurotransmitter gene expression, behavior, brain regional volumes, and neurochemistry in mice. Alcohol. Clin. Exp. Res. 35, 671–688.

Crews, F. T., He, J., and Hodge, C. (2007). Adolescent cortical development: a critical period of vulnerability for addiction. Pharmacol. Biochem. Behav. 86, 189–199.

Crews, F. T., Mdzinarishvili, A., Kim, D., He, J., and Nixon, K. (2006a). Neurogenesis in adolescent brain is potently inhibited by ethanol. Neuroscience 137, 437–445.

Crews, F. T., Nixon, K., Kim, D., Joseph, J., Shukitt-Hale, B., Qin, L., and Zou, J. (2006b). BHT blocks NF-kappaB activation and ethanol-induced brain damage. Alcohol. Clin. Exp. Res. 30, 1938–1949.

Crews, F. T., and Nixon, K. (2003). Alcohol, neural stem cells, and adult neurogenesis. Alcohol Res. Health 27, 197–204.

De Bellis, M. D., Narasimhan, A., Thatcher, D. L., Keshavan, M. S., Soloff, P., and Clark, D. B. (2005). Prefrontal cortex, thalamus, and cerebellar volumes in adolescents and young adults with adolescent-onset alcohol use disorders and comorbid mental disorders. Alcohol. Clin. Exp. Res. 29, 1590–1600.

Dolganiuc, A., Bakis, G., Kodys, K., Mandrekar, P., and Szabo, G. (2006). Acute ethanol treatment modulates toll-like receptor-4 association with lipid rafts. Alcohol. Clin. Exp. Res. 30, 76–85.

Dranovsky, A., and Hen, R. (2006). Hippocampal neurogenesis: regulation by stress and antidepressants. Biol. Psychiatry 59, 1136–1143.

Duka, T., Gentry, J., Malcolm, R., Ripley, T. L., Borlikova, G., Stephens, D. N., Veatch, L. M., Becker, H. C., and Crews, F. T. (2004). Consequences of multiple withdrawals from alcohol. Alcohol. Clin. Exp. Res. 28, 233–246.

Eisenberger, N. I., Berkman, E. T., Inagaki, T. K., Rameson, L. T., Mashal, N. M., and Irwin, M. R. (2010). Inflammation-induced anhedonia: endotoxin reduces ventral striatum responses to reward. Biol. Psychiatry 68, 748–754.

Ernst, M., Romeo, R. D., and Andersen, S. L. (2009). Neurobiology of the development of motivated behaviors in adolescence: a window into a neural systems model. Pharmacol. Biochem. Behav. 93, 199–211.

Faden, V. B. (2006). Trends in initiation of alcohol use in the United States 1975 to 2003. Alcohol. Clin. Exp. Res. 30, 1011–1022.

Fagen, R. M. (1976). "Exercise, play, and physical training in animals," in Perspectives in Ethology, Vol. 2, eds P. P. G. Bateson and P. M. Klopfer (New York, NY: Plenum Press), 189–219.

Galef, B. G. Jr. (1977). "Mechanisms for the social transmission of food preferences from adult to weanling rats," in Learning Mechanisms in Food Selection, eds. L. M. Barker, M. Best, and M. Domjan (Waco, TX: Baylor University Press), 123–148.

Garg, A. D., Nowis, D., Golab, J., Vandenabeele, P., Krysko, D. V., and Agostinis, P. (2010). Immunogenic cell death, DAMPs, and anticancer therapeutics: an emerging amalgamation. Biochim. Biophys. Acta 1805, 53–71.

Ghosh, S., and Hayden, M. S. (2008). New regulators of NF-kappaB in inflammation. Nat. Rev. Immunol. 8, 837–848.

Giedd, J. N. (2004). Structural magnetic resonance imaging of the adolescent brain. Ann. N. Y. Acad. Sci. 1021, 77–85.

Giedd, J. N., Blumenthal, J., Jeffries, N. O., Castellanos, F. X., Liu, H., Zijdenbos, A., Paus, T., Evans, A. C., and Rapoport, J. L. (1999). Brain development during childhood and adolescence: a longitudinal MRI study. Nat. Neurosci. 2, 861–863.

Gould, E., Woolf, N. J., and Butcher, L. L. (1991). Postnatal development of cholinergic neurons in the rat: I. Forebrain. Brain Res. Bull. 27, 767–789.

Graeber, M. B. (2010). Changing face of microglia. Science 330, 783–788.

Grant, B. F., and Dawson, D. A. (1998). Age of onset of drug use and its association with DSM-IV drug abuse and dependence: results from the National Longitudinal Alcohol Epidemiologic Survey. J. Subst. Abuse 10, 163–173.

Gregus, A., Wintink, A. J., Davis, A. C., and Kalynchuk, L. E. (2005). Effect of repeated corticosterone injections and restraint stress on anxiety and depression-like behavior in male rats. Behav. Brain Res. 156, 105–114.

Gruber, A. J., Calhoun, Gwendolyn, G., Shusterman, I., Schoenbaum, G., Roesch, M. R., and O'Donnell, P. (2010). More is less: a disinhibited prefrontal cortex impairs cognitive flexibility. J. Neurosci. 30, 17102–17110.

He, J., and Crews, F. T. (2007). Neurogenesis decreases during brain maturation from adolescence to adulthood. Pharmacol. Biochem. Behav. 86, 327–333.

He, J., and Crews, F. T. (2008). Increased MCP-1 and microglia in various regions of the human alcoholic brain. Exp. Neurol. 210, 349–358.

Huang, W., Tang, Y., and Li, L. (2010). HMGB1, a potent proinflammatory cytokine in sepsis. Cytokine 51, 119–126.

Hutchinson, M. R., Zhang, Y., Brown, K., Coats, B. D., Shridhar, M., Sholar, P. W., Patel, S. J., Crysdale, N. Y., Harrison, J. A., Maier, S. F., Rice, K. C., and Watkins, L. R. (2008). Non-stereoselective reversal of neuropathic pain by naloxone and naltrexone: involvement of toll-like receptor 4 (TLR4). Eur. J. Neurosci. 28, 20–29.

Hutchinson, M. R., Zhang, Y., Shridhar, M., Evans, J. H., Buchanan, M. M., Zhao, T. X., Slivka, P. F., Coats, B. D., Rezvani, N., Wieseler, J., Hughes, T. S., Landgraf, K. E., Chan, S., Fong, S., Phipps, S., Falke, J. J., Leinwand, L. A., Maier, S. F., Yin, H., Rice, K. C., and Watkins, L. R. (2010). Evidence that opioids may have toll-like receptor 4 and MD-2 effects. Brain Behav. Immun. 24, 83–95.

Huttenlocher, P. R. (1984). Synapse elimination and plasticity in developing human cerebral cortex. Am. J. Ment. Defic. 88, 488–496.

Jentsch, J. D., and Taylor, J. R. (1999). Impulsivity resulting from frontostriatal dysfunction in drug abuse: implications for the control of behavior by reward-related stimuli. Psychopharmacology (Berl.) 146, 373–390.

Johnson, S. A., Fournier, N. M., and Kalynchuk, L. E. (2006). Effect of different doses of corticosterone on depression-like behavior and HPA axis responses to a novel stressor. Behav. Brain Res. 168, 280–288.

Kalsbeek, A., Voorn, P., Buijs, R. M., Pool, C. W., and Uylings, H. B. (1988). Development of the dopaminergic innervation in the prefrontal cortex of the rat. J. Comp. Neurol. 269, 58–72.

Kelley, K. W., and Dantzer, R. (2011). Alcoholism and inflammation: neuroimmunology of behavioral and mood disorders. Brain Behav. Immun. doi: 10.1016/j.bbi.2010.12.013. [Epub ahead of print].

Kellogg, C. K., Awatramani, G. B., and Piekut, D. T. (1998). Adolescent development alters stressor-induced Fos immunoreactivity in rat brain. Neuroscience 83, 681–689.

Kempermann, G. (2002). Why new neurons? Possible functions for adult hippocampal neurogenesis. J. Neurosci. 22, 635–638.

Knapp, D. J., and Crews, F. T. (1999). Induction of cyclooxygenase-2 in brain during acute and chronic ethanol treatment and ethanol withdrawal. Alcohol. Clin. Exp. Res. 23, 633–643.

Koo, J. W., and Duman, R. S. (2008). IL-1beta is an essential mediator of the antineurogenic and anhedonic effects of stress. Proc. Natl. Acad. Sci. U.S.A. 105, 751–756.

Koo, J. W., Russo, S. J., Ferguson, D., Nestler, E. J., and Duman, R. S. (2011). Nuclear factor-kappa B is a critical mediator of stress-impaired neurogenesis and depressive behavior. Proc. Natl. Acad. Sci. U.S.A. 107, 2669–2674.

Koob, G. F., and Volkow, N. D. (2010). Neurocircuitry of addiction. Neuropsychopharmacology 35, 217–238.

Kostovic, I. (1990). Structural and histochemical reorganization of the human prefrontal cortex during perinatal and postnatal life. Prog. Brain Res. 85, 223–240.

Liu, B., Du, L., and Hong, J. S. (2000a). Naloxone protects rat dopaminergic neurons against inflammatory damage through inhibition of microglia activation and superoxide generation. J. Pharmacol. Exp. Ther. 293, 607–617.

Liu, B., Jiang, J. W., Wilson, B. C., Du, L., Yang, S. N., Wang, J. Y., Wu, G. C., Cao, X. D., and Hong, J. S. (2000b). Systemic infusion of naloxone reduces degeneration of rat substantia nigral dopaminergic neurons induced by intranigral injection of lipopolysaccharide. J. Pharmacol. Exp. Ther. 295, 125–132.

Liu, J., Lewohl, J. M., Harris, R. A., Iyer, V. R., Dodd, P. R., Randall, P. K., and Mayfield, R. D. (2006). Patterns of gene expression in the frontal cortex discriminate alcoholic from nonalcoholic individuals. *Neuropsychopharmacology* 31, 1574–1582.

Loftis, J. M., Choi, D., Hoffman, W., and Huckans, M. S. (2010). Methamphetamine causes persistent immune dysregulation: a cross-species, translational report. *Neurotox. Res.* doi: 10.1007/s12640-010-9223-x. [Epub ahead of print].

Madrigal, B., Puebla, P., Caballero, E., Pelaez, R., Gravalos, D. G., and Medarde, M. (2001). Synthesis of imidazo[4,5-d]oxazolo[3,4-a]pyridines. New heterocyclic analogues of lignans. *Arch. Pharm. (Weinheim)* 334, 177–179.

Madrigal, J. L., Garcia-Bueno, B., Moro, M. A., Lizasoain, I., Lorenzo, P., and Leza, J. C. (2003). Relationship between cyclooxygenase-2 and nitric oxide synthase-2 in rat cortex after stress. *Eur. J. Neurosci.* 18, 1701–1705.

Malberg, J. E., and Duman, R. S. (2003). Cell proliferation in adult hippocampus is decreased by inescapable stress: reversal by fluoxetine treatment. *Neuropsychopharmacology* 28, 1562–1571.

Malberg, J. E., Eisch, A. J., Nestler, E. J., and Duman, R. S. (2000). Chronic antidepressant treatment increases neurogenesis in adult rat hippocampus. *J. Neurosci.* 20, 9104–9110.

Maroso, M., Balosso, S., Ravizza, T., Liu, J., Aronica, E., Iyer, A. M., Rossetti, C., Moteni, M., Casalgrandi, M., Manfredi, A. A., Bianchi, M. E., and Vezzani, A. (2010). Toll-like receptor 4 and high-mobility group box-1 are involved in ictogenesis and can be targeted to reduce seizures. *Nat. Med.* 16, 413–419.

Monti, P. M., Miranda, R. Jr., Nixon, K., Sher, K. J., Swartzwelder, H. S., Tapert, S. F., White, A., and Crews, F. T. (2005). Adolescence: booze, brains, and behavior. *Alcohol. Clin. Exp. Res.* 29, 207–220.

Mulligan, M. K., Ponomarev, I., Hitzemann, R. J., Belknap, J. K., Tabakoff, B., Harris, R. A., Crabbe, J. C., Blednov, Y. A., Grahame, N. J., Phillips, T. J., Finn, D. A., Hoffman, P. L., Iyer, V. R., Koob, G. F., and Bergeson, S. E. (2006). Toward understanding the genetics of alcohol drinking through transcriptome meta-analysis. *Proc. Natl. Acad. Sci. U.S.A.* 103, 6368–6373.

Munhoz, C. D., Sorrells, S. F., Caso, J. R., Scavone, C., and Sapolsky, R. M. (2010). Glucocorticoids exacerbate lipopolysaccharide-induced signaling in the frontal cortex and hippocampus in a dose-dependent manner. *J. Neurosci.* 30, 13690–13698.

Obernier, J. A., White, A. M., Swartzwelder, H. S., and Crews, F. T. (2002). Cognitive deficits and CNS damage after a 4-day binge ethanol exposure in rats. *Pharmacol. Biochem. Behav.* 72, 521–532.

O'Connor, M. F., Irwin, M. R., Seldon, J., Kwan, L., and Ganz, P. A. (2007). Pro-inflammatory cytokines and depression in a familial cancer registry. *Psychooncology* 16, 499–501.

Okvist, A., Johansson, S., Kuzmin, A., Bazov, I., Merino-Martinez, R., Ponomarev, I., Mayfield, R. D., Harris, R. A., Sheedy, D., Garrick, T., Harper, C., Hurd, Y. L., Terenius, L., Ekstrom, T. J., Bakalkin, G., and Yakovleva, T. (2007). Neuroadaptations in human chronic alcoholics: dysregulation of the NF-kappaB system. *PLoS ONE* 2, e930. doi: 10.1371/journal.pone.0000930

Pahl, H. L. (1999). Activators and target genes of Rel/NF-kappaB transcription factors. *Oncogene* 18, 6853–6866.

Pascual, M., Blanco, A. M., Cauli, O., Minarro, J., and Guerri, C. (2007). Intermittent ethanol exposure induces inflammatory brain damage and causes long-term behavioural alterations in adolescent rats. *Eur. J. Neurosci.* 25, 541–550.

Pascual, M., Boix, J., Felipo, V., and Guerri, C. (2009). Repeated alcohol administration during adolescence causes changes in the mesolimbic dopaminergic and glutamatergic systems and promotes alcohol intake in the adult rat. *J. Neurochem.* 108, 920–931.

Peleg-Oren, N., Saint-Jean, G., Cardenas, G. A., Tammara, H., and Pierre, C. (2009). Drinking alcohol before age 13 and negative outcomes in late adolescence. *Alcohol. Clin. Exp. Res.* 3, 1966–1972.

Qin, L., Block, M. L., Liu, Y., Bienstock, R. J., Pei, Z., Zhang, W., Wu, X., Wilson, B., Burka, T., and Hong, J. (2005). Microglial NADPH oxidase is a novel target for femtomolar neuroprotection against oxidative stress. *FASEB J.* 19, 550–557.

Qin, L., He, J., Hanes, R. N., Pluzarev, O., Hong, J. S., and Crews, F. T. (2008). Increased systemic and brain cytokine production and neuroinflammation by endotoxin following ethanol treatment. *J. Neuroinflammation* 5, 10.

Qin, L., Wu, X., Block, M. L., Liu, Y., Breese, G. R., Hong, J. S., Knapp, D. J., and Crews, F. T. (2007). Systemic LPS causes chronic neuroinflammation and progressive neurodegeneration. *Glia* 55, 453–462.

Raison, C. L., Borisov, A. S., Majer, M., Drake, D. F., Pagnoni, G., Woolwine, B. J., Vogt, G. J., Massung, B., and Miller, A. H. (2009). Activation of central nervous system inflammatory pathways by interferon-alpha: relationship to monoamines and depression. *Biol. Psychiatry* 65, 296–303.

Reissner, K. J., and Kalivas, P. W. (2010). Using glutamate homeostasis as a target for treating addictive disorders. *Behav. Pharmacol.* 21, 514–522.

Robinson, T. E., and Berridge, K. C. (2003). Addiction. *Annu. Rev. Psychol.* 54, 25–53.

Rosenberg, D. R., and Lewis, D. A. (1994). Changes in the dopaminergic innervation of monkey prefrontal cortex during late postnatal development: a tyrosine hydroxylase immunohistochemical study. *Biol. Psychiatry* 36, 272–277.

Russo, S. J., Mazei-Robison, M. S., Ables, J. L., and Nestler, E. J. (2009). Neurotrophic factors and structural plasticity in addiction. *Neuropharmacology* 56, 73–82.

Santarelli, L., Saxe, M., Gross, C., Surget, A., Battaglia, F., Dulawa, S., Weisstaub, N., Lee, J., Duman, R., Arancio, O., Belzung, C., and Hen, R. (2003). Requirement of hippocampal neurogenesis for the behavioral effects of antidepressants. *Science* 301, 805–809.

Schoenbaum, G., Roesch, M. R., and Stalnaker, T. A. (2006). Orbitofrontal cortex, decision-making, and drug addiction. *Trends Neurosci.* 29, 116–124.

Schoenbaum, G., Saddoris, M. P., Ramus, S. J., Shaham, Y., and Setlow, B. (2004). Cocaine-experienced rats exhibit learning deficits in a task sensitive to orbitofrontal cortex lesions. *Eur. J. Neurosci.* 19, 1997–2002.

Schoenbaum, G., and Shaham, Y. (2008). The role of orbitofrontal cortex in drug addiction: a review of preclinical studies. *Biol. Psychiatry* 63, 256–262.

Shors, T. J., Miesegaes, G., Beylin, A., Zhao, M., Rydel, T., and Gould, E. (2001). Neurogenesis in the adult in involved in the formation of trace memories. *Nature* 410, 372–376.

Silveri, M. M., and Spear, L. P. (1998). Decreased sensitivity to the hypnotic effects of ethanol early in ontogeny. *Alcohol. Clin. Exp. Res.* 22, 670–676.

Smith, P. K. (1982). Does play matter? Functional and evolutionary aspects of animal and human play. *Behav. Brain Sci.* 5, 139–184.

Sowell, E. R., Thompson, P. M., Holmes, C. J., Jernigan, T. L., and Toga, A. W. (1999). In vivo evidence for post-adolescent brain maturation in frontal and striatal regions. *Nat. Neurosci.* 2, 859–861.

Sowell, E. R., Thompson, P. M., Tessner, K. D., and Toga, A. W. (2001). Mapping continued brain growth and gray matter density reduction in dorsal frontal cortex: inverse relationships during postadolescent brain maturation. *J. Neurosci.* 22, 8819–8829.

Spanagel, R., Rosenwasser, A. M., Schumann, G., and Sarker, D. K. (2005). Alcohol consumption and the body's biological clock. *Alcohol. Clin. Exp. Res.* 29, 1550–1557.

Spear, L. P. (2000). The adolescent brain and age-related behavioral manifestations. *Neurosci. Biobehav. Rev.* 24, 417–463.

Stalnaker, T. A., Takahashi, Y., Roesch, M. R., and Schoenbaum, G. (2009). Neural substrates of cognitive inflexibility after chronic cocaine exposure. *Neuropharmacology* 56, 63–72.

Stevenson, J. R., Schroeder, J. P., Nixon, K., Besheer, J., Crews, F. T., and Hodge, C. W. (2009). Abstinence following alcohol drinking produces depression-like behavior and reduced hippocampal neurogenesis in mice. *Neuropsychopharmacology* 34, 1209–1222.

Swann, J. W., Pierson, M. G., Smith, K. L., and Lee, C. L. (1999). Developmental neuroplasticity: roles in early life seizures and chronic epilepsy. *Adv. Neurol.* 79, 203–216.

Tamm, L., Menon, V., and Reiss, A. L. (2002). Maturation of brain function associated with response inhibition. *J. Am. Acad. Child Adolesc. Psychiatry* 41, 1231–1238.

Tanapat, P., Hastings, N. B., Rydel, T. A., Galea, L. A., and Gould, E. (2001). Exposure to fox odor inhibits cell proliferation in the hippocampus of adult rats via an adrenal hormone-dependent mechanism. *J. Comp. Neurol.* 437, 496–504.

Tarazi, F. I., Tomasini, E. C., and Baldessarini, R. J. (1998a). Postnatal development of dopamine D4-like receptors in rat forebrain regions: comparison with D2-like receptors. *Brain Res. Dev. Brain Res.* 110, 227–233.

Tarazi, F. I., Tomasini, E. C., and Baldessarini, R. J. (1998b). Postnatal development of dopamine and serotonin transporters in rat caudate-putamen and nucleus accumbens septi. *Neurosci. Lett.* 254, 21–24.

Teicher, M. H., Andersen, S. L., and Hostetter, J. C. Jr. (1995). Evidence for dopamine receptor pruning between adolescence and adulthood in striatum but not nucleus accumbens. *Brain Res. Dev. Brain Res.* 89, 167–172.

Townshend, J. M., and Duka, T. (2003). Mixed emotions: alcoholics' impairments in the recognition of specific emotional facial expressions. *Neuropsychologia* 41, 773–782.

van Eden, C. G., Kros, J. M., and Uylings, H. B. (1990). The development of the rat prefrontal cortex. Its size and development of connections with thalamus, spinal cord and other cortical areas. *Prog. Brain Res.* 85, 169–183.

Videbech, P., and Ravnkilde, B. (2004). Hippocampal volume and depression: meta-analysis of MRI studies. *Am. J. Psychiatry* 161, 1957–1966.

Walker, E. F., Walder, D. J., and Reynolds, F. (2001). Developmental changes in cortisol secretion in normal and at-risk youth. *Dev. Psychopathol.* 13, 721–732.

Ward, R. J., Colivicchi, M. A., Allen, R., Schol, F., Lallemand, F., de Witte, P., Ballini, C., Corte, L. D., and Dexter, D. (2009). Neuroinflammation induced in the hippocampus of "binge drinking" rats may be mediated by elevated extracellular glutamate content. *J. Neurochem.* 111, 1119–1128.

Waters, N. S., Klintsova, A. Y., and Foster, T. C. (1997). Insensitivity of the hippocampus to environmental stimulation during postnatal development. *J. Neurosci.* 17, 7967–7973.

Weissenborn, R., and Duka, T. (2003). Acute alcohol effects on cognition function in social drinkers: their relationship to drinking habits. *Psychopharmacology (Berl.)* 165, 306–312.

Wills, T. A., Vaccaro, D., and McNamara, G. (1994). Novelty seeking, risk taking, and related constructs as predictors of adolescent substance use: an application of Cloninger's theory. *J. Subst. Abuse* 6, 1–20.

Yang, L., Seifert, A., Wu, D., Wang, X., Rankovic, V., Schroder, H., Brandenburg, L. O., Hollt, V., and Koch, T. (2010). Role of phospholipase D2/phosphatidic acid signal transduction in micro- and delta-opioid receptor endocytosis. *Mol. Pharmacol.* 78, 105–113.

Zecevic, N., Bourgeois, J. P., and Rakic, P. (1989). Changes in synaptic density in motor cortex of rhesus monkey during fetal and postnatal life. *Brain Res. Dev. Brain Res.* 50, 11–32.

Zehr, J. L., Todd, B. J., Schulz, K. M., McCarthy, M. M., and Sisk, C. L. (2006). Dendritic pruning of the medial amygdala during pubertal development of the Syrian hamster. *J. Neurobiol.* 66, 578–590.

Zou, J. Y., and Crews, F. T. (2005). TNF alpha potentiates glutamate neurotoxicity by inhibiting glutamate uptake in organotypic brain slice cultures: Neuroprotection by NF kappa B inhibition. *Brain Res.* 1034, 11–24.

Zou, J., and Crews, F. T. (2006). CREB and NF-kappaB transcription factors regulate sensitivity to excitotoxic and oxidative stress induced neuronal cell death. *Cell. Mol. Neurobiol.* 26, 385–405.

Zou, J., and Crews, F. T. (2010). Induction of innate immune gene expression cascades in brain slice cultures by ethanol: key role of NF-kappaB and proinflammatory cytokines. *Alcohol. Clin. Exp. Res.* 34, 777–789.

Use of high resolution 3D diffusion tensor imaging to study brain white matter development in live neonatal rats

Yu Cai[1,2], Matthew S. McMurray[3], Ipek Oguz[3,4], Hong Yuan[1,2], Martin A. Styner[3,4], Weili Lin[1,2], Josephine M. Johns[3,4] and Hongyu An[1,2]*

[1] Department of Radiology, University of North Carolina at Chapel Hill, Chapel Hill, NC, USA
[2] Biomedical Research Imaging Center, University of North Carolina at Chapel Hill, Chapel Hill, NC, USA
[3] Department of Psychology, University of North Carolina at Chapel Hill, Chapel Hill, NC, USA
[4] Department of Psychiatry, University of North Carolina at Chapel Hill, Chapel Hill, NC, USA

*Correspondence:
Hongyu An, Department of Radiology, University of North Carolina at Chapel Hill, 106 Mason Farm Road, CB#7515, Chapel Hill, NC 27599, USA.
e-mail: hongyuan@med.unc.edu

High resolution diffusion tensor imaging (DTI) can provide important information on brain development, yet it is challenging in live neonatal rats due to the small size of neonatal brain and motion-sensitive nature of DTI. Imaging in live neonatal rats has clear advantages over fixed brain scans, as longitudinal and functional studies would be feasible to understand neuro-developmental abnormalities. In this study, we developed imaging strategies that can be used to obtain high resolution 3D DTI images in live neonatal rats at postnatal day 5 (PND5) and PND14, using only 3 h of imaging acquisition time. An optimized 3D DTI pulse sequence and appropriate animal setup to minimize physiological motion artifacts are the keys to successful high resolution 3D DTI imaging. Thus, a 3D rapid acquisition relaxation enhancement DTI sequence with twin navigator echoes was implemented to accelerate imaging acquisition time and minimize motion artifacts. It has been suggested that neonatal mammals possess a unique ability to tolerate mild-to-moderate hypothermia and hypoxia without long term impact. Thus, we additionally utilized this ability to minimize motion artifacts in magnetic resonance images by carefully suppressing the respiratory rate to around 15/min for PND5 and 30/min for PND14 using mild-to-moderate hypothermia. These imaging strategies have been successfully implemented to study how the effect of cocaine exposure in dams might affect brain development in their rat pups. Image quality resulting from this *in vivo* DTI study was comparable to *ex vivo* scans. fractional anisotropy values were also similar between the live and fixed brain scans. The capability of acquiring high quality *in vivo* DTI imaging offers a valuable opportunity to study many neurological disorders in brain development in an authentic living environment.

Keywords: magnetic resonance imaging, diffusion tensor imaging, brain development, white matter, neonatal rats

INTRODUCTION

High resolution non-invasive imaging on live neonatal rodents is a highly desirable tool in neurological development studies, as it can provide full representation of 3D neuroanatomy and allow for longitudinal studies. The spatio-temporal maturation pattern of the rodent brain obtained using such neuroimaging methods affords valuable information in the identification of normal, as well as abnormal, brain developmental features. Magnetic resonance (MR) diffusion tensor imaging (DTI) is a quantitative and non-invasive imaging technique reflecting the magnitude and direction of water molecule diffusion in tissues. DTI offers a unique non-invasive window into the process of brain maturation (Le Bihan et al., 1986; Basser and Pierpaoli, 1996) using a set of water diffusion related parameters, including fractional anisotropy (FA), radial diffusivity (RD), axial diffusivity (AD), and mean diffusivity (MD). FA reflects water diffusion anisotropy due to the differences among diffusitivities along the three principal directions. As a result of the presence of orderly arranged axon and myelin sheaths within white matter fiber tracts, FA values are usually higher in white matter structures than surrounding brain regions. MD is an averaged measure of local water diffusivity.

Due to the presence of myelin sheaths and microstructural components of axons in white matter, water molecules move more freely along than perpendicularly to the long axis of the white matter fiber. This phenomenon is known as anisotropic diffusion. Though anisotropic diffusion can still be detected in a white matter dysmyelination mouse model (shiverer mice), it is significantly lower in the fixed brains of shiverer mice than that of wild-type (Tyszka et al., 2006). It has been suggested that both myelination and intact axon structures contribute to diffusion anisotropy (Mori et al., 2001; Neil et al., 2002; Zhang et al., 2003; Tyszka et al., 2006). Thus, data gleaned from DTI is directly linked to the anatomic organization and microstructural features of white matter fiber tracts (Basser et al., 1994); information that cannot be obtained through conventional MRI T1 or T2 images.

Aside from traditional DTI techniques, 3D high resolution DTI MRI (Adolph, 1948) on intact rodent brains provides a 3D characterization of tissue samples in a non-destructive way and therefore is free from sectioning-related artifacts (Mori et al., 2001) when compared to histological methods. Moreover, unlike the labor intensive histological methods, high resolution 3D DTI of the whole brain is obtained during one scan session and can be "sliced" in any orientation desired. Therefore, it potentially plays an important role in neonatal developmental studies (Neil et al., 1998; Mori et al., 2001; Zhang et al., 2003; Bockhorst et al., 2008). Since DTI MR imaging utilizes strong magnetic gradients to generate imaging contrast based on small water molecule diffusion, it is inherently extremely sensitive to motion induced artifacts. Furthermore, in order to acquire high resolution DTI images, historically, long acquisition times (>10 h) have to be utilized for both diffusion and spatial encoding. These two major limitations make 3D DTI imaging difficult for live animals (Schick, 1997; Mori and van Zijl, 1998; Xue et al., 1999; Mori et al., 2001).

Thus far, most studies have been performed in *ex vivo* fixed brain specimen (Zhang et al., 2003, 2005; Verma et al., 2005; Tyszka et al., 2006; Huang et al., 2008; Aggarwal et al., 2010; Jiang and Johnson, 2010). DTI imaging on live neonatal rodents offers many advantages over fixed brain specimen scans. First, it provides information in an authentic physiological environment without the effects of brain fixation. Second, it allows for a longitudinal follow-up study to probe the temporal change of brain development or disease progress in the same animals, leading to more statistical power without the need of sacrificing a large number of animals.

Currently, efforts have been made toward DTI imaging of live rodents. However, most of these studies are multi-slice 2D DTI imaging-based, using either conventional spin echo or echo planar imaging (EPI) spin echo sequences (Sun et al., 2003, 2005; Chahboune et al., 2007, 2009; Bockhorst et al., 2008; Kim et al., 2009). Compared with 3D acquisition mode, it is difficult to achieve less than 0.5 mm through-plane resolution in such images, due to the limitation of the radio-frequency (RF) excitation slice profile in 2D acquisition. For perspective, it has been demonstrated that 0.5 mm is in the range of the width of corpus callosum (from 0.327 to 0.751 mm) of 3-month Purdue-Wistar rats (Fitch et al., 1990). Many studies have shown that spatial resolution can affect the accuracy of FA calculation (Kim et al., 2006). Additionally, partial-volume-effects can lead to an underestimation of FA, and thus inaccurate assessment of spatio-temporal changes of white matter. This problem, which is exacerbated particularly in the neonatal rodent brain due to its small size, can be mitigated by high resolution 3D imaging. Thus far, only a few studies have successfully performed 3D DTI imaging in live adult rodent brains using a DTI rapid acquisition relaxation enhancement (RARE) based approach (Xue et al., 1999; Aggarwal et al., 2010). Due to the high respiratory rates of neonatals, it is even more challenging to achieve high resolution DTI in neonatal rat pups.

In this study, we have investigated tactics which may facilitate the acquisition of high resolution 3D DTI imaging in neonatal rats. We have found that an optimized 3D DTI RARE method, with motion and eddy current artifacts correction using twin navigator echoes phase correction strategy (Xue et al., 1999), can allow for a 3D DTI acquisition within a few hours (~3 h). It has been suggested that mammalian neonatal can tolerate mild-to-moderate hypothermia and hypoxia when compared to their adult counterparts (Adolph, 1969; Singer, 1999). Thus, we used mild-to-moderate hypothermia to minimize motion artifacts in MR images by carefully suppressing the respiratory rate to 15/min for postnatal day 5 (PND5) and 30/min for PND14. In this paper, we explored the feasibility of acquiring high resolution 3D DTI images in live neonatal rats at two different ages using these strategies. Image quality and various DTI parameters of the live neonatal rat scans were compared with those of postmortem fixed brain scans at the same ages.

MATERIALS AND METHODS
MRI PULSE SEQUENCE

Conventional 3D Stejskal–Tanner spin echo DTI acquisition can achieve high resolution images. However, the long acquisition time (10 h or more) and highly motion-sensitive nature limit its usage mainly on postmortem imaging. Two major DTI acquisition approaches, diffusion weighed EPI/SPIRAL (DW–EPI/SPIRAL) and diffusion weighed rapid acquisition relaxation enhancement (DW–RARE) methods, can be employed to accelerate the acquisition time by a factor of 2–10 when compared to the conventional diffusion weighed spin echo pulse sequence (Turner and Lebihan, 1990; Muller et al., 1994; Schick, 1997; Mori and van Zijl, 1998; Pipe et al., 2002; Liu et al., 2004; Frank et al., 2010). By refocusing the echoes using a series of 180° RF pulses, the advantage of DW–RARE over the DW–EPI/SPIRAL pulse sequence is that it is less sensitive to signal loss and image distortion caused by the field inhomogeneity, a feature that is critically important for small-animal high resolution 3D DTI study using high magnetic fields (Pipe et al., 2002; Deng et al., 2008; Sarlls and Pierpaoli, 2008). However, motion artifacts augmented by the diffusion sensitizing gradients may degrade image quality through the different magnetization pathways generated by multiple 180° RF pulses for the DW–RARE method. Proper strategies need to be taken to minimize such artifacts.

Similar to the approach proposed by Mori and van Zijl (1998), a 3D DTI RARE sequence with twin navigator echoes was implemented on a Bruker horizontal bore 9.4 T scanner (BioSpec 9.4/30 USR, Bruker Biospin, Billerica, MA, USA). A pair of diffusion gradients was applied around the first 180° RF pulse. The strength and direction of diffusion gradients were set according to the input b value and diffusion directions. Moreover, to remove the stimulated echo pathways that did not have correct diffusion encoding, crusher gradients with varying magnitudes and polarities were applied around each 180° refocusing RF pulse. The bandwidth of the 180° refocus RF pulse was set at two to three times larger than that of the excitation 90° RF pulse to minimize the stimulated echoes induced by the imperfect refocus pulse. Two navigator echoes were acquired after the imaging echoes to correct for motion and eddy current artifacts (Mori and van Zijl, 1998). The acquisition parameters were: TR = 700 ms; the first RARE echo was assigned to the k-space center, effective TE = 23.662 ms; RARE echo spacing = 11.9 ms.

The total imaging time is inversely proportionate to the RARE factor. However, we cannot use a very high RARE factor in this DTI RARE sequence due to the fact that the stimulated echo pathway in high RARE factor readout becomes more complex and difficult to be removed, leading to the poor image quality. Using phantom studies, we empirically determined that a RARE factor of three yields a good trade-off between acquisition speed and sharpness of images for *in vivo* neonatal animal scans.

Diffusion gradient duration δ = 6.5 ms, diffusion gradient separation Δ = 12.72 ms, field of view (FOV) = 27 mm × 19.2 mm × 11 mm, matrix size = 180 × 128 × 55, the resolution = 0.15 mm × 0.15 mm × 0.2 mm, readout direction: H–F, phase encoding direction: L–R, slab encoding direction: A–P. The twin navigator echoes were used to correct for the phase incoherence between the odd and even echoes to alleviate the motion and eddy current effects (Mori and van Zijl, 1998). A 72-mm volume coil and a surface coil were used for RF transmission and signal receiving, respectively, under an actively decoupled cross-coil routine mode. Finally, the data was interpolated to the final matrix size 360 × 256 × 128 to achieve a nominal spatial resolution around 0.075 mm × 0.075 mm × 0.1 mm.

IN VIVO ANIMAL SCAN

This methods described were designed for a study (P01DA022446) to determine how the effect of prenatal cocaine exposure may affect a rat pup's brain development. The animal scanning protocol was approved by Institutional Animal Care and Use Committee (IACUC) of University of North Carolina at Chapel Hill. Twelve Sprague-Dawley PND5 (average weight 9.6 ± 1.1 g) and 30 PND14 (average weight 32.3 ± 2.3 g) rats were studied. Male and female subjects were in pairs from the same litter. Anesthesia was induced using 3% isoflurane mixed with oxygen. For maintaining anesthesia in neonatal rats, isoflurane level was adjusted in the range of 0.6–1.5 to keep the respiratory rate within a target range. The body surface of PND5 pups was covered in 100% pure petroleum jelly (Vi-Jon Laboratories, Inc, St. Louis, MO 63114, USA) to prevent skin dehydration during image acquisition. The lower jaw of PND5 pups was secured to reduce the bulk of the motion, and reinforced by padding around the head. The room temperature of the MR scanner room was set at 22°C. Animal respiration and surface body temperature were continuously monitored using a MR compatible small-animal monitoring system SAII 1025L (SAII Instruments, Inc, Stony Brook, NY 11790, USA). In this study, body surface temperatures were obtained from abdomen region, and maintained in the range of 24–26°C and 33°C for PND5 and PND14 pups, respectively, using a circulating water heating system. Thus, since the normal body surface temperature of rat pups ranges from 35 to 37°C, the PND5 and PND14 pups were under moderate and mild hypothermic conditions, respectively. Respiratory rates were maintained at about 15/min and 30/min in PND5 and PND14 pups, respectively. A mouse head surface coil and a rat head phase array surface coil were used for imaging PND5 and PND14 rat pups, respectively. Six non-collinear diffusion encoding directions with $b = 1000$ s/mm^2 images and one baseline reference $b = 0$ image were acquired for the *in vivo* DTI scans. The diffusion b values were set to 1000 s/mm^2 for the *in vivo* scans. The total scan time was 3 h 10 min, which is reduced by a factor of three compared to conventional DW–SE pulse sequences used to acquire the same resolution DTI images.

POSTMORTEM FIXED BRAIN SCAN

Tissues were collected from both PND5 and PND14 rats following standard cardiac puncture perfusions while under anesthesia [150 g/kg sodium pentobarbital (sigma)], first with 1.5 mL/min phosphate-buffered saline (PBS) followed by 1.5 mL/min 4% paraformaldehyde. The intact head was then excised and placed in 4% paraformaldehyde. The specimens were placed in PBS solution and stored at 4°C at least 12 h before MR imaging. All fixed tissue was equilibrated to room temperature for several hours prior to imaging of the whole head. The sample temperatures were measured to be 21 ± 0.2°C. Similar acquisition parameters of 3D DTI RARE pulse sequence were used for DTI acquisition in fixed brain specimen. In total, one baseline reference scan and 21 diffusion encoding directions were utilized. Since the paraformaldehyde fixation reduces water mobility in tissue (Sun et al., 2003, 2005), a higher b value ($b = 1600$ s/mm^2) was utilized for the postmortem fixed brain DTI. The fixed brains were scanned at room temperature and the total image acquisition time was about 10 h.

COMPARISON BETWEEN *IN VIVO* AND *EX VIVO* SCANS

Since the postmortem scans were free of physiological motion-related artifacts, these scans were used to quantitatively evaluate the image quality of the *in vivo* scans. Two independent raters performed their evaluation by examining the extent of motion artifact, signal loss in images, overall noise, and other artifacts in multiple brain regions. Using the fixed brain specimen DTI scans as references, *in vivo* DTI images with very little motion artifact, negligible ringing artifact, and little or no signal loss were rated good, or otherwise rated poor. Scan successful rate was defined as the ratio of good data set to total data set.

The signal to noise ratio (SNR) in the $b = 0$ reference and diffusion scans was computed and compared between images acquired from the *in vivo* and *ex vivo* scans. The chemical fixation procedure changed many tissue MR properties, including T1, T2, and ADC, leading to altered MR signal intensity in the images of the fixed postmortem brains (Sun et al., 2003, 2005; Yong-Hing et al., 2005; Shepherd et al., 2009). Taking these factors into consideration in the SNR comparison, we computed the adjusted SNR for the *ex vivo* fixed brain as SNR$_{adjusted}$ = $S_{adjusted}/\sigma$, where σ is the SD of the background Gaussian noise, and $S_{adjusted}$ is the adjusted MR signal. The adjust MR signal is computed as

$$S_{adjusted} = S\left(\frac{M0_{live}}{M0_{fixed}}\right) e^{b \cdot D_{fixed}} e^{-b \cdot D_{live}} e^{\frac{TE}{T2_{fixed}}} e^{-\frac{TE}{T2_{live}}}$$
$$\times \frac{1 - e^{-\frac{TR}{T1_{live}}}}{1 - e^{-\frac{TR}{T1_{fixed}}}},$$

where S is the measured MR signal from the postmortem brain, and the subscripts "fixed" and "live" refer to the MR properties for the fixed and live tissues, respectively.

Assuming a D_{live} of 1×10^{-3} mm^2/s, a $T1_{live}$ of 1800 ms, a $T2_{live}$ of 40 ms and a proton density $M0_{live}$ of 1.0 for the *in vivo* scans, and a D_{fixed} of 0.3×10^{-3} mm^2/s, a $T1_{fixed}$ of 1400 ms, a $T2_{fixed}$ of 32 ms and a proton density $M0_{fixed}$ of 0.85 for the *ex vivo* scans using previously published literature values (de Graaf et al., 2006; Shepherd et al., 2009), we computed SNR$_{adjusted}$ for the *ex vivo* images. A two tail *t*-test was used to compare FA, MD, and SNR between the *in vivo* and *ex vivo* scans.

All DTI data were processed using DTI Studio software (www.mristudio.org). MD and FA were computed using ROIs ranging from 20 to 24 pixels (0.0113–0.0135 mm³), placed in the genu of corpus callosum (gcc), body of corpus callosum (bcc), splenium of corpus callosum (scc). DTI tractography was performed using the gcc ROI as the seed point, and the tracking algorithm was terminated when the FA value was below 0.25. The allowed maximum turn angle for adjacent voxels was set to 70° to minimize the occurrence of spurious fiber orientations caused by noise.

RESULTS

All PND5 and PND14 rat pups recovered 10–30 min after MR scans (∼3.5 h) with a zero mortality rate. Representative *in vivo* images and *ex vivo* brain DTI images are demonstrated in **Figure 1** and the computed diffusion indices, such as FA and MD are shown in **Figure 2**. The two independent raters had the same ratings in 40 out of a total of 42 scans (a 95.2% agreement). For the two cases that two raters initially disagreed, consensus was reached after discussion. After reaching consensus, images acquired from 10 out of 12 PND5 and 27 out of 30 PND14 rats were rated as "good," resulting in success rates of 83 and 90% for the PND5 and PND14 pups, respectively. Though the overall image quality of the *in vivo* scans was comparable to that of the *ex vivo* scans, more ringing artifacts were observed in the $b=0$ and diffusion weighted raw images as demonstrated in **Figure 1**. However, these remaining artifacts have very little effect on DTI indices as shown in **Figure 2**.

As shown in **Figure 2**, major white matter fibers depicted in the FA maps were similar between the *in vivo* and the *ex vivo* scans. Conversely, the contrast between gray and white matter was more pronounced in the *ex vivo* than in the *in vivo* MD images, suggesting that MD had a greater reduction within white matter during the chemical fixation.

Figure 3 demonstrates the efficacy of motion correction using the twin navigator echoes. Due primarily to respiration and pulsatile motion of large blood vessels near the ventral side, it was expected that more motion artifact might occur in slices close to the ventral side (**Figure 3C**) when compared to the dorsal side of the head (**Figure 3A**). After the twin navigator echo motion correction, signal loss was recovered, and the background noise was reduced as marked by the arrows in **Figures 3B,D**. Though DTI image quality has been improved after the dual echo navigator correction, some residual motion artifacts can still be observed.

Tables 1 and **2** shows the FA and MD values from the *in vivo* and *ex vivo* scans in several anatomical regions: gcc, bcc, scc. There was no statistically significant difference in the FA value between the *in vivo* and the *ex vivo* scans, while MD values were significantly lower ($P < 0.05$) in the *ex vivo* scans, in agreement with previous findings (Sun et al., 2003, 2005). Moreover, there was no

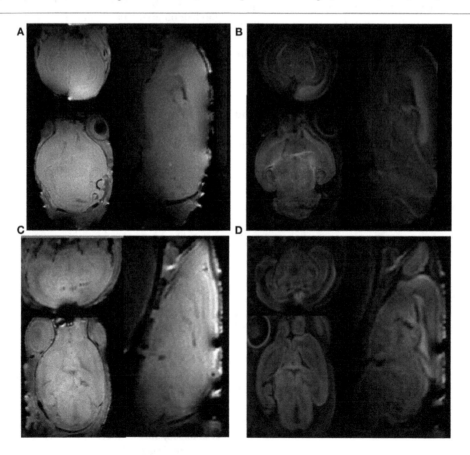

FIGURE 1 | The comparison of $b=0$ and diffusion weighted images between the *ex vivo* scan and the *in vivo* scans. (A) *Ex vivo* baseline $b=0$ image; **(B)** *ex vivo* diffusion weighted image; **(C)** *in vivo* baseline $b=0$ image; **(D)** *in vivo* diffusion weighted image. The axial, sagittal, and coronal plane images are shown clockwise.

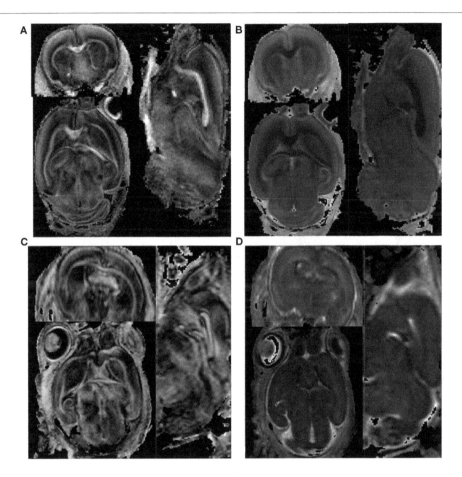

FIGURE 2 | The comparison of FA and MD maps between the *ex vivo* and the *in vivo* scan. (A) *Ex vivo* baseline image. (B) *Ex vivo* diffusion weighted image (C) *in vivo* baseline image (D) *in vivo* diffusion weighted image. The axial, sagittal, and coronal plane images are shown clockwise.

significant difference between the SNR of the *in vivo* scans and the adjusted SNR of the *ex vivo* scans for both the baseline and diffusion weighted images, as shown in **Table 3**.

Figure 4 shows the fiber tracking results in live and postmortem fixed brain DTI images. The major fiber bundle of corpus callosum can be readily obtained in PND5 and PND14 live DTI images. The tracked fibers showed very similar patterns between the *in vivo* and the *ex vivo* scans for both the PND5 and PND14 groups.

DISCUSSION

Recent studies have shown that a Periodically Rotated Overlapping ParallEL Lines with Enhanced Reconstruction (PROPELLER) and its recent modified form with split acquisition of fast spin echo signal for diffusion imaging (SPLICE) pulse sequence techniques (Schick, 1997; Deng et al., 2008) are intrinsically motion insensitive because these methods are self-navigated. These techniques have been successfully applied for abdominal DTI study. Though this is a very promising technique, it has several limitations. First, 1.5 times longer image acquisition time is needed for PROPELLER acquisition compared with conventional sampling for a 2D acquisition (Pipe et al., 2002). To achieve a high resolution 3D DTI, blade sampling needs to be performed on a 3D sphere, resulting in a dramatically increased image acquisition time. Second, non-Cartesian k-space sampling is utilized in PROPELLER and SPLICE methods. The k-space regridding is usually required for image reconstruction and any system imperfection will cause image blurring by degrading the point spread function of k-space. In contrast, the DTI RARE sequence uses multiple 180° pulses to refocus the signal and a Cartesian k-space sampling is obtained. This approach is not sensitive to geometric distortion and signal reduction caused by background susceptibility artifacts. The image reconstruction is straightforward and rapid. The disadvantage of DTI RARE is its sensitivity to motion artifacts. By physically suppressing the respiratory motion using hypothermia together with twin navigator echo motion correction, we have demonstrated that high quality DTI images can be obtained *in vivo* from rat pups. In our study, the experimentally measured SNR of *in vivo* scans is only slightly lower than that of the *ex vivo* scans, further indicating that the image quality of the *in vivo* rat pup scans are comparable to that of the postmortem fixed *ex vivo* brain scans.

DIFFUSION ENCODING DIRECTIONS

In this study, we used 21 and 6 non-collinear diffusion gradient directions for the *ex vivo* and *in vivo* scans, respectively. More diffusion encoding directions could be used for the *in vivo* study if a longer DTI image acquisition time was possible. Six diffusion

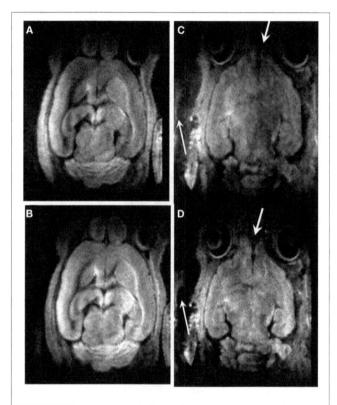

FIGURE 3 | The comparison before and after twin navigator echo correction. (A) A slice of the dorsal side before (A) and after (B) correction; (C) a slice of the ventral side before (C) and after (D) correction. Motion artifacts were minimized after the twin navigator echo correction as marked by the arrow.

Table 1 | Fractional anisotropy comparison between the *in vivo* and the *ex vivo* scans for PND5 and PND14 rat pups.

	PND5 (*in vivo*)	PND5 (*ex vivo*)	PND14 (*in vivo*)	PND14 (*ex vivo*)
GCC	0.73 ± 0.034	0.74 ± 0.022	0.78 ± 0.053	0.80 ± 0.029
BCC	0.55 ± 0.039	0.56 ± 0.028	0.56 ± 0.086	0.58 ± 0.042
SCC	0.79 ± 0.037	0.80 ± 0.019	0.81 ± 0.045	0.81 ± 0.021

Fractional anisotropy values were not significantly different between the in vivo and ex vivo scans.

Table 2 | Mean diffusivity (unit: 10^{-3} mm^2/s) comparison between *in vivo* and *ex vivo* scans for PND5 and PND14 scans.

	PND5 (*in vivo*)	PND5 (*ex vivo*)	PND14 (*in vivo*)	PND14 (*ex vivo*)
GCC	0.970 ± 0.053*	0.284 ± 0.022	0.734 ± 0.047*	0.233 ± 0.018
BCC	1.120 ± 0.089*	0.394 ± 0.047	0.884 ± 0.086*	0.344 ± 0.031
SCC	0.930 ± 0.055*	0.293 ± 0.026	0.865 ± 0.045*	0.277 ± 0.028

Significant differences were found in MD between the in vivo and the ex vivo scans ($P < 0.05$).*

Table 3 | Signal to noise ratio comparison between the *in vivo* and the *ex vivo* DTI scan.

	SNR for *in vivo*	SNR$_{adjusted}$ for *ex vivo* scans
$b = 0$ reference images	24.3 ± 3.4	29.4 ± 2.39
Diffusion weighted images	8.3 ± 3.4	10.447 ± 0.865

No significant difference was observed between the in vivo SNR and the adjusted SNR of the postmortem fixed ex vivo scans in both baseline and diffusion images.

encoding directions is the least number of directions for DTI computation assuming a simple ellipsoid tensor model. It does not provide sufficient information to resolve fiber crossing in DTI. The high angular resolution diffusion imaging (HARDI) approach has been proposed to overcome this problem by using a large number of diffusion encoding directions at an expense of increasing the imaging acquisition time (Tuch et al., 2002). We only performed a six diffusion encoding acquisition for *in vivo* scans due to the following reasons. First, we needed to obtain high resolution 3D DTI images with a time constraint of a few hours to reduce the risk of damaging the very young rat pups. Second, based on the established white matter atlas in both human and rodents (Chuang et al., 2011; Nowinski et al., 2011), the white matter tracks in rodent brain do not have as many fiber crossing regions as those in human brain. Third, our study mainly focused on major white matter regions in which fiber crossing is less likely to be found. We qualitatively compared the tracked fiber within major white matter regions such as corpus callosum between the *in vivo* and the *ex vivo* scans. We have found that major white matter fibers in both PND5 and PND14 pups can be readily obtained from the *in vivo* scans using less than one-third of the data acquisition time/diffusion encoding directions when compared to the *ex vivo* fixed brain scans. This suggests that the imaging acquisition tactics developed in this study can be utilized to acquire DTI images in live rat pups reliably and consistently.

MOTION CORRECTION

We adopted the twin navigator echo navigator method developed by Mori and van Zijl (1998) to alleviate the motion effect in our 3D DTI RARE sequence. This approach assumes a constant phase variation between the odd and even echoes induced by motion or eddy current. As demonstrated in **Figure 3**, image quality has been improved with recovered signal and reduced noise after the correction. However, since the assumption of constant phase variation between odd and even echoes did not always hold true in the *in vivo* scans, residual motion artifacts were still observed, as shown in **Figure 3**. To further minimize the motion artifacts, 2D navigator correction (Porter and Heidemann, 2009) may be explored in the future.

We did not use respiratory gating to minimize motion effects for several reasons. The TR of the 3D DTI RARE sequence was kept relatively short (700 ms) to achieve a 3-h total acquisition time and respiratory gating may lengthen image acquisition quite substantially. The respiratory rate of a neonatal rat pup may change during the 3-h acquisition window, leading to variations in the effective TR. If TR is short (as in our study), these variations are not negligible, and can result in signal variations and inaccurate calculation of DTI indices. In our study, we found that respiration

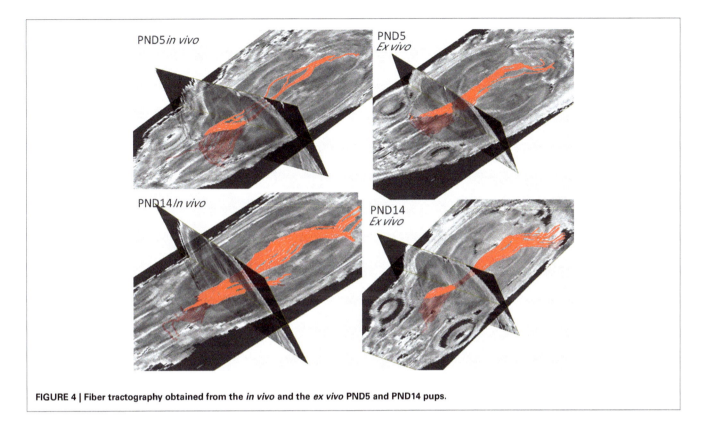

FIGURE 4 | Fiber tractography obtained from the *in vivo* and the *ex vivo* PND5 and PND14 pups.

gating did not yield good quality images if the respiratory rate is high. On the other hand, suppressing respiratory rates without gating was adequate to achieve virtually motion artifacts free images.

It is more challenging to acquire high quality 3D DTI images in live PND5 pups compared to PND14 rats. It has been suggested that mammalian neonatal can tolerate severe hypoxia and hypothermia for a longer time compared to their adult counterparts (Adolph, 1969; Singer, 1999). In a study investigating the survival rate of neonatal rats in a pure nitrogen environment (Adolph, 1969), Adolph demonstrated that 0 to 5-day-old rats could survive in such an environment for 1–2 h when the colonic temperature was cooled down to 8–10°C, while in 11 to 16-day-old rats, the optimal body temperature for survival increased to 20°C and endurance time decreased to 0.5 h. These findings provided the base of utilizing hypothermia for PND5 DTI. The neuroprotective effects of the mild-to-moderate hypothermia have been firmly established (Adolph, 1969; Blackmon and Stark, 2006). Additionally, hypothermia reduces the metabolic rate and further minimizes physiological motion. In our study, we found that a low level of isoflurane (0.6–0.8%) in conjunction with hypothermia was sufficient to keep most PND5 pups under anesthesia and to maintain a respiratory rate around 15/min.

OTHER ISSUES

The direct advantage of improving the resolution is to reduce the partial volume effect, making the diffusion indices calculation more accurate. Lee et al. (2006) reported much lower FA values in major white matter using low resolution DTI images (∼1 mm in plane and 0.5 through-plane resolution) at 1.5 T. They correctly ascribe it to the partial volume effect. The mean FA values of corpus callosum in our study are higher than those in a brain development study to investigate the temporal change of DTI indices from PND0 to PND56 rats reported by Bockhorst et al. (2008) using a spatial resolution of 0.27 mm × 0.27 mm × 0.5 mm.

A higher RARE factor could further increase the speed of image acquisition. However, the stimulated echo pathway becomes more complex and more difficult to be removed along with an increase of RARE factor, leading to the poor image quality. In an empirical phantom study, we found that a RARE factor of three was a good trade-off between acquisition speed and sharpness of images for *in vivo* neonatal animal scans (data not shown). To further improve the speed of the image acquisition, a 3D diffusion weighed gradient and spin echo (3D DW–GRASE) could be implemented. The GRASE sequence is a combination of segmented EPI and fast spin echo, interleaving the short EPI echo readout train with RF refocusing pulses. A 3D DW–GRASE provides a compromise between signal loss due to the field inhomogeneity in gradient echoes and the interference of stimulated echoes by refocus RF pulses in spin echoes. Aggarwal et al. (2010) have explored a DW–GRASE approach that yields a four times acceleration using two refocus pulses and two gradient echoes.

CONCLUSION

In this study, we have demonstrated that an optimized 3D DTI RARE approach and an appropriate animal setup minimizing respiration motion are the keys to achieving high quality 3D DTI images in live animals. Taking advantage of the distinct physiological characteristic that neonatal rats can survive low body temperatures, we have demonstrated that mild-to-moderate hypothermia can be utilized to suppress physiological motion artifacts to achieve good quality DTI images.

ACKNOWLEDGMENTS

The work described was supported in part by awards P01DA022446 (Josephine M. Johns) and F31DA026251 (Martin A. Styner) from the National Institutes on Drug Abuse. The content is solely the responsibility of the authors and does not necessarily represent the official views of the National Institutes on Drug Abuse or the National Institutes of Health. We thank Drs. Susumu Mori and Jiangyang Zhang for their valuable suggestions regarding the MR pulse sequence. NICHD P30 HD03110 awarded to J. Piven.

REFERENCES

Adolph, E. (1948). Tolerance to cold and anoxia in infant rats. *Am. J. Physiol.* 155, 366–377.

Adolph, E. F. (1969). Regulations during survival without oxygen in infant mammals. *Respir. Physiol.* 7, 356–368.

Aggarwal, M., Mori, S., Shimogori, T., Blackshaw, S., and Zhang, J. Y. (2010). Three-dimensional diffusion tensor microimaging for anatomical characterization of the mouse brain. *Magn. Reson. Med.* 64, 249–261.

Basser, P. J., Mattiello, J., and LeBihan, D. (1994). MR diffusion tensor spectroscopy and imaging. *Biophys. J.* 66, 259–267.

Basser, P. J., and Pierpaoli, C. (1996). Microstructural and physiological features of tissues elucidated by quantitative-diffusion-tensor MRI. *J. Magn. Reson. B.* 111, 209–219.

Blackmon, L. R., and Stark, A. R. (2006). Hypothermia: a neuroprotective therapy for neonatal hypoxic-ischemic encephalopathy. *Pediatrics* 117, 942–948.

Bockhorst, K. H., Narayana, P. A., Liu, R., Vijjula, P. A., Ramu, J., Kamel, M., Wosik, J., Bockhorst, T., Hahn, K., Hasan, K. M., and Perez-Polo, J. R. (2008). Early postnatal development of rat brain: in vivo diffusion tensor imaging. *J. Neurosci. Res.* 86, 1520–1528.

Chahboune, H., Ment, L. R., Stewart, W. B., Ma, X. X., Rothman, D. L., and Hyder, F. (2007). Neurodevelopment of c57b/l6 mouse brain assessed by in vivo diffusion tensor imaging. *NMR Biomed.* 20, 375–382.

Chahboune, H., Ment, L. R., Stewart, W. B., Rothman, D. L., Vaccarino, F. M., Hyder, F., and Schwartz, M. L. (2009). Hypoxic injury during neonatal development in murine brain: correlation between in vivo DTI findings and behavioral assessment. *Cereb. Cortex* 19, 2891–2901.

Chuang, N., Mori, S., Yamamoto, A., Jiang, H., Ye, X., Xu, X., Richards, L. J., Nathans, J., Miller, M. I., Toga, A. W., Sidman, R. L., and Zhang, J. (2011). An MRI-based atlas and database of the developing mouse brain. *Neuroimage* 54, 80–89.

de Graaf, R. A., Brown, P. B., McIntyre, S., Nixon, T. W., Behar, K. L., and Rothman, D. L. (2006). High magnetic field water and metabolite proton t1 and t2 relaxation in rat brain in vivo. *Magn. Reson. Med.* 56, 386–394.

Deng, J., Omary, R. A., and Larson, A. C. (2008). Multishot diffusion-weighted splice propeller MRI of the abdomen. *Magn. Reson. Med.* 59, 947–953.

Fitch, R. H., Berrebi, A. S., Cowell, P. E., Schrott, L. M., and Denenberg, V. H. (1990). Corpus callosum: effects of neonatal hormones on sexual dimorphism in the rat. *Brain Res.* 515, 111–116.

Frank, L. R., Jung, Y., Inati, S., Tyszka, J. M., and Wong, E. C. (2010). High efficiency, low distortion 3d diffusion tensor imaging with variable density spiral fast spin echoes (3d dw vds rare). *Neuroimage* 49, 1510–1523.

Huang, H., Yamamoto, A., Hossain, M. A., Younes, L., and Mori, S. (2008). Quantitative cortical mapping of fractional anisotropy in developing rat brains. *J. Neurosci.* 28, 1427–1433.

Jiang, Y., and Johnson, G. A. (2010). Microscopic diffusion tensor imaging of the mouse brain. *Neuroimage* 50, 465–471.

Kim, J. H., Haldar, J., Liang, Z. P., and Song, S. K. (2009). Diffusion tensor imaging of mouse brain stem and cervical spinal cord. *J. Neurosci. Methods* 176, 186–191.

Kim, M., Ronen, I., Ugurbil, K., and Kim, D. S. (2006). Spatial resolution dependence of dti tractography in human occipito-callosal region. *Neuroimage* 32, 1243–1249.

Le Bihan, D., Breton, E., Lallemand, D., Grenier, P., Cabanis, E., and Laval-Jeantet, M. (1986). MR imaging of intravoxel incoherent motions: application to diffusion and perfusion in neurologic disorders. *Radiology* 161, 401–407.

Lee, F. K., Fang, M. R., Antonio, G. E., Yeung, D. K., Chan, E. T., Zhang, L. H., Yew, D. T., and Ahuja, A. T. (2006). Diffusion tensor imaging (DTI) of rodent brains in vivo using a 1.5t clinical MR scanner. *J. Magn. Reson. Imaging* 23, 747–751.

Liu, C. L., Bammer, R., Kim, D. H., and Moseley, M. E. (2004). Self-navigated interleaved spiral (snails): application to high-resolution diffusion tensor imaging. *Magn. Reson. Med.* 52, 1388–1396.

Mori, S., Itoh, R., Zhang, J. Y., Kaufmann, W. E., van Zijl, P. C. M., Solaiyappan, M., and Yarowsky, P. (2001). Diffusion tensor imaging of the developing mouse brain. *Magn. Reson. Med.* 46, 18–23.

Mori, S., and van Zijl, P. C. M. (1998). A motion correction scheme by twin-echo navigation for diffusion-weighted magnetic resonance imaging with multiple RF echo acquisition. *Magn. Reson. Med.* 40, 511–516.

Muller, M. F., Prasad, P., Siewert, B., Nissenbaum, M. A., Raptopoulos, V., and Edelman, R. R. (1994). Abdominal diffusion mapping with use of a whole-body echo-planar system. *Radiology* 190, 475–478.

Neil, J., Miller, J., Mukherjee, P., and Huppi, P. S. (2002). Diffusion tensor imaging of normal and injured developing human brain – a technical review. *NMR Biomed.* 15, 543–552.

Neil, J. J., Shiran, S. I., McKinstry, R. C., Schefft, G. L., Snyder, A. Z., Almli, C. R., Akbudak, E., Aronovitz, J. A., Miller, J. P., Lee, B. C. P., and Conturo, T. E. (1998). Normal brain in human newborns: apparent diffusion coefficient and diffusion anisotropy measured by using diffusion tensor MR imaging. *Radiology* 209, 57–66.

Nowinski, W. L., Chua, B. C., Yang, G. L., and Qian, G. Y. (2011). Three-dimensional interactive and stereotactic human brain atlas of white matter tracts. *Neuroinformatics*.

Pipe, J. G., Farthing, V. G., and Forbes, K. P. (2002). Multishot diffusion-weighted FSE using propeller MRI. *Magn. Reson. Med.* 47, 42–52.

Porter, D. A., and Heidemann, R. M. (2009). High resolution diffusion-weighted imaging using readout-segmented echo-planar imaging, parallel imaging and a two-dimensional navigator-based reacquisition. *Magn. Reson. Med.* 62, 468–475.

Sarlls, J. E., and Pierpaoli, C. (2008). Diffusion-weighted radial fast spin-echo for high-resolution diffusion tensor imaging at 3t. *Magn. Reson. Med.* 60, 270–276.

Schick, F. (1997). Splice: sub-second diffusion-sensitive MR imaging using a modified fast spin-echo acquisition made. *Magn. Reson. Med.* 38, 638–644.

Shepherd, T. M., Thelwall, P. E., Stanisz, G. J., and Blackband, S. J. (2009). Aldehyde fixative solutions alter the water relaxation and diffusion properties of nervous tissue. *Magn. Reson. Med.* 62, 26–34.

Singer, D. (1999). Neonatal tolerance to hypoxia: a comparative-physiological approach. *Comp. Biochem. Physiol. A Mol. Integr. Physiol.* 123, 221–234.

Sun, S. W., Neil, J. J., Liang, H. F., He, Y. Y., Schmidt, R. E., Hsu, C. Y., and Song, S. K. (2005). Formalin fixation alters water diffusion coefficient magnitude but not anisotropy in infracted brain. *Magn. Reson. Med.* 53, 1447–1451.

Sun, S. W., Neil, J. J., and Song, S. K. (2003). Relative indices of water diffusion anisotropy are equivalent in live and formalin-fixed mouse brains. *Magn. Reson. Med.* 50, 743–748.

Tuch, D. S., Reese, T. G., Wiegell, M. R., Makris, N., Belliveau, J. W., and Wedeen, V. J. (2002). High angular resolution diffusion imaging reveals intravoxel white matter fiber heterogeneity. *Magn. Reson. Med.* 48, 577–582.

Turner, R., and Lebihan, D. (1990). Single-shot diffusion imaging at 2.0 tesla. *J. Magn. Reson.* 86, 445–452.

Tyszka, J. M., Readhead, C., Bearer, E. L., Pautler, R. G., and Jacobs, R. E. (2006). Statistical diffusion tensor histology reveals regional dysmyelination effects in the shiverer mouse mutant. *Neuroimage* 29, 1058–1065.

Verma, R., Mori, S., Shen, D. G., Yarowsky, P., Zhang, J. Y., and Davatzikos, C. (2005). Spatiotemporal maturation patterns of murine brain quantified by diffusion tensor MRI and deformation-based morphometry. *Proc. Natl. Acad. Sci. U.S.A.* 102, 6978–6983.

Xue, R., van Zijl, P. C. M., Crain, B. J., Solaiyappan, M., and Mori, S.

(1999). In vivo three-dimensional reconstruction of rat brain axonal projections by diffusion tensor imaging. *Magn. Reson. Med.* 42, 1123–1127.

Yong-Hing, C. J., Obenaus, A., Stryker, R., Tong, K., and Sarty, G. E. (2005). Magnetic resonance imaging and mathematical modeling of progressive formalin fixation of the human brain. *Magn. Reson. Med.* 54, 324–332.

Zhang, J. Y., Miller, M. I., Plachez, C., Richards, L. J., Yarowsky, P., van Zijl, P., and Mori, S. (2005). Mapping postnatal mouse brain development with diffusion tensor microimaging. *Neuroimage* 26, 1042–1051.

Zhang, J. Y., Richards, L. J., Yarowsky, P., Huang, H., van Zijl, P. C. M., and Mori, S. (2003). Three-dimensional anatomical characterization of the developing mouse brain by diffusion tensor microimaging. *Neuroimage* 20, 1639–1648.

Maternal neural responses to infant cries and faces: Relationships with substance use

Nicole Landi[1,2]*, Jessica Montoya[3], Hedy Kober[3], Helena J. V. Rutherford[1], W. Einar Mencl[2], Patrick D. Worhunsky[3], Marc N. Potenza[1,3,4] and Linda C. Mayes[1]

[1] Yale Child Study Center, Yale University School of Medicine, New Haven, CT, USA
[2] Haskins Laboratories, New Haven, CT, USA
[3] Department of Psychiatry, Yale University School of Medicine, New Haven, CT, USA
[4] Department of Neurobiology, Yale University School of Medicine, New Haven, CT, USA

Correspondence:
Nicole Landi, E 74 Yale Child Study Center, 230 South Frontage Road, New Haven, CT 06511, USA.
e-mail: nicole.landi@yale.edu

Substance abuse in pregnant and recently post-partum women is a major public health concern because of effects on the infant and on the ability of the adult to care for the infant. In addition to the negative health effects of teratogenic substances on fetal development, substance use can contribute to difficulties associated with the social and behavioral aspects of parenting. Neural circuits associated with parenting behavior overlap with circuits involved in addiction (e.g., frontal, striatal, and limbic systems) and thus may be co-opted for the craving/reward cycle associated with substance use and abuse and be less available for parenting. The current study investigates the degree to which neural circuits associated with parenting are disrupted in mothers who are substance-using. Specifically, we used functional magnetic resonance imaging to examine the neural response to emotional infant cues (faces and cries) in substance-using compared to non-using mothers. In response to both faces (of varying emotional valence) and cries (of varying distress levels), substance-using mothers evidenced reduced neural activation in regions that have been previously implicated in reward and motivation as well as regions involved in cognitive control. Specifically, in response to faces, substance users showed reduced activation in prefrontal regions, including the dorsolateral and ventromedial prefrontal cortices, as well as visual processing (occipital lobes) and limbic regions (parahippocampus and amygdala). Similarly, in response to infant cries, substance-using mothers showed reduced activation relative to non-using mothers in prefrontal regions, auditory sensory processing regions, insula and limbic regions (parahippocampus and amygdala). These findings suggest that infant stimuli may be less salient for substance-using mothers, and such reduced saliency may impair developing infant-caregiver attachment and the ability of mothers to respond appropriately to their infants.

Keywords: fMRI, emotion, cry, parenting

INTRODUCTION

In 2007, The National Survey on Drug Use and Health (NSDUH) found that 5.2% of pregnant women aged 15–44 years reported using illicit drugs during pregnancy; in addition, 11.6% reported alcohol use and 16.4% reported tobacco use. While drug, alcohol and tobacco abuse are a significant public health concern for all individuals, use of these substances during pregnancy and the post-partum period may have particularly detrimental consequences in mothers. This may be both because of the direct impact of teratogenic substances on infant development, and because the effects of drug abuse on maternal behavior and brain function may negatively impact the post-partum parenting environment.

Data indicate that maternal substance use and abuse are associated with poor parenting measures. Substance-abusing mothers have a two-fold increase in the removal of their children from their care (U.S. Dept. of Health and Human Services, National Center for Health Statistics, and National Health Interview Survey, 1999). Interview and self-report assessments reveal differences in child-related attitudes of substance-using mothers compared to non-substance-using mothers; specifically, substance-using mothers demonstrate less understanding about their child's development and use harsher discipline (Mayes and Sean, 2002). Mothers identified as cocaine users during pregnancy were observed as responding more passively and spending more time disengaged from their newborn compared to drug-free mothers (Gottwald and Thurman, 1994). A similar pattern in maladaptive interactions was also observed in substance-using mothers parenting their child beyond infancy and into toddlerhood (Johnson et al., 2002; Molitor and Mayes, 2010).

At a neurobiological level, alterations in reward and motivational circuitry contribute to substance use, abuse and addiction (Volkow and Li, 2004; Everitt and Robbins, 2005). It has been suggested that as a consequence, decisions are made to use substances at the expense of other behaviors (e.g., relating to parenting;

Chambers et al., 2007). Specifically, in the addictive cycle, the reward system may be "co-opted" for purposes of maintaining habitual use behavior; in this process, other more adaptive rewards may not hold the same value for users if they are not part of the conditioned reward/motivation link associated with substance use. Importantly, these more adaptive rewards include social affiliation and relationships, and this kind of co-optation may have profound implications for parenting behaviors among addicted adults. Moreover, key neural regions associated with motivation and reward, including the prefrontal cortex and amygdala, are also engaged when parents perceive and/or interact with infant cues (for a review of this literature see Rutherford et al., 2011). Thus, we suggest that in addition to overt negative behavioral patterns associated with addiction that may cause difficulty in parenting (e.g., increased irritability), drug, alcohol and tobacco use may have a direct impact on maternal infant interactions in the post-partum and a direct effect on those neural systems that have been identified as important for maternal behavior.

To address this question directly, our current investigation focuses on identifying the differences between substance-using and non-using mothers in neural circuitry involved in early maternal infant attachment. Specifically, we investigate the neural response to infant expressions of emotion in recently post-partum substance-using and non-substance-using mothers. Infant-caregiver attachment is forged during early development when cries and facial expressions are the primary means of infant communication with their caregiver. The way in which a caregiver interprets and responds to these cues can directly influence the quality of the attachment between caregiver and infant, as evidenced by the adverse developmental outcomes when infant-caregiver interactions are compromised by depression or substance abuse in caregivers (Murray, 1992; Mayes et al., 1997; Network NICHD Early Child Care Research, 1999). In the current study we seek to further investigate the substance-using maternal brain response using fMRI to these early expressions of infant emotion (specifically, cries and facial expressions) relative to non-using mothers during the first three post-partum months.

PREVIOUS fMRI INVESTIGATIONS OF RESPONSE TO EMOTIONAL STIMULI IN SUBSTANCE USERS

Although there exists a fairly large literature of adult processing of emotional stimuli in both parents and non-parents (reviewed below), there is relatively little extant investigating of processing of human emotional stimuli in substance-using adults. To date, most fMRI work in this area has focused on presenting participants with craving relevant stimuli such as drug paraphernalia. These studies typically identify in association with drug cues increased activation in regions such as the anterior cingulate cortex (ACC), dorsolateral prefrontal cortex (dlPFC), orbiotofrontal cortex, amygdala and temporal regions (Breiter et al., 1997; Maas et al., 1998; Childress et al., 1999; Wexler et al., 2001). With respect to processing emotionally laden stimuli not directly associated with drug use/misuse, one fMRI study (Asenio et al., 2010) showed groups of cocaine-using and non-using subjects images from the International Affective Picture System (IAPS). These pictures are designed to elicit unpleasant, neutral, or pleasant emotions. The data revealed greater activation for controls in the pleasant condition in the superior and inferior frontal lobules (bilaterally) the anterior nucleus of the thalamus, dorsomedial prefrontal cortex (dmPFC), ACC, and right striatum. There were no group differences for negative or neutral stimuli. However, other studies have found relatively diminished activation of cortical and subcortical regions in cocaine dependent versus control subjects during the processing of simulated interpersonal interactions of sad content, with some of the regions overlapping with those relatively overactivated in cocaine dependent subjects in response to drug cues (Wexler et al., 2001). Taken together, these findings suggest that regions that may respond to rewarding stimuli (such as positive emotion or arousal) or to negative emotions (sad interpersonal interactions) are relatively deactivated in substance users compared to non-users, but that some of these regions can be activated to a greater degree in response to craving inducing stimuli.

PREVIOUS fMRI INVESTIGATIONS OF MATERNAL RESPONSE TO INFANT EMOTION (FACES AND CRIES)

Prior fMRI studies that have examined the neural response to infant cries in parents and have compared cries to non-cry acoustic stimuli (e.g., white noise), and have found greater recruitment of regions associated with auditory processing and emotional processing/regulation during the perception of cries relative to a control sound (Lorberbaum et al., 2002; Seifritz et al., 2003; Swain et al., 2007; Swain and Lorberbaum, 2008). These regions that include the hypothalamus, midbrain, basal ganglia, ACC, prefrontal cortex, and thalamus are common areas of activation associated with parental responses to infant cries in fMRI paradigms, as well as being commonly associated with motivation and reward-processing. Additionally, observed increases in activation in the insula and prefrontal cortex for cries relative to white noise suggest that circuitry associated with social cognition and empathic processes may also be relevant to parental responsiveness to cries. Notably, neural responses to cries appear to be modulated by time since delivery; mothers showed greater cingulate, amygdala, and insula activation at 2–4 weeks post-partum when listening to their own relative to another baby's cry, whereas at 3–4 months post-partum no greater activity was seen in these regions. Instead, increased activity in the medial prefrontal cortex was observed for own baby cry relative to other baby cry (Swain et al., 2003, 2004a). These findings suggest that experience with an infant over the first several months post-partum may influence the neural response to cries, and that this may reflect the functional re-organization of sensitivity to infant cues in parents.

With respect to processing of facial expression/emotion the mesocorticolimbic circuitry has been implicated in maternal responses to infant faces. For example, studies have found increased activity in the striatum, as well as increased activity in the medial prefrontal cortex, occipital cortex, insula, ACC, and in some studies amygdala and parahippocampus, when mothers view images of infants faces (Bartels and Zeki, 2004; Leibenluft et al., 2004; Nitschke et al., 2004; Strathearn et al., 2008). Furthermore, a recent fMRI study identified maternal brain responses to infant facial affective states (happy, neutral, and sad) in dopamine-associated reward-processing areas when first-time mothers viewed images of their own infants compared to unknown infants expressing comparable affective expressions (Strathearn et al., 2008). Specifically, these authors found that happy, but not neutral or sad own-infant faces, significantly activated nigrostriatal brain regions interconnected by dopaminergic neurons, including the substantia nigra and dorsal putamen. In addition, a region-of-interest (ROI) analysis in this region revealed that activation was related to positive infant affect (happy > neutral > sad) for each own–unknown infant face contrast.

The present study extends this work on maternal perception of infant cries and facial expression by examining how substance use status may relate to maternal neural response to audio and visual cues of different infant emotions. Specifically, we examine neural response to cries of varying distress levels and to faces displaying happy, sad or neutral emotion in mothers using cocaine, marijuana, tobacco, alcohol, amphetamines, heroin, opiates, or a combination of these substances (see substance use status below) relative to a group of age-matched mothers who were not users of any of these substances. We include cries of varying distress levels and faces displaying a range of emotion in order to examine systems responsible for distinguishing between different infant emotional states and needs (Wolff, 1969). Given what we know about disruptions in mother–infant interactions in substance-using populations, we predicted that substance-using mothers (compared to non-substance-using mothers) will show reduced activation in regions previously identified as being relevant for parenting (active while parents view infant faces and listening to infant cries), including sensory processing regions (visual for faces, auditory for cries), emotional processing regions such as the amygdala, insula and striatum, as well as regions involved in cognitive control such as the prefrontal cortex and cingulate.

MATERIALS AND METHODS
PARTICIPANTS
All participants provided informed consent and data were collected approximately 2 months into the post-partum period (range was 1–3 months). Substance use status was determined by a combination of self-report data and urine toxicology (see below). Sixty-two participants were initially scanned (31 substance-using and 31 non-using participants); 8 subjects were excluded due to excessive motion (5 substance-using and 3 non-using), leaving 26 substance-using and 28 non-using mothers in the sample.

Substance-using mothers
Twenty-six-English-speaking, right-handed recently post-partum mothers who used one or more teratogenic substances (see substance use status below) with normal or corrected-to-normal vision, between the ages of 18 and 42 years inclusive ($M = 25.58$ $SD = 5.64$), participated. Racial/ethnic composition included 5 Caucasian, 16 African American, and 5 Hispanic women.

Non-using mothers
Twenty-eight-English-speaking, right-handed recently post-partum mothers participated. These individuals were free of tobacco or illicit substance use, had normal or corrected-to-normal vision, and were between the ages of 17 and 42 years inclusive ($M = 29$, $SD = 5.89$). Racial/ethnic composition included 19 Caucasian, 1 Asian American, 5 African American, 1 woman of mixed race (African American and Caucasian) and 2 Hispanic women.

Additional participant information
With regard to socioeconomic status, we gathered data on maternal education level. All mothers in the non-using group had completed high school and many had completed four or more years of college (mean number of years of education = 17; SD = 3.45). In the substance-using group, 12 of the 26 had completed education through to at least high school, with 3 having gone on to college (mean years of education = 12; SD = 1.80). Seventy-eight percentage of the non-using participants were first-time mothers and 30% of the substance-using participants were first-time mothers. The mean number of children in the home for the substance-using group was 2 (SD = 0.97), and the mean number of children in the non-using group was 1 (SD = 0.89).

All participants were paid $80 and given a small gift for the baby (e.g., baby blanket, baby supplies, baby toy, or baby chair) for their participation. Participants had no neurological impairment or head injury. Written, informed consent was obtained in accordance with the Yale School of Medicine Institutional Review Board. This study has an associated certificate of confidentiality from NIDA.

Substance use status
Participants were recruited through rehabilitation facilities, maternity wards, and flyers posted on local busses and gathering spots. Substance use status was determined by a combination of self-report data and urine toxicology. Women were considered substance-using if they used any teratogenic substance (including tobacco, heroin, marijuana, opiates, cocaine, alcohol) during pregnancy and/or into the post-partum period (see **Table 1**). Because some women were in active drug treatment ($N = 2$), they may not have been using at the time of their MRI; however, if they reported substance use, they were included in the substance-using group. Conversely, if participants did not self-report use but tested positive for any of the above named substances they were included in the substance-using group as well (17 of the 26 substance-using women tested positive (urine toxicity) for one or more substances on the day of the scan). For alcohol and tobacco use, the Fagerstrom test for nicotine dependence (FTND) and alcohol use disorder identification test (AUDIT) were collected. See **Table 1** for a breakdown of particular substance use by participant.

STIMULI
Auditory stimuli
Cry stimuli were 2-s segments generated from those used by Green and Gustafson (1983). The cries came from infants who ranged in age from 27 to 32 days. All infants were healthy at birth and healthy at their 1-month checkups. Cries were recorded in the infant's home before the infants were fed. Detailed information about the recording procedure has been reported elsewhere (Green and Gustafson, 1983). For the current experiment, we chose four 2-s segments from two different infants that we determined (by two experimenters) to be either of high- or low-distress, resulting in both a high- and low-distress exemplar from each infant. Distress level was verified by an independent group of 10 female participants (ages 19–24; none of the participants had children) who rated the cries for distress level. Participants rated each cry on a scale of 1–10, with 1 representing "calm" and 10 representing

Table 1 | Substance use breakdown including the number of women using particular substances, the percentage who were identified by self-report and the percentage who were identified by urine toxicology on the day of the scan.

Substances used	N	Self-report (%)	Positive toxicology (%)
Tobacco only	10	10	90
Marijuana only	4	0	100
Alcohol only	2	100	0
Non-disclosed drugs	4	100	0
Heroin, tobacco, and cocaine	1	100	0
Alcohol and tobacco	2	100	100
Alcohol, tobacco, and other non-disclosed drugs	1	100	0
Tobacco and heroin	1	0	100
Amphetamines and tobacco	1	0	100

"distressed". High-distress cries were rated as significantly more distressed ($M = 8.06$, $SD = 1.3$) than low-distress cries ($M = 3.54$, $SD = 0.82$; $t = 11.52$, $p < 0.001$). In addition to cries, participants in the MRI study also heard a "neutral" 220-Hz pure tone. Additional information on the acoustic properties of the cries and neutral stimuli are contained in the Appendix.

Visual stimuli
Photographs of infant faces between the ages of 5 and 10 months were used; these images, initially used by Strathearn and McClure (2002), were modified to include only the baby's head and not the full body. The stimulus set consisted of 21 images from each of six infants, resulting in a total of 126 images. Infant stimuli were balanced for both gender and race and included Caucasian and African American babies. The infant face images displayed affective states of happy, neutral, and sad. The size, luminance, and contrast were kept constant for all face stimuli, and faces were presented on a gray background. Prior to imaging, face stimuli were rated by an independent group of 11 participants who were not mothers on a scale of 1 (happy) to 10 (distressed). A repeated measures ANOVA of the infant face ratings of subjective responses to the three types of emotional facial cues (happy, neutral, sad) was significant $F(2, 20) = 146.43$, $p < 0.001$. Pair-wise comparisons showed that happy faces ($M = 2.19$, $SD = 0.75$) were rated as significantly less distressed (Mean difference $= -1.55$, $SD = 1.15$, $p = 0.006$) than neutral faces ($M = 3.74$, $SD = 143$). Neutral faces were rated as significantly less distressed (Mean difference $= -4.16$, $SD = 1.28$, $p < 0.001$) than sad faces ($M = 7.90$, $SD = 0.34$).

DESIGN
The stimuli were presented using E-Prime software (Version 1.2; Psychology Software Tools Inc., Pittsburgh, PA, USA). The auditory stimuli were delivered via headphones with no visual display. The visual stimuli were displayed foveally at the fixation point for 1000 ms and followed by a fixation cross. Subjects received seven functional runs, each consisting of 42 trials (six trials of each condition of interest and six one-back memory trials). The conditions of interest were high-distress cry, low-distress cry, neutral tone, happy face, sad face, and neutral face. Trials were presented in a different randomized order in each functional run, with the constraints that the one-back catch trials could not be presented on the first trial, or immediately repeated. The duration of the inter-trial-interval (ITI) was jittered (4000–14000 ms) to allow event-related analysis and to minimize stimulus expectation.

During each run, subjects were asked to attend to the stimulus sequence of faces and cries. For the one-back memory trials (14% of total trials), subjects were presented with a row of question marks and either a visual stimulus (infant face) was presented above the question marks or an auditory stimulus (cry or tone) was delivered via the headphones. The question marks cued the subject to make a yes/no decision via a stimulus response box as to whether the current stimulus was identical to the stimulus of the preceding trial (i.e., a one-back memory task). No action was required of participants on non-catch trials. Analysis of catch trial data revealed an accuracy rate of 84% correct for non-using mothers and 70% for substance-using mothers. The rare catch trials were included to enhance and assess subjects' attention during task performance and were modeled but not included in further analyses.

DATA ACQUISITION
Data were acquired with a Siemens Trio 3T magnetic resonance imaging system (Siemens AG, Erlangen, Germany) using a standard 12-channel head coil. Localizer images were acquired for prescribing the functional image volumes, aligning the eighth slice parallel to the plane transecting the anterior and posterior commissures. Functional images were collected using a gradient echo, echoplanar sequence [repetition time (TR) = 2000 ms; echo time (TE) = 30 ms; flip angle = 80°, field of view (FOV) 20 cm × 20 cm, 64 × 64 matrix, 3.4 mm × 3.4 mm in-plane resolution, 4 mm slice thickness, 32 slices]. Each stimulus run consisted of 163 volumes, including an initial rest period of 12 s (to achieve signal stability) that was removed from analyses.

IMAGE ANALYSIS
Preprocessing
Functional data were preprocessed using SPM5 (Wellcome Functional Imaging Laboratory, London, UK), following our prior published methods (e.g., Kober et al., 2010). This included slice-time correction to the first slice of each volume; SPM's two-pass realign-to-mean strategy (which ultimately realigns all functional images to a mean functional image); coregistration of the anatomical image and the average of these realigned functional images; coregistration of all functional images using the parameters obtained from coregistration of the mean image; application of the SPM Unified Segmentation process to the anatomical scan, using prior information from the International Consortium for Brain Mapping (ICBM) Tissue Probabilistic Atlas and estimation of non-linear warping parameters (e.g., Ashburner and Friston, 2005); warping the functional images to the Montreal Neurological Institute (MNI) template space; reslicing into isometric 3 mm × 3 mm × 3 mm voxels; subsequent smoothing of functional images using a 6 mm isometric Gaussian kernel. Participants who could not be properly warped using the segmentation routine ($N = 6$) were separately normalized to the MNI structural

brain without segmentation. All images were inspected for motion in excess of one voxel (3 mm × 3 mm × 3 mm); eight participants were excluded from the analysis for excessive motion (in excess of one voxel).

GLM data analysis

Once the functional images were preprocessed, first-level robust regression was performed using the standard general linear model but with iteratively reweighted least squares using the bisquare weighting function for robustness (Wager et al., 2005; Kober et al., 2010), as implemented in MATLAB 7.3 (Mathworks, Natick, MA, USA; robust.m). Motion parameters and high-pass filter parameters were added as additional regressors of no interest. Once conditions were estimated using percent signal change for each participant, a second-level, random effects analysis was performed to estimate group activity and to compare activity between-groups, using NeuroElf (NeuroElf.net) and following our prior methods. We then used Monte-Carlo simulation implemented in Alpha Sim to identify voxels that survived whole-brain correction. Clusters were considered significant at a corrected $p < 0.05$ threshold at an uncorrected voxel-level threshold of $p < 0.005$ at each tail and a cluster of 25. Anatomical labels of all results were confirmed using the Talairach Daemon toolbox as well as manually, using a human brain atlas (Talairach and Tornoux, 1988).

RESULTS

Our primary interest was to compare activity elicited in response to infant cries and faces in substance-free mothers and substance-using mothers. We therefore performed between-group comparisons for activity during each condition. Consistent with our hypotheses, we found relatively increased activity in non-using mothers relative to substance-using mothers for both face and cry stimuli. We now discuss the non-using relative to substance-using findings for each condition (faces, cries) in turn.

FACES

Figures 1A–C shows the contrast of substance non-using > substance-using mothers in response to happy, sad and neutral faces respectively.

Happy expressions

In response to happy infant faces we observed greater activation for non-using mothers relative to substance-using mothers in prefrontal regions including ventromedial prefrontal cortex (vmPFC), the right dlPFC/middle frontal gyrus (MFG) and dmPFC (including medial and superior frontal gyri). We also observed greater activity for non-using relative to substance-using mothers in visual processing regions, such as the middle occipital gyrus, as well as in limbic regions including the right hippocampus/parahippocampus as well as in the cerebellum. We observed only one small region of increased activation for substance-using relative to non-using in the left posterior parahippocampal gyrus (see **Table 2**).

Sad expressions

In response to sad infant faces, multiple and extensive regions distinguished non-using from substance-using mothers.

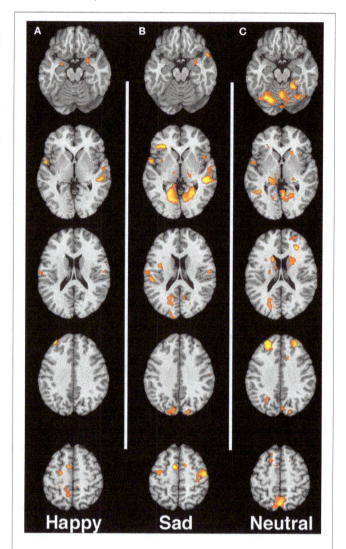

FIGURE 1 | (A–C) Contrast of non-using > substance-using mothers for happy, sad, and neutral faces, respectively. Images are shown in neurological convention, with the left hemisphere on the left side of each image. Slices are at MNI z-coordinate locations −19, −1, +17, +35, and +53 mm.

Substance-using mothers tended to show less activation in response to sad infant faces. In this condition, we observed greater activation for non-using relative to substance-using mothers in extensive regions of cortex, including prefrontal regions such as the right and left dlPFC/MFG, medial orbitofrontal cortex, right inferior frontal gyrus (IFG), sensorimotor regions, the middle/superior temporal gyrus and posterior cingulate cortex (PCC). In addition we observed greater activation for non-users in visual processing regions such as the right occipital gyrus/cuneus, and in limbic regions, including the right amygdala and parahippocampal gyrus (see **Table 3**). There were no areas that showed greater activation for substance-using relative to non-using mothers.

Neutral expressions

For the neutral faces, we again observed greater activity for the non-using relative to the substance-using in several prefrontal

Table 2 | x, y, z coordinates, max activation, and cluster size for the contrast of non-using > substance-using mothers, and substance-using > non-using mothers for happy infant faces.

x	y	z	k	Max	Region
					NU > SU
10	−39	63	57	4.314	R. postcentral gyrus/superior parietal
32	37	26	48	3.974	R. middle frontal gyrus/dlPFC
−8	14	54	50	3.923	L. medial/superior frontal gyrus/dmPFC
7	42	−12	46	3.811	R. vmPFC
30	−89	3	28	3.683	R. middle occipital gyrus
27	−34	2	57	3.591	R. hippocampus/parahippocampus
−29	−71	−12	35	3.220	L. cerebellum (declive)
					SU > NU
−34	−55	6	26	−4.358	L. posterior parahippocampal gyrus

regions including the dmPFC/medial and superior frontal gyri, vmPFC, dlPFC, and right IFG, in sensorimotor regions, visual processing areas such as the cuneus/PCC and in limbic/striatal regions including the right amygdala/parahippocampal gyrus/globus pallidus (see **Table 4**). Again, there were no areas that showed greater activation for substance-using relative to non-using mothers.

CRIES

Figures 2A,B shows the neural response for the contrast of non-using mothers > substance-using mothers for high and low-distress cries respectively.

Low-distress cries

In response to low-distress infant cries, non-using mothers showed greater activation in auditory sensory processing regions including right superior/middle temporal gyri, and prefrontal regions such as the medial frontal gyrus/pre-SMA, sensorimotor regions, as well as regions involved in emotional processing, memory and empathy such as the insula, thalamus, and bilateral amygdala/parahippocampal gyrus (See **Table 5**).

High-distress cries

In response to high-distress cries, fewer regions differentiated non-using from substance-using groups. Increased activation for non-using relative to substance-using mothers was seen in the left superior/MFG, sensorimotor regions, insula, mid cingulate gyrus/precuneus and bilateral amygdala/parahippocampal gyrus (see **Table 6**; see also **Table 7** for neural response to the tone).

DISCUSSION

In the study presented here, we used fMRI to investigate whether substance use during pregnancy or in the recent post-partum relates to neural response to infant cries and faces in post-partum mothers. We found generally reduced activation for substance-using mothers relative to non-using mothers when processing such infant-related sensory stimuli in areas that have previously been identified in parenting studies and emotional processing more generally. To our knowledge, this study provides the first empirical evidence to suggest that the neural circuitry recruited when processing infant faces and cries is altered in mothers who use substances of abuse.

Across happy, sad, and neutral face conditions, we observed greater activity for non-using relative to substance-using mothers in prefrontal regions (e.g., dlPFC, vmPFC), visual processing regions (e.g., occipital cortex) and limbic regions (e.g., hippocampus/amygdala). These regions comprise a network underscoring social, emotional and visual sensory processing, and have been previously implicated in studies exploring the neural response to facial affect (e.g., Hariri et al., 2000; Gur et al., 2002). Additionally, many of these regions overlap with those observed to be active in previous studies of parental response to infant faces such as the medial prefrontal cortex, occipital cortex, hippocampus and amygdala (e.g., Strathearn et al., 2008). However, we also note that some regions previously identified in response to infant faces, particularly in the striatum (e.g., the caudate and putamen) did not discriminate substance-using from non-using mothers in our study. Nevertheless, the generally reduced activity in substance-using relative to non-using mothers in response to infant facial expression of emotion supports the hypothesis that the neural systems associated with emotional processing of infant cues in substance-using mothers may be less responsive relative to those in non-using mothers.

With respect to cries, we also observed a large network of sensory and emotional processing regions that were more active for non-using mothers relative to substance-using mothers. For both low and high-distress cries we observed greater activation for non-using relative to substance-using mothers in auditory sensory processing regions (STG/MTG) as well as in sensorimotor/precentral gyrus, prefrontal and limbic regions (amygdala and parahippocampus bilaterally), as well as the insula. Again, many of these areas, including the amygdala, insula, MTG/STG as well as prefrontal regions, overlap with those previously identified as active for mothers in responses to infants cries (Swain et al., 2003, 2004a). Notably, we did not observe substance-related differences in all previously identified regions associated with cry perception (e.g., ACC). As with our findings for faces, these data indicate potential alterations in neural systems responsible for processing infant cries in substance-using mothers. These findings are consistent with the behavioral literature of negative parenting outcomes in situations of substance use, and may help to explain why appropriate interaction with the infant may be difficult for substance-using mothers.

Taken together, the data suggest generally reduced neural responsiveness to infant cues in substance-using compared to non-using mothers. We suggest that such reduced neural responsiveness may lead to difficulty in subsequent behavioral maternal response to the infant, and in the formation of infant-caregiver attachment. In turn, this resulting difficulty may underlie some of the parenting difficulties observed in substance-using parents. Specifically, we suggest that reduced activation may reflect reduced saliency of infant cues themselves, which may lead to late or inappropriate parental response to the infants needs. This in turn could lead to a consequent failure to comfort the infant and thus an impaired ability to build an appropriate infant-caregiver relationship. In this way, substance use may lead to a cycle of inappropriate behavioral and neurobiological responses, involving altered neurobiological

Table 3 | x, y, z coordinates, max activation, and cluster size for the contrast of non-using > substance-using mothers for sad infant faces.

				NU > SU	
x	y	z	k	Max	Region
−18	−66	−27	246	5.638743	L. cerebellum
−55	−61	−21	112	5.250342	L. cerebellum (declive)
45	−33	−3	251	4.97915	R. middle/superior temporal gyrus, inferior parietal lobule
−35	31	6	2594	4.880452	Inferior frontal gyrus (Brodmann area 46)
−35	31	6	199	4.880452	Inferior frontal gyrus (Brodmann area 46)
−47	29	4	7	4.652219	Inferior frontal gyrus (Brodmann area 45)
35	−33	−22	41	4.351667	R. culmen
−16	−42	49	254	4.30304	L. precuneus
−31	16	25	317	4.287189	L. middle frontal gyrus
27	−19	−11	59	4.26608	R. parahippocampal gyrus
−28	−32	67	30	4.211668	L. postcentral gyrus
−7	9	23	167	4.207603	L. anterior cingulate
−11	−23	1	80	4.18913	L. thalamus
10	−36	63	139	4.188221	R. paracentral lobule
−32	1	25	20	4.163018	L. precentral gyrus
13	−48	58	31	4.15905	R. precentral gyrus
12	−21	1	114	4.098029	R. precuneus
−9	−47	65	53	4.082886	L. postcentral gyrus
10	2	25	22	4.068956	R. cingulate gyrus
23	−35	−15	38	4.068416	R. culmen
−22	28	47	145	4.026933	L. superior frontal gyrus
27	−23	0	21	4.006106	R. lentiform nucleus
−50	−38	7	79	3.97014	L. superior temporal gyrus
−48	−49	14	24	3.926296	L. superior temporal gyrus
21	−30	2	6	3.916912	R. thalamus
−52	7	21	46	3.860483	L. inferior frontal gyrus
7	−36	49	6	3.820081	R. paracentral lobule
−7	−12	71	22	3.819647	L. medial frontal gyrus
−15	20	37	81	3.807613	L. cingulate gyrus
−8	17	60	41	3.807233	L. superior frontal gyrus
−3	−6	33	58	3.759351	L. cingulate gyrus
14	5	42	52	3.757323	R. cingulate gyrus
−43	29	−12	12	3.745067	L. inferior frontal gyrus
−25	13	52	21	3.742426	L. middle frontal gyrus
−7	3	47	41	3.697044	L. cingulate gyrus
40	−25	23	28	3.686666	R. insula
19	−5	14	95	3.643686	R. lentiform nucleus
16	−18	33	43	3.586584	R. cingulate gyrus
12	−15	16	7	3.543675	R. thalamus
−18	−31	8	54	3.508624	L. thalamus (pulvinar)
−34	−31	11	34	3.479951	L. superior temporal gyrus
−16	−26	71	15	3.451032	L. precentral gyrus
34	−13	24	16	3.426919	R. insula
7	−9	41	5	3.412857	R. cingulate gyrus
−3	−20	41	11	3.382658	L. paracentral lobule
−18	17	29	5	3.353571	L. cingulate gyrus
31	−26	9	5	3.331212	R. insula
−18	−18	12	28	3.325903	L. thalamus
−12	−9	10	9	3.296702	L. thalamus
15	−26	9	6	3.292171	R. thalamus
−3	−52	46	5	3.113006	L. precuneus
33	5	25	146	4.78171	R. middle frontal gyrus/precentral

(Continued)

Table 3 | Continued

x	y	z	k	NU > SU Max	Region
−13	−92	−8	179	4.573222	L. occipital/lingual gyrus/cuneus/precuneus
−49	−82	−3	35	4.387002	L. inferior occipital gyrus
−29	−10	50	62	4.316063	L. dorsolateral prefrontal cortex/precentral gyrus
−20	−15	−18	88	4.314709	L. amygdala/parahippocampal
3	−56	17	164	4.240038	R. posterior cingulate/cuneus
25	−40	−38	44	4.140538	R. cerebellum
32	37	26	102	4.1223	R. dorsolateral prefrontal cortex/middle frontal gyrus
−36	−28	37	94	4.072572	L. postcentral gyrus
−7	42	−18	61	4.009093	L. medial orbitofrontal cortex
53	−76	−12	65	3.959023	R. lateral occipital/cerebellum
−23	38	28	39	3.956656	L. superior frontal gyrus
−18	−40	−37	159	3.918909	L. cerebellum/posterior parahippocampal gyrus
−45	−63	4	26	3.895407	L. middle temporal gyrus
19	−9	−14	39	3.870903	R. amygdala/parahippocampal
33	−89	3	125	3.849272	R. occipital/cuneus
9	−80	−21	25	3.817537	R. cerebellum (declive)
58	9	7	50	3.796894	R. inferior frontal gyrus
55	−3	47	42	3.668281	R. dorsolateral prefrontal cortex/precentral gyrus
53	−49	4	57	3.591696	R. middle temporal gyrus
17	12	−15	42	3.587929	R. orbital gyrus
38	−9	50	33	3.587715	R. precentral gyrus
−57	−35	38	83	3.414358	L. inferior parietal lobule
37	−64	−15	25	3.365405	R. cerebellum (declive)
32	−19	67	26	3.33502	R. precentral gyrus

responses to infant sensory stimuli early in motherhood. Indeed extant work has demonstrated that the ability of mothers to detect signal differences in cries at the sensory level is important for providing an appropriate response to infant actions, which has implications for mother–child attachment (e.g., Donnovan et al., 2007).

Somewhat surprisingly, we found almost no regions that were more active for substance-using relative to non-using mothers. We might have expected that substance-using mothers would have shown heightened activation in stress related circuits, reflecting the idea that infant cues are less rewarding and more stressful for substance-using mothers, particularly for negative or

Table 4 | x, y, z coordinates, max activation, and cluster size for the contrast of non-using > substance-using mothers for neutral infant faces.

x	y	z	k	NU > SU Max	Region
−12	20	49	153	4.883	L. medial/superior frontal gyrus
37	−23	61	231	4.463	R. precentral/postcentral gyus; SMA
9	−75	24	475	4.448	R. posterior cingulate cortex/cuneus
−40	27	4	168	4.318	L. inferior frontal gyrus
−7	40	−12	145	4.145	L. ventromedial prefrontal cortex/medial orbitofrontal gyrus, subgenual ACC
3	−36	52	328	4.004	R. postcentral gyrus/mid cingulate cortex, precuneus
−16	44	30	35	3.810	L. superior/medial frontal gyrus, dmPFC
7	5	25	31	3.746	R. mid cingulate gyrus
−34	−60	−15	42	3.673	L. cerebellum (declive)
36	−80	28	28	3.669	R. superior occipital gyrus
11	11	52	31	3.631	R. medial frontal gyrus
−32	−66	−31	35	3.627	L. cerebellum
−49	−1	38	26	3.584	L. dlPFC
36	17	−20	47	3.529	R. inferior frontal gyrus/superior temporal gyrus
−61	−37	7	29	3.389	L. posterior middle temporal gyrus
25	−9	−1	28	3.379	R. amygdala/parahippocampal/globus pallidus

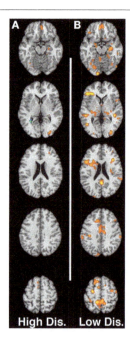

FIGURE 2 | (A,B) Contrast of non-using > substance-using for low-distress and high-distress cries respectively. Slices are at MNI z-coordinate locations −16, +2, +20, +38, and +56 mm.

upsetting stimuli (e.g., cries). For example, Sinha et al. (2005) have found that cocaine dependant but currently abstinent participants showed increased activation of corticolimbic circuitry (caudate and dorsal striatum) for stressful stimuli relative to healthy controls. Instead, we observed only one small region of increased activity in the left parahippocampus for happy faces. This null finding may be due to the nature of the stimuli and the populations being explored; that is, response to emotional or stressful stimuli may be particularly blunted in the presence of substance use, possibly via the mechanism of co-opting of motivation/reward circuitry. Alternatively, it is possible that the system is simply less responsive overall, or that the pattern of responding in substance-using mothers is far more variable; future research will be necessary to directly address these possibilities. Such research could possibly include images that are likely to elicit increased response in substance users, such as paraphernalia, or stimuli that are more stressful than infant cries.

One of the important limitations of the present study is the heterogeneity of substances that were used by the mothers in our sample. Indeed the consequences of different substances of abuse vary at neurochemical as well as behavioral levels. In this sample, we are focusing on the impact of an addictive process on the response to what would be expected to be salient cues. Future studies should examine the potential impact of specific substances (and the quantity/frequency of their use) on the neural responses to infant stimuli, as well as investigate groups of parents (both mothers and fathers) with specific addictions. We also note differences between the groups in terms of maternal education and number of children in the home, as well as racial distribution across the groups as potential limitations of the current study; these factors are very difficult to match in studies of substance use, particularly in the case of SES/maternal education and race, as substance users tend to have lower SES than non-users, and are more often members of minority groups. We acknowledge that these factors may influence the results as they may influence home environments and parenting styles and thus should be examined further in future research. Nevertheless, the result of this study represent an important and novel step in identifying the impact of substance use on maternal responding.

Table 5 | x, y, z coordinates, max activation, and cluster size for the contrast of non-using > substance-using mothers for low-distress infant cries.

					NU > SU
x	y	z	k	Max	Region
50	−37	2	227	4.927	R. superior/middle temporal gyrus
−24	−4	−17	48	4.734	L. amygdala/parahippocampal gyrus
−34	28	6	108	4.604	L. inferior frontal gyrus
−11	3	50	75	4.328	L. medial frontal gyrus/pre-SMA/dorsal cingulate gyrus
22	−59	3	523	4.254	R. lingual gyrus/fusiform gyrus/cuneus/middle occipital gyrus
−52	−30	21	83	4.252	Posterior insula/postcentral gyrus
51	−17	49	247	4.228	R. postcentral gyrus
−18	−53	−4	647	4.158	L. lingual gyrus/fusiform gyrus/posterior parahippocampal/cuneus/middle occipital gyrus
−57	−1	6	119	4.023	L. mid/anterior insula/precentral gyrus
51	−68	−6	29	4.017	R. lateral middle occipital gyrus
53	8	−12	219	3.955	R. amygdala/parahippocampal/middle temporal/superior temporal gyrus
−37	−11	43	145	3.893	L. precentral gyrus
−18	−20	9	24	3.818	L. thalamus
−19	−29	67	32	3.779	L. precentral gyrus
15	−21	7	29	3.718	R. thalamus
25	−35	44	29	3.543	R. postcentral gyrus
47	7	6	24	3.524	R. insula
14	2	47	60	3.397	R. medial frontal gyrus/pre-SMA/dorsal cingulate/gyrus

Table 6 | x, y, z coordinates, max activation, and cluster size for the contrast of non-using > substance-using mothers for high-distress infant cries.

				NU > SU	
x	y	z	k	Max	Region
−41	42	33	27	4.459	L. superior/middle frontal gyrus/dlPFC
−54	−3	6	38	4.295	L. precentral gyrus/mid insula
50	−34	0	65	4.219	R. middle temporal gyrus
−64	−19	15	29	4.107	L. postcentral gyrus
−26	−12	53	87	4.037	L. precentral gyrus
13	−18	41	273	4.001	R. mid cingulate/precuneus
62	−25	20	49	3.923	R. postcentral gyrus
66	−1	16	35	3.683	R. precentral gyrus
−11	3	50	39	3.630	L. medial frontal gyrus/pre-SMA/dorsal cingulate gyrus
28	0	−12	49	3.540	R. amygdala/parahippocampal gyrus
53	−20	3	33	3.538	R. superior temporal gyrus
−24	−7	−12	23	3.366	L. amygdala/parahippocampal gyrus
13	−33	63	31	3.288	R. postcentral gyrus
−22	−26	61	31	3.097	L. postcentral gyrus

Table 7 | x, y, z coordinates, max activation, and cluster size for the contrast of non-using > substance-using mothers for the pure tone.

				NU > SU	
x	y	z	k	Max	Regions
−29	43	31	168	5.294	L. superior frontal gyrus
32	34	27	246	5.044	R. superior/middle frontal gyrus/dlPFC
−21	−29	−1	247	4.975	L. thalamus/midbrain/posterior cingulate
−7	−80	−6	1583	4.694	L. cerebellum/lingual/occipital gyrus
−35	31	9	37	4.578	L. inferior/middle frontal gyrus
15	−86	35	585	4.485	R. precuneus/cuneus/posterior cingulate cortex
−8	11	66	64	4.426	L. superior/medial frontal gyrus
25	7	60	97	4.247	R. superior/anterior cingulate gyrus
−43	−52	1	40	4.072	L. inferior temporal gyrus
−20	14	14	87	3.989	L. dorsal caudate
23	10	17	132	3.930	R. dorsal caudate
−47	−57	43	27	3.739	Inferior temporal gyrus
−54	0	6	26	3.555	Superior temporal/insula
27	−25	0	57	3.520	Lateral ventral thalamus
−34	−87	−1	26	3.318	Middle occipital gyrus
−22	−12	17	25	3.316	Thalamus
−22	14	49	37	3.313	Superior frontal gyrus

It will be important for future work to further explore individual differences among substance-using and non-using mothers in order to better understand the underlying contributing factors responsible for behavioral and neurobiological differences associated with parenting under conditions of substance use. For instance, substance-using mothers report higher levels of stress than non-substance-using mothers (Kelley, 1998), and maternal stress is considered to be an important mediator of parenting, as well as child outcomes (Suchman and Luthar, 2001). Substance-abusing mothers may also be more likely to have undergone emotional or physical trauma and like stress, this may impact their parenting. Future studies investigating possible contributions related to stress and trauma, as well as domains that might be influenced by stress and trauma exposure (e.g., mood and attention) warrant direct investigation. Moreover, additional research on the neural circuitry associated with response to emotion under conditions of substance use/addiction in mothers will be necessary to determine whether our observed findings are specific to infant emotion and social cues or reflect a more general reduced sensitivity in circuits involved in emotion processing. Because the current investigation focused on infant emotional stimuli, it is not possible to determine if the observed effects of substance use on brain activation would generalize to other types of relevant stimuli. One additional area for future exploration, which has been explored in non-abusing parents, is the degree to which processing of images or cries of one's own infant mediates neural responses. With respect to substance use, it would be helpful to determine whether some of the differences we observed between substance users and non-users are alleviated when mothers view their own relative to an unknown infant; it is possible that viewing or listening to one's own infant will be more salient, thus mitigating our observed altered response. Exploring these factors along with better understanding the specificity of the response to infant emotion/cues compared to other social/emotional cues and the effects of specific drugs and degrees of addiction will go a long way toward furthering our understanding of parenting under conditions of substance use and abuse.

Finally, one important implication from our findings of altered neural circuitry in response to infant cues in substance-using post-partum mothers is that interventions that focus on improving mother–child interactions rather than simply on eliminating substance use may be equally important for improving mother–child attachment in the presence of substance use. Specifically, increasing the amount and quality of appropriate mother–child interaction in the post-partum may help to retune the circuitry involved in reward/motivation and parenting. Recent work focusing on mother–child interactions in substance-using mothers to increase maternal mindfulness of the baby has had positive results, including improvements in observed mother–toddler interactions (e.g., Suchman et al., 2008). Future work that examines functional neural activity before and after this style of intervention would be useful for determining whether improvements in observed behavior correspond with changes in the underlying neural circuitry and more generally if there is significant plasticity in the neural circuitry for parenting in substance-abusing mothers.

ACKNOWLEDGMENTS

This work was supported by the NIH (NIDA) grants P01 DA022446 and R01 DA026437. This publication was also made possible by CTSA Grant Number UL1 RR024139 from the National Center for Research Resources (NCRR), a component of the National Institutes of Health (NIH), and NIH roadmap for Medical Research. Its contents are solely the responsibility of the authors and do not necessarily represent the official view of any of the funding agencies. The authors report that they have no financial conflicts of interest with respect to the content of this manuscript. Dr. Potenza has received financial support or compensation for the following: Dr. Potenza has consulted for and advised Boehringer Ingelheim; has consulted for and has financial interests in Somaxon; has received research support from the National Institutes of Health, Veteran's Administration, Mohegan Sun Casino, the National Center for Responsible Gaming and its affiliated Institute for Research on Gambling Disorders, and Forest Laboratories, Ortho-McNeil, Oy-Control/Biotie, Glaxo-SmithKline and Psyadon pharmaceuticals; has participated in surveys, mailings or telephone consultations related to drug addiction, impulse control disorders or other health topics; has consulted for law offices and the federal public defender's office in issues related to impulse control disorders; provides clinical care in the Connecticut Department of Mental Health and Addiction Services Problem Gambling Services Program; has performed grant reviews for the National Institutes of Health and other agencies; has guest-edited journal sections; has given academic lectures in grand rounds, CME events and other clinical or scientific venues; and has generated books or book chapters for publishers of mental health texts. The other authors reported no biomedical financial interests or other conflicts of interest. We also thank Dr. James Green for sharing his cry stimuli with us, Max Greger-Moser for assisting with collection of cry rating data, Marion Mayes for coordinating visits and working with participants and Kara Holcomb for overseeing the fMRI visits with participants.

REFERENCES

Asenio, S., Romero, M. J., Palu, C., Sanchez, A., Senebre, I., Morales, J., Carcelen, R., and Romero, F. (2010). Altered neural response of the appetitive emotional system in cocaine addiction: an fRMI study. *Addict. Biol.* 15, 504–516.

Ashburner, J., and Friston, K. J. (2005). Unified segmentation. *Neuroimage* 26, 839–851.

Bartels, A., and Zeki, S. (2004). The neural correlates of maternal and romantic love. *Neuroimage* 21, 1155–1166.

Breiter, H. C., Gollub, R. L., Weisskoff, R. M., Kennedy, D. N., Makris, N., Berke, J. D., Goodman, J. M., Kantor, H. L., Gastfriend, D. R., Riorden, J. P., Mathew, R. T., Rosen, B. R., and Hyman, S. E. (1997). Acute effects of cocaine on human brain activity and emotion. *Neuron* 19, 591–611.

Chambers, R. A., Bickel, W. K., and Potenza, M. N. (2007). A scale-free systems theory of motivation and addiction. *Neurosci. Biobehav. Rev.* 31, 1017–1045.

Childress, A. R., Mozley, P. D., McElgin, W., Fitzgerald, J., Reivich, M., and O'Brien, C. P. (1999). Limbic activation during cue-induced cocaine craving. *Am. J. Psychiatry* 156, 11–18.

Donnovan, W., Leavitt, L., Taylor, N., and Border, J. (2007). Maternal sensory sensitivity, mother-infant 9-month interacton, infant attachment status: predictors of mother-toddler interaction at 24 months. *Infant Behav. Dev.* 30, 336–352.

Everitt, B. J., and Robbins, T. W. (2005). Neural systems of reinforcement for drug addiction: from actions to habits to compulsion. *Nat. Neurosci.* 8, 1481–1489.

Gottwald, S. R., and Thurman, S. K. (1994). The effects of prenatal cocaine exposure on mother-infant interaction and infant arousal in the newborn period. *Topics Early Child. Spec. Educ.* 14, 217–231.

Green, J. A., and Gustafson, G. E. (1983). Individual recognition of human infants on the basis of cries alone. *Dev. Psychobiol.* 16, 485–493.

Gur, R. C., Schroeder, L., Turner, T., McGrath, C., Chan, R. M., Turetsky, B. I., Alsop, D., Maldjian, J., and Gur, R. E. (2002). Brain activation during facial emotion processing. *Neuroimage* 16, 651–662.

Hariri, A. R., Bookheimer, S. Y., and Mazziotta, J. C. (2000). Modulating emotional responses: effects of a neocortical network on the limbic system. *NeuroReport* 11, 43–48.

Johnson, A. L., Morrow, C. E., Accornero, V. H., Xue, L., Anthony, J. C., and Bandstra, E. S. (2002). Maternal cocaine use: estimated effects on mother-child play interactions in the preschool period. *J. Dev. Behav. Pediatr.* 23, 191–202.

Kelley, S. J. (1998). Stress and coping behaviors of substance-abusing mothers. *J. Soc. Pediatr. Nurs.* 3, 103–110.

Kober, H., Mende-Siedlecki, P., Kross, E., Weber, J., Mischel, W., Hart, C., and Ochsner, K. N. (2010). Prefrontal striatal pathway underlies cognitive regulation of craving. *Proc. Natl. Acad. Sci. U.S.A.* 107, 14811–14816.

Leibenluft, E., Gobbini, M. I., Harrison, T., and Haxby, J. V. (2004). Mothers' neural activation in response to pictures of their children and other children. *Biol. Psychiatry* 56, 225–232.

Lorberbaum, J. P., Newman, J. D., Horwitz, A. R., Dubno, J. R., Lydiard, R. B., Hamner, M. B., Bohning, D. E., and George, M. S. (2002). A potential role for thalamocingulate circuitry in human maternal behavior. *Biol. Psychiatry* 51, 431–445.

Maas, L. C., Lukas, S. E., Kaufman, M. J., Weiss, R. D., Daniels, S. L., Rogers, V. W., Kukes, T. J., and Renshaw, P. F. (1998). Functional magnetic resonance imaging of human brain activation during cue-induced cocaine craving. *Am. J. Psychiatry* 155, 124–126.

Mayes, L. C., Feldman, R., Granger, R. H., Haynes, O. M., Bornstein, M. H., and Schottenfeld, R. (1997). The effects of polydrug use with and without cocaine on mother-infant interaction at 3 and 6 months. *Infant Behav. Dev.* 20, 489–502.

Mayes, L. C., and Sean T. D. (2002). "Substance abuse and parenting," in *Handbook of Parenting. Vol. 4. Social Conditions and Applied Parenting*, 2nd Edn, ed. M. H. Bornstein (Mahwah, NJ: Lawrence Erlbaum Associates Publishers), 329–359.

Molitor, A., and Mayes, L. C. (2010). Problematic dyadic interaction among toddlers and their polydrug-cocaine-using mothers. *Infant Ment. Health J.* 31, 121–140.

Murray, L. (1992). The impact of postnatal depression on infant development. *J. Child Psychol. Psychiatry* 33, 543–561.

Network NICHD Early Child Care Research. (1999). Child care and mother-child interaction in the first 3 years of life. *Dev. Psychol.* 35, 1399–1413.

Nitschke, J. B., Nelson, E. E., Rusch, B. D., Fox, A. S., Oakes, T. R., and Davidson, R. J. (2004). Orbitofrontal cortex tracks positive mood in mothers viewing pictures of their newborn infants. *Neuroimage* 21, 583–592.

Rutherford, H., Williams, S., Moy, S., Mayes, L., and Johns, J. (2011). Disruption of maternal parenting circuitry by addictive process: rewiring of reward and stress systems.

Seifritz, E., Esposito, F., Neuhoff, J. G., Luthi, A., Mustovic, H., Dammann, G., von Bardeleben, U., Radue, E. W., Cirillo, S., Tedeschi, G., and Di Salle, F. (2003). Differential sex-independent amygdala response to infant crying and laughing in parents versus nonparents. *Biol. Psychiatry* 54, 1367–1375.

Sinha, R., Lacadie, C., Skudlarski, P., Fulbright, R. K., Rounsaville, B. J., Kosten, T. R., and Wexler, B. E. (2005). Neural activity associated with stress-induced cocaine craving: a functional magnetic imaging study. *Psychopharmacology (Berl.)* 183, 171–180.

Strathearn, L., Li, J., Fonagy, P., and Montague, P. R. (2008). What's in a smile? Maternal brain responses to infant facial cues. *Pediatrics* 122, 40–51.

Strathearn, L., and McClure, S. M. (2002). *A Functional MRI Study of Maternal Responses to Infant Facial Cues*. Program No. 517.2.2002 Abstract Viewer/Itinerary Planner, Washington, DC: Social Neuroscience. [Abstract Online].

Suchman, N., Decoste, C., Castiglioni, N., Legow, N., and Mayes, L. (2008). The mothers and toddlers program: preliminary findings from an attachment-based parenting intervention for substance-abusing mothers. *Psychoanal. Psychol.* 25, 499–517.

Suchman, N. E., and Luthar, S. S. (2001). The mediating role of parenting stress in methadone-maintained mothers' parenting. *Parent. Sci. Pract.* 1, 285–315.

Swain, J. E., Leckman, J. F., Mayes, L. C., Feldman, R., Constable, R. T., and Schultz, R. (2003). "The neural circuitry of parent-infant attachment in the early postpartum," in *American College of Neuropsychopharmacology 42nd Annual Meeting*, San Juan.

Swain, J. E., Leckman, J. F., Mayes, L. C., Feldman, R., Constable, R. T., and Schultz, R. T. (2004a). Neural substrates of human parent-infant attachment in the postpartum. *Biol. Psychiatry* 55, 153s.

Swain, J. E., Mayes, L. C., and Leckman, J. F. (2004b). The development of parent-infant attachment through dynamic and interactive signaling loops of care and cry. *Behav. Brain Sci.* 27, 472–473.

Swain, J. E., and Lorberbaum, J. P. (2008). "Imaging the parental brain," in *Neurobiology of the Parental Brain*, ed. R. S. Bridges (London: Elsevier), 83–110.

Swain, J. E., Lorberbaum, J. P., Kose, S., and Strathearn, L. (2007). Brain basis of early parent–infant interactions: psychology, physiology, and in vivo functional neuroimaging studies. *J. Child Psychol. Psychiatry* 48, 262–287.

Talairach, J., and Tornoux, P. (1988). *Co-planar Stereotaxic Atlas of the Human Brain: 3-Dimensional Proportional System: An Approach to Cerebral Imaging*. Stuttgart: Georg Thieme.

U.S. Dept. of Health and Human Services, National Center for Health Statistics, and National Health Interview Survey. (1999). ICPSR version. Hyattsville, MD: U.S. Dept. of Health and Human Services, National Center for Health Statistics 1999; Ann Arbor, MI: Inter-university Consortium for Political and Social Research 2002.

Volkow, N. D., and Li, T. K. (2004). Drug addiction: the neurobiology of behaviour gone awry. *Nat. Rev. Neurosci.* 5, 963–970.

Wager, T. D., Keller, M. C., Lacey, S. C., and Jonides, J. (2005). Increased sensitivity in neuroimaging analyses using robust regression. *Neuroimage* 26, 99–113.

Wexler, B. E., Gottschalk, C. H., Fulbright, R. F., Prohovnik, I., Lacadie, C. M., Rounsaville, B. J., and Gore, J. C. (2001). fMRI of cocaine craving. *Am. J. Psychiatry* 158, 86–95.

Wolff, P. H. (1969). "The natural history of crying and other vocalizations in early infancy," in *Determinants of Infant Behaviour IV*, ed. B. M Foss (London: Methuen), 81–109.

Prenatal stress alters progestogens to mediate susceptibility to sex-typical, stress-sensitive disorders, such as drug abuse

Cheryl A. Frye[1,2,3,4]*, Jason J. Paris[1], Danielle M. Osborne[1], Joannalee C. Campbell[5] and Tod E. Kippin[5]

[1] Department of Psychology, University at Albany-State University of New York, Albany, NY, USA
[2] Department of Biological Sciences, University at Albany-State University of New York, Albany, NY, USA
[3] The Centers for Life Sciences, University at Albany-State University of New York, Albany, NY, USA
[4] Neuroscience Research, University at Albany-State University of New York, Albany, NY, USA
[5] Department of Psychology, University of California, Santa Barbara, CA, USA

*Correspondence:
Cheryl A. Frye, Life Sciences 1049, The University at Albany-State University of New York, Albany, NY 12222, USA.
e-mail: cafrye@albany.edu

Maternal–offspring interactions begin prior to birth. Experiences of the mother during gestation play a powerful role in determining the developmental programming of the central nervous system. In particular, stress during gestation alters developmental programming of the offspring resulting in susceptibility to sex-typical and stress-sensitive neurodevelopmental, neuropsychiatric, and neurodegenerative disorders. However, neither these effects, nor the underlying mechanisms, are well understood. Our hypothesis is that allopregnanolone, during gestation, plays a particularly vital role in mitigating effects of stress on the developing fetus and may mediate, in part, alterations apparent throughout the lifespan. Specifically, altered balance between glucocorticoids and progestogens during critical periods of development (stemming from psychological, immunological, and/or endocrinological stressors during gestation) may permanently influence behavior, brain morphology, and/or neuroendocrine-sensitive processes. 5α-reduced progestogens are integral in the developmental programming of sex-typical, stress-sensitive, and/or disorder-relevant phenotypes. Prenatal stress (PNS) may alter these responses and dysregulate allopregnanolone and its normative effects on stress axis function. As an example of a neurodevelopmental, neuropsychiatric, and/or neurodegenerative process, this review focuses on responsiveness to drugs of abuse, which is sensitive to PNS and progestogen milieu. This review explores the notion that allopregnanolone may effect, or be influenced by, PNS, with consequences for neurodevelopmental-, neuropsychiatric-, and/or neurodegenerative-relevant processes, such as addiction.

Keywords: addiction, alcohol, allopregnanolone, cocaine, dopamine, prenatal stress, serotonin, sex differences

INTRODUCTION

From the moment of conception, mothers provide a supportive environment for offspring development. Mother–fetus interactions during this period are largely mediated by hormonal communication. Progestogens, pro-gestational hormones, such as progesterone (P_4) and its 5α-reduced/3α-hydroxylated metabolite, allopregnanolone (AlloP), may play an important role in developmental programming of offspring, which can have pervasive effects throughout the lifespan. How responses to specific challenges, during critical periods of development, alter the vulnerability or phenotype of offspring, and the potential mediation of AlloP, is the subject of this review. This review discusses findings regarding *in utero* maternal–offspring interactions via prenatal stress (PNS), which may influence drug effects and addiction, as well as other neurodevelopment-, neuropsychiatric-, and/or neurodegenerative-relevant processes in people and animal models. The emphasis on PNS and vulnerability to substance use and addiction may be one example of behavioral programming that can be influenced by pervasive changes in neuroendocrine milieu. The impact of PNS on addiction and drug effects is discussed. Next, how addiction-relevant brain circuits are changed by PNS is covered. Then, the role of stress and neuroendocrine regulation, as mediators of these effects are summarized. In particular, the role of progestogens, which mediate the stress axis and exert activating and/or organizing functions, are emphasized. The broader context and the role of AlloP mediating neurodevelopmental, neuropsychiatric, and/or neurodegenerative functions, that are relevant for drug abuse, are integrated. Thus, this review focuses on putative neuroendocrine mechanisms by which PNS may confer vulnerability to addiction and/or its related sequelae.

IMPACT OF PRENATAL STRESS ON ANIMAL MODELS OF ADDICTION AND VULNERABILITY

Prenatal stress increases the vulnerability to engagement in drug of abuse consumption. Several studies have revealed that PNS heightens the response to, and/or seeking of, stimulant drugs. Enhanced psychomotor activation in response to stimulants occurs in adult PNS male rats following challenge with amphetamine (Deminiere et al., 1992), cocaine (Kippin et al., 2008), or nicotine (Koehl et al., 2000), as well as in adolescent females (males were not examined in this report) following challenge with methylenedioxymethamphetamine (Morley-Fletcher et al., 2004). Further, greater behavioral sensitization has been observed in adult PNS males following repeated amphetamine injections (Henry et al., 1995) and in adult PNS females, but not males, following repeated cocaine injections (Thomas et al., 2009). Additionally, PNS appears to alter amphetamine-induced directional biases in adult female and male rats (Weinstock and Fride, 1989). Thus, PNS-induced changes in developmental programming impact subsequent psychomotor stimulant responses in both males and females, yet, PNS males may exhibit a more robust response to amphetamines.

Despite having different mechanisms of action, PNS can increase intake and seeking behavior of several drugs of abuse, including amphetamines, cocaine, and alcohol. Adult PNS male rats trained to self-administer amphetamine (30 μl/infusion, IV) or cocaine (escalating 0.3–0.5 mg/kg/infusion, IV) exhibit higher intakes, as well as response rates, relative to controls (Deminiere et al., 1992; Thomas et al., 2009). PNS may also influence the response to alcohol and increase alcohol-seeking behavior. Adult PNS rats show blunted effects of alcohol on autonomic measures, including body temperature, and behavioral measures (DeTurck and Pohorecky, 1987). Moreover, PNS consistently increases the intake and response rate during operant self-administration of alcohol in male mice (Campbell et al., 2009), while the impact of PNS on female intake and response rates is more variable (Campbell et al., 2010). Interestingly, sex differences have been observed in these effects. No effect of PNS was observed on the intake or response rates in females self-administering cocaine (escalating 0.3–0.5 mg/kg/infusion, IV), despite these animals exhibiting enhanced psychomotor stimulant sensitization compared to control females (Thomas et al., 2009). In comparison, another study (Kippin et al., 2008) using a higher, but constant, dose of cocaine (1.0 mg/kg), revealed a non-significant trend toward increased intake in PNS relative to control males. Moreover, these PNS males exhibited significantly greater responding under extinction conditions and greater cocaine-primed (5 and 10 mg/kg) reinstatement of cocaine-seeking behavior compared to controls (Kippin et al., 2008). Further, observations of a PNS-induced blunted response to alcohol and an increased motivation for alcohol, resemble the widely supported observations that an initially blunted response to alcohol challenge is highly correlated with vulnerability to alcohol abuse and alcoholism development in humans (reviewed in Schuckit, 2009). Overall, the pre-clinical data indicate that PNS interacts with stress exposure and sex to impact subsequent drug-seeking behavior to increase addiction vulnerability to a variety of drugs of abuse.

Given the divergent mechanisms of action between drugs of abuse, PNS may play a broader role to influence reward by perturbing targets and substrates that are important for pharmacological reinforcement. Indeed, PNS produces a variety of age-dependent alterations in cellular connectivity and plasticity in limbic-corticostriatal regions that may be associated with reward. PNS studies report decreased spine densities in CA1 and CA3 regions of the hippocampus among adult rats (Martinez-Tellez et al., 2009). Our own data demonstrate reduced synaptic spine density in dorsal hippocampus of adolescent (28- to 30-day-old) rats exposed to variable PNS stressors (Paris and Frye, 2011b). The limbic system, comprising interconnected circuits in the cortex, amygdala, and hippocampus, along with the striatum and brainstem monoamine modulatory systems, appears to exhibit similar activation by reward and different classes of abuse drugs. Glutamatergic signaling, both between limbic structures and in projections to striatal and brainstem structures, are also widely implicated in reward and addiction processes (see, e.g., Gass and Olive, 2008; Kalivas et al., 2009; Volkow et al., 2010). PNS increases NMDA receptor binding in medial and dorsal prefrontal cortex (PFC), CA1, dorsal striatum (dSTR), and nucleus accumbens (NAcc), as well as, group III metabotropic glutamate receptor binding in both the medial and dorsal PFC (Berger et al., 2002; Barros et al., 2004). We have observed that PNS also decreases basal extracellular levels of glutamate measured by conventional microdialysis in the NAcc, but not in the PFC, of male rats (Kippin et al., 2008).

Prenatal stress also produces changes in the serotonin and norepinephrine monoamine systems throughout limbo-corticostriatal circuitry. PNS increases serotonin and 5-HIAA total content in the dSTR (Gerardin et al., 2005) and PNS males, but not females, show significantly lower levels of 5-HT1A receptor binding in the ventral hippocampus (Van den Hove et al., 2006). PNS rats also exhibit decreased basal extracellular levels of serotonin measured by conventional microdialysis in the NAcc, but not in the PFC (Kippin et al., 2008). Conversely, basal levels of norepinephrine are lower in the NAcc of adolescent, but not adult, PNS rats (Silvagni et al., 2008) and in the PFC of both adult and adolescent PNS rats (Carboni et al., 2010). Given the roles of serotonin and norepinephrine in the regulation of dopamine systems and addiction (see, e.g., Goodman, 2008; Sofuoglu and Sewell, 2009), actions within these areas are widely believed to mediate the reinforcing properties of abused drugs, as well as play critical roles in addiction processes (reviewed in, e.g., McBride and Li, 1998; Lapish et al., 2006; Feltenstein and See, 2008; Koob and Volkow, 2010). Neuroplastic changes that are promoted by prolonged drug use may exert effects that are long-term and pervasive (Tindell et al., 2005). Within these reward circuits, PNS may also have pervasive effects to reduce the spine density of the medium spiny cells of the NAcc in adult, but not pre-adolescent, male rats (Martinez-Tellez et al., 2009). Thus, PNS has effects to alter the morphology and neurotransmitter activity of the rodent brain, which may have pervasive effects to influence reward responding throughout life.

Changes in neural structure and activity associated with PNS interact with drugs of abuse to influence their effects. In addition to PNS-induced changes under basal conditions, neurotransmitter responses are further altered with drug administration in PNS rodents. Cocaine-naïve and -experienced PNS males exhibit both greater dopamine and glutamate release in the NAcc, but not PFC, during acute cocaine challenge (Kippin et al., 2008). Acute amphetamine, but not nicotine, challenge produces greater dopamine release in the NAcc in both PNS adolescent and adult rats compared to controls (Silvagni et al., 2008), whereas amphetamine challenge also produces lower dopamine release in the PFC of adult PNS offspring (Carboni et al., 2010). Conversely, both amphetamine and nicotine challenge produced greater norepinephrine release in the NAcc of adult, but not adolescent, PNS rats (Silvagni et al., 2008). Amphetamine and nicotine challenge produced larger and smaller, respectively, norepinephrine release in the PFC of adult, but not adolescent, PNS rats (Carboni et al., 2010). Thus, PNS alters the circuitry mediating addiction-related behaviors in both drug-naïve and -experienced individuals under both basal and drug challenge conditions. However, the precise roles of these basal and drug-induced alterations to elevate drug-seeking behavior or drug-induced plasticity remain to be clarified. Moreover, how PNS alters natural reward processes is of interest.

IMPACT OF PRENATAL STRESS ON ANIMAL MODELS OF NATURAL REWARD

Natural rewards, as well as pharmacological rewards, via drugs of abuse, interact with PNS to affect the mesocorticolimbic and nigrostriatal dopamine systems. Actions of these systems are involved in providing incentive salience to stimuli and inducing, or maintaining, the performance of goal-directed behavior (e.g., Ikemoto and Panksepp, 1999; Salamone et al., 2009). The midbrain ventral tegmental area (VTA) is an important region involved in endogenously rewarding behavior and has been considered to be among the most important regions underlying pharmacological and natural reward (Nestler and Carlezon, 2006). The VTA receives glutamatergic inputs from the hippocampus, PFC, and amygdala, as well as monoaminergic inputs from the dorsal raphe, locus coeruleus, and hypothalamus and projects dopaminergic efferents to GABAergic neurons in the NAcc (reviewed in Nestler and Carlezon, 2006). Among rodents, engaging in mating is rewarding and can condition a place preference (Frye et al., 1998; Paredes and Vazquez, 1999; Meerts and Clark, 2007). In the VTA, actions at dopamine type 1-like receptors facilitate (while actions at dopamine type 2-like receptors inhibit) mating in female rodents (Frye et al., 2004, 2006a; Sumida et al., 2005; Frye and Walf, 2008b). Dopamine is a necessary component involved in the motivational processes that facilitate mating among female rats (Becker et al., 2001). Some of these actions may be progestogen-dependent. Microinfusion of AlloP to the VTA enhances mating in female rodents in minutes (Frye et al., 2006a, 2008). Blocking D1 receptors attenuates AlloP's intra-VTA actions to enhance mating among female rats (Frye et al., 2004, 2006a). Indeed, PNS alters mating responses in adult female rats (Frye and Orecki, 2002) and increases total dopamine content in the dSTR (Gerardin et al., 2005), and NAcc (Alonso et al., 1994, 1997; McArthur et al., 2005). Notably, dopaminergic pharmacotherapy can bolster the motivational aspects of reward in animal models (Tindell et al., 2005).

Actions of AlloP in the VTA of the midbrain are profound and mediate goal-directed behaviors including those involved in natural reward, such as engagement in mating. For example, in adult female rats or hamsters, AlloP mediates approach and consummatory aspects of mating behavior, which are integral for conception to occur (Frye et al., 2006a). The proportion, intensity, and duration of lordosis responding (a stereotypical posture essential for mating behavior of rodents to occur) can be modulated by AlloP (Frye et al., 2006a). Midbrain dopamine cell bodies in the VTA project to limbic structures, including the amygdalar areas, hippocampus, and NAcc, as well as to areas of the PFC, and cell bodies in the substantia nigra innervate dSTR regions and other motor structures (reviewed in Haber and Fudge, 1997; Horvitz, 2000). Together, dopaminergic VTA projections makeup the mesolimbic dopamine system. Connections between the VTA and NAcc modulate the valence of pharmacological and natural reward and the motivation to engage rewarding stimuli (Koob and Le Moal, 2001; Kelley and Berridge, 2002; Wise, 2004). Investigation into the ability of AlloP, and other neurosteroids, to mediate altered neural function associated with heightened vulnerability to drug abuse (as well as other disorders) may lead to novel therapeutic avenues for the management of addiction-related problems. Thus, PNS alterations in levels of AlloP may partly mediate the lifelong alterations in the mesocorticolimbic dopamine system and perhaps other components of addiction circuitry involved in PNS-induced elevations of drug/alcohol-seeking behavior.

PRENATAL STRESS-INDUCED ALTERATIONS IN NEUROCHEMISTRY AND ALLOPREGNANOLONE MAY BE ASSOCIATED WITH CHANGES IN ADDICTION-RELATED BEHAVIOR

Prenatal stress influences the circuitry of addiction, as well as AlloP, in adulthood. Although direct evidence is not available, we hypothesize that these endpoints are functionally inter-related. Indirect support for this hypothesis stems from separate lines of research indicating that: (1) PNS impacts cortico-limbic circuitry and its midbrain monoamine modulatory systems; (2) PNS alters hormonal milieu, including levels of AlloP, in a sex-dependent fashion; (3) AlloP modulates drug/alcohol-seeking behavior; and (4) AlloP has direct effects on "addiction circuitry" that are behaviorally relevant.

PRENATAL STRESS ALTERS ALLOPREGNANOLONE

Prenatal stress can influence endogenous AlloP concentrations of rodents. There are several models of PNS that are used in rats, which typically involve applying stressful stimuli during gestational days (GDs) 17–21, which is a critical period of hippocampal development in rats. Psychological stress can involve exposing pregnant dams to either a chronic predictable stressor (such as restraint thrice daily for 45 min), or chronic unpredictable stressors (including forced swim, restraint, cold exposure, overnight fasting, light, and social crowding). We have previously observed perinatal psychosocial stressors, such as early maternal separation, reduce the ratio of P_4 to its 5α-reduced metabolites, dihydroprogesterone (DHP), and AlloP, in whole brain of postnatal day 2 rats, and dysregulate DHP and AlloP formation in whole brain of postnatal day 9 rats (Kehoe et al., 2000). We have recently investigated similar effects among juvenile rats. Among male and female offspring (between 28 and 30 days of age), stress resulted in decreased maternal AlloP levels during gestation, and reduced cognitive performance among offspring in an object recognition task, compared to controls (**Table 1**). These data are in concordance with findings wherein perinatal isolation is observed to increase circulating concentrations of the stress hormone, corticosterone, concurrent with reduced whole brain AlloP in rats (McCormick et al., 2002). Together, these data support the notion that early developmental stress can result in programmatic changes in neuroendocrine status with later consequences for cognition.

Table 1 | Summarized results (mean ± SEM) adapted from recent prenatal stress (PNS) studies in our lab, which indicate the effects of PNS via psychological stress [exposure to physical restraint (restraint) or unpredictable variable stress (variable) which included forced swim, restraint, cold exposure, overnight fasting, light, and social crowding], immune challenge [exposure to lipopolysaccharide (LPS, 30 μg/kg; dams only), or interleukin-1β (IL-1β, 1 μg/rat)], finasteride administration (50 mg/kg), or minimal handling/vehicle (control) on gestational days 17–21 (n = 4–8 dams/group; n = 17–30 offspring/group) has on maternal/fetal allopregnanolone and dependent cognitive behaviors (object recognition performance) of male and female rats (data are collapsed on the variable of sex).

Challenge at GD17-21	How?	Dams' plasma AlloP at parturition (ng/ml)	Offspring (male and female) Hippo AlloP (ng/g)	Novel obj recognition (% time with Object)	Reference
Control (nothing, vehicle)	Handling, IP Saline, SC oil	2.2 ± 0.8	1.8 ± 0.2	53 ± 4%	•Paris and Frye (2011a,b), Paris et al. (2011, under review)
Psychological (restraint, variable)	Thrice daily	0.7 ± 0.2*	1.0 ± 0.4	31 ± 9%*	•Paris and Frye (2011a), Paris and Frye (2011b)
Immune (LPS-dams only, IL-1β)	LPS (30 μg/kg, IP); IL-1β (1 μg/day, IP)	1.2 ± 0.1*	1.5 ± 0.6 (IL-1β only)	27 ± 9%* (IL-1β only)	• Paris et al. (under review)
Endocrine (finasteride)	50 mg/kg	0.5 ± 0.3*	0.5 ± 0.2*	22 ± 7%*	•Paris et al. (2011)

*Indicates significantly different from control group, p < 0.05.

MECHANISMS OF PRENATAL STRESS: EVIDENCE FOR CRUCIAL INTERACTIONS BETWEEN GLUCOCORTICOIDS AND PROGESTOGENS

There are pervasive effects of stress on developmental programming and functions throughout the lifespan; however, the mechanisms underlying these effects are not fully understood. There exists extensive evidence supporting a critical role for glucocorticoids in the programming effects of PNS, as well as, indications that glucocorticoids may be acting, in part, through alterations of other hormonal systems. We are interested in elucidating the extent to which AlloP may influence such responses through its actions on the stress axis. Changes in AlloP via PNS may be one mechanism by which PNS alters HPA axis-sensitive behaviors, such as drug use. Thus, findings regarding the stress axis and its interactions with AlloP on people, and in animal models, are summarized below.

THE STRESS RESPONSE

In response to acute stressors, there are changes in autonomic and neuroendocrine processes which may subserve adaptive behaviors. Irrespective of the type of stress experienced, the autonomic and neuroendocrine responses are ubiquitous and rapid. Catecholamines, epinephrine, and norepinephrine, heighten arousal by dilating pupils, increasing heart rate and respiration, and preparing for energy mobilization (reviewed in Wortsman, 2002). The sustained neuroendocrine response is mediated by the HPA axis. The HPA is comprised of the paraventricular nucleus (PVN) of the hypothalamus, the anterior pituitary (adenohypophysis), and the adrenals (reviewed in Turnbull and Rivier, 1997). The PVN synthesizes and releases corticotropin-releasing factor (CRF) to the adenohypophysis, where it promotes the release of adrenocorticotropic hormone (ACTH) into the periphery. ACTH stimulates the adrenal cortex to release glucocorticoids (i.e., cortisol in humans and corticosterone in most rodents), which have actions peripherally and centrally (reviewed in George and Koob, 2010).

Activation of these systems subserve behavioral responding (i.e., flight-or-flight) to acute stress, and may function to consolidate information surrounding salient events. Termination of the stress response occurs via negative feedback by glucocorticoid actions in the hypothalamus and pituitary (Herman et al., 1996) and also by AlloP (Patchev et al., 1994; Patchev and Almeida, 1996). Under chronic stress, the HPA feedback systems that typically act to restore (para)sympathetic tone are dysregulated and stressors may elicit a greater, lesser, or more prolonged HPA response than is typical.

Prenatal corticosterone exposure alone mirrors the effects of PNS on increased basal dopamine metabolism in both the dSTR and NAcc in male and female offspring (Diaz et al., 1995) suggesting that these processes may be influenced by HPA activation. Notably, PNS changes the expression and/or binding potential of dopamine D1 and D2 receptors, the dopamine transporter, as well as, the number of tyrosine hydroxylase-positive cells within the mesocorticolimbic dopamine system, including the NAcc, medial PFC, and hippocampal subregions (Alonso et al., 1994; Henry et al., 1995; Berger et al., 2002; McArthur et al., 2005; Son et al., 2007), which are important targets of the VTA (Nestler and Carlezon, 2006). As such, PNS may exert organizational effects to perturb the trajectory of the developing mesolimbic dopamine system. Indeed, perinatal stress (via early maternal separation) is observed to attenuate motor and dopamine responses to stress among adolescent rats (McCormick et al., 2002). Thus, there is evidence for PNS-induced changes in the structural and functional integrity of the dopamine reward circuitry among rodents.

PROGESTOGEN MODULATION OF THE HPA AXIS RESPONSE

There are differences in how females and males respond to stress and/or HPA activation, which may have bearing on the organizing effects of progestogens and/or responses to PNS. In response to stress, women typically have higher circulating cortisol levels and are more sensitive to glucocorticoid secretion than are men (Ellermeier and Westphal, 1995; Jezová et al., 1996; Ferrini et al., 1997; Hinojosa-Laborde et al., 1999; Rhodes and Rubin, 1999; Rohleder et al., 2001); however, females also demonstrate greater physiological and behavioral resiliency to negative/long-term effects of stress (Uno et al., 1989; Mizoguchi et al., 1992; Brown et al., 1996; Galea et al., 1997; Bowman et al., 2001, 2002; Beck and Luine, 2002; Conrad et al., 2003; Kitraki et al., 2004; McFadden et al., 2011). These sex differences in stress responding may be mediated by circulating levels of progestogens and/or their neurosteroid metabolites.

Progesterone, via actions of its metabolites, can suppress HPA axis activation. Progesterone can be 5α-reduced to form DHP, which can be 3α-hydroxylated to form the neuroactive metabolite, AlloP. Unlike progesterone and DHP, physiological concentrations of AlloP have little affinity for intracellular progestin receptors (Iswari et al., 1986). Rather, AlloP is a potent positive modulator of inhibitory $GABA_A$ receptors (Majewska et al., 1986), which may underlie its effects to dampen the HPA axis response (Purdy et al., 1991; Barbaccia et al., 1998). As such, it is progesterone's metabolism to AlloP, in response to stress, that promotes direct actions in hypothalamus to reduce CRF transcription and peptide precursors of the HPA mediated response (Patchev et al., 1994; Patchev and Almeida, 1996). These actions of AlloP partly underlie actions of progestogens to dampen HPA responsiveness in pregnancy; thereby, reducing fetal glucocorticoid exposure (Brunton et al., 2009). During pregnancy of people, the fetus can mount HPA responses by the second trimester, independent of the mother's HPA response (Gitau et al., 2001). Among female rats, PNS is associated with increased circulating corticosterone levels later in life (Walf and Frye, 2007). The extent to which stress-promoted maternal and/or fetal AlloP formation may account for physiological and behavioral stress phenotypes is of interest.

ALLOPREGNANOLONE NORMALLY INHIBITS THE HPA AXIS RESPONSE TO STRESS DURING PREGNANCY

AlloP's role in attenuating stress axis response extends to maintaining gestation, protection of the fetus, and/or possible organizing effects. Among pregnant women and rodents, circulatory AlloP is elevated throughout gestation and its decline precedes parturition (Concas et al., 1999; Gilbert-Evans et al., 2005; Paris and Frye, 2008). During early pregnancy, progestogens are secreted from the corpora lutea until the placenta becomes a source of progestogens (Concas et al., 1998). Circulating levels of P_4 and AlloP co-vary and increase together during the first half of gestation. However, P_4 levels decline prior to AlloP, later in pregnancy. Among rats, P_4 levels peak between GD 10–15; whereas, AlloP asymptotes later in pregnancy (GD19; Concas et al., 1998) and declines to estrous levels around GD21 (Concas et al., 1998). During pregnancy, ACTH, corticosterone, and PVN CRF levels are lower, and oxytocin neurons are inhibited, such that stimuli that evoke a stress response in virgin rats do not elicit the same stress response in pregnant rats (Atkinson and Waddell, 1995; Johnstone et al., 2000; Brunton and Russell, 2003; Brunton et al., 2006a,b, 2005; Ma et al., 2005). In the developing offspring, central AlloP is observed as early as embryonic day 14 in rats (Kellogg and Frye, 1999), while postnatal AlloP increases in response to stressors on GD 6 (Kehoe et al., 2000; McCormick et al., 2002). Inhibiting AlloP formation with a 5α-reductase inhibitor, finasteride, in late pregnancy restores HPA activation of ACTH, corticosterone, CRF, and oxytocin which can result in termination of pregnancy (Antonijevic et al., 2000; Brussaard and Herbison, 2000; Grobin and Morrow, 2001; Russell et al., 2003; Chanrachakul et al., 2005; Brunton and Russell, 2008a,b, 2010; Brunton et al., 2009). Thus, AlloP during gestation influences stress responding and gestational outcomes. Notably, administration of AlloP prenatally, counteracts the effects of PNS on anxiety-like tasks, indicating its role in neuropsychiatric-relevant behaviors (Zimmerberg and Blaskey, 1998).

AlloP during perinatal development may influence sex-typical differences in stress responding. We, and others, have utilized models of PNS in order to assess AlloP's developmental effects prior to parturition. Epidemiological studies of people, and experimental investigations using rodents, provide evidence that PNS can confer vulnerability to stress-related disorders that persist into adulthood. Behavioral and neurobiological aberrations associated with PNS may be sex-typical (i.e., predominant in one sex and/or related to changes in sex hormones), stress-sensitive (i.e., related to HPA activation and/or changes in stress hormones), and/or disorder-relevant (i.e., associated with the etiology or pathology of a neurodevelopmental, neuropsychiatric, and/or neurodegenerative disorder) functions. Although acute stress can be adaptive in adults through enhancing autonomic, neuroendocrine, and behavioral outputs that subserve species-typical adaptive responses (e.g., fight-or-flight), developmental stress can be pathological and detrimental to mothers and offspring. Typically, during late gestation, maternal stress responding is dampened. This stress hyporesponsive period, which is well-documented in rodents, may limit the deleterious developmental programming effects of PNS. The period of stress hyporesponsiveness coincides with elevations in AlloP (Paris and Frye, 2008; Brunton et al., 2009), which can be protective to the offspring (Frye and Bayon, 1998; Yawno et al., 2009), and dampen HPA axis reactivity (Patchev et al., 1994, 1996; Patchev and Almeida, 1996; Paris and Frye, 2008; Frye, 2009). There are PNS-induced alterations in neurosteroid levels which may play a direct role in programming the developing fetus (Kehoe et al., 2000; McCormick et al., 2002). This has led to our hypothesis that some effects of PNS may involve 5α-reduced progestogens influence on developmental programming of sex-typical, stress-sensitive, and/or disorder-relevant phenotypes. Additionally, postnatal perturbation of maternal–infant interactions may have profound effects on stress responding and AlloP formation in offspring that are sex-dependent. We have found that maternal separation during postnatal days two through nine produces increases in central AlloP in offspring and these effects are greater in males (Kehoe et al., 2000). Thus, AlloP formation during early postnatal development may play an important role in programming of stress responses, and may present as a mechanism of PNS pervasive effects to influence drug reward and related sequelae.

ALLOPREGNANOLONE INFLUENCES DRUG RESPONDING AND HAS POTENTIAL LINKS TO PRENATAL STRESS EFFECTS

Pharmacological stimuli, such as drugs of abuse, activate the HPA robustly, as do the physical, psychological, and immune challenges described heretofore. We have presented evidence that PNS can alter responses to drugs of abuse, and that there are sex differences in response to PNS in these measures. Additionally, there is evidence consistent with the notion that PNS alters HPA function as well as AlloP levels, and that changes in AlloP can alter subsequent drug intake behaviors, also in a sex-dependent way. Causal relationships have not been established between perturbation of endogenous AlloP formation via PNS and later drug-seeking behavior. Rather, separate lines of research have revealed PNS to alter susceptibility to drug abuse/responding and AlloP formation in adolescence and adulthood. Adolescents are vulnerable to substance use, which is co-morbid with neuropsychiatric disorders and neurodegeneration. An important question for future investigation is what role progestogen formation may play in conferring vulnerability to natural or pharmacological reward. In support, progestogens, including AlloP, have been shown to modulate responding to many drugs of abuse. It is beyond the scope of this review to provide an in depth analysis of progestogen interactions with all drugs of abuse, such as depressants (i.e., alcohol), stimulants (i.e., cocaine, amphetamine, nicotine), and opiates. Thus, we focus on recent findings surrounding progestogens and drug abuse, and provide specific references for the complex interactions between AlloP and other steroid hormones with drugs, including alcohol and cocaine.

In addition to organizational effects of progestogens suggested by PNS, activational effects of progestogens are observed, which can differ across the sexes (another indication of potential organizing actions of hormones). There are sex differences in response to drugs of abuse, which may be partly mediated by progestogens and other sex steroids. Women are more likely than men to initiate drug use, demonstrate binge use, experience greater cravings, and relapse to greater use (Brady and Randall, 1999; Robbins et al., 1999; Mann et al., 2005; Gallop et al., 2007; Becker and Hu, 2008). Some evidence for hormonal mediation of drug use among pre-menopausal women is observed during cyclical hormonal fluctuations. In response to alcohol, women in the luteal phase (when circulatory progestogens are typically low) have increased positive effects of alcohol (Evans and Levin, 2011), decreased elimination, and blood alcohol clearance, which correlates with P_4 levels (Sutker et al., 1987), lower AlloP levels (Nyberg et al., 2005), and feelings of anxiety and stress (Howell et al., 2010), the latter of which is co-morbid with cocaine use (Morton, 1999; Torres and Ortega, 2003; Poling et al., 2007; Rubin et al., 2007). In people, alcohol consumption decreases circulating P_4 and AlloP levels in men (Pierucci-Lagha et al., 2006) and in women in the luteal phase (Nyberg et al., 2005). Nicotine effects, like alcohol, may vary based on hormone condition. During the luteal phase, number of cigarets smoked, nicotine craving, and positive subjective effects of smoking, increased in women (Mello et al., 1987; Snively et al., 2000; Franklin et al., 2004). Thus, low endogenous progestogen profile may yield vulnerability to alcohol's hedonic effects among naturally cycling women.

Animal models also show sex differences in substance use which may be influenced by hormonal milieu. Female rats and monkeys acquire, maintain, and escalate drug use, extinction, and reinstatement more readily than do males (see, e.g., Anker and Carroll, 2010). More targeted analyses have been conducted in rodents in response to alcohol that may be mediated by sex and duration of exposure. Notably, PNS can perturb hormone-sensitive behaviors across the estrous cycle of rats, which has been observed via reduced engagement in copulatory behaviors when rats are naturally sexually receptive (Frye and Orecki, 2002). When orally consumed, ethanol increased brain AlloP in male, but not female mice, an effect not observed when ethanol was injected (Finn et al., 2004). However, when alcohol is administered to facilitate alcohol-dependence, exposure may decrease cortical levels of AlloP in male, but not female, rats (Janis et al., 1998). As such, effects of alcohol on neurosteroid formation are biphasic and complex; a linear relationship between alcohol-enhanced neurosteroidogenesis and reward is unlikely. In support, cynomolgus monkeys that were trained to discriminate alcohol from water, demonstrated an enhanced ability to also discriminate AlloP when in the luteal (vs. follicular) phase of the menstrual cycle; however, cycle differences in discrimination were not observed for alcohol (Green et al., 1999). Neurosteroids, including $3\alpha,5\alpha$-tetrahydrodeoxycorticosterone and 3α-androstanediol, can be enhanced with alcohol administration and/or implicated in some alcohol effects (Paris and Frye, 2009; Serra et al., 2007. Indeed, AlloP and 3α-androstanediol may promote hedonic effects in males, given that male rats will orally self-administer AlloP preferentially over water (Sinnott et al., 2002a), and male hamsters will orally self-administer 3α-androstanediol over water (Frye et al., 2007). However, any effects that neurosteroid mechanisms may contribute to the reinforcing properties of alcohol are likely sex- and dose-dependent, given that AlloP injections have been observed to dose-dependently increase oral alcohol consumption among male, but not female, mice (Sinnott et al., 2002b). In addition to pregnane and androstane neurosteroids, estradiol may also contribute to sex differences to increase, while progestogens decrease, drug effects among females compared to males (Becker and Hu, 2008; Anker and Carroll, 2010). However, estradiol has been observed to not be altered in adult cycling female rats that have been exposed to PNS (Walf and Frye, 2007), which may suggest that it is a less likely mechanism for PNS-mediated changes in drug use. As such, there are complex interactions between sex hormones and many different drugs of abuse. These interactions may influence aspects of drugs abuse. For further review of alcohol's reinforcing interactions with AlloP (see Morrow et al., 2001; Finn et al., 2008; Helms and Grant, 2011). For evidence of other gonadal hormone contributions to alcohol's reinforcing effects (see Devaud et al., 2006).

Much research surrounding progestogens' effects on drug abuse have focused on cocaine. Autonomic, pleasurable effects, stress-induced cravings, and self-administration for cocaine are reduced when hormone levels are high in women during the luteal phase (Sofuoglu et al., 1999; Evans et al., 2002; Evans and Foltin, 2006; Sinha et al., 2007) and in rats during the proestrus phase (Hecht et al., 1999; Feltenstein and See, 2007). Administration of P_4 to women attenuates subjective and HPA axis autonomic effects of cocaine and reduces craving (Sofuoglu et al., 2002, 2004; Evans and Foltin, 2006). Indeed, suppression of HPA axis responding following craving may be associated with some of cocaine's hedonic effects. Rodents will voluntarily self-administer either corticosterone (DeRoche et al., 1993) or AlloP (Sinnott et al., 2002a).

We, and others, have found that P_4 and AlloP levels of males and females are elevated in plasma, striatum, and hippocampus following cocaine administration, along with enhanced psychomotor behavior (Quinones-Jenab et al., 2008). Some of these effects may be dependent on estrous cycle phase, given that threshold for dose-dependent psychomotor activation to cocaine was increased among diestrous, compared to proestrus, female rats (Kohtz et al., 2010). Moreover, AlloP may influence some of cocaine's reinforcing effects. Pretreatment with AlloP diminishes escalating self-administration of cocaine in rats (Larsen et al., 2007; Anker et al., 2010). Progesterone reduced cocaine-primed reinstatement of cocaine-seeking behavior in female, but not male, rats and this effect was attenuated by finasteride and mimicked by AlloP administration (Anker et al., 2009). Although other gonadal hormones, such as estradiol have been investigated for their role on cocaine effects (for review see Segarra et al., 2009), it is P_4 that has been utilized for clinical applications. Indeed, oral P_4 has been investigated as a potential treatment for cocaine dependence (Reed et al., 2011); however, despite the need for further investigations, that study did not yield discriminating effects of P_4 on self-administration. Therefore, drug effects and addiction behaviors that are increased by exposure to PNS, in particular, cocaine, are mediated by progestogens, including AlloP, which may indicate a possible mechanisms for further exploration into the neurodevelopmental impact and mechanisms of PNS on maternal–fetal interactions and later offspring behavior.

NEURODEVELOPMENTAL, NEUROPSYCHIATRIC, AND NEURODEGENERATIVE SEQUELAE ASSOCIATED WITH PRENATAL STRESS AND/OR DRUG USE AND MAY BE PROGESTOGEN-SENSITIVE

Neurodevelopmental, neuropsychiatric, and/or neurodegenerative disorders are co-morbid with drug use and are characterized by gender/sex differences and sensitivity to stress that may be influenced by progestogens. There is emerging consensus for similar neurobiological factors to underlie disorders that share similar features and/or endophenotypes. Thus, findings regarding the impact of gestational stress on people and animals, and the influence of progestogens in these processes, are summarized below.

IMPACT OF PRENATAL STRESS ON DEVELOPMENTAL DISORDERS IN PEOPLE AND ANIMAL MODELS

There are neurodevelopmental consequences of prenatal and perinatal stress that can be observed in juvenile (pre-pubertal) offspring. Despite the relative protection of the uterine environment, the fetus can be affected by environmental stressors that the mother experiences (Schlotz and Phillips, 2009). Like most stress challenges, *in utero* adaptation to environmental stressors may be an important aspect of organismal preparation for survival; however, enhancements in the chronicity, or saliency, of such stressors may also promote adverse effects. In people, PNS via chronic psychological and/or physical stress (such as those associated with low socio-economic status, poor coping skills, and maternal physical abuse) are associated with preterm birth and low birth-weight offspring (Facchinetti et al., 2007; Rodrigues et al., 2008; Giurgescu, 2009; Latendresse, 2009). Early birth under these conditions may lead to impairments in social, cognitive, and emotional behavior, which are observable when children are of school-age (Talge et al., 2010; Kerstjens et al., 2011; Lind et al., 2011). Among infants who are born preterm, there are also aberrations in cortico-limbic volume and/or sulci/gyri folding may be associated with neurodevelopmental disabilities, compared to antenatally age-matched controls (reviewed in Lodygensky et al., 2010). Moreover, the severity of premature birth may predict poorer neurodevelopmental outcomes (Talge et al., 2010). In addition to chronic stress, salient stress exposure during pregnancy can promote similar outcomes. After hurricane Katrina, over a two-fold increase in the incidence of preterm births was reported among pregnant women who were residing in a severely hit area, compared to those in less damaged areas (Xiong et al., 2008). Similarly, offspring born to women enlisted in the military that were deployed to a combat zone while pregnant, have a greater incidence of preterm birth and neurodevelopmental disorders, such as a major birth defect or malignancy (Ryan et al., 2011). Thus, chronic and/or salient PNS may promote neurodevelopmental disorder among people.

Prenatal stress exerts neurodevelopmental effects that can be modeled in rodents. In particular, the cortico-limbic brain regions may be a target for PNS. Compared to controls, pre-adolescent male rats that were born to dams that underwent physical restraint (2 h/day from GD 11 to birth), exhibited increased CA1, but decreased CA3, spine densities, while adult PNS male offspring had reduced spine densities in both areas (Martinez-Tellez et al., 2009). Long-term neurodevelopmental effects of PNS on the hippocampus may be particularly salient among females, given that a single exposure of PNS on GD18 can reduce adult dentate gyrus volume in female, but not male, rats (Schmitz et al., 2002). PNS is also observed to reduce spine density in PFC (Murmu et al., 2006; Michelsen et al., 2007). Over the course of development, the volumes of amygdalar sub-nuclei (an extension of the limbic system) tend to diverge among male PNS vs. control rats. By early adulthood PNS individuals may begin to match controls on some measures of nuclei volume (Kraszpulski et al., 2006), and may even surpass controls in the region of the lateral nucleus later in adulthood (Salm et al., 2004). The production of new neurons in the adult hippocampus is also reduced following PNS (e.g., Lemaire et al., 2000; Coe et al., 2003; Odagiri et al., 2008). Further, PNS or prenatal corticosterone treatment alter the levels of trophic factors and synapse-regulating proteins in limbic and cortical structures in an age-dependent fashion that may be responsible for the observed changes in dendritic spine densities (Fumagalli et al., 2004, 2005; Burton et al., 2007; Afadlal et al., 2010; Jutapakdeegul et al., 2010). Accordingly, these effects may have important consequences for early social and emotional development given the role of cortico-limbic function in regulating decision making and affect. In support, female PNS rats that are juvenile (~30 days of age) have increased anxiety-like behavior and decreased weight compared to control females (Baker et al., 2008). Male and female PNS juvenile offspring also show decreased social play behavior and reduced psychomotor activity (Kleinhaus et al., 2010). Additionally, PNS can affect male and female juvenile cognitive function in Y-maze, T-maze, and passive avoidance, the latter of which revealed females to have decreased performance compared to males (Gué et al., 2004). In rats, perinatal isolation has also been observed to worsen adult performance in the Morris water maze (Frisone et al., 2002). In people, this time period is equivalent to adolescence, which is characterized by the emergence of sex-typical, stress-sensitive behavioral disorders (i.e., autism, attention deficit hyperactivity disorder; McCormick and Mathews, 2007), novelty/drug seeking, and substance abuse (reviewed in Kroll, 2007; Bukstein, 2008). These findings suggest that aberrations in cortico-limbic brain regions may be present in adolescence and pervasive, at least until adulthood, following a history of PNS.

The HPA axis is activated in response to stressors, such as the physical and psychological stressors described above; however, one method to activate HPA axis activity in pregnancy is via immune challenge. This methodology is clinically relevant given that up to 40% of preterm births are associated with immune challenge/infection (Goldenberg et al., 2008). Administration of the bacterial endotoxin, lipopolysaccharide (LPS), or the cytokine, interleukin-1β (IL-1β), in late gestation mimics infection/inflammation (Hermus and Sweep, 1990; Johnson et al., 1997; Turnbull and Rivier, 1999) and activates adrenergic synapses in the hypothalamus (Besedovsky and del Rey, 1992; Ericsson et al., 1994; Givalois et al., 1995; Turnbull et al., 1998; Brunton et al., 2005) and placenta (Paintlia et al., 2008). We have observed these regimens to reduce circulating AlloP in dams at the time of parturition (**Table 1**). Offspring that were gestationally exposed to immune challenge spent a significantly lower percentage of time with a novel object compared to controls (**Table 1**), which may indicate reduced cognitive performance. Given AlloP's importance in dampening HPA response during pregnancy, and the results from studies indicating decreased maternal AlloP following gestational stress (Frye and Walf, 2004; Paris and Frye, 2011a), we have investigated the necessity of maternal AlloP for these effects by administering finasteride (50 mg/kg) to dams in late gestation. Indeed, gestational finasteride produced similar effects to that of gestational stressors, resulting in reduced offspring cognitive behavior (**Table 1**). Notably, we have observed adolescent rats to spend less time with a novel object than do adult rats, irrespective of gestational manipulations. These data may imply a neophobic aspect to this task, that is not observed in adults, which may explain some of the aversion observed among adolescent rats exposed to gestational stressors (Paris and Frye, 2011a). These data support the notion that maternally derived 5α-reduced steroids play an important role in the neurodevelopmental programming of late-gestating offspring. This does not preclude finasteride interacting with other steroid hormones; given that finasteride also inhibits formation of androstane and glucocorticoid metabolites (reviewed in Finn et al., 2006) and further study of AlloP add-back will assess the ability of AlloP to rescue these effects.

Involvement of the HPA axis is further implied in studies of perinatal perturbation. Deficiencies in AlloP formation that are observed in plasma, via perinatal stress (lithium chloride injection), at 10 and 60 days of age are ameliorated by 90 days of age (Frye et al., 2006b). These data indicate that some perinatal reprogramming effects on the endocrine system may be transient; however, in these experiments, hippocampus AlloP remained perturbed at 60 and 90 days of age, suggesting that perturbation of central steroid formation may be pervasive throughout life (Frye et al., 2006b). These investigations imply that chronic HPA perturbation may be less severe in rodent models when manipulations occur later in development. An intriguing hypothesis for future consideration is that AlloP can have organizational effects in pre- or perinatal development which may be associated with its actions as a trophic factor throughout life. We have previously observed AlloP to be neuroprotective in rats, particularly when the HPA axis is perturbed (Rhodes et al., 2004). Thus, PNS can result in perturbed maternal and offspring AlloP levels and increased HPA responses, which may have effects on fetal neurodevelopment, neuropsychiatric-relevant behavior, and may reduce later neuroprotective capacity.

IMPACT OF PRENATAL STRESS ON NEUROPSYCHIATRIC DISORDERS IN PEOPLE AND NEUROPSYCHIATRIC-RELEVANT BEHAVIOR IN RODENTS

Among people, some findings suggests that stress during gestation may influence the etiopathology of neuropsychiatric processes. Those exposed to inordinate stressors during gestation, particularly during mid-gestation, are more likely to be diagnosed with schizophrenia, anxiety disorders, and depressive disorders (as reviewed in Bertram and Hanson, 2002; Matthews et al., 2002; Huizink et al., 2004; Seckl and Meaney, 2004; King, 2011). Children whose mothers experienced psychological stress during pregnancy show less social behavior, which is an early symptom of schizophrenia (Done et al., 1994). Adolescent children of women who had lost husbands during WWII while pregnant, suffered from higher rates of mood disorders and schizophrenia (Huttunen and Niskanen, 1978). There is also a significant correlation between the maternal experience of famine during the second and third trimesters and affective disorders in the adult children of those women (Brown et al., 2000).

Some of these effects may be due to perturbations in AlloP formation or actions. Women diagnosed with depression and/or premenstrual dysphoric disorder have decreased AlloP sensitivity (Freeman et al., 2002; Girdler and Klatzkin, 2007; Gracias et al., 2009) and do not experience the expected increase in AlloP following stress (Klatzkin et al., 2006). Women suffering from post-traumatic stress disorder (PTSD) have decreased AlloP levels in cerebrospinal fluid (Rasmusson et al., 2006). Men with PTSD, who have a greater psychological distress to trauma-relevant stimuli have lower levels of AlloP (Casada and Roache, 2004; Frye, 2009). Moreover, reduced 5α-reductase activity (as determined by cortisol metabolism) was associated with symptom severity among individuals afflicted with treatment-resistant PTSD following the World Trade Center attacks in 2001 (Yehuda et al., 2009). Post-mortem brain AlloP levels were also decreased in a combined male/female sample of schizophrenic patients (Marx et al., 2006). As such, stress during human fetal development, and/or later chronic stress, may promote sex-typical, stress-sensitive disorders in adulthood, where AlloP varies with the incidence or expression of these disorders.

Findings from animal models suggest that PNS influences the developmental trajectory of neuropsychiatric-relevant function. Rodent models of PNS, specifically stress during late gestation, can produce behavioral sequelae later in life that were initially characterized by hyper-responsiveness to stressors. These responses have since been typified as maladaptive and/or early symptoms of behavioral disturbances. Offspring of PNS dams can be behaviorally inhibited, as is observed in response to maternal separation, wherein PNS pups vocalize and move less than do their non-PNS counterparts (Morgan et al., 1999). Male PNS juvenile rats demonstrate less social behavior and rough-and-tumble play than do control males (Ohkawa, 1987; Ward and Stehm, 1991). PNS increases anxiety-like behavior, indicated by spending less time on the open arms of an elevated plus maze (Fride et al., 1985; Zimmerberg and Blaskey, 1998) and/or more defecation in a novel environment (Wakshlak and Weinstock, 1990; Poltyrev et al., 1996; Vallée et al., 1997). PNS also increases depressive behavior, such as learned helplessness in the inescapable footshock paradigm, and increases anhedonia in the sucrose consumption model (Keshet and Weinstock, 1995; Secoli and Teixeira, 1998). Females, in particular, may be more vulnerable to some effects of PNS on depressive behavior as indicated by greater immobility in the forced swim test and less responsiveness to the anti-depressive effects of hormonal intervention, compared to their male counterparts (Drago et al., 1999; Frye and Wawrzycki, 2003). Aberrations in affective-like behavior may persist in female rats throughout life; adult females exposed to PNS demonstrate less struggling behavior (indicative of depression-like phenotype) in the forced swim test when pregnant (albeit not statistically significant), and significantly less struggling behavior when post-partum, compared to controls (Frye and Walf, 2004). While, it is not clear that AlloP formation/perturbation plays a role in the etiology of neuropsychiatric disorder, converging pre-clinical and clinical evidence support investigation of this premise, and provide evidence of the therapeutic efficacy of AlloP. For instance, AlloP add-back, concomitant with PNS, has been demonstrated to ameliorate, or reverse, anxiety-like behaviors produced by PNS (Zimmerberg and Blaskey, 1998). AlloP has demonstrated efficacy in improving neurodevelopmental disorders in mouse models of Niemann Pick disease (Mellon et al., 2008). Moreover, AlloP enhancement is associated with improvement in neuropsychiatric disorders, such as premenstrual dysphoric disorder among women (Freeman et al., 2002; Gracias et al., 2009).

IMPACT OF PRENATAL STRESS ON NEURODEGENERATION IN ANIMAL MODELS

Prenatal stress may promote neurodegenerative processes. Depression is associated with neurodegeneration in the hippocampus, concomitant with increased circulatory glucocorticoids (stress hormones), which may be facilitated by PNS. In adults, and rodent models, depression is associated with decreased neurogenesis in dentate gyrus and increased plasma glucocorticoid formation (Manji et al., 2001; Sapolsky, 2001). Early corticosterone exposure is necessary for dentate gyrus development of rodents and species-typical cognitive function (He et al., 2009) and glucocorticoid production from the adrenals promotes cell survival in the brain. Indeed, removal of the adrenals in rats increases cell death in the granule layer and dentate gyrus of the hippocampus (Frye and McCormick, 2000a,b; Rhodes et al., 2004). Moreover, co-administration of the 5α-reductase inhibitor, finasteride, with P_4 reinstatement attenuates these effects in ovariectomized females (Rhodes et al., 2004), suggesting that adrenally derived, 5α-reduced progestogens have important trophic effects to maintain limbic integrity. These data support lines of research that utilize murine models of Alzheimer's disease. In support, APPswe + PSEN1Δe9 mice that present with central plaques and neurofibrillary tangles (an Alzheimer's disease-like phenotype) have decrements in hippocampally mediated behavioral tasks, compared to wild-type mice, and are deficient in their conversion of P_4 to AlloP (Frye and Walf, 2008a). Thus, progestogens, such as AlloP, may have important trophic and neuroprotective effects throughout life.

Chronic stress exposure can promote neural degeneration (reviewed in Schoenfeld and Gould, 2011), as can exposure to a salient, acute stressors. For instance, a single episode of maternal restraint during a critical period for limbic development (GD18) reduces the number of granule cells in CA1-3 of adult female (but not male) offspring (Schmitz et al., 2002). Female PNS rats also exhibit age-dependent reductions in hippocampal neurogenesis (Koehl et al., 2009) and repeated maternal restraint, not only reduces the production of adult-born neurons, but also the number of adult neural stem cells (Kippin et al., 2004). These cells are critical for limiting the damage induced by central insults (Li et al., 2010). Thus, PNS effects may also promote later degenerative processes, and/or reduce proliferative processes, in the rodent brain, predisposing organisms to neurodevelopmental/affective disorder. Unfortunately, the greater incidence of morbidity and mortality among PNS offspring limits what is known about the influence of PNS on neurodegeneration throughout development. However, PNS is also notably associated with vulnerability to substance use and addiction. Indeed, adolescents are uniquely vulnerable to engagement in drugs of abuse, which is co-morbid with neuropsychiatric disorder and can promote/facilitate neurodegenerative processes. While, PNS can alter fetal programming of the neuroendocrine axis, altering AlloP formation, direct evidence for involvement of AlloP formation, via PNS, in the etiology of neurodevelopmental and/or neurodegenerative disorders is not clearly established. However, AlloP administration is associated with improvement in rodent models of neurodegenerative disorders including Alzheimer's disease (Wang et al., 2010), ischemic brain insult (Sayeed et al., 2006), and traumatic brain injury (Djebaili et al., 2005). Further, AlloP formation is perturbed in a mouse model of Alzheimer's disease and P administration improves cognitive performance (Frye and Walf, 2008a) and reduces depressive-like behavior (Frye and Walf, 2009) in a mouse model.

CONCLUSION

In conclusion, PNS may influence fetal programming, promoting vulnerability to drug seeking/use as well as some co-morbid neurodevelopmental, neuropsychiatric, and/or neurodegenerative disorders. These sequelae may be partly associated with secondary effects of PNS to alter natural reward processes, promoting vulnerability to substance abuse, and addiction. Thus, for its role in modulating drug salience, endogenous reward, developmental-, neuropsychiatric-, and neurodegenerative-relevant sequelae, AlloP remains an intriguing target for investigation. The extent to which regulation/actions of AlloP contribute to the etiopathophysiology of various sex-typical, stress-sensitive, neurodevelopmental, neuropsychiatric, and/or neurodegenerative disorders that have their origins in early puerperal, mother–infant interactions is an open and critical question.

ACKNOWLEDGMENTS

This work was supported by funding from NIMH (MH06769801), NIAAA (INIA-Stress pilot project; U01AA01364-9), NIDA (DA077525; DA027115), NSF (IBN03-16083; IOS-0957148), and the National Alliance for Research on Schizophrenia and Affective Disorders.

REFERENCES

Afadlal, S., Polaboon, N., Surakul, P., Govitrapong, P., and Jutapakdeegul, N. (2010). Prenatal stress alters presynaptic marker proteins in the hippocampus of rat pups. *Neurosci. Lett.* 470, 24–27.

Alonso, S. J., Navarro, E., and Rodriguez, M. (1994). Permanent dopaminergic alterations in then accumbens after prenatal stress. *Pharmacol. Biochem. Behav.* 49, 353–358.

Alonso, S. J., Navarro, E., Santana, C., and Rodriguez, M. (1997). Motor lateralization, behavioral despair and dopaminergic brain asymmetry after prenatal stress. *Pharmacol. Biochem. Behav.* 58, 443–448.

Anker, J. J., and Carroll, M. E. (2010). The role of progestins in the behavioral effects of cocaine and other drugs of abuse: human and animal research. *Neurosci. Biobehav. Rev.* 35, 315–333.

Anker, J. J., Holtz, N. A., Zlebnik, N., and Carroll, M. E. (2009). Effects of allopregnanolone on the reinstatement of cocaine-seeking behavior in male and female rats. *Psychopharmacology (Berl.)* 203, 63–72.

Anker, J. J., Zlebnik, N. E., and Carroll, M. E. (2010). Differential effects of allopregnanolone on the escalation of cocaine self-administration and sucrose intake in female rats. *Psychopharmacology (Berl.)* 212, 419–429.

Antonijevic, I. A., Russell, J. A., Bicknell, R. J., Leng, G., and Douglas, A. J. (2000). Effect of progesterone on the activation of neurones of the supraoptic nucleus during parturition. *J. Reprod. Fertil.* 120, 367–376.

Atkinson, H. C., and Waddell, B. J. (1995). The hypothalamic-pituitary-adrenal axis in rat pregnancy and lactation: circadian variation and interrelationship of plasma adrenocorticotropin and corticosterone. *Endocrinology* 136, 512–520.

Baker, S., Chebli, M., Rees, S., Lemarec, N., Godbout, R., and Bielajew, C. (2008). Effects of gestational stress: 1. Evaluation of maternal and juvenile offspring behavior. *Brain Res.* 1213, 98–110.

Barbaccia, M. L., Concas, A., Serra, M., and Biggio, G. (1998). Stress and neurosteroids in adult and aged rats. *Exp. Gerontol.* 33, 697–712.

Barros, V. G., Berger, M. A., Martijena, I. D., Sarchi, M. I., Pérez, A. A., Molina, V. A., Tarazi, F. I., and Antonelli, M. C. (2004). Early adoption modifies the effects of prenatal stress on dopamine and glutamate receptors in adult rat brain. *J. Neurosci. Res.* 76, 488–496.

Beck, K. D., and Luine, V. N. (2002). Sex differences in behavioral and neurochemical profiles after chronic stress: role of housing conditions. *Physiol. Behav.* 75, 661–673.

Becker, J. B., and Hu, M. (2008). Sex differences in drug abuse. *Front. Neuroendocrinol.* 29, 36–47.

Becker, J. B., Rudick, C. N., and Jenkins, W. J. (2001). The role of dopamine in the nucleus accumbens and striatum during sexual behavior in the female rat. *J. Neurosci.* 21, 3236–3241.

Berger, M. A., Barros, V. G., Sarchi, M. I., Tarazi, F. I., and Antonelli, M. C. (2002). Long-term effects of prenatal stress on dopamine and glutamate receptors in adult rat brain. *Neurochem. Res.* 27, 1525–1533.

Bertram, C. E., and Hanson, M. A. (2002). Prenatal programming of postnatal endocrine responses by glucocorticoids. *Reproduction* 124, 459–467.

Besedovsky, H. O., and del Rey, A. (1992). Immune-neuroendocrine circuits: integrative role of cytokines. *Front. Neuroendocrinol.* 13, 61–94.

Bowman, R. E., Ferguson, D., and Luine, V. N. (2002). Effects of chronic restraint stress and estradiol on open field activity, spatial memory, and monoaminergic neurotransmitters in ovariectomized rats. *Neuroscience* 113, 401–410.

Bowman, R. E., Zrull, M. C., and Luine, V. N. (2001). Chronic restraint stress enhances radial arm maze performance in female rats. *Brain Res.* 904, 279–289.

Brady, K. T., and Randall, C. L. (1999). Gender differences in substance use disorders. *Psychiatr. Clin. North Am.* 22, 241–252.

Brown, A. S., van Os, J., Driessens, C., Hoek, H. W., and Susser, E. S. (2000). Further evidence of relation between prenatal famine and major affective disorder. *Am. J. Psychiatry* 157, 190–195.

Brown, L. L., Siegel, H., and Etgen, A. M. (1996). Global sex differences in stress-induced activation of cerebral metabolism revealed by 2-deoxyglucose autoradiography. *Horm. Behav.* 30, 611–617.

Brunton, P. J., McKay, A. J., Ochedalski, T., Piastowska, A., Rebas, E., Lachowicz, A., and Russell, J. A. (2009). Central opioid inhibition of neuroendocrine stress responses in pregnancy in the rat is induced by the neurosteroid allopregnanolone. *J. Neurosci.* 29, 6449–6460.

Brunton, P. J., Meddle, S. L., Ma, S., Ochedalski, T., Douglas, A. J., and Russell, J. A. (2005). Endogenous opioids and attenuated hypothalamic-pituitary-adrenal axis responses to immune challenge in pregnant rats. *J. Neurosci.* 25, 5117–5126.

Brunton, P. J., and Russell, J. A. (2003). Hypothalamic-pituitary-adrenal responses to centrally administered orexin-A are suppressed in pregnant rats. *J. Neuroendocrinol.* 15, 633–637.

Brunton, P. J., and Russell, J. A. (2008a). Attenuated hypothalamo-pituitary-adrenal axis responses to immune challenge during pregnancy: the neurosteroid opioid connection. *J. Physiol.* 586, 369–375.

Brunton, P. J., and Russell, J. A. (2008b). Keeping oxytocin neurons under control during stress in pregnancy. *Prog. Brain Res.* 170, 365–377.

Brunton, P. J., and Russell, J. A. (2010). Prenatal social stress in the rat programmes neuroendocrine and behavioural responses to stress in the adult offspring: sex-specific effects. *J. Neuroendocrinol.* 22, 258–271.

Brunton, P. J., Sabatier, N., Leng, G., and Russell, J. A. (2006a). Suppressed oxytocin neuron responses to immune challenge in late pregnant rats: a role for endogenous opioids. *Eur. J. Neurosci.* 23, 1241–1247.

Brunton, P. J., Bales, J., and Russell, J. A. (2006b). Neuroendocrine stress but not feeding responses to centrally administered neuropeptide Y are suppressed in pregnant rats. *Endocrinology* 147, 3737–3745.

Brussaard, A. B., and Herbison, A. E. (2000). Long-term plasticity of postsynaptic GABAA-receptor function in the adult brain: insights from the oxytocin neurone. *Trends Neurosci.* 23, 190–195.

Bukstein, O. (2008). Substance abuse in patients with attention-deficit/hyperactivity disorder. *Medscape J. Med.* 10, 24.

Burton, C. L., Chatterjee, D., Chatterjee-Chakraborty, M., Lovic, V., Grella, S. L., Steiner, M., and Fleming, A. S. (2007). Prenatal restraint stress and motherless rearing disrupts expression of plasticity markers and stress-induced corticosterone release in adult female Sprague-Dawley rats. *Brain Res.* 1158, 28–38.

Campbell, J. C., Dunn, C. P., Nayak, R. R., Cornateanu, R. J., and Kippin, T. E. (2010). *Prenatal Stress Produces Sex-Specific Effects on Alcohol Reinforcement and Intake in C57Bl/6J Mice.* San Antonio, TX: Research Society on Alcoholism.

Campbell, J. C., Szumlinski, K. K., and Kippin, T. E. (2009). Contribution of early environmental stress to alcoholism vulnerability. *Alcohol* 43, 547–554.

Carboni, E., Barros, V. G., Ibba, M., Silvagni, A., Mura, C., and Antonelli, M. C. (2010). Prenatal restraint stress: an in vivo microdialysis study on catecholamine release in the rat prefrontal cortex. *Neuroscience* 168, 156–166.

Casada, J. H., and Roache, J. D. (2004). Neurosteroids in PTSD. *International Society for Traumatic Stress Studies Annual Meeting*, New Orleans, LA.

Chanrachakul, B., Broughton Pipkin, F., Warren, A. Y., Arulkumaran, S., and Khan, R. N. (2005). Progesterone enhances the tocolytic effect of ritodrine in isolated pregnant human myometrium. *Am. J. Obstet Gynecol.* 192, 458–463.

Coe, C. L., Kramer, M., Czéh, B., Gould, E., Reeves, A. J., Kirschbaum, C., and Fuchs, E. (2003). Prenatal stress diminishes neurogenesis in the dentate gyrus of juvenile rhesus monkeys. *Biol. Psychiatry* 54, 1025–1034.

Concas, A., Follesa, P., Barbaccia, M. L., Purdy, R. H., and Biggio, G. (1999). Physiological modulation of GABA(A) receptor plasticity by progesterone metabolites. *Eur. J. Pharmacol.* 375, 225–235.

Concas, A., Mostallino, M. C., Porcu, P., Follesa, P., Barbaccia, M. L., Trabucchi, M., Purdy, R. H., Grisenti, P., and Biggio, G. (1998). Role of brain allopregnanolone in the plasticity of gamma-aminobutyric acid type A receptor in rat brain during pregnancy and after delivery. *Proc. Natl. Acad. Sci. U.S.A.* 95, 13284–13289.

Conrad, C. D., Grote, K. A., Hobbs, R. J., and Ferayorni, A. (2003). Sex differences in spatial and non-spatial Y-maze performance after chronic stress. *Neurobiol. Learn. Mem.* 79, 32–40.

Deminiere, J. M., Piazza, P. V., Guegan, G., Abrous, N., Maccari, S., Le Moal, M., and Simon, H. (1992). Increased locomotor response to novelty and propensity to intravenous amphetamine self-administration in adult offspring of stressed mothers. *Brain Res.* 586, 135–139.

DeRoche, V., Piazza, P. V., Deminiere, J. M., Le Moal, M., and Simon, H. (1993). Rats orally self-administer corticosterone. *Brain Res.* 622, 315–320.

DeTurck, K. H., and Pohorecky, L. A. (1987). Ethanol sensitivity in rats: effect of prenatal stress. *Physiol. Behav.* 40, 407–410.

Devaud, L. L., Risinger, F. O., and Selvage, D. (2006). Impact of the hormonal milieu on the neurobiology of alcohol dependence and withdrawal. *J. Gen. Psychol.* 133, 337–356.

Diaz, R., Ogren, S. O., Blum, M., and Fuxe, K. (1995). Prenatal corticosterone increases spontaneous and d-amphetamine induced locomotor activity and brain dopamine metabolism in prepubertal male and female rats. *Neuroscience* 66, 467–473.

Djebaili, M., Guo, Q., Pettus, E. H., Hoffman, S. W., and Stein, D. G. (2005). The neurosteroids progesterone and allopregnanolone reduce cell death, gliosis, and functional deficits after traumatic brain injury in rats. *J. Neurotrauma* 22, 106–118.

Done, D. J., Crow, T. J., Johnstone, E. C., and Sacker, A. (1994). Childhood antecedents of schizophrenia and affective illness: social adjustment at ages 7 and 11. *BMJ* 309, 699–703.

Drago, F., Di Leo, F., and Giardina, L. (1999). Prenatal stress induces body weight deficit and behavioural alterations in rats: the effect of diazepam. *Eur. Neuropsychopharmacol.* 9, 239–245.

Ellermeier, W., and Westphal, W. (1995). Gender differences in pain ratings and pupil reactions to painful pressure stimuli. *Pain* 61, 435–439.

Ericsson, A., Kovács, K. J., and Sawchenko, P. E. (1994). A functional anatomical analysis of central pathways subserving the effects of interleukin-1 on stress-related neuroendocrine neurons. *J. Neurosci.* 14, 897–913.

Evans, S. M., and Foltin, R. W. (2006). Exogenous progesterone attenuates the subjective effects of smoked cocaine in women, but not in men. *Neuropsychopharmacology* 31, 659–674.

Evans, S. M., Haney, M., and Foltin, R. W. (2002). The effects of smoked cocaine during the follicular and luteal phases of the menstrual cycle in women. *Psychopharmacology (Berl.)* 159, 397–406.

Evans, S. M., and Levin, F. R. (2011). Response to alcohol in women: role of the menstrual cycle and a family history of alcoholism. *Drug Alcohol Depend.* 114, 18–30.

Facchinetti, F., Ottolini, F., Fazzio, M., Rigatelli, M., and Volpe, A. (2007). Psychosocial factors associated with preterm uterine contractions. *Psychother. Psychosom.* 76, 391–394.

Feltenstein, M. W., and See, R. E. (2007). Plasma progesterone levels and cocaine-seeking in freely cycling female rats across the estrous cycle. *Drug Alcohol Depend.* 89, 183–189.

Feltenstein, M. W., and See, R. E. (2008). The neurocircuitry of addiction: an overview. *Br. J. Pharmacol.* 154, 261–274.

Ferrini, M. G., Grillo, C. A., Piroli, G., de Kloet, E. R., and De Nicola, A. F. (1997). Sex difference in glucocorticoid regulation of vasopressin mRNA in the paraventricular hypothalamic nucleus. *Cell. Mol. Neurobiol.* 17, 671–686.

Finn, D. A., Beadles-Bohling, A. S., Beckley, E. H., Ford, M. M., Gililland, K. R., Gorin-Meyer, R. E., and Wiren, K. M. (2006). A new look at the 5α-reductase inhibitor finasteride. *CNS Drug Rev.* 12, 53–76.

Finn, D. A., Mark, G. P., Fretwell, A. M., Gililland-Kaufman, K. R., Strong, M. N., and Ford, M. M. (2008). Reinstatement of ethanol and sucrose seeking by the neurosteroid allopregnanolone in C57BL/6 mice. *Psychopharmacology (Berl.)* 201, 423–433.

Finn, D. A., Sinnott, R. S., Ford, M. M., Long, S. L., Tanchuck, M. A., and Phillips, T. J. (2004). Sex differences in the effect of ethanol injection and consumption on brain allopregnanolone levels in C57BL/6 mice. *Neuroscience* 123, 813–819.

Franklin, T. R., Napier, K., Ehrman, R., Gariti, P., O'Brien, C. P., and Childress, A. R. (2004). Retrospective study: influence of menstrual cycle on cue-induced cigarette craving. *Nicotine Tob. Res.* 6, 171–175.

Freeman, E. W., Frye, C. A., Rickels, K., Martin, P. A., and Smith, S. S. (2002). Allopregnanolone levels and symptom improvement in severe premenstrual syndrome. *J. Clin. Psychopharmacol.* 22, 516–520.

Fride, E., Dan, Y., Gavish, M., and Weinstock, M. (1985). Prenatal stress impairs maternal behavior in a conflict situation and reduces hippocampal benzodiazepine receptors. *Life Sci.* 36, 2103–2109.

Frisone, D. F., Frye, C. A., and Zimmerberg, B. (2002). Social isolation stress during the third week of life has age-dependent effects on spatial learning in rats. *Behav. Brain Res.* 128, 153–160.

Frye, C. A. (2009). "Neurosteroids-from basic research to clinical perspectives," in *Hormones/Behavior Relations of Clinical Importance*, eds R. T. Rubin and D. W. Pfaff (San Diego: Academic Press), 395–416.

Frye, C. A., Babson, A., and Walf, A. A. (2007). Self-administration of 3α-androstanediol increases locomotion and analgesia and decreases aggressive behavior of male hamsters. *Pharmacol. Biochem. Behav.* 86, 415–421.

Frye, C. A., and Bayon, L. E. (1998). Seizure activity is increased in endocrine states characterized by decline in endogenous levels of the neurosteroid 3α,5α-THP. *Neuroendocrinology* 68, 272–280.

Frye, C. A., Bayon, L. E., Pursnani, N. K., and Purdy, R. H. (1998). The neurosteroids, progesterone and 3α,5α-THP, enhance sexual motivation, receptivity, and proceptivity in female rats. *Brain Res.* 808, 72–83.

Frye, C. A., and McCormick, C. M. (2000a). The neurosteroid, 3α-androstanediol, prevents inhibitory avoidance deficits and pyknotic cells in the granule layer of the dentate gyrus induced by adrenalectomy in rats. *Brain Res.* 855, 166–170.

Frye, C. A., and McCormick, C. M. (2000b). Androgens are neuroprotective in the dentate gyrus of adrenalectomized female rats. *Stress* 3, 185–194.

Frye, C. A., and Orecki, Z. A. (2002). Prenatal stress alters reproductive responses of rats in behavioral estrus and paced mating of hormone-primed rats. *Horm. Behav.* 42, 472–483.

Frye, C. A., Paris, J. J., and Rhodes, M. E. (2008). Estrogen is necessary for 5α-pregnan-3α-ol-20-one (3α,5α-THP) infusion to the ventral tegmental area to facilitate social and sexual, but neither exploratory nor affective behavior of ovariectomized rats. *Pharmacol. Biochem. Behav.* 91, 261–270.

Frye, C. A., and Rhodes, M. E. (2006). Progestin concentrations are increased following paced mating in midbrain, hippocampus, diencephalon, and cortex of rats in behavioral estrus, but only in midbrain of diestrous rats. *Neuroendocrinology* 83, 336–347.

Frye, C. A., Rhodes, M. E., Petralia, S. M., Walf, A. A., Sumida, K., and Edinger, K. L. (2006a). 3α-hydroxy-5α-pregnan-20-one in the midbrain ventral tegmental area mediates social, sexual, and affective behaviors. *Neuroscience* 138, 1007–1014.

Frye, C. A., Rhodes, M. E., Raol, Y. H., and Brooks-Kayal, A. R. (2006b). Early postnatal stimulation alters pregnane neurosteroids in the hippocampus. *Psychopharmacology (Berl.)* 186, 343–350.

Frye, C. A., and Walf, A. A. (2004). Hippocampal 3α,5α-THP may alter depressive behavior of pregnant and lactating rats. *Pharmacol. Biochem. Behav.* 78, 531–540.

Frye, C. A., and Walf, A. A. (2008a). Effects of progesterone administration and APPswe+PSEN1Deltae9 mutation for cognitive performance of mid-aged mice. *Neurobiol. Learn. Mem.* 89, 17–26.

Frye, C. A., and Walf, A. A. (2008b). Membrane actions of progestins at dopamine type 1-like and GABA(A) receptors involve downstream signal transduction pathways. *Steroids* 73, 906–913.

Frye, C. A., and Walf, A. A. (2009). Progesterone reduces depression-like behavior in a murine model of Alzheimer's Disease. *Age (Dordr.)* 31, 143–153.

Frye, C. A., Walf, A. A., and Sumida, K. (2004). Progestins' actions in the VTA to facilitate lordosis involve dopamine-like type 1 and 2 receptors. *Pharmacol. Biochem. Behav.* 78, 405–418.

Frye, C. A., and Wawrzycki, J. (2003). Effect of prenatal stress and gonadal hormone condition on depressive behaviors of female and male rats. *Horm. Behav.* 44, 319–326.

Fumagalli, F., Bedogni, F., Perez, J., Racagni, G., and Riva, M. A. (2004). Corticostriatal brain-derived neurotrophic factor dysregulation in adult rats following prenatal stress. *Eur. J. Neurosci.* 20, 1348–1354.

Fumagalli, F., Bedogni, F., Slotkin, T. A., Racagni, G., and Riva, M. A. (2005). Prenatal stress elicits regionally selective changes in basal FGF-2 gene expression in adulthood and alters the adult response to acute or chronic stress. *Neurobiol. Dis.* 20, 731–737.

Galea, L. A., McEwen, B. S., Tanapat, P., Deak, T., Spencer, R. L., and Dhabhar, F. S. (1997). Sex differences in dendritic atrophy of CA3 pyramidal neurons in response to chronic restraint stress. *Neuroscience* 81, 689–697.

Gallop, R. J., Crits-Christoph, P., Ten Have, T. R., Barber, J. P., Frank, A., Griffin, M. L., and Thase, M. E. (2007). Differential transitions between cocaine use and abstinence for men and women. *J. Consult. Clin. Psychol.* 75, 95–103.

Gass, J. T., and Olive, M. F. (2008). Glutamatergic substrates of drug addiction and alcoholism. *Biochem. Pharmacol.* 75, 218–265.

George, O., and Koob, G. F. (2010). Individual differences in prefrontal cortex function and the transition from drug use to drug dependence. *Neurosci. Biobehav. Rev.* 35, 232–247.

Gerardin, D. C., Pereira, O. C., Kempinas, W. G., Florio, J. C., Moreira, E. G., and Bernardi, M. M. (2005). Sexual behavior, neuroendocrine, and neurochemical aspects in male rats exposed prenatally to stress. *Physiol. Behav.* 84, 97–104.

Gilbert Evans, S. E., Ross, L. E., Sellers, E. M., Purdy, R. H., and Romach, M. K. (2005). 3α-reduced neuroactive steroids and their precursors during pregnancy and the postpartum period. *Gynecol. Endocrinol.* 21, 268–279.

Girdler, S. S., and Klatzkin, R. (2007). Neurosteroids in the context of stress: implications for depressive disorders. *Pharmacol. Ther.* 116, 125–139.

Gitau, R., Fisk, N. M., Teixeira, J. M., Cameron, A., and Glover, V. (2001). Fetal hypothalamic-pituitary-adrenal stress responses to invasive procedures are independent of maternal responses. *J. Clin. Endocrinol. Metab.* 86, 104–109.

Giurgescu, C. (2009). Are maternal cortisol levels related to preterm birth? *J. Obstet. Gynecol. Neonatal. Nurs.* 38, 377–390.

Givalois, L., Gaillet, S., Mekaouche, M., Ixart, C., Bristow, A. F., Siaud, P., Szafarczyk, A., Malaval, F., Assenmacher, I., and Barbanel, G. (1995). Deletion of the ventral noradrenergic bundle obliterates the early ACTH response after systemic LPS, independently from the plasma IL-1β surge. *Endocrine* 3, 481–485.

Goldenberg, R. L., Culhane, J. F., Iams, J. D., and Romero, R. (2008). Epidemiology and causes of preterm birth. *Lancet* 371, 75–84.

Goodman, A. (2008). Neurobiology of addiction. An integrative review. *Biochem. Pharmacol.* 75, 266–322.

Gracias, C. R., Freeman, E. W., Sammel, M. D., Lin, H., Sheng, L., and Frye, C. A. (2009). Allopregnanolone levels before and after selective serotonin reuptake inhibitor treatment of premenstrual symptoms. *J. Clin. Psychopharmacol.* 29, 403–405.

Green, K. L., Azarov, A. V., Szeliga, K. T., Purdy, R. H., and Grant, K. A. (1999). The influence of menstrual cycle phase on sensitivity to ethanol-like discriminative stimulus effects of GABA(A)-positive modulators. *Pharmacol. Biochem. Behav.* 64, 379–383.

Grobin, A. C., and Morrow, A. L. (2001). 3α-hydroxy-5α-pregnan-20-one levels and GABA(A) receptor-mediated 36Cl(−) flux across development in rat cerebral cortex. *Brain Res. Dev. Brain Res.* 131, 31–39.

Gué, M., Bravard, A., Meunier, J., Veyrier, R., Gaillet, S., Recasens, M., and Maurice, T. (2004). Sex differences in learning deficits induced by prenatal stress in juvenile rats. *Behav. Brain Res.* 150, 149–157.

Haber, S. N., and Fudge, J. L. (1997). The primate substantia nigra and VTA: integrative circuitry and function. *Crit. Rev. Neurobiol.* 11, 323–342.

He, W. B., Zhao, M., Machida, T., and Chen, N. H. (2009). Effect of corticosterone on developing hippocampus: short-term and long-term outcomes. *Hippocampus* 19, 338–349.

Hecht, G. S., Spear, N. E., and Spear, L. P. (1999). Changes in progressive ratio responding for intravenous cocaine throughout the reproductive process in female rats. *Dev. Psychobiol.* 35, 136–145.

Helms, C. M., and Grant, K. A. (2011). The effect of age on the discriminative stimulus effects of ethanol and its GABA(A) receptor mediation in cynomolgus monkeys. *Psychopharmacology (Berl.)* 216, 333–343.

Henry, C., Guegant, G., Cador, M., Arnauld, E., Arsaut, J., Le Moal, M., and Demotes-Mainard, J. (1995). Prenatal stress in rats facilitates amphetamine-induced sensitization and induces long-lasting changes in dopamine receptors in the nucleus accumbens. *Brain Res.* 685, 179–186.

Herman, J. P., Prewitt, C. M., and Cullinan, W. E. (1996). Neuronal circuit regulation of the hypothalamo-pituitary-adrenocortical stress axis. *Crit. Rev. Neurobiol.* 10, 371–394.

Hermus, A. R., and Sweep, C. G. (1990). Cytokines and the hypothalamic-pituitary-adrenal axis. *J. Steroid Biochem. Mol. Biol.* 37, 867–871.

Hinojosa-Laborde, C., Chapa, I., Lange, D., and Haywood, J. R. (1999). Gender differences in sympathetic nervous system regulation. *Clin. Exp. Pharmacol. Physiol.* 26, 122–126.

Horvitz, J. C. (2000). Mesolimbocortical and nigrostriatal dopamine responses to salient non-reward events. *Neuroscience* 96, 651–656.

Howell, A. N., Leyro, T. M., Hogan, J., Buckner, J. D., and Zvolensky, M. J. (2010). Anxiety sensitivity, distress tolerance, and discomfort intolerance in relation to coping and conformity motives for alcohol use and alcohol use problems among young adult drinkers. *Addict. Behav.* 35, 1144–1147.

Huizink, A. C., Mulder, E. J., and Buitelaar, J. K. (2004). Prenatal stress and risk for psychopathology: specific effects or induction of general susceptibility? *Psychol. Bull.* 130, 115–142.

Huttunen, M. O., and Niskanen, P. (1978). Prenatal loss of father and psychiatric disorders. *Arch. Gen. Psychiatry* 35, 429–431.

Ikemoto, S., and Panksepp, J. (1999). The role of nucleus accumbens dopamine in motivated behavior: a unifying interpretation with special reference to reward-seeking. *Brain Res. Brain Res. Rev.* 31, 6–41.

Iswari, S., Colas, A. E., and Karavolas, H. J. (1986). Binding of 5α-dihydroprogesterone and other progestins to female rat anterior pituitary nuclear extracts. *Steroids* 47, 189–203.

Janis, G. C., Devaud, L. L., Mitsuyama, H., and Morrow, A. L. (1998). Effects of chronic ethanol consumption and withdrawal on the neuroactive steroid 3α-hydroxy-5α-pregnan-20-one in male and female rats. *Alcohol. Clin. Exp. Res.* 22, 2055–2061.

Jezová, D., Juránková, E., Mosnárová, A., Kriska, M., and Skultétyová, I. (1996). Neuroendocrine response during stress with relation to gender differences. *Acta Neurobiol. Exp. (Wars)* 56, 779–785.

Johnson, R. W., Gheusi, G., Segreti, S., Dantzer, R., and Kelley, K. W. (1997). C3H/HeJ mice are refractory to lipopolysaccharide in the brain. *Brain Res.* 752, 219–226.

Johnstone, H. A., Wigger, A., Douglas, A. J., Neumann, I. D., Landgraf, R., Seckl, J. R., and Russell, J. A. (2000). Attenuation of hypothalamic-pituitary-adrenal axis stress responses in late pregnancy: changes in feedforward and feedback mechanisms. *J. Neuroendocrinol.* 12, 811–822.

Jutapakdeegul, N., Afadlal, S., Polaboon, N., Phansuwan-Pujito, P., and Govitrapong, P. (2010). Repeated restraint stress and corticosterone injections during late pregnancy alter GAP-43 expression in the hippocampus and prefrontal cortex of rat pups. *Int. J. Dev. Neurosci.* 28, 83–90.

Kalivas, P. W., Lalumiere, R. T., Knackstedt, L., and Shen, H. (2009). Glutamate transmission in addiction. *Neuropharmacology* 56, 169–173.

Kehoe, P., Mallinson, K., McCormick, C. M., and Frye, C. A. (2000). Central allopregnanolone is increased in rat pups in response to repeated, short episodes of neonatal isolation. *Brain Res. Dev. Brain Res.* 124, 133–136.

Kelley, A. E. and Berridge, K. C. (2002). The neuroscience of natural rewards: relevance to addictive drugs. *J. Neurosci.* 22, 3306–3311.

Kellogg, C. K., and Frye, C. A. (1999). Endogenous levels of 5α-reduced progestins and androgens in fetal vs. adult rat brains. *Dev. Brain Res.* 115, 17–24.

Kerstjens, J. M., de Winter, A. F., Bocca-Tjeertes, I. F., Ten Vergert, E. M., Reijneveld, S. A., and Bos, A. F. (2011). Developmental delay in moderately preterm-born children at school entry. *J. Pediatr.* 159, 92–98.

Keshet, G. I., and Weinstock, M. (1995). Maternal naltrexone prevents morphological and behavioral alterations induced in rats by prenatal stress. *Pharmacol. Biochem. Behav.* 50, 413–419.

King, C. R. (2011). A novel embryological theory of autism causation involving endogenous biochemicals capable of initiating cellular gene transcription: a possible link between twelve autism risk factors and the autism 'epidemic'. *Med. Hypotheses* 76, 653–660.

Kippin, T. E., Cain, S. W., Maszum, Z., and Ralph, M. M. (2004). Neural stem cells show bidirectional experience-dependent plasticity in the perinatal mammalian brain. *J. Neurosci.* 24, 2832–2836.

Kippin, T. E., Szumlinski, K. K., Kapasova, Z., Rezner, B., and See, R. E. (2008). Prenatal stress enhances responsiveness to cocaine. *Neuropsychopharmacology* 33, 769–782.

Kitraki, E., Kremmyda, O., Youlatos, D., Alexis, M. N., and Kittas, C. (2004). Gender-dependent alterations in corticosteroid receptor status and spatial performance following 21 days of restraint stress. *Neuroscience* 125, 47–55.

Klatzkin, R. R., Morrow, A. L., Light, K. C., Pedersen, C. A., and Girdler, S. S. (2006). Histories of depression, allopregnanolone responses to stress, and premenstrual symptoms in women. *Biol. Psychol.* 71, 2–11.

Kleinhaus, K., Steinfeld, S., Balaban, J., Goodman, L., Craft, T. S., and Malaspina, D., Myers, M. M., and Moore, H. (2010). Effects of excessive glucocorticoid receptor stimulation during early gestation on psychomotor and social behavior in the rat. *Dev. Psychobiol.* 52, 121–132.

Koehl, M., Bjijou, Y., Le Moal, M., and Cador, M. (2000). Nicotine-induced locomotor activity is increased by preexposure of rats to prenatal stress. *Brain Res.* 882, 196–200.

Koehl, M., Lemaire, V., Le Moal, M., and Abrous, D. N. (2009). Age-dependent effect of prenatal stress on hippocampal cell proliferation in female rats. *Eur. J. Neurosci.* 29, 635–640.

Kohtz, A. S., Paris, J. J., and Frye, C. A. (2010). Low doses of cocaine decrease, and high doses increase, anxiety-like behavior and brain progestogen levels among intact rats. *Horm. Behav.* 57, 474–480.

Koob, G. F., and Le Moal, M. (2001). Drug addiction, dysregulation of reward, and allostasis. *Neuropsychopharmacology* 24, 97–129.

Koob, G. F., and Volkow, N. D. (2010). Neurocircuitry of addiction. *Neuropsychopharacology* 35, 217–238.

Kraszpulski, M., Dickerson, P. A., and Salm, A. K. (2006). Prenatal stress affects the developmental trajectory of the rat amygdala. *Stress* 9, 85–95.

Kroll, J. L. (2007). New directions in the conceptualization of psychotic disorders. *Curr. Opin. Psychiatry* 20, 573–577.

Lapish, C. C., Seamans, J. K., and Chandler, L. J. (2006). Glutamate-dopamine cotransmission and reward processing in addiction. *Alcohol. Clin. Exp. Res.* 30, 1451–1465.

Larsen, E. B., Anker, J. J., Gliddon, L. A., Fons, K. S., and Carroll, M. E. (2007). Effects of estrogen and progesterone on the escalation of cocaine self-administration in female rats during extended access. *Exp. Clin. Psychopharmacol.* 15, 461–471.

Latendresse, G. (2009). The interaction between chronic stress and pregnancy: preterm birth from a biobehavioral perspective. *J. Midwifery Womens Health* 54, 8–17.

Lemaire, V., Koehl, M., Le Moal, M., and Abrous, D. N. (2000). Prenatal stress produces learning deficits associated with an inhibition of neurogenesis in the hippocampus. *Proc. Natl. Acad. Sci. U.S.A.* 97, 11032–11037.

Li, H., Li, Q. H., Zhu, Z. L., Chen, R., Cheng, D. X., Cai, Q., Jia, N., and Song, L. (2007). Prenatal restraint stress decreases neurogranin expression in rat offspring hippocampus. *Sheng Li Xue Bao* 59, 299–304.

Lind, A., Korkman, M., Lehtonen, L., Lapinleimu, H., Parkkola, R., Matomäki, J., Haataja, L., and PIPARI Study Group. (2011). Cognitive and neuropsychological outcomes at 5 years of age in preterm children born in the 2000s. *Dev. Med. Child Neurol.* 53, 256–362.

Lodygensky, G. A., Vasung, L., Sizonenko, S. V., and Hüppi, P. S. (2010). Neuroimaging of cortical development and brain connectivity in human newborns and animal models. *J. Anat.* 217, 418–428.

Ma, S., Shipston, M. J., Morilak, D., and Russell, J. A. (2005). Reduced hypothalamic vasopressin secretion underlies attenuated adrenocorticotropin stress responses in pregnant rats. *Endocrinology* 146, 1626–1637.

Majewska, M. D., Harrison, N. L., Schwartz, R. D., Barker, J. L., and Paul, S. M. (1986). Steroid hormone metabolites are barbiturate-like modulators of the GABA receptor. *Science* 232, 1004–1007.

Manji, H. K., Drevets, W. C., and Charney, D. S. (2001). The cellular neurobiology of depression. *Nat. Med.* 7, 541–547.

Mann, K., Ackermann, K., Croissant, B., Mundle, G., Nakovics, H., and Diehl, A. (2005). Neuroimaging of gender differences in alcohol dependence: are women more vulnerable? *Alcohol. Clin. Exp. Res.* 29, 896–901.

Martinez-Tellez, R. I., Hernandez-Torres, E., Gamboa, C., and Flores, G. (2009). Prenatal stress alters spine density and dendritic length of nucleus accumbens and hippocampus neurons in rat offspring. *Synapse* 63, 794–804.

Marx, C. E., Stevens, R. D., Shampine, L. J., Uzunova, V., Trost, W. T., Butterfield, M. I., Massing, M. W., Hamer, R. M., Morrow, A. L., and Lieberman, J. A. (2006). Neuroactive steroids are altered in schizophrenia and bipolar disorder: relevance to pathophysiology and therapeutics. *Neuropsychopharmacology* 31, 1249–1263.

Matthews, S. G., Owen, D., Banjanin, S., and Andrews, M. H. (2002). Glucocorticoids, hypothalamo-pituitary-adrenal (HPA) development, and life after birth. *Endocr. Res.* 28, 709–718.

McArthur, S., McHale, E., Dalley, J. W., Buckingham, J. C., and Gillies, G. E. (2005). Altered mesencephalic dopaminergic populations in adulthood as a consequence of brief perinatal glucocorticoid exposure. *J. Neuroendocrinol.* 17, 475–482.

McBride, W. J., and Li, T. K. (1998). Animal models of alcoholism: neurobiology of high alcohol-drinking behavior in rodents. *Crit. Rev. Neurobiol.* 12, 339–369.

McCormick, C. M., Kehoe, P., Mallinson, K., Cecchi, L., and Frye, C. A. (2002). Neonatal isolation alters stress hormone and mesolimbic dopamine release in juvenile rats. *Pharmacol. Biochem. Behav.* 73, 77–85.

McCormick, C. M., and Mathews, I. Z. (2007). HPA function in adolescence: role of sex hormones in its regulation and the enduring consequences of exposure to stressors. *Pharmacol. Biochem. Behav.* 86, 220–233.

McFadden, L. M., Paris, J. J., Mitzelfelt, M. S., McDonough, S., Frye, C. A., and Matuszewich, L. (2011). Sex-dependent effects of chronic unpredictable stress in the water maze. *Physiol. Behav.* 102, 266–275.

Meerts, S. H. and Clark, A. S. (2007). Female rats exhibit a conditioned place preference for nonpaced mating. *Horm. Behav.* 51, 89–94.

Mello, N. K., Mendelson, J. H., and Palmieri, S. L. (1987). Cigarette smoking by women: interactions with alcohol use. *Psychopharmacology (Berl.)* 93, 8–15.

Mellon, S. H., Gong, W., and Schonemann, M. D. (2008). Endogenous and synthetic neurosteroids in treatment of Niemann-Pick type C disease. *Brain Res. Rev.* 57, 410–420.

Michelsen, K. A., van den Hove, D. L., Schmitz, C., Segers, O., Prickaerts, J., and Steinbusch, H. W. (2007). Prenatal stress and subsequent exposure to chronic mild stress influence dendritic spine density and morphology in the rat medial prefrontal cortex. *BMC Neurosci.* 8, 107. doi:10.1186/1471-2202-8-107

Mizoguchi, K., Kunishita, T., Chui, D. H., and Tabira, T. (1992). Stress induces neuronal death in the hippocampus of castrated rats. *Neurosci. Lett.* 138, 157–160.

Morgan, K. N., Thayer, J. E., and Frye, C. A. (1999). Prenatal stress suppresses rat pup ultrasonic vocalization and myoclonic twitching in response to separation. *Dev. Psychobiol.* 34, 205–215.

Morley-Fletcher, S., Puopolo, M., Gentili, S., Gerra, G., Macchia, T., and Laviola, G. (2004). Prenatal stress affects 3,4-methylenedioxymethamphetamine pharmacokinetics and drug-induced motor alterations in adolescent female rats. *Eur. J. Pharmacol.* 489, 89–92.

Morrow, A. L., VanDoren, M. J., Fleming, R., and Penland, S. (2001). Ethanol and neurosteroid interactions in the brain. *Int. Rev. Neurobiol.* 46, 349–377.

Morton, W. A. (1999). Cocaine and psychiatric symptoms. *Prim. Care Companion J. Clin. Psychiatry* 1, 109–113.

Murmu, M. S., Salomon, S., Biala, Y., Weinstock, M., Braun, K., and Bock, J. (2006). Changes of spine density and dendritic complexity in the prefrontal cortex in offspring of mothers exposed to stress during pregnancy. *Eur. J. Neurosci.* 24, 1477–1487.

Nestler, E. J., and Carlezon, W. A. Jr. (2006). The mesolimbic dopamine reward circuit in depression. *Biol. Psychiatry* 59, 1151–1159.

Nyberg, S., Andersson, A., Zingmark, E., Wahlström, G., Bäckström, T., and Sundström-Poromaa, I. (2005). The effect of a low dose of alcohol on allopregnanolone serum concentrations across the menstrual cycle in women with severe premenstrual syndrome and controls. *Psychoneuroendocrinology* 30, 892–901.

Odagiri, K., Abe, H., Kawagoe, C., Takeda, R., Ikeda, T., Matsuo, H., Nonaka, H., Ebihara, K., Nishimori, T., Ishizuka, Y., Hashiguchi, H., and Ishida, Y. (2008). Psychological prenatal stress reduced the number of BrdU immunopositive cells in the dorsal hippocampus without affecting the open field behavior of male and female rats at one month of age. *Neurosci. Lett.* 446, 25–29.

Ohkawa, T. (1987). Sexual differentiation of social play and copulatory behavior in prenatally stressed male and female offspring of the rat: the influence of simultaneous treatment by tyrosine during exposure to prenatal stress. *Nippon Naibunpi Gakkai Zasshi* 63, 823–835.

Paredes, R. G., and Vazquez, B. (1999). What do female rats like about sex? Paced mating. *Behav. Brain Res.* 105, 117–127.

Paintlia, M. K., Paintlia, A. S., Singh, A. K., and Singh, I. (2008). Attenuation of lipopolysaccharide-induced inflammatory response and phospholipids metabolism at the feto-maternal interface by N-acetyl cysteine. *Pediatr. Res.* 64, 334–339.

Paris, J. J., Brunton, P. J., Russell, J. A., Walf, A. A., and Frye, C. A. (2011). Inhibition of 5α-reductase activity in late pregnancy decreases gestational length and fecundity and impairs object memory and central progestogen milieu of juvenile rat offspring. *J. Neuroendocrinol.* doi: 10.1111/j.1365-2826.2011.02219.x.

Paris, J. J., and Frye, C. A. (2008). Estrous cycle, pregnancy, and parity enhance performance of rats in object recognition or object placement tasks. *Reproduction* 136, 105–115.

Paris, J. J., and Frye, C. A. (2009). Alcohol dose-dependently enhances 3α-androstanediol formation in frontal cortex of male rats concomitant with aggression. *Open Neuropsychopharmacol. J.* 2, 1–10.

Paris, J. J., and Frye, C. A. (2011a). Juvenile offspring of rats exposed to restraint stress in late gestation have impaired cognitive performance and dysregulated progestogen formation. *Stress* 14, 23–32.

Paris, J. J., and Frye, C. A. (2011b). Gestational exposure to variable stressors produces decrements in cognitive and neural development of juvenile male and female rats. *Curr. Top. Med. Chem.* 11, 1706–1713.

Patchev, V. K., and Almeida, O. F. (1996). Gonadal steroids exert facilitating and "buffering" effects on glucocorticoid-mediated transcriptional regulation of corticotropin-releasing hormone and corticosteroid receptor genes in rat brain. *J. Neurosci.* 16, 7077–7084.

Patchev, V. K., Hassan, A. H., Holsboer, D. F., and Almeida, O. F. (1996). The neurosteroid tetrahydroprogesterone attenuates the endocrine response to stress and exerts glucocorticoid-like effects on vasopressin gene transcription in the rat hypothalamus. *Neuropsychopharmacology* 15, 533–540.

Patchev, V. K., Shoaib, M., Holsboer, F., and Almeida, O. F. (1994). The neurosteroid tetrahydroprogesterone counteracts corticotropin-releasing hormone-induced anxiety and alters the release and gene expression of corticotropin-releasing hormone in the rat hypothalamus. *Neuroscience* 62, 265–271.

Pierucci-Lagha, A., Covault, J., Feinn, R., Khisti, R. T., Morrow, A. L., Marx, C. E., Shampine, L. J., and Kranzler, H. R. (2006). Subjective effects and changes in steroid hormone concentrations in humans following acute consumption of alcohol. *Psychopharmacology (Berl.)* 186, 451–461.

Poling, J., Kosten, T. R., and Sofuoglu, M. (2007). Treatment outcome predictors for cocaine dependence. *Am. J. Drug Alcohol Abuse* 33, 191–206.

Poltyrev, T., Keshet, G. I., Kay, G., and Weinstock, M. (1996). Role of experimental conditions in determining differences in exploratory behavior of prenatally stressed rats. *Dev. Psychobiol.* 29, 453–462.

Purdy, R. H., Morrow, A. L., Moore, P. H. Jr., and Paul, S. M. (1991). Stress-induced elevations of gamma-aminobutyric acid type A receptor-active steroids in the rat brain. *Proc. Natl. Acad. Sci. U.S.A.* 88, 4553–4557.

Quinones-Jenab, V., Minerly, A. C., Niyomchia, T., Akahvan, A., Jenab, S., and Frye, C. A. (2008). Progesterone and allopregnanolone are induced by cocaine in serum and brain tissues of male and female rats. *Pharmacol. Biochem. Behav.* 89, 292–297.

Rasmusson, A. M., Pinna, G., Paliwal, P., Weisman, D., Gottschalk, C., Charney, D., Krystal, J., and Guidotti, A. (2006). Decreased cerebrospinal fluid allopregnanolone levels in women with posttraumatic stress disorder. *Biol. Psychiatry* 60, 704–713.

Reed, S. C., Evans, S. M., Bedi, G., Rubin, E., and Foltin, R. W. (2011). The effects of oral micronized progesterone on smoked cocaine self-administration in women. *Horm. Behav.* 59, 227–235.

Rhodes, M. E., McCormick, C. M., and Frye, C. A. (2004). 3α,5α-THP mediates progestins' effects to protect against adrenalectomy-induced cell death in the dentate gyrus of female and male rats. *Pharmacol. Biochem. Behav.* 78, 505–512.

Rhodes, M. E., and Rubin, R. T. (1999). Functional sex differences ('sexual diergism') of central nervous system cholinergic systems, vasopressin, and hypothalamic-pituitary-adrenal axis activity in mammals: a selective review. *Brain Res. Brain Res. Rev.* 30, 135–152.

Robbins, S. J., Ehrman, R. N., Childress, A. R., and O'Brien, C. P. (1999). Comparing levels of cocaine cue reactivity in male and female outpatients. *Drug Alcohol Depend.* 53, 223–230.

Rodrigues, T., Rocha, L., and Barros, H. (2008). Physical abuse during pregnancy and preterm delivery. *Am. J. Obstet. Gynecol.* 198, 171.e1–e6.

Rohleder, N., Schommer, N. C., Hellhammer, D. H., Engel, R., and Kirschbaum, C. (2001). Sex differences in glucocorticoid sensitivity of proinflammatory cytokine production after psychosocial stress. *Psychosom. Med.* 63, 966–972.

Rubin, E., Aharonovich, E., Bisaga, A., Levin, F. R., Raby, W. N., and Nunes, E. V. (2007). Early abstinence in cocaine dependence: influence of comorbid major depression. *Am. J. Addict.* 16, 283–290.

Russell, J. A., Leng, G., and Douglas, A. J. (2003). The magnocellular oxytocin system, the fount of maternity: adaptations in pregnancy. *Front. Neuroendocrinol.* 24, 27–61.

Ryan, M. A., Jacobson, I. G., Sevick, C. J., Smith, T. C., Gumbs, G. R., Conlin, A. M., and United States Department of Defense Birth and Infant Health Registry. (2011). Health outcomes among infants born to women deployed to United States military operations during pregnancy. *Birth Defects Res. A Clin. Mol. Teratol.* 91, 117–124.

Salamone, J. D., Correa, M., Farrar, A. M., Nunes, E. J., and Pardo, M. (2009). Dopamine, behavioral economics, and effort. *Front. Behav. Neurosci.* 3:13. doi:10.3389/neuro.08.013.2009

Salm, A. K., Pavelko, M., Krouse, E. M., Webster, W., Kraszpulski, M., and Birkle, D. (2004). Lateral amygdaloid nucleus expansion in adult rats is associated with exposure to prenatal stress. *Dev. Brain Res.* 148, 159–167.

Sapolsky, R. M. (2001). Depression, antidepressants, and the shrinking hippocampus. *Proc. Natl. Acad. Sci. U.S.A.* 98, 12320–12322.

Sayeed, I., Guo, Q., Hoffman, S. W., and Stein, D. G. (2006). Allopregnanolone, a progesterone metabolite, is more effective than progesterone in reducing cortical infarct volume after transient middle cerebral artery occlusion. *Ann. Emerg. Med.* 47, 381–389.

Schlotz, W., and Phillips, D. I. (2009). Fetal origins of mental health: evidence and mechanisms. *Brain Behav. Immun.* 23, 905–916.

Schmitz, C., Rhodes, M. E., Bludau, M., Kaplan, S., Ong, P., Ueffing, I., Vehoff, J., Korr, H., and Frye, C. A. (2002). Depression: reduced number of granule cells in the hippocampus of female, but not male, rats due to prenatal restraint stress. *Mol. Psychiatry* 7, 810–813.

Schoenfeld, T. J., and Gould, E. (2011). Stress, stress hormones, and adult neurogenesis. *Exp. Neurol.* doi:10.1016/j.expneurol.2011.01.008

Schuckit, M. A. (2009). An overview of genetic influences in alcoholism. *J. Subst. Abuse Treat.* 36, S5–S14.

Seckl, J. R., and Meaney, M. J. (2004). Glucocorticoid programming. *Ann. N. Y. Acad. Sci.* 1032, 63–84.

Secoli, S. R., and Teixeira, N. A. (1998). Chronic prenatal stress affects development and behavioral depression in rats. *Stress* 2, 273–280.

Segarra, A. C., Agosto-Rivera, J. L., Febo, M., Lugo-Escobar, N., Menéndez-Delmestre, R., Puig-Ramos, A., and Torres-Diaz, Y. M. (2009). Estradiol: a key biological substrate mediating the response to cocaine in female rats. *Horm. Behav.* 58, 33–43.

Serra, M., Sanna, E., Mostallino, M. C., and Biggio, G. (2007). Social isolation stress and neuroactive steroids. *Eur. Neuropsychopharmacol.* 17, 1–11.

Silvagni, A., Barros, V. G., Mura, C., Antonelli, M. C., and Carboni, E. (2008). Prenatal restraint stress differentially modifies basal and stimulated dopamine and noradrenaline release in the nucleus accumbens shell: an 'in vivo' microdialysis study in adolescent and young adult rats. *Eur. J. Neurosci.* 28, 744–758.

Sinha, R., Fox, H., Hong, K. I., Sofuoglu, M., Morgan, P. T., and Bergquist, K. T. (2007). Sex steroid hormones, stress response, and drug craving in cocaine-dependent women: implications for relapse susceptibility. *Exp. Clin. Psychopharmacol.* 15, 445–452.

Sinnott, R. S., Mark, G. P., and Finn, D. A. (2002a). Reinforcing effects of the neurosteroid allopregnanolone in rats. *Pharmacol. Biochem. Behav.* 72, 923–929.

Sinnott, R. S., Phillips, T. J., and Finn, D. A. (2002b). Alteration of voluntary ethanol and saccharin consumption by the neurosteroid allopregnanolone in mice. *Psychopharmacology (Berl.)* 162, 438–447.

Snively, T. A., Ahijevych, K. L., Bernhard, L. A., and Wewers, M. E. (2000). Smoking behavior, dysphoric states and the menstrual cycle: results from single smoking sessions and the natural environment. *Psychoneuroendocrinology* 25, 677–691.

Sofuoglu, M., Babb, D. A., and Hatsukami, D. K. (2002). Effects of progesterone treatment on smoked cocaine response in women. *Pharmacol. Biochem. Behav.* 72, 431–435.

Sofuoglu, M., Dudish-Poulsen, S., Nelson, D., Pentel, P. R., and Hatsukami, D. K. (1999). Sex and menstrual cycle differences in the subjective effects from smoked cocaine in humans. *Exp. Clin. Psychopharmacol.* 7, 274–283.

Sofuoglu, M., Mitchell, E., and Kosten, T. R. (2004). Effects of progesterone treatment on cocaine responses in male and female cocaine users. *Pharmacol. Biochem. Behav.* 78, 699–705.

Sofuoglu, M., and Sewell, R. A. (2009). Norepinephrine and stimulant addiction. *Addict. Biol.* 14, 119–219.

Son, G. H., Chung, S., Geum, D., Kang, S. S., Choi, W. S., Kim, K., and Choi, S. (2007). Hyperactivity and alteration of the midbrain dopaminergic system in maternally stressed male mice offspring. *Biochem. Biophys. Res. Commun.* 352, 823–829.

Sumida, K., Walf, A. A., and Frye, C. A. (2005). Progestin-facilitated lordosis of hamsters may involve dopamine-like type 1 receptors in the ventral tegmental area. *Behav. Brain Res.* 161, 1–7.

Sutker, P. B., Goist, K. C. Jr., and King, A. R. (1987). Acute alcohol intoxication in women: relationship to dose and menstrual cycle phase. *Alcohol. Clin. Exp. Res.* 11, 74–79.

Talge, N. M., Holzman, C., Wang, J., Lucia, V., Gardiner, J., and Breslau, N. (2010). Late-preterm birth and its association with cognitive and socioemotional outcomes at 6 years of age. *Pediatrics* 126, 1124–1131.

Thomas, M. B., Hu, M., Lee, T. M., Bhatnagar, S., and Becker, J. B. (2009). Sex-specific susceptibility to cocaine in rats with a history of prenatal stress. *Physiol. Behav.* 97, 270–277.

Tindell, A. J., Berridge, K. C., Zhang, J., Peciña, S., and Aldridge, J. W. (2005). Ventral pallidal neurons code incentive motivation: amplification by mesolimbic sensitization and amphetamine. *Eur. J. Neurosci.* 22, 2617–2634.

Torres, J. M., and Ortega, E. (2003). Alcohol intoxication increases allopregnanolone levels in female adolescent humans. *Neuropsychopharmacology* 28, 1207–1209.

Turnbull, A. V., Lee, S., and Rivier, C. (1998). Mechanisms of hypothalamic-pituitary-adrenal axis stimulation by immune signals in the adult rat. *Ann. N. Y. Acad. Sci.* 840, 434–443.

Turnbull, A. V., and Rivier, C. (1997). Corticotropin-releasing factor (CRF) and endocrine responses to stress: CRF receptors, binding protein, and related peptides. *Proc. Soc. Exp. Biol. Med.* 215, 1–10.

Turnbull, A. V., and Rivier, C. L. (1999). Sprague-Dawley rats obtained from different vendors exhibit distinct adrenocorticotropin responses to inflammatory stimuli. *Neuroendocrinology* 70, 186–195.

Uno, H., Tarara, R., Else, J. G., Suleman, M. A., and Sapolsky, R. M. (1989). Hippocampal damage associated with prolonged and fatal stress in primates. *J. Neurosci.* 9, 1705–1711.

Vallée, M., Mayo, W., Dellu, F., Le Moal, M., Simon, H., and Maccari, S. (1997). Prenatal stress induces high anxiety and postnatal handling induces low anxiety in adult offspring: correlation with stress-induced corticosterone secretion. *J. Neurosci.* 17, 2626–2636.

Van den Hove, D. L., Lauder, J. M., Scheepens, A., Prickaerts, J., Blanco, C. E., and Steinbusch, H. W. (2006). Prenatal stress in the rat alters 5-HT1A receptor binding in the ventral hippocampus. *Brain Res.* 1090, 29–34.

Volkow, N. D., Wang, G. J., Fowler, J. S., Tomasi, D., Telang, F., and Baler, R. (2010). Addiction: decreased reward sensitivity and increased expectation sensitivity conspire to overwhelm the brain's control circuit. *Bioessays* 32, 748–755.

Wakshlak, A., and Weinstock, M. (1990). Neonatal handling reverses behavioral abnormalities induced in rats by prenatal stress. *Physiol. Behav.* 48, 289–292.

Walf, A. A., and Frye, C. A. (2007). Estradiol decreases anxiety behavior and enhances inhibitory avoidance and gestational stress produces opposite effects. *Stress* 10, 251–260.

Wang, J. M., Singh, C., Liu, L., Irwin, R. W., Chen, S., Chung, E. J., Thompson, R. F., and Brinton, R. D. (2010). Allopregnanolone reverses neurogenic and cognitive deficits in mouse model of Alzheimer's disease. *Proc. Natl. Acad. Sci. U.S.A.* 107, 6498–6503.

Ward, I. L., and Stehm, K. E. (1991). Prenatal stress feminizes juvenile play patterns in male rats. *Physiol. Behav.* 50, 601–605.

Weinstock, M., and Fride, E. (1989). Alterations in behavioral and striatal dopamine asymmetries induced by prenatal stress. *Pharmacol. Biochem. Behav.* 32, 425–430.

Wise, R. A. (2004). Drive, incentive, and reinforcement: the antecedents and consequences of motivation. *Nebr. Symp. Motiv.* 50, 159–195.

Wortsman, J. (2002). Role of epinephrine in acute stress. *Endocrinol. Metab. Clin. North Am.* 31, 79–106.

Xiong, X., Harville, E. W., Mattison, D. R., Elkind-Hirsch, K., Pridjian, G., and Buekens, P. (2008). Exposure to Hurricane Katrina, posttraumatic stress disorder and birth outcomes. *Am. J. Med. Sci.* 336, 111–115.

Yawno, T., Hirst, J. J., Castillo-Melendez, M., and Walker, D. W. (2009). Role of neurosteroids in regulating cell death and proliferation in the late gestation fetal brain. *Neuroscience* 163, 838–847.

Yehuda, R., Bierer, L. M., Sarapas, C., Makotkine, I., Andrew, R., and Seckl, J. R. (2009). Cortisol metabolic predictors of response to psychotherapy for symptoms of PTSD in survivors of the World Trade Center attacks on September 11, 2001. *Psychoneuroendocrinology* 34, 1304–1313.

Zimmerberg, B., and Blaskey, L. G. (1998). Prenatal stress effects are partially ameliorated by prenatal administration of the neurosteroid allopregnanolone. *Pharmacol. Biochem. Behav.* 59, 819–827.

Maternal genetic mutations as gestational and early life influences in producing psychiatric disease-like phenotypes in mice

Georgia Gleason, Bojana Zupan and Miklos Toth*

Department of Pharmacology, Weill Medical College of Cornell University, New York, NY, USA

*Correspondence:
Miklos Toth, Weill Medical College of Cornell University, 1300 York Avenue, New York, NY, USA.
e-mail: mtoth@med.cornell.edu

Risk factors for psychiatric disorders have traditionally been classified as genetic or environmental. Risk (candidate) genes, although typically possessing small effects, represent a clear starting point to elucidate downstream cellular/molecular pathways of disease. Environmental effects, especially during development, can also lead to altered behavior and increased risk for disease. An important environmental factor is the mother, demonstrated by the negative effects elicited by maternal gestational stress and altered maternal care. These maternal effects can also have a genetic basis (e.g., maternal genetic variability and mutations). The focus of this review is "maternal genotype effects" that influence the emotional development of the offspring resulting in life-long psychiatric disease-like phenotypes. We have recently found that genetic inactivation of the serotonin 1A receptor (5-HT1AR) and the *fmr1* gene (encoding the fragile X mental retardation protein) in mouse dams results in psychiatric disease-like phenotypes in their genetically unaffected offspring. 5-HT1AR deficiency in dams results in anxiety and increased stress responsiveness in their offspring. Offspring of 5-HT1AR deficient dams display altered development of the hippocampus, which could be linked to their anxiety-like phenotype. Maternal inactivation of *fmr1*, like its inactivation in the offspring, results in a hyperactivity-like condition and is associated with receptor alterations in the striatum. These data indicate a high sensitivity of the offspring to maternal mutations and suggest that maternal genotype effects can increase the impact of genetic risk factors in a population by increasing the risk of the genetically normal offspring as well as by enhancing the effects of offspring mutations.

Keywords: anxiety, fragile X, transgenerational, epigenetic, maternal

MATERNAL GENOTYPE EFFECTS CAN CONTRIBUTE TO THE HIGH HERITABILITY OF PSYCHIATRIC DISEASES

A large number of studies indicate that the pre/postnatal maternal environment can increase the offspring's risk for psychopathology. Although some of these maternal effects may have a genetic basis or are at least influenced by genes, only a few examples of "maternal genotype effects" are currently known/confirmed in humans and in animal models (Doolin et al., 2002; Rouse and Azen, 2004). A classical example is maternal phenylketonuria (high blood phenylalanine levels due to the lack of phenylalanine hydroxylase) that leads to mental retardation, seizures, microcephaly, and growth retardation in the offspring. Also, maternal mutations in methionine biosynthesis (G allele of methionine synthase A2756G and methionine synthase reductase A66G polymorphisms) can lead to spina bifida in the offspring. Reports also indicate that maternal genotype effects contribute not only to neurological disorders but also to common psychiatric conditions such as autism and attention deficit hyperactivity disorder (ADHD). Glutathione S-transferases (GST), a protective factor against reactive oxygen species, is expressed in multiple forms and polymorphic variants. Maternal transmission disequilibrium tests showed that the Val allele of the Ile105Val (A313G) polymorphism in *GSTP1* (a pi class GST) is overtransmitted to mothers of autistic children (Williams et al., 2007). The variation at position 105 affects thermostability and catalytic activity suggesting that a change in enzyme activity in mothers during pregnancy may be related to the increased likelihood of autism in their children. By using a similar approach, maternal (but not offspring or paternal) *TPH1* (tryptophan hydroxylase) mutations have been shown to increase the risk for ADHD (Halmoy et al., 2011). There are additional examples supporting the effect of maternal mutations on gestational development, but they are all based on statistical data from relatively small populations that will need to be replicated (Johnson, 2003). On the other hand, the list of maternal genes that affect offspring development could be expanded to include those that have an effect on maternal behavior prepartum and during early postnatal life. Experimental data in animals clearly show a significant impact of maternal care on the development of psychiatric disease-like conditions (Meaney, 2001). Also, clinical studies indicate that maternal anxiety, depression, and ADHD increase the risk of psychopathology (Halligan et al., 2004, 2007; Murray and Johnston, 2006; Davis and Tremont, 2007; Van den Bergh et al., 2008; Yehuda et al., 2008; Figueiredo and Costa, 2009; Brummelte and Galea, 2010; Murray et al., 2010). Although it is possible that these postnatal maternal effects may also have a genetic component, no maternal mutations have been identified in either human or animal models.

Since most association studies do not include the mother's genotype, it is likely that the prevalence of maternal genotype effects is greatly underestimated in pedigrees and in populations.

Indeed, maternal genotype effects could significantly contribute to the high heritability of common disorders including psychiatric diseases. It is striking that despite the high heritability in these disorders (proportion of variability in a population attributable to genetic variation among individuals), only a small percentage of the risk can be explained by identified genetic variants, a phenomenon often referred to as missing heritability (Manolio et al., 2009). Since they are apparent at the pedigree and population level but not detectable at the genetic level, maternal genotype effects could be one of the mechanisms that explain "missing heritability." Therefore, maternal genotype effects may have major significance in understanding and treating common diseases, including psychiatric conditions discussed in this review.

ANIMAL MODELS CAN HELP IDENTIFY MECHANISMS UNDERLYING MATERNAL GENOTYPE EFFECTS

Although an altered prenatal environment due to maternal genetic variability has been shown as a risk factor in psychiatric diseases such as autism and ADHD (Williams et al., 2007; Halmoy et al., 2011), the underlying disease mechanisms are difficult to identify because of the limitations associated with human studies. Animal (rodent) models have been invaluable tools in studying diseases, especially at the mechanistic level. Many rat and mouse lines are considered inbred – or lacking genetic differences between individuals – and therefore genetic mutations/modifications in the dams are not likely modified by between-subject genetic background variability. In addition to the highly controllable genetic background, rodent models allow for high degree of control of environmental factors. This control is of critical importance because environmental influences could interfere with the maternal genotype effect. Lastly, the advantages of rodent models include the availability of methods to determine if a particular behavioral change in the offspring is dependent on prenatal and/or postnatal parental or maternal environment. Cross-fostering, a procedure in which rodent pups are placed with a foster mother within the first postnatal day, can be used to determine whether a phenotype requires a postnatal maternal contribution, which may be either behavioral or physiological, transmitted through maternal milk. The advantages of animal models are clearly demonstrated in a work that explored the effect of a maternal mutation in *Peg-3* (paternally expressed gene 3). The maternal allele of this gene is imprinted and silenced and therefore the offspring of mutant mothers and wild-type (WT) fathers are essentially WT (expressing the paternal allele) allowing to study the maternal genotype effect without the interference of or interaction with the mutation in the offspring. The offspring of mutant mothers displayed increased neophobia and decreased exploration, although these effects were seen only in females (Champagne et al., 2009). Furthermore, an association was found between the offspring behavioral abnormalities and the reduced postpartum maternal care of *Peg-3* KO dams (Curley et al., 2008).

To demonstrate the feasibility of mouse models in studying maternal genotype effects and their mechanisms, we present our research on two maternal mutations that alter specific behavioral phenotypes and correlated cellular or pharmacologic properties in the genetically unaffected offspring.

MATERNAL SEROTONIN 1A RECEPTOR AND OFFSPRING ANXIETY

The serotonin (5-HT1A) receptor has been implicated in anxiety and depression through receptor binding and pharmacological studies (Drevets et al., 1999; Lemonde et al., 2003; Strobel et al., 2003; Neumeister et al., 2004). The 5-HT1A receptor knockout mouse model demonstrates increased anxiety-related behavior in several behavioral assays, on multiple genetic backgrounds (Heisler et al., 1998; Parks et al., 1998; Ramboz et al., 1998). However, the interpretation of the anxiety phenotype of 5-HT1A receptor KO mice is complicated by the fact that following a typical heterozygote × heterozygote (H × H) breeding, the offspring is exposed to a receptor deficient maternal environment. Considering the association between the 5-HT1A receptor and depression (Van den Hove et al., 2006; Spinelli et al., 2010), including postpartum depression (Moses-Kolko et al., 2008), and the importance of maternal care on the normal emotional development of the offspring, the maternal receptor genotype itself may modulate anxiety-like behavior in the WT offspring and/or could interact with the null allele in the KO offspring, making the dissociation between the maternal and offspring genotype effects on offspring anxiety levels difficult. By studying maternal–offspring 5-HT1A receptor genotype interactions, Weller et al. (2003) found reduced adult anxiety when the behavior of the H offspring of KO dams were compared to that of the WT dams suggesting an anxiolytic-like effect of the maternal KO alleles on offspring behavior. Since the offspring themselves were receptor deficient, the effect of maternal receptor deficiency as a single factor on offspring behavior could not be determined.

We recently showed that partial or complete 5-HT1A receptor deficiency in Swiss Webster (SW) mouse dams can cause increased anxiety-related behavior and enhanced stress reactivity in their offspring, independently of offspring genotype (Gleason et al., 2010; **Figure 1**) Genetically WT offspring of 5-HT1A receptor deficient mice displayed increased anxiety-related behavior in the elevated plus maze. This phenotype was found to require prenatal maternal 5-HT1A receptor deficiency, as mice which developed from WT embryos implanted into 5-HT1A receptor deficient mothers and raised by either 5-HT1A deficient or WT mothers after birth displayed increased anxiety-related behavior (**Figure 1**). This phenotype was also shown to be dependent on strain background (Gleason et al., 2010). In contrast, increased anxiety-related behavior in the open field, a less stressful assay for unconditioned anxiety, was found to be dependent on offspring 5-HT1A receptor genotype. Finally, we demonstrated that maternal 5-HT1A receptor deficiency leads to reduced immobility time in the Porsolt Forced Swim Test, which can be interpreted as a lack of normal coping skills and an increase in reactivity to inescapable stress. The development of this phenotype is independent of offspring genotype and requires both prenatal and postnatal maternal receptor deficit, as shown by embryo transfer and cross-fostering experiments.

In addition, we examined early postnatal development of the ventral dentate gyrus of the hippocampus in mice exposed to maternal 5-HT1A receptor deficiency, because the ventral hippocampus and this time period have been linked to the development of anxiety (Gross et al., 2002; Bannerman et al., 2003). We identified several developmental changes that correlate with later life anxiety-related behavior, including an increased volume of the ventral granule cell layer (GCL) during the first postnatal week, which normalized by the age of 4 weeks (in the absence of changes in the number of

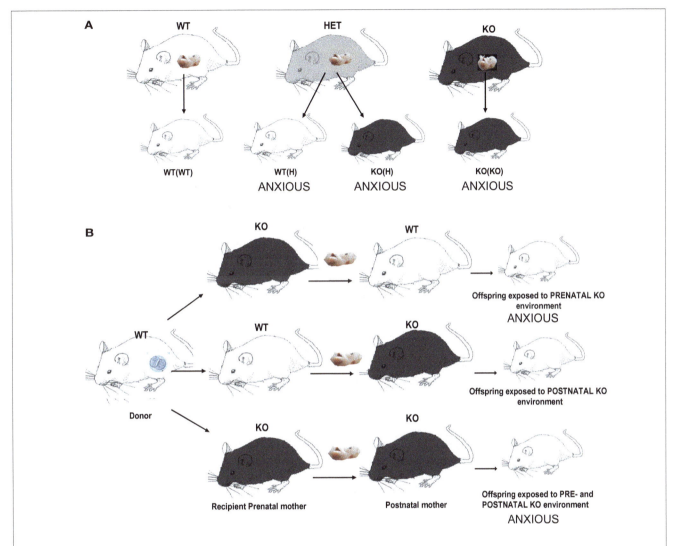

FIGURE 1 | Diagram showing breeding and embryonic cross-fostering schemes for the 5-HT1A receptor deficient line. (A) WT mice are bred together to generate WT(WT) control animals with neither a maternal nor an offspring 5-HT1A receptor effect. Homozygous 5-HT1A receptor knockout mice are bred together to generate KO(KO) mice with both a maternal and an offspring 5-HT1A receptor genotype effect, which display increased anxiety-related behavior in the elevated plus maze. WT and 5-HT1A receptor homozygous knockout mice are bred together to generate 5-HT1A receptor heterozygotes, which are intercrossed to generate both WT(H) and KO(H) mice, both of which also display increased anxiety-related behavior. WT(H) mice have a maternal but not offspring 5-HT1A receptor genotype effect, while KO(H) mice have both a maternal and offspring 5-HT1A receptor genotype effect. (B) WT embryos (indicated by the oocyte in the donor) are implanted into WT and 5-HT1A receptor homozygous KO pseudopregnant mothers. Within 24 h after birth, pups are cross-fostered to WT or 5-HT1A receptor homozygous KO mothers, resulting in offspring raised with a prenatal, postnatal, or combined pre and postnatal maternal KO environment. Mice with either a prenatal or combined pre and postnatal maternal 5-HT1A receptor genotype effect exhibit increased anxiety-related behavior.

proliferating cells) and a maturational delay of developing neurons in the ventral GCL at postnatal day 7. To provide a possible link between the developmental delay in the ventral dentate gyrus and the maternal 5-HT1A receptor mediated anxiety-related behavior, we examined the effect of inactivating a candidate gene involved in neuronal precursor maturation, $p16^{Ink4a}$. We found that deletion of this gene phenocopies both the ventral GCL volume increase in the first postnatal week, and the increased anxiety-related behavior in the elevated plus maze. These data indicate that the maternal 5-HT1A receptor deficit alters hippocampal development in the offspring, and that these developmental changes could contribute to the increased anxiety-like behavior in the elevated plus maze (**Figure 2**).

It is important to note that the offspring were more sensitive to the maternal than to their own receptor gene dosage as a partial maternal receptor deficit was sufficient to elicit a full anxiety phenotype while a strong anxiety phenotype developed only in the homozygote knockout offspring (in the absence of maternal effect). The significance of this finding is that while a complete loss of the receptor has not been observed in humans, a 40–50% reduction in receptor binding, associated with stress and psychiatric disease, is relatively common (Lesch et al., 1992; Lopez et al., 1998; Drevets et al., 1999, 2007; Mann, 1999; Arango et al., 2001; Moses-Kolko et al., 2008). Therefore, a maternal 5-HT1AR deficit could be more relevant than an offspring deficit to human anxiety.

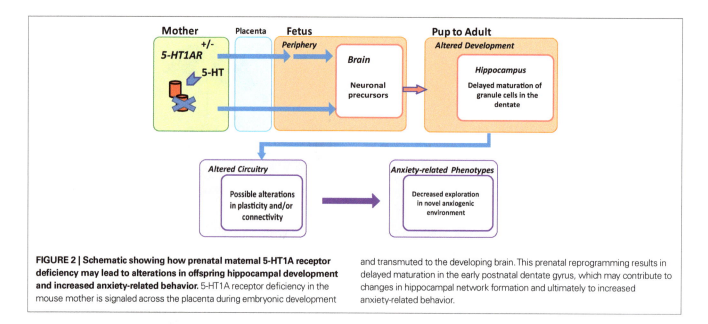

FIGURE 2 | Schematic showing how prenatal maternal 5-HT1A receptor deficiency may lead to alterations in offspring hippocampal development and increased anxiety-related behavior. 5-HT1A receptor deficiency in the mouse mother is signaled across the placenta during embryonic development and transmuted to the developing brain. This prenatal reprogramming results in delayed maturation in the early postnatal dentate gyrus, which may contribute to changes in hippocampal network formation and ultimately to increased anxiety-related behavior.

MATERNAL FRAGILE X MENTAL RETARDATION PROTEIN AND OFFSPRING HYPERACTIVITY

Our second mouse model of human disease is produced by the inactivation of the *fmr1* gene encoding the fragile X mental retardation protein (FMRP). This model reproduces key behavioral features of the human fragile X syndrome (FXS; Consortium TD-BFX, 1994). FMRP is an RNA binding protein that affects multiple stages of RNA translation and is involved in the regulation of both local and global protein synthesis (Kao et al., 2010). Mice lacking Fmrp exhibit a number of FXS-like phenotypes including locomotor hyperactivity, sensory hyper-reactivity, cognitive defect, and macroorchidism (D'Hooge et al., 1997; Peier et al., 2000; Chen and Toth, 2001; Spencer et al., 2005; Yun et al., 2006). In addition, Fmrp deficient mice reproduce some of the autistic-like behaviors seen in FXS. Interestingly, the manifestation of autistic-like behaviors is genetic background dependent, consistent with the observation that autistic behaviors in FXS vary considerably, presumably as a result of genetic modifiers (Spencer et al., 2011).

Although FMRP has been identified as the singular cause of FXS, a typical Mendelian disease, we found that the maternal Fmrp deficit can contribute to the development of some of the disease-associated phenotypes. Specifically, we found that the genetically unaffected adult male offspring of heterozygote *fmr1* KO dams displayed increased constitutive locomotor activity and that the combination of maternal and offspring genotype effects in the FXS mouse model had an additive effect on locomotor activity (Zupan and Toth, 2008a). This finding suggests that even a partial deficit in Fmrp in the dam has long-term effects on offspring behavior and is sufficient to induce a disease-like phenotype. Other FXS-associated phenotypes such as macroorchidism and sensory hypersensitivity were unaffected by the maternal genotype and present only if *fmr1* was mutated in the offspring.

Locomotor activity is regulated in part by the activity of mesolimbic dopamine neurons originating in the ventral tegmental area and projecting to the ventral striatum (Koob and Swerdlow, 1988; Szczypka et al., 2001). Hyperactivity has been linked to low tonic dopamine activity promoted by D2 autoreceptors and high phasic dopamine neurotransmission (Grace, 2001). Activation of D2 autoreceptors, by reducing the amount of DA released into the synapse (presynaptically) and reducing the excitability of the DA neurons (in the somatodendritic compartment), inhibits locomotor activity in rodents (Starke et al., 1989; Cory-Slechta et al., 1996; Usiello et al., 2000; **Figure 3**). When we probed the dopamine system using quinpirole at a D2 autoreceptor preferring dose, we found that the hyperactive offspring of FMRP deficient dams, regardless of their own genotype, had attenuated behavioral responses to quinpirole. This indicates a functional downregulation of the D2 autoreceptor that can explain or contribute to the hyperactivity phenotype (**Figure 4**). While the functional D2 receptor downregulation was not affected by the offspring genotype, the KO offspring of heterozygote *fmr1* KO dams had a higher level of hyperactivity than their WT offspring indicating that only the maternally induced component of the hyperactivity may be explained by the downregulation of presynaptic D2 receptors. In addition to the D2 autoreceptors, the presynaptic $GABA_B$ receptors also inhibit DA release while receptors located somatodendritically reduce the firing rate of DA neurons (Engberg et al., 1993; Smolders et al., 1995; Madden and Johnson, 1998; Labouebe et al., 2007; **Figure 3**). Administration of the $GABA_B$ agonist baclofen at doses that had no sedative effects resulted in a more prominent reduction in locomotor activity in the offspring of *fmr1* heterozygote KO dams as compared to offspring of WT dams (Zupan and Toth, 2008b; **Figure 4**). Again, this change was maternal but not offspring genotype dependent. This indicated a maternal genotype-dependent sensitization of the $GABA_B$ receptor in the offspring that may compensate for the hyperactivity related to the D2 receptor downregulation. Taken together, these data indicate that the maternal genotype effect can be linked not only to behavioral alterations but also to neurochemical changes which can ultimately help elucidate the underlying mechanisms.

Fmrp has been directly linked to FXS, as the sole cause of this Mendelian disorder. However, FMRP, at least in the mouse model, may have an additional function as its partial or complete deficit in the mother results in hyperactivity in the offspring that can be further increased by the offspring's own mutation. This raises the possibility that in affected sons of mothers with full *fmr1* mutation some of the behavioral phenotypes may be caused by a non-genetic mechanism related to the mother's mutation and that genetically non-affected sons may also acquire some vulnerability to mental disorder. Interestingly, FMRP levels were found to be reduced in conditions unrelated to FXS such as autism, schizophrenia, bipolar disorder, and major depressive disorder (Fatemi and Folsom, 2011; Fatemi et al., 2010). Because the offspring are highly sensitive to even a partial reduction in FMRP, we speculate that these non-FXS conditions, via maternal effects, can expand the impact of FMRP in the human population.

POSSIBLE MEDIATORS OF MATERNAL GENOTYPE EFFECTS

Maternal effects, unrelated to the genetic transfer of any genetic variation or mutation, are in principle either behavioral, in particular during the postnatal period, or are related to maternal substances that reach or signal to the developing brain during pre and/or postnatal life.

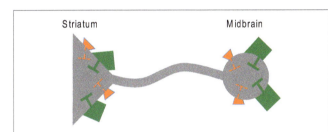

FIGURE 3 | Illustration of dopamine D2 autoreceptors (orange) and GABA$_B$ receptors (green) on somatodendritic and presynaptic sites of a mesolimbic dopamine neuron. Maternal *fmr1* insufficiency resulted in reduced D2 autoreceptor and enhanced GABA$_B$ receptor function in adult male offspring as measured by the locomotor response following quinpirole and baclofen administration, respectively.

First we discuss maternal genotype effects which are likely mediated by the behavioral interaction between mother and infant. Then we will discuss potential mediators of the maternal genotype effect that act during prenatal but also postnatal life.

INFLUENCE OF MATERNAL CARE AND BEHAVIOR ON THE OFFSPRING

Several genes have been identified as being required for normal maternal care, and mutations in these genes lead to phenotypes including impaired pup retrieval, failure of pups to thrive, and increased pup mortality. Some of these maternal mutations lead to severe impairment of maternal behavior and subsequent reductions in pup survival or impaired somatic development, and thus are not directly relevant to maternal genotype related psychiatric conditions. Nevertheless, we briefly summarize these genes below because they could provide insights to mother–infant interaction mechanisms. FosB null mouse dams exhibit impaired nurturing behavior (time crouching over pups, failure to maintain pups in a huddle), and impaired pup retrieval (Brown et al., 1996; Kuroda et al., 2008). CREBαδ null mouse dams also exhibit impaired pup retrieval, and CREBαδ heterozygous pups fail to thrive (Jin et al., 2005). Dams carrying a null allele of *Peg-3* show reduced nurturing behavior toward their offspring and associated reductions in offspring survival, as well as reduced lactation, which was correlated with a reduction in the number of oxytocin neurons in the hypothalamus (Li et al., 1999). In a follow-up study, Curley et al. (2004, 2008) examined the effect of Peg-3 maternal and/or offspring deficiency on offspring development, and demonstrated that pups born to WT mothers who inherited a mutant Peg-3 allele exhibit reduced suckling activity and weight gain, and that their mothers ate less during pregnancy, indicating impaired fetal–maternal signaling. Peg-3 mutant mothers of WT pups also failed to increase caloric intake during pregnancy and had reduced milk let-down, while their offspring gained weight less rapidly and entered puberty later. When both mother and pup

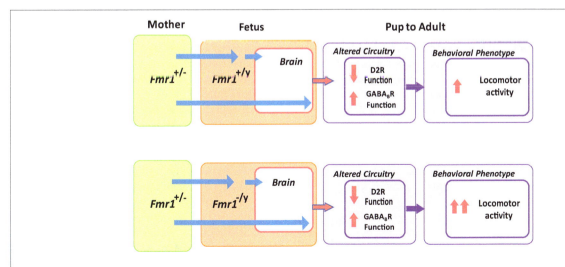

FIGURE 4 | Maternal and offspring *fmr1* genotype effects on locomotor activity. Locomotor activity is increased in genetically unaffected animals due to maternal FMRP deficit, and this behavioral effect is further enhanced by the offspring's own lack of FMRP. Maternal FMRP deficit increases GABA$_B$ receptor and decreases D2 autoreceptor function and this effect is not further modified by the offspring's own *fmr1* expression suggesting that these neurochemical changes are specifically associated with the maternal deficit in FMRP.

were mutant for Peg-3, these abnormalities were additive, and led to substantially increased pup mortality. Other genes implicated in maternal behavior include *Mest/Peg1* (Lefebvre et al., 1998), the prolactin receptor gene (Lucas et al., 1998), the corticotropin-releasing factor I gene (Gammie et al., 2007), *Pet-1*, encoding a serotonergic transcription factor (Lerch-Haner et al., 2008), the brain vasopressin gene (Bosch and Neumann, 2008), the oxytocin and the oxytocin receptor genes (Takayanagi et al., 2005), and *CD38* (Jin et al., 2007).

As discussed earlier, thus far there have been few animal models in which specific maternal mutations were found to contribute to offspring behavioral changes that are reminiscent of psychiatric-like conditions. Instead, research has focused mostly on strain differences, innate variability within rodent strains, or rodents selectively bred for behavioral traits. For instance, there is a line of Wistar rats selectively bred for anxiety (high anxiety behavior and low anxiety behavior rats; Liebsch et al., 1998), in which high anxiety rats have been shown to display reduced levels of maternal behavior relative to low anxiety rats (Kessler et al., 2011). However, these rat lines are bred to maximize phenotypic variability, and as such have a large number of genetic differences, making it difficult to determine which genetic changes are relevant to the observed behavioral changes.

Meaney and colleagues have compiled an extensive body of work demonstrating how innate variability in maternal behavior in Long–Evans rats can lead to altered offspring behavior. A large cohort of rats was phenotyped for natural variations in maternal behavior, and two subpopulations were identified, the 10% displaying the most licking–grooming and arched back nursing (High LG–ABN), as well as the 10% displaying the lowest frequency of these behaviors (Low LG–ABN; Liu et al., 1997). The offspring of high LG–ABN rats were found to display reduced fearfulness, reduced hypothalamic–pituitary–adrenal (HPA) axis responses to stress, and decreased startle response, as well as increased hippocampal glucocorticoid receptor expression. When rats were cross-fostered at birth, their adult behavioral phenotypes and their own maternal behavior resembled that of their foster mothers, indicating a postnatal and transgenerational effect (Francis et al., 1999). Again, the selection procedure segregated two different populations that likely differ in multiple genetic mutations or polymorphisms. The variability in maternal behavior was found to selectively alter the epigenome of the offspring by differential methylation of the glucocorticoid receptor promoter during the first postnatal week, an effect which persisted into adulthood and was reversible through cross-fostering (Weaver et al., 2004). The group differences in epigenetic modification, glucocorticoid receptor expression, and HPA responses to stress could be removed through central infusion of a histone deacetylase inhibitor into the adult offspring (Weaver et al., 2004).

A similar approach was also used with mouse strains showing genetic and phenotypic heterogeneity. For instance, the C57/Bl6 (B6) mouse displays greater licking/grooming behavior, reduced anxiety-related behavior, increased learning ability in the Morris water maze (MWM), and increased pre-pulse inhibition (PPI) of acoustic startle, relative to the BalbC. When BalbC zygotes were implanted into B6 hosts and raised by B6 foster mothers dams during both the prenatal and postnatal period, elevated plus maze, open field, and MWM behavior were shown to be no different from that of B6 mice raised by B6 mothers (Francis et al., 2003). Carola et al. (2008) used the maternal care variability in this strains to create mice that are genetically identical (B6/BalbC heterozygotes), but nonetheless display different maternal behavior based on maternal strain. They then utilized B6/BalbC heterozygote dams with either B6 or BalbC like behavior to study the effect of maternal behavior on offspring behavior. These data, although revealing no maternal genes, again indicate the importance of the maternal genotype on the behavior of genetically unrelated offspring producing psychiatric disease-like conditions.

MATERNAL CYTOKINES

Maternal cytokines have been proposed as potential mediators that signal across the placenta to the developing embryo, either directly, or through induction of fetal cytokines. Although we have no direct evidence that the maternal genotype effects in the 5-HT1A receptor and Fmrp deficient mouse lines or in other models of maternal genotype effects would be mediated by cytokines, these molecules are plausible candidates because they can cross the placenta and blood–brain barrier and because cytokine receptors are abundant in the brain, providing a means to convey the maternal genotype effects to developing neurons. Both the 5-HT1A receptor and FMRP are expressed in immune cells and could alter their functions, including cytokine production and secretion. Indeed, the 5-HT1A receptor is prominently expressed in the immune system and we and others have shown that 5-HT, via the 5-HT1A receptor, has chemotactic activity for eosinophils and mast cells (Boehme et al., 2004; Kushnir-Sukhov et al., 2006). Regarding FMRP, significant differences in the plasma levels of a number of cytokines, including IL-1alpha, were reported between FXS individuals and controls (Ashwood et al., 2011).

The evidence for the ability of cytokines to alter offspring brain development and function comes from studies in which the maternal immune system is challenged, resulting in offspring behavioral abnormalities (Smith et al., 2007; Patterson, 2009). Maternal infection and inflammation during pregnancy have long been implicated as potential predisposing factors to offspring psychiatric disorders, including schizophrenia and autism. For instance, retrospective studies examining maternal medical records have shown that maternal infection increases the risk of schizophrenia in offspring (2× for respiratory infection, 8× for influenza infection; Brown et al., 1996; Byrne et al., 2007). Schizophrenia in offspring has also been associated with elevated cytokines and anti-influenza antibodies in archived maternal serum (Brown et al., 2004a,b). A Danish registry study recently showed that maternal hospital admission due to either viral infection in the first trimester or bacterial infection in the second trimester was significantly associated with the diagnosis of Autism Spectrum Disorder in offspring (Atladottir et al., 2010). Animal models that have been used to test the link between maternal inflammation and offspring psychiatric-like phenotypes include administration of lipopolysaccharide (LPS), polyinosinic polycytidylic acid [Poly(I:C)] or antibodies, or direct exposure to pathogens such as influenza, all of which induce an immune response in the dam, which may directly or via the induction of fetal cytokines have profound consequences for the developing fetus (reviewed in Boksa, 2010).

Poly(I:C) is a synthetic dsRNA that acts through the toll-like receptor (TLR) 3 (Cunningham et al., 2007). The injection of Poly(I:C) into rodent dams during gestation has been shown to lead to a panoply of schizophrenia-related behavioral abnormalities in their offspring including deficits in PPI, social interaction, latent inhibition, working memory, and novel object exploration (Patterson, 2009). In addition, maternal Poly(I:C) exposure induces a range of histological and structural changes in systems relevant to schizophrenia, including increased $GABA_A$ receptor α2 immunoreactivity and dopamine hyperfunction, ventricular enlargement, reduced NMDA receptor expression in the hippocampus, and reduced dopamine D1 and D2 receptor expression in the prefrontal cortex (Patterson, 2009). These neurochemical changes may underlie the behavioral abnormalities. Extending the Poly(I:C) model of maternal immune activation, Abazyan et al. (2010) exposed an *mhDISC1* mutant mouse to Poly(I:C) at gestational day 9 (GD9), which increased the anxiety-related behaviors, depression-like responses, and altered social behaviors in adults as compared to mutant mice of uninfected dams. Polymorphisms in the *DISC1* gene have been linked to increased risk of several psychiatric diseases, including schizophrenia, major depression, bipolar disorder, autism, and Asperger's syndrome (Millar et al., 2000, 2001; Blackwood et al., 2001; Kilpinen et al., 2008) and DISC1 mutant animals display a range of cellular and behavioral phenotypes relevant to schizophrenia (Clapcote et al., 2007; Hikida et al., 2007; Kvajo et al., 2008; Pletnikov et al., 2008; Shen et al., 2008). Importantly, Poly(I:C) treatment altered cytokine levels in the fetal brain in a genotype-dependent manner indicating that offspring mutations can increase the maternal effect presumably via the induction of fetal cytokines. Tuberous sclerosis (TSC) is a genetic condition in which 40–50% of affected individuals display autism spectrum disorder (Ehninger et al., 2010). These authors exposed a mouse mutant for Tsc2 to gestational immune activation, and demonstrated that this mutation increases in *utero* mortality after Poly(I:C) injection, and that the combined genetic and environmental factors lead to abnormalities in social interaction in surviving offspring (Ehninger et al., 2010).

CONCLUSION

The high heritability of psychiatric disorders is likely explained by a number of mechanisms including the inheritance of rare alleles with high penetrance and various combinations of low penetrance alleles. Here we describe another mechanism that could also significantly contribute to the heritability of these disorders. Specifically, here we show that maternal mutations alone or in combination with offspring mutations can result in anxiety and hyperactivity in the offspring. The importance of maternal genotype effects is twofold. First, it can increase the severity of the phenotype caused by the offspring genotype. Second, maternal genotype effects can produce disease-like phenotypes in genetically unaffected individuals. This finding expands the population vulnerable to psychiatric disease. Since conventional association studies do not include the maternal genome, the identification of maternal genotype effects is difficult. Efforts to incorporate parental genomes into large scale genome-wide association studies (Kong et al., 2009), could eventually help to estimate the overall impact of maternal genotypes in increasing risk for mental disorders.

REFERENCES

Abazyan, B., Nomura, J., Kannan, G., Ishizuka, K., Tamashiro, K. L., Nucifora, F., Pogorelov, V., Ladenheim, B., Yang, C., Krasnova, I. N., Cadet, J. L., Pardo, C., Mori, S., Kamiya, A., Vogel, M. W., Sawa, A., Ross, C. A., and Pletnikov, M. V. (2010). Prenatal interaction of mutant DISC1 and immune activation produces adult psychopathology. *Biol. Psychiatry* 68, 1172–1181.

Arango, V., Underwood, M. D., Boldrini, M., Tamir, H., Kassir, S. A., Hsiung, S., Chen, J. J., and Mann, J. J. (2001). Serotonin 1A receptors, serotonin transporter binding and serotonin transporter mRNA expression in the brainstem of depressed suicide victims. *Neuropsychopharmacology* 25, 892–903.

Ashwood, P., Nguyen, D. V., Hessl, D., Hagerman, R. J., and Tassone, F. (2011). Plasma cytokine profiles in Fragile X subjects: is there a role for cytokines in the pathogenesis? *Brain Behav. Immun.* 24, 898–902.

Atladottir, H. O., Thorsen, P., Schendel, D. E., Ostergaard, L., Lemcke, S., and Parner, E. T. (2010). Association of hospitalization for infection in childhood with diagnosis of autism spectrum disorders: a Danish cohort study. *Arch. Pediatr. Adolesc. Med.* 164, 470–477.

Bannerman, D. M., Grubb, M., Deacon, R. M., Yee, B. K., Feldon, J., and Rawlins, J. N. (2003). Ventral hippocampal lesions affect anxiety but not spatial learning. *Behav. Brain Res.* 139, 197–213.

Blackwood, D. H., Fordyce, A., Walker, M. T., St Clair, D. M., Porteous, D. J., and Muir, W. J. (2001). Schizophrenia and affective disorders – cosegregation with a translocation at chromosome 1q42 that directly disrupts brain-expressed genes: clinical and P300 findings in a family. *Am. J. Hum. Genet.* 69, 428–433.

Boehme, S. A., Lio, F. M., Sikora, L., Pandit, T. S., Lavrador, K., Rao, S. P., and Sriramarao, P. (2004). Cutting edge: serotonin is a chemotactic factor for eosinophils and functions additively with eotaxin. *J. Immunol.* 173, 3599–3603.

Boksa, P. (2010). Effects of prenatal infection on brain development and behavior: a review of findings from animal models. *Brain Behav. Immun.* 24, 881–897.

Bosch, O. J., and Neumann, I. D. (2008). Brain vasopressin is an important regulator of maternal behavior independent of dams' trait anxiety. *Proc. Natl. Acad. Sci. U.S.A.* 105, 17139–17144.

Brown, A. S., Begg, M. D., Gravenstein, S., Schaefer, C. A., Wyatt, R. J., Bresnahan, M., Babulas, V. P., and Susser, E. S. (2004a). Serologic evidence of prenatal influenza in the etiology of schizophrenia. *Arch. Gen. Psychiatry* 61, 774–780.

Brown, A. S., Hooton, J., Schaefer, C. A., Zhang, H., Petkova, E., Babulas, V., Perrin, M., Gorman, J. M., and Susser, E. S. (2004b). Elevated maternal interleukin-8 levels and risk of schizophrenia in adult offspring. *Am. J. Psychiatry* 161, 889–895.

Brown, J. R., Ye, H., Bronson, R. T., Dikkes, P., and Greenberg, M. E. (1996). A defect in nurturing in mice lacking the immediate early gene fosB. *Cell* 86, 297–309.

Brummelte, S., and Galea, L. A. (2010). Depression during pregnancy and postpartum: contribution of stress and ovarian hormones. *Prog. Neuropsychopharmacol. Biol. Psychiatry* 34, 766–776.

Byrne, M., Agerbo, E., Bennedsen, B., Eaton, W. W., and Mortensen, P. B. (2007). Obstetric conditions and risk of first admission with schizophrenia: a Danish national register based study. *Schizophr. Res.* 97, 51–59.

Carola, V., Frazzetto, G., Pascucci, T., Audero, E., Puglisi-Allegra, S., Cabib, S., Lesch, K. P., and Gross, C. (2008). Identifying molecular substrates in a mouse model of the serotonin transporter × environment risk factor for anxiety and depression. *Biol. Psychiatry* 63, 840–846.

Champagne, F. A., Curley, J. P., Swaney, W. T., Hasen, N. S., and Keverne, E. B. (2009). Paternal influence on female behavior: the role of Peg3 in exploration, olfaction, and neuroendocrine regulation of maternal behavior of female mice. *Behav. Neurosci.* 123, 469–480.

Chen, L., and Toth, M. (2001). Fragile X mice develop sensory hyperreactivity to auditory stimuli. *Neuroscience* 103, 1043–1050.

Clapcote, S. J., Lipina, T. V., Millar, J. K., Mackie, S., Christie, S., Ogawa, F., Lerch, J. P., Trimble, K., Uchiyama, M., Sakuraba, Y., Kaneda, H., Shiroishi, T., Houslay, M. D., Henkelman, R. M.,

Sled, J. G., Gondo, Y., Porteous, D. J., and Roder, J. C. (2007). Behavioral phenotypes of Disc1 missense mutations in mice. *Neuron* 54, 387–402.

Consortium TD-BFX. (1994). Fmr1 knockout mice: a model to study fragile X mental retardation. *Cell* 78, 23–33.

Cory-Slechta, D. A., Zuch, C. L., and Fox, R. A. (1996). Comparison of the stimulus properties of a pre- vs. a putative postsynaptic dose of quinpirole. *Pharmacol. Biochem. Behav.* 55, 423–432.

Cunningham, C., Campion, S., Teeling, J., Felton, L., and Perry, V. H. (2007). The sickness behaviour and CNS inflammatory mediator profile induced by systemic challenge of mice with synthetic double-stranded RNA (poly I:C). *Brain Behav. Immun.* 21, 490–502.

Curley, J. P., Barton, S., Surani, A., and Keverne, E. B. (2004). Coadaptation in mother and infant regulated by a paternally expressed imprinted gene. *Proc. Biol. Sci.* 271, 1303–1309.

Curley, J. P., Champagne, F. A., Bateson, P., Keverne, E. B., and Curley, K. O. Jr. (2008). Transgenerational effects of impaired maternal care on behaviour of offspring and grandoffspring. *Anim. Behav.* 75, 1551–1561.

Davis, J. D., and Tremont, G. (2007). Neuropsychiatric aspects of hypothyroidism and treatment reversibility. *Minerva Endocrinol.* 32, 49–65.

D'Hooge, R., Nagels, G., Franck, F., Bakker, C. E., Reyniers, E., Storm, K., Kooy, R. F., Oostra, B. A., Willems, P. J., and De Deyn, P. P. (1997). Mildly impaired water maze performance in male Fmr1 knockout mice. *Neuroscience* 76, 367–376.

Doolin, M. T., Barbaux, S., McDonnell, M., Hoess, K., Whitehead, A. S., and Mitchell, L. E. (2002). Maternal genetic effects, exerted by genes involved in homocysteine remethylation, influence the risk of spina bifida. *Am. J. Hum. Genet.* 71, 1222–1226.

Drevets, W. C., Frank, E., Price, J. C., Kupfer, D. J., Holt, D., Greer, P. J., Huang, Y., Gautier, C., and Mathis, C. (1999). PET imaging of serotonin 1A receptor binding in depression. *Biol. Psychiatry* 46, 1375–1387.

Drevets, W. C., Thase, M. E., Moses-Kolko, E. L., Price, J., Frank, E., Kupfer, D. J., and Mathis, C. (2007). Serotonin-1A receptor imaging in recurrent depression: replication and literature review. *Nucl. Med. Biol.* 34, 865–877.

Ehninger, D., Sano, Y., de Vries, P. J., Dies, K., Franz, D., Geschwind, D. H., Kaur, M., Lee, Y. S., Li, W., Lowe, J. K., Nakagawa, J. A., Sahin, M., Smith, K., Whittemore, V., and Silva, A. J. (2010). Gestational immune activation and Tsc2 haploinsufficiency cooperate to disrupt fetal survival and may perturb social behavior in adult mice. *Mol. Psychiatry*, [Epub ahead of print].

Engberg, G., Kling-Petersen, T., and Nissbrandt, H. (1993). GABAB-receptor activation alters the firing pattern of dopamine neurons in the rat substantia nigra. *Synapse* 15, 229–238.

Fatemi, S. H., and Folsom, T. D. (2011). The role of fragile X mental retardation protein in major mental disorders. *Neuropharmacology* 60, 1221–1226.

Fatemi, S. H., Kneeland, R. E., Liesch, S. B., and Folsom, T. D. (2010). Fragile X mental retardation protein levels are decreased in major psychiatric disorders. *Schizophr. Res.* 124, 246–247.

Figueiredo, B., and Costa, R. (2009). Mother's stress, mood and emotional involvement with the infant: 3 months before and 3 months after childbirth. *Arch. Womens Ment. Health* 12, 143–153.

Francis, D., Diorio, J., Liu, D., and Meaney, M. J. (1999). Nongenomic transmission across generations of maternal behavior and stress responses in the rat. *Science* 286, 1155–1158.

Francis, D. D., Szegda, K., Campbell, G., Martin, W. D., and Insel, T. R. (2003). Epigenetic sources of behavioral differences in mice. *Nat. Neurosci.* 6, 445–446.

Gammie, S. C., Bethea, E. D., and Stevenson, S. A. (2007). Altered maternal profiles in corticotropin-releasing factor receptor 1 deficient mice. *BMC Neurosci.* 8, 17. doi: 10.1186/1471-2202-8-17

Gleason, G., Liu, B., Bruening, S., Zupan, B., Auerbach, A., Mark, W., Oh, J. E., Gal-Toth, J., Lee, F., and Toth, M. (2010). The serotonin1A receptor gene as a genetic and prenatal maternal environmental factor in anxiety. *Proc. Natl. Acad. Sci. U.S.A.* 107, 7592–7597.

Grace, A. (2001). "Psychostimulant actions on dopamine and limbic system function: relevance to the pathophysiology and treatment of ADHD," in *Stimulant Drugs and ADHD: Basic and Clinical Neuroscience*, eds M. V. Solanto, A. F. T. Arnsten, and F. X. Castellanos (New York: Oxford University Press), 134–155.

Gross, C., Zhuang, X., Stark, K., Ramboz, S., Oosting, R., Kirby, L., Santarelli, L., Beck, S., and Hen, R. (2002). Serotonin1A receptor acts during development to establish normal anxiety-like behaviour in the adult. *Nature* 416, 396–400.

Halligan, S. L., Herbert, J., Goodyer, I., and Murray, L. (2007). Disturbances in morning cortisol secretion in association with maternal postnatal depression predict subsequent depressive symptomatology in adolescents. *Biol. Psychiatry* 62, 40–46.

Halligan, S. L., Herbert, J., Goodyer, I. M., and Murray, L. (2004). Exposure to postnatal depression predicts elevated cortisol in adolescent offspring. *Biol. Psychiatry* 55, 376–381.

Halmoy, A., Johansson, S., Winge, I., McKinney, J. A., Knappskog, P. M., and Haavik, J. (2011). Attention-deficit/hyperactivity disorder symptoms in offspring of mothers with impaired serotonin production. *Arch. Gen. Psychiatry* 67, 1033–1043.

Heisler, L. K., Chu, H. M., Brennan, T. J., Danao, J. A., Bajwa, P., Parsons, L. H., and Tecott, L. H. (1998). Elevated anxiety and antidepressant-like responses in serotonin 5-HT1A receptor mutant mice. *Proc. Natl. Acad. Sci. U.S.A.* 95, 15049–15054.

Hikida, T., Jaaro-Peled, H., Seshadri, S., Oishi, K., Hookway, C., Kong, S., Wu, D., Xue, R., Andrade, M., Tankou, S., Mori, S., Gallagher, M., Ishizuka, K., Pletnikov, M., Kida, S., and Sawa, A. (2007). Dominant-negative DISC1 transgenic mice display schizophrenia-associated phenotypes detected by measures translatable to humans. *Proc. Natl. Acad. Sci. U.S.A.* 104, 14501–14506.

Jin, D., Liu, H. X., Hirai, H., Torashima, T., Nagai, T., Lopatina, O., Shnayder, N. A., Yamada, K., Noda, M., Seike, T., Fujita, K., Takasawa, S., Yokoyama, S., Koizumi, K., Shiraishi, Y., Tanaka, S., Hashii, M., Yoshihara, T., Higashida, K., Islam, M. S., Yamada, N., Hayashi, K., Noguchi, N., Kato, I., Okamoto, H., Matsushima, A., Salmina, A., Munesue, T., Shimizu, N., Mochida, S., Asano, M., and Higashida, H. (2007). CD38 is critical for social behaviour by regulating oxytocin secretion. *Nature* 446, 41–45.

Jin, S. H., Blendy, J. A., and Thomas, S. A. (2005). Cyclic AMP response element-binding protein is required for normal maternal nurturing behavior. *Neuroscience* 133, 647–655.

Johnson, W. G. (2003). Teratogenic alleles and neurodevelopmental disorders. *Bioessays* 25, 464–477.

Kao, D. I., Aldridge, G. M., Weiler, I. J., and Greenough, W. T. (2010). Altered mRNA transport, docking, and protein translation in neurons lacking fragile X mental retardation protein. *Proc. Natl. Acad. Sci. U.S.A.* 107, 15601–15606.

Kessler, M. S., Bosch, O. J., Bunck, M., Landgraf, R., and Neumann, I. D. (2011). Maternal care differs in mice bred for high vs. low trait anxiety: impact of brain vasopressin and cross-fostering. *Soc. Neurosci.* 6, 156–168.

Kilpinen, H., Ylisaukko-Oja, T., Hennah, W., Palo, O. M., Varilo, T., Vanhala, R., Nieminen-von Wendt, T., von Wendt, L., Paunio, T., and Peltonen, L. (2008). Association of DISC1 with autism and Asperger syndrome. *Mol. Psychiatry* 13, 187–196.

Kong, A., Steinthorsdottir, V., Masson, G., Thorleifsson, G., Sulem, P., Besenbacher, S., Jonasdottir, A., Sigurdsson, A., Kristinsson, K. T., Jonasdottir, A., Frigge, M. L., Gylfason, A., Olason, P. I., Gudjonsson, S. A., Sverrisson, S., Stacey, S. N., Sigurgeirsson, B., Benediktsdottir, K. R., Sigurdsson, H., Jonsson, T., Benediktsson, R., Olafsson, J. H., Johannsson, O. T., Hreidarsson, A. B., Sigurdsson, G., Ferguson-Smith, A. C., Gudbjartsson, D. F., Thorsteinsdottir, U., and Stefansson, K. (2009). Parental origin of sequence variants associated with complex diseases. *Nature* 462, 868–874.

Koob, G. F., and Swerdlow, N. R. (1988). The functional output of the mesolimbic dopamine system. *Ann. N. Y. Acad. Sci.* 537, 216–227.

Kuroda, K. O., Meaney, M. J., Uetani, N., and Kato, T. (2008). Neurobehavioral basis of the impaired nurturing in mice lacking the immediate early gene FosB. *Brain Res.* 1211, 57–71.

Kushnir-Sukhov, N. M., Gilfillan, A. M., Coleman, J. W., Brown, J. M., Bruening, S., Toth, M., and Metcalfe, D. D. (2006). 5-hydroxytryptamine induces mast cell adhesion and migration. *J. Immunol.* 177, 6422–6432.

Kvajo, M., McKellar, H., Arguello, P. A., Drew, L. J., Moore, H., MacDermott, A. B., Karayiorgou, M., and Gogos, J. A. (2008). A mutation in mouse Disc1 that models a schizophrenia risk allele leads to specific alterations in neuronal architecture and cognition. *Proc. Natl. Acad. Sci. U.S.A.* 105, 7076–7081.

Labouebe, G., Lomazzi, M., Cruz, H. G., Creton, C., Lujan, R., Li, M., Yanagawa, Y., Obata, K., Watanabe, M., Wickman, K., Boyer, S. B., Slesinger, P. A., and Luscher, C. (2007). RGS2 modulates coupling between GABAB receptors and GIRK channels in dopamine neurons of the ventral tegmental area. *Nat. Neurosci.* 10, 1559–1568.

Lefebvre, L., Viville, S., Barton, S. C., Ishino, F., Keverne, E. B., and Surani, M. A. (1998). Abnormal maternal behaviour and growth retardation associated with loss of the imprinted gene Mest. *Nat. Genet.* 20, 163–169.

Lemonde, S., Turecki, G., Bakish, D., Du, L., Hrdina, P. D., Bown, C. D., Sequeira, A., Kushwaha, N., Morris, S. J., Basak, A., Ou, X. M., and Albert,

P. R. (2003). Impaired repression at a 5-hydroxytryptamine 1A receptor gene polymorphism associated with major depression and suicide. *J. Neurosci.* 23, 8788–8799.

Lerch-Haner, J. K., Frierson, D., Crawford, L. K., Beck, S. G., and Deneris, E. S. (2008). Serotonergic transcriptional programming determines maternal behavior and offspring survival. *Nat. Neurosci.* 11, 1001–1003.

Lesch, K. P., Wiesmann, M., Hoh, A., Muller, T., Disselkamp-Tietze, J., Osterheider, M., and Schulte, H. M. (1992). 5-HT1A receptor-effector system responsivity in panic disorder. *Psychopharmacology (Berl.)* 106, 111–117.

Li, L., Keverne, E. B., Aparicio, S. A., Ishino, F., Barton, S. C., and Surani, M. A. (1999). Regulation of maternal behavior and offspring growth by paternally expressed Peg3. *Science* 284, 330–333.

Liebsch, G., Montkowski, A., Holsboer, F., and Landgraf, R. (1998). Behavioural profiles of two Wistar rat lines selectively bred for high or low anxiety-related behaviour. *Behav. Brain Res.* 94, 301–310.

Liu, D., Diorio, J., Tannenbaum, B., Caldji, C., Francis, D., Freedman, A., Sharma, S., Pearson, D., Plotsky, P. M., and Meaney, M. J. (1997). Maternal care, hippocampal glucocorticoid receptors, and hypothalamic-pituitary-adrenal responses to stress. *Science* 277, 1659–1662.

Lopez, J. F., Chalmers, D. T., Little, K. Y., and Watson, S. J. (1998). A.E. Bennett Research Award. Regulation of serotonin1A, glucocorticoid, and mineralocorticoid receptor in rat and human hippocampus: implications for the neurobiology of depression. *Biol. Psychiatry* 43, 547–573.

Lucas, B. K., Ormandy, C. J., Binart, N., Bridges, R. S., and Kelly, P. A. (1998). Null mutation of the prolactin receptor gene produces a defect in maternal behavior. *Endocrinology* 139, 4102–4107.

Madden, T. E., and Johnson, S. W. (1998). Gamma-hydroxybutyrate is a GABAB receptor agonist that increases a potassium conductance in rat ventral tegmental dopamine neurons. *J. Pharmacol. Exp. Ther.* 287, 261–265.

Mann, J. J. (1999). Role of the serotonergic system in the pathogenesis of major depression and suicidal behavior. *Neuropsychopharmacology* 21, 99S–105S.

Manolio, T. A., Collins, F. S., Cox, N. J., Goldstein, D. B., Hindorff, L. A., Hunter, D. J., McCarthy, M. I., Ramos, E. M., Cardon, L. R., Chakravarti, A., Cho, J. H., Guttmacher, A. E., Kong, A., Kruglyak, L., Mardis, E., Rotimi, C. N., Slatkin, M., Valle, D., Whittemore, A. S., Boehnke, M., Clark, A. G., Eichler, E. E., Gibson, G., Haines, J. L., Mackay, T. F., McCarroll, S. A., and Visscher, P. M. (2009). Finding the missing heritability of complex diseases. *Nature* 461, 747–753.

Meaney, M. J. (2001). Maternal care, gene expression, and the transmission of individual differences in stress reactivity across generations. *Annu. Rev. Neurosci.* 24, 1161–1192.

Millar, J. K., Christie, S., Anderson, S., Lawson, D., Hsiao-Wei Loh, D., Devon, R. S., Arveiler, B., Muir, W. J., Blackwood, D. H., and Porteous, D. J. (2001). Genomic structure and localisation within a linkage hotspot of disrupted in Schizophrenia 1, a gene disrupted by a translocation segregating with schizophrenia. *Mol. Psychiatry* 6, 173–178.

Millar, J. K., Wilson-Annan, J. C., Anderson, S., Christie, S., Taylor, M. S., Semple, C. A., Devon, R. S., St Clair, D. M., Muir, W. J., Blackwood, D. H., and Porteous, D. J. (2000). Disruption of two novel genes by a translocation co-segregating with schizophrenia. *Hum. Mol. Genet.* 9, 1415–1423.

Moses-Kolko, E. L., Wisner, K. L., Price, J. C., Berga, S. L., Drevets, W. C., Hanusa, B. H., Loucks, T. L., and Meltzer, C. C. (2008). Serotonin 1A receptor reductions in postpartum depression: a positron emission tomography study. *Fertil. Steril.* 89, 685–692.

Murray, C., and Johnston, C. (2006). Parenting in mothers with and without attention-deficit/hyperactivity disorder. *J. Abnorm. Psychol.* 115, 52–61.

Murray, L., Halligan, S. L., Goodyer, I., and Herbert, J. (2010). Disturbances in early parenting of depressed mothers and cortisol secretion in offspring: a preliminary study. *J. Affect. Disord.* 122, 218–223.

Neumeister, A., Bain, E., Nugent, A. C., Carson, R. E., Bonne, O., Luckenbaugh, D. A., Eckelman, W., Herscovitch, P., Charney, D. S., and Drevets, W. C. (2004). Reduced serotonin type 1A receptor binding in panic disorder. *J. Neurosci.* 24, 589–591.

Parks, C. L., Robinson, P. S., Sibille, E., Shenk, T., and Toth, M. (1998). Increased anxiety of mice lacking the serotonin1A receptor. *Proc. Natl. Acad. Sci. U.S.A.* 95, 10734–10739.

Patterson, P. H. (2009). Immune involvement in schizophrenia and autism: etiology, pathology and animal models. *Behav. Brain Res.* 204, 313–321.

Peier, A. M., McIlwain, K. L., Kenneson, A., Warren, S. T., Paylor, R., and Nelson, D. L. (2000). (Over)correction of FMR1 deficiency with YAC transgenics: behavioral and physical features. *Hum. Mol. Genet.* 9, 1145–1159.

Pletnikov, M. V., Ayhan, Y., Nikolskaia, O., Xu, Y., Ovanesov, M. V., Huang, H., Mori, S., Moran, T. H., and Ross, C. A. (2008). Inducible expression of mutant human DISC1 in mice is associated with brain and behavioral abnormalities reminiscent of schizophrenia. *Mol. Psychiatry* 13, 173–186.

Ramboz, S., Oosting, R., Amara, D. A., Kung, H. F., Blier, P., Mendelsohn, M., Mann, J. J., Brunner, D., and Hen, R. (1998). Serotonin receptor 1A knockout: an animal model of anxiety-related disorder. *Proc. Natl. Acad. Sci. U.S.A.* 95, 14476–14481.

Rouse, B., and Azen, C. (2004). Effect of high maternal blood phenylalanine on offspring congenital anomalies and developmental outcome at ages 4 and 6 years: the importance of strict dietary control preconception and throughout pregnancy. *J. Pediatr.* 144, 235–239.

Shen, S., Lang, B., Nakamoto, C., Zhang, F., Pu, J., Kuan, S. L., Chatzi, C., He, S., Mackie, I., Brandon, N. J., Marquis, K. L., Day, M., Hurko, O., McCaig, C. D., Riedel, G., and St Clair, D. (2008). Schizophrenia-related neural and behavioral phenotypes in transgenic mice expressing truncated Disc1. *J. Neurosci.* 28, 10893–10904.

Smith, S. E., Li, J., Garbett, K., Mirnics, K., and Patterson, P. H. (2007). Maternal immune activation alters fetal brain development through interleukin-6. *J. Neurosci.* 27, 10695–10702.

Smolders, I., De Klippel, N., Sarre, S., Ebinger, G., and Michotte, Y. (1995). Tonic GABA-ergic modulation of striatal dopamine release studied by in vivo microdialysis in the freely moving rat. *Eur. J. Pharmacol.* 284, 83–91.

Spencer, C. M., Alekseyenko, O., Hamilton, S. M., Thomas, A. M., Serysheva, E., Yuva-Paylor, L. A., and Paylor, R. (2011). Modifying behavioral phenotypes in Fmr1KO mice: genetic background differences reveal autistic-like responses. *Autism Res.* 4, 40–56.

Spencer, C. M., Alekseyenko, O., Serysheva, E., Yuva-Paylor, L. A., and Paylor, R. (2005). Altered anxiety-related and social behaviors in the Fmr1 knockout mouse model of fragile X syndrome. *Genes Brain Behav.* 4, 420–430.

Spinelli, S., Chefer, S., Carson, R. E., Jagoda, E., Lang, L., Heilig, M., Barr, C. S., Suomi, S. J., Higley, J. D., and Stein, E. A. (2010). Effects of early-life stress on serotonin(1A) receptors in juvenile Rhesus monkeys measured by positron emission tomography. *Biol. Psychiatry* 67, 1146–1153.

Starke, K., Gothert, M., and Kilbinger, H. (1989). Modulation of neurotransmitter release by presynaptic autoreceptors. *Physiol. Rev.* 69, 864–989.

Strobel, A., Gutknecht, L., Rothe, C., Reif, A., Mossner, R., Zeng, Y., Brocke, B., and Lesch, K. P. (2003). Allelic variation in 5-HT1A receptor expression is associated with anxiety- and depression-related personality traits. *J. Neural Transm.* 110, 1445–1453.

Szczypka, M. S., Kwok, K., Brot, M. D., Marck, B. T., Matsumoto, A. M., Donahue, B. A., and Palmiter, R. D. (2001). Dopamine production in the caudate putamen restores feeding in dopamine-deficient mice. *Neuron* 30, 819–828.

Takayanagi, Y., Yoshida, M., Bielsky, I. F., Ross, H. E., Kawamata, M., Onaka, T., Yanagisawa, T., Kimura, T., Matzuk, M. M., Young, L. J., and Nishimori, K. (2005). Pervasive social deficits, but normal parturition, in oxytocin receptor-deficient mice. *Proc. Natl. Acad. Sci. U.S.A.* 102, 16096–16101.

Usiello, A., Baik, J. H., Rouge-Pont, F., Picetti, R., Dierich, A., LeMeur, M., Piazza, P. V., and Borrelli, E. (2000). Distinct functions of the two isoforms of dopamine D2 receptors. *Nature* 408, 199–203.

Van den Bergh, B. R., Van Calster, B., Smits, T., Van Huffel, S., and Lagae, L. (2008). Antenatal maternal anxiety is related to HPA-axis dysregulation and self-reported depressive symptoms in adolescence: a prospective study on the fetal origins of depressed mood. *Neuropsychopharmacology* 33, 536–545.

Van den Hove, D. L., Lauder, J. M., Scheepens, A., Prickaerts, J., Blanco, C. E., and Steinbusch, H. W. (2006). Prenatal stress in the rat alters 5-HT1A receptor binding in the ventral hippocampus. *Brain Res.* 1090, 29–34.

Weaver, I. C., Cervoni, N., Champagne, F. A., D'Alessio, A. C., Sharma, S., Seckl, J. R., Dymov, S., Szyf, M., and Meaney, M. J. (2004). Epigenetic programming by maternal behavior. *Nat. Neurosci.* 7, 847–854.

Weller, A., Leguisamo, A. C., Towns, L., Ramboz, S., Bagiella, E., Hofer, M., Hen, R., and Brunner, D. (2003). Maternal effects in infant and adult phenotypes of 5HT1A and 5HT1B receptor knockout mice. *Dev. Psychobiol.* 42, 194–205.

Williams, T. A., Mars, A. E., Buyske, S. G., Stenroos, E. S., Wang, R., Factura-Santiago, M. F., Lambert, G. H., and Johnson, W. G. (2007). Risk of autistic disorder in affected offspring of mothers with a glutathione S-transferase P1 haplotype. *Arch. Pediatr. Adolesc. Med.* 161, 356–361.

Yehuda, R., Bell, A., Bierer, L. M., and Schmeidler, J. (2008). Maternal, not paternal, PTSD is related to increased risk for PTSD in offspring of Holocaust survivors. *J. Psychiatr. Res.* 42, 1104–1111.

Yun, S. W., Platholi, J., Flaherty, M. S., Fu, W., Kottmann, A. H., and Toth, M. (2006). Fmrp is required for the establishment of the startle response during the critical period of auditory development. *Brain Res.* 1110, 159–165.

Zupan, B., and Toth, M. (2008a). Wild-type male offspring of fmr-1(+/−) mothers exhibit characteristics of the fragile X phenotype. *Neuropsychopharmacology* 33, 2667–2675.

Zupan, B., and Toth, M. (2008b). Inactivation of the maternal fragile X gene results in sensitization of GABAB receptor function in the offspring. *J. Pharmacol. Exp. Ther.* 327, 820–826.

Epigenetics of early child development

Chris Murgatroyd* and Dietmar Spengler

Max Planck Institute of Psychiatry, Munich, Germany

*Correspondence:
Chris Murgatroyd, Max Planck Institute of Psychiatry, Kraepelinstrasse 2-10, 80804 Munich, Germany.
e-mail: murgatroyd@mpipsykl.mpg.de

Comprehensive clinical studies show that adverse conditions in early life can severely impact the developing brain and increase vulnerability to mood disorders later in life. During early postnatal life the brain exhibits high plasticity which allows environmental signals to alter the trajectories of rapidly developing circuits. Adversity in early life is able to shape the experience-dependent maturation of stress-regulating pathways underlying emotional functions and endocrine responses to stress, such as the hypothalamo–pituitary–adrenal (HPA) system, leading to long-lasting altered stress responsivity during adulthood. To date, the study of gene–environment interactions in the human population has been dominated by epidemiology. However, recent research in the neuroscience field is now advancing clinical studies by addressing specifically the mechanisms by which gene–environment interactions can predispose individuals toward psychopathology. To this end, appropriate animal models are being developed in which early environmental factors can be manipulated in a controlled manner. Here we will review recent studies performed with the common aim of understanding the effects of the early environment in shaping brain development and discuss the newly developing role of epigenetic mechanisms in translating early life conditions into long-lasting changes in gene expression underpinning brain functions. Particularly, we argue that epigenetic mechanisms can mediate the gene–environment dialog in early life and give rise to persistent epigenetic programming of adult physiology and dysfunction eventually resulting in disease. Understanding how early life experiences can give rise to lasting epigenetic marks conferring increased risk for mental disorders, how they are maintained and how they could be reversed, is increasingly becoming a focus of modern psychiatry and should pave new guidelines for timely therapeutic interventions.

Keywords: epigenetics, DNA methylation, chromatin, hypothalamo–pituitary–adrenal axis, brain, early life

INTRODUCTION

The close relationship between the quality of early life and mental health in later life is a longstanding certainty (Gluckman et al., 2008). Many studies in humans, primates, and rodents illustrate that aspects of the early environment can lead to dramatic changes in physical and mental development compromising cardiovascular and metabolic diseases, altered cognition, mood, and behavior. In particular, adverse conditions during early life periods of development can shape individual differences in vulnerability to stress-related disorders throughout life (for review see Heim and Nemeroff, 2002), dependent on the degree of "match" and "mismatch" between early and later life environments.

These findings raise the intriguing question of how these experiences become incorporated at the cellular and molecular level in the brain architecture leading to long-term alterations in various functions ultimately culminating in an increased risk to mental disease. Developmental plasticity defines an organism's ability to adapt to the environment during early life and to implement long-lasting changes in sets of key biological programs on the assumption that the environmental conditions during this early period will persist throughout later life (for review see Hochberg et al., 2010). Adverse maternal experience during early life might profoundly influence the experience-dependent maturation of structures underlying emotional functions and endocrine responses to stress, such as the hypothalamo–pituitary–adrenal (HPA) system – an integral component of the body's stress response – leading to increased stress responsivity in adulthood (for review see Seckl and Meaney, 2004). Indeed, depressed patients with a history of childhood abuse or neglect are often characterized by hyperactivity of the HPA axis (for review see Heim and Nemeroff, 2002).

To understand gene–environment interactions in human populations, and to elucidate the pathways through which programming in response to early life experiences is mediated, researchers in the neuroscience field rely on animal models in which the early environment can be manipulated in a controlled fashion. Current work suggests that so-called epigenetic mechanisms of gene regulation, which alter the activity of genes without changing the order of their DNA sequence, could explain how early life experiences can leave indelible chemical marks on the brain and influence both physical and mental health later in life even when the initial trigger is long gone (for review see Dudley et al., 2011).

In this review we highlight recent animal and human studies addressing epigenetic regulation of gene expression in sustaining the effects of early life experiences. Hereby, we focus on clinical and animal studies that have investigated how biological stress systems, particularly the HPA axis, are shaped by adversity and then provide a description of what we know about the function of epigenetic systems and their roles in brain development and disease. The dynamic nature of epigenetic mechanisms may have important implications when considering the possibility of therapeutic interventions, wherefore we conclude on current evidences of this new research field for the treatment of mental diseases.

CHILDHOOD DECIDES

Sigmund Freud postulated that the trauma of birth – disrupting the physical symbiosis between fetus and mother – becomes a central force in our adult life. This fear and experience of abandonment is a deep-rooted subject in psychology. According to Bowlby (1982), attachment processes are central to understanding anxiety, as illustrated in his decades long studies of children and their attachments to their caregivers, where infants demonstrate distress upon impending departure of the mother as soon as they are old enough to sense signs that she is leaving – around 6–9 months (Sartre, 1964).

It has been suggested that a mother's external regulation of the infant's developing immature emotional systems during selected critical periods may represent the essential factor influencing the experience-dependent growth of brain areas and structures important in regulating mood and behavior. Attachment behaviors could therefore be considered a biological system, interrelated with the fear and stress system, evolved specifically to increase the likelihood of infant–parent proximity which, in turn ensures increased chances of survival of the infant. Indeed, the attachment system is activated especially in times of stress, and the availability of an attachment figure such as the mother, has a great influence in reducing a child's fearfulness (for review see Schore, 2000). However, frequent or prolonged bouts of abandonment can lead to the stress becoming a part of the infant's and, later, the adult's personality. Unfortunately, such situations are all too common where infants are inhibited from forming attachments by either being raised without the stimulation and attention of a regular caregiver, or suffering abuse or extreme neglect; conservative estimates suggest that each year in the United States, more than 1,000,000 children are exposed to such conditions (Sedlak and Broadhurst, 1996). The possible short-term effects of this are anger, despair, detachment, and temporary delay in intellectual development while long-term effects can include psychosomatic disorders, and increased risk of depression or anxiety.

Studies of institutionally reared children have been instrumental in understanding the long-term consequences of childhood social deprivation and have revealed the presence of cognitive, social, and physical deficits (e.g., Rutter, 1998), with good reason to consider emotional neglect as the major precipitating factor (for review see Tarullo and Gunnar, 2006). These observations are consistent with the view that early social interactions play a significant role in the development of basic affective processes, supporting learning through connections between cues, situations, and emotional experiences. In support, post-institutionalized children demonstrate significant difficulty matching appropriate facial expressions to happy, sad, and fearful scenarios (Fries and Pollak, 2004). Reports on post-institutionalized children from Romania reveal the development of difficulties in forming emotional attachments to adoptive caregivers, providing further validation for the attachment disorder construct; moreover, these children display irregular glucose metabolic rates in brain regions controlling cognitive and emotional functions, and an increased HPA axis activity associated with the length of time spent in this type of postnatal environment (e.g., O'Connor and Rutter, 2000). These findings are supported by longitudinal studies of abuse and neglect that indicate increased risk of cognitive impairment, social and emotional difficulties, and risk of mental and physical disease, with those later manifesting post-traumatic stress disorder showing smaller cerebellar and cerebral volumes correlating with earlier onsets and increased durations of abuse (e.g., De Bellis and Kuchibhatla, 2006). Furthermore, in adulthood, the experience of childhood abuse or neglect is tightly associated with increased HPA axis activity (e.g., Carpenter et al., 2010).

EARLY LIFE ADVERSITY SHAPES THE HPA AXIS

On exposure to a stressor a body activates stress systems to prepare for events that may threaten well-being or survival. The autonomic nervous system initiates a rapid and relatively short-lived "fight-or-flight" response while the HPA axis is slower, instigating a more protracted response. The HPA axis is therefore core to the long-term regulation of systems controlling stress responsivity.

Following exposure to a stressor, the neuropeptides corticotropin-releasing hormone (CRH) and arginine vasopressin (AVP) are released from the paraventricular nucleus (PVN) of the hypothalamus into the portal vessel system. These neuropeptides bind to and activate specific receptors (the CRHR1 and V1b receptors for CRH and AVP, respectively) on anterior pituitary corticotroph cells stimulating the release of adrenocorticotrophic hormone (ACTH) which then acts on the adrenal cortex to synthesize and release glucocorticoid hormones (cortisol in primates and corticosterone in rats). Glucocorticoids mobilize glucose from energy stores and increase cardiovascular tone, among further widespread effects. Feedback loops, primarily mediated by the PVN and pituitary corticotroph cells, through glucocorticoid receptors (GR) restrain responsiveness of the HPA axis to reset the system to baseline activity (**Figure 1**; for review see De Kloet et al., 1998). In short, the forward loop prepares the organism to anticipate and respond optimally to a threat, while the feedback loop ensures returning efficiently to a homeostatic balance when it is no longer challenged.

Following periods of sustained stress, negative feedback control of the HPA axis can become dysregulated and this may underlie the development of disorders such as major depression (for review see Holsboer, 2000). Indeed, altered activity of this circuit is one of the most commonly observed neuroendocrine symptoms in patients suffering from major depressive disorder (MDD) and dysregulation of cortisol secretion can be found in as many as 80% of depressed patients if subjects are clustered into different age ranges (Heuser et al., 1994).

In clinical studies early life stress has been shown to be a strong predictor of impaired inhibitory feedback regulation of the HPA axis (Heim et al., 2008) as deduced by dexamethasone/CRH challenge tests. Clinical findings give strong evidence to assume that depression is characterized by a hypothalamic overdrive of CRH and/or AVP systems. Postmortem studies of brain tissue reveal elevated CRH (Raadsheer et al., 1994) and AVP (e.g., Meynen et al., 2006) in the hypothalamus of depressed individuals. In cerebrospinal fluid increased concentrations of CRH have been reported to associate with depression, PTSD and obsessive–compulsive disorder (e.g., Bremner et al., 1997;) while higher plasma

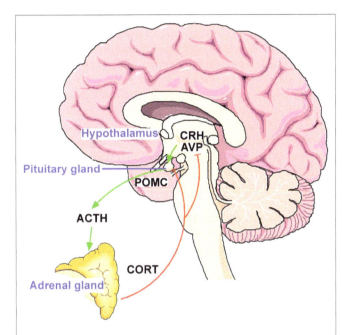

FIGURE 1 | The hypothalamo–pituitary–adrenal (HPA) stress axis. The neuropeptides corticotropin-releasing hormone (CRH) and arginine vasopressin (AVP) are expressed in the parvocellular neurons of the hypothalamic nucleus paraventricularis. The joint release of CRH and AVP into the portal blood vessels leads to potent stimulation of anterior pituitary ACTH secretion and in turn of corticosterone from the adrenal glands. The activational effects of the HPA axis are counteracted by the inhibitory effects of glucocorticoid receptors expressed in the hippocampus, hypothalamus, and anterior pituitary.

levels of AVP have been noted in depression (e.g., Goekoop et al., 2006). Receptors for the hormones also appear to be altered in depression with reduced CRH binding sites being detected in the frontal cortex (Nemeroff et al., 1988) and reduced ACTH responses to CRH (Rupprecht et al., 1989). A recent study further suggested that variations in the CRH receptor1 gene moderated the effect of childhood maltreatment on cortisol responses to a dexamethasone/CRH test (Tyrka et al., 2009) and mutation screens have linked polymorphisms in the V1b and AVP genes with childhood-onset depression (e.g., Dempster et al., 2009), supporting previous preclinical work in which selective inbreeding of rodents for high levels of anxiety-like behavior inadvertently enriches for alterations in the *AVP* gene (Murgatroyd et al., 2004; Kessler et al., 2007; Bunck et al., 2009).

Studies in rodent models demonstrate that exposure to chronic stress can dramatically alter the balance between AVP and CRH control of the HPA axis. For instance, repeated exposure to a stressor leads to enhanced expression of AVP in the PVN, an increase in the number of CRH-containing neurons that co-express AVP and elevation of V1b receptor mRNA in the pituitary – data consistent with the hypothesis that under circumstances of sustained stress AVP becomes the driving force in regulation of the HPA axis (Aguilera and Rabadan-Diehl, 2000). In further support, *in vitro* studies have shown that stimulation of ACTH release by AVP is less sensitive to negative feedback control by glucocorticoids in comparison with ACTH responses to CRH (e.g., Bilezikjian et al., 1987). Conclusively, these data suggest a reduction in the sensitivity of GR-mediated negative feedback regulation of the HPA axis in depression, which would appear to result from a shift toward increased AVP secretion.

MODELING EARLY ADVERSE EXPERIENCES

Given that early life stress may lead to enduring dysregulation of the HPA axis and the close link between HPA dysfunction and major depression it has been suggested that early life stress may predispose individuals to psychiatric diseases in later life. Evidently there are ethical limitations to conducting prospective early life stress experiments in human participants. Therefore, animal models are invaluable in gaining insight into the behavioral and physiological mechanisms underlying the long-term effects of early experiences on emotional reactivity and the stress response.

Rodents are particularly well suited to studies of the effects of early life experience as it is possible to rear them in large numbers and under controlled environmental conditions. Even quite subtle alterations in the experience of rats during the early postnatal or prenatal periods can provoke long enduring consequences in behavioral and endocrine phenotypes (for review see Holmes et al., 2005). Acknowledging attachment theories, many of these models investigate adverse early life factors by focusing on the preeminent mother–infant relationship.

EARLY LIFE STRESS

One of the most widely studied models for early life stress is maternal separation (MS) in which rodents are separated for around 3 h per day for the first 2 weeks of life. Whether the exact psychological cause of the effects of postnatal MS stress results as a direct effect of the pup itself, or indirectly though the manipulation of the mother is still not completely understood: either simulating maternal stroking and feeding during the separation period or providing the dams with a foster litter during the period of separation from their own pups can both dampen the effects of MS on later stress hyper-reactivity (e.g., van Oers et al., 1999; Huot et al., 2004). This procedure can result in persistent increases in anxiety-related behaviors and life-long hyperactivity of the HPA axis in response to stressors (for review see Holmes et al., 2005). Early life stress can also induce long-term effects on hippocampal associated cognitive function and memory (e.g., Eiland and McEwen, 2010) with growing evidence suggesting that the paradigm can disrupt development of neural systems mediating reward-related behaviors, as evident from increases in voluntary ethanol consumption and exaggerated responses to psychostimulants (e.g., Lopez et al., 2010), supporting the concept that maternal and infant attachment is a reward-mediated behavior (e.g., Moles et al., 2004).

Elucidation of neuroendocrine changes underlying the persistent effects of early life stress in rodents has become a major research area. A growing number of reports has documented permanent increases in neurotransmission and hypothalamic expression of CRH (e.g., Vazquez et al., 2006) and AVP (e.g., Veenema et al., 2006) following early life stress. In addition, the ability of hippocampal GRs to attenuate HPA axis may be persistently disrupted; rats subjected to postnatal MS exhibit significantly reduced expression of forebrain GRs and an impairment of the synthetic glucocorticoid dexamethasone to suppress HPA axis activity in adults (e.g., Ladd et al., 2004).

EARLY LIFE CARE

Shorter periods of separation in rodents (e.g., 15 min) or "handling," appear to evoke qualitative changes in maternal care and have consequently been found to elicit effects on behavioral and stress-related responses that are opposite to MS, i.e., reduced anxiety and attenuated HPA axis responses to stress when tested as adults (for review see Fernández-Teruel et al., 2002). This result would support the so called "maternal mediation" hypothesis (Smotherman et al., 1974) whereby the "emotional state" of the mother imprints the one of the offspring.

Indeed, there appears to be a direct relationship between variations in the levels of maternal care and the development of individual differences in the behavioral and neuroendocrine responses to stress of the offspring. In particular, high levels of maternal care appear to be directly associated with reduced behavioral and neuroendocrine responses to novelty in the offspring (Liu et al., 1997). Data from rodent models indicate that the long-term effects of handling appear to depend upon changes in the differentiation of those neurons known to curtail the stress response (Meaney et al., 1996). These alterations include increases in GR expression in the hippocampus, a region strongly implicated in glucocorticoid feedback regulation and reduced levels of hypothalamic CRH (Plotsky and Meaney, 1993).

HIGHER PRIMATE MODELS

Primates are particularly interesting for studying the role of environmental influences during early life; most psychopathology revolves around social functions and, compared to rodents, non-human primates display complex social behaviors and structures resembling humans. The mother–infant bond in primates is the most fundamental early relationship and, as such, primate infants demonstrate remarkable similarities to humans upon separation from their mother, with chronic and sustained separation in infanthood leading to anxiety-like behaviors, cognitive impairments and long-term alterations in the HPA axis (e.g., Sanchez et al., 2010). It is also possible to deploy more subtle manipulations in early life experience in primates. One study, increased stress experiences of the mother through unpredictable disruption of food availability during foraging. Such hardship led to infants developing increased concentrations of cerebrospinal fluid CRH, reduced cortisol levels and fearful behaviors when compared to control infants. Furthermore, when followed into young adulthood, concentrations of CRH remained elevated, indicating that even relatively brief disturbances of the maternal–infant relationship can establish long-lasting changes in stress response systems in monkeys (Coplan et al., 2001).

NEW ANSWERS TO OLD QUESTIONS

The aforementioned studies demonstrate that various aspects of the early environment can lead to dramatic changes in neurodevelopmental trajectories and lead to differential risk of physical and psychiatric disorders. However, the question remains as to how early life exposure to stress is able to evoke such persistent alterations in neuronal substrates, hormonal regulation, and behavioral responses in the adult?

Cells of a multicellular organism are genetically identical but structurally and functionally distinct owing to the differential expression of genes. Many of these differences in gene expression arise during development and are subsequently retained through mitosis. The term epigenetics is now commonly used to describe the study of stable alterations in gene expression potential that arise during development, differentiation and under the influence of the environment (for review see Jaenisch and Bird, 2003). In contrast to DNA sequence that is identical in all tissues, the patterns of epigenetic marks are tissue-specific. Hence, a genome can be considered to contain two layers of information: the DNA sequence inherited from our parents which are conserved throughout life and mostly identical in all cells and tissues of our body, and epigenetic marks (i.e., chromatin and DNA methylation patterns) which are cell- and tissue-specific.

Epigenetic regulation of gene expression therefore allows the integration of intrinsic and environmental signals in the genome, thus facilitating the adaptation of an organism to changing environment through alterations in gene activity. In this way, epigenetics could be thought of as conferring additional plasticity to the hard-coded genome. In the context of the early life environment, epigenetic changes offer a plausible mechanism by which early experiences could be integrated into the genome to program adult hormonal and behavioral responses.

The epigenome refers to the ensemble of coordinated epigenetic marks that govern accessibility of the DNA to the machinery driving gene expression; inaccessible genes become silenced whereas accessible genes are actively transcribed. Although the understanding of the interplay between epigenetic modifications is still evolving, the modification of core histones that package the DNA into chromatin and methylation of DNA at the cytosine side-chain in cytosine–guanine (CpG) dinucleotides represent the best-understood epigenetic marks (**Figure 2**).

HISTONE SIGNATURES

Chromatin refers to a complex of DNA wrapped around histone proteins to form nucleosomes. These histone proteins are extensively modified at their N-terminal tails by methylation, phosphorylation, acetylation, and ubiquitination as part of a histone signature serving to define accessibility to the DNA; densely packaged "closed" chromatin is termed heterochromatin while accessible "open" chromatin is termed euchromatin (Jenuwein and Allis, 2001). Histone acetylation is known to be a predominant signal for active chromatin configurations while some specific histone methylation reactions are associated with either gene silencing or activation. Key to this chromatin remodeling are histone-modifying enzymes such as histone acetyltransferases (HAT) that acetylate histone tails, histone deacetylases (HDAC) which deacetylate and histone demethylases that remove methylation. These histone-modifying enzymes are generally recruited through interactions with specific transcription factors that recognize and bind to certain cis-acting sequences in genes. In this way, signaling pathways registering environmental conditions and governing transcription factor activities, could serve as conduits for linking experiences to epigenetic modifications of genes.

DNA METHYLATION – THE SOUND OF SILENCE

DNA methylation refers to the chemical transfer of a methyl group to the 5 position of cytosine rings, usually in the context of CpG dinucleotide sequences, and generally results in gene

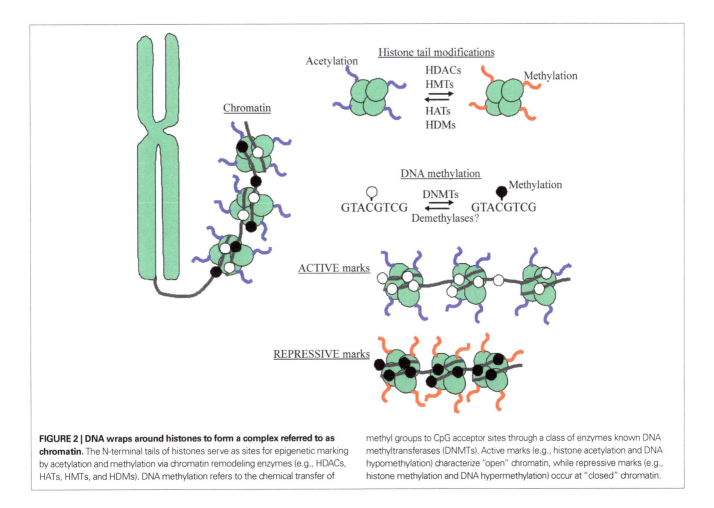

FIGURE 2 | DNA wraps around histones to form a complex referred to as chromatin. The N-terminal tails of histones serve as sites for epigenetic marking by acetylation and methylation via chromatin remodeling enzymes (e.g., HDACs, HATs, HMTs, and HDMs). DNA methylation refers to the chemical transfer of methyl groups to CpG acceptor sites through a class of enzymes known DNA methyltransferases (DNMTs). Active marks (e.g., histone acetylation and DNA hypomethylation) characterize "open" chromatin, while repressive marks (e.g., histone methylation and DNA hypermethylation) occur at "closed" chromatin.

silencing. Since DNA methylation represents a covalent bond, it is thought to be more stable than other epigenetic marks. Such CpG sequences are conspicuously under-represented in mammalian genomes with over 85% of these locating to repetitive sequences scattered throughout the genome and being heavily hypermethylated, possibly playing a crucial role in silencing these elements and thereby maintaining integrity of the genome. The remaining ~15%, of CpG dinucleotides typically cluster within GC-rich regions known as "CpG islands" that locate within or around the promoters of approximately 40% of genes in the genome (for review see Illingworth and Bird, 2009). Accounting for ~1% of the genome, these CpG islands are largely unmethylated in the normal somatic cells while regions showing lower CpG density are more frequently methylated (Weber et al., 2007). In general, patterns of methylation tend to correlate with chromatin structure, i.e., active regions of the chromatin are associated with hypomethylated DNA whereas hypermethylated DNA is packaged in inactive chromatin (Razin and Cedar, 1977).

In mitotically active cells DNA methylation is not copied by the DNA replication machinery, but maintained by DNA methyltransferase enzymes (DNMTs) that use S-adenosylmethionine as a methyl donor. The DNA methylation machinery first has to establish new cell-type-specific DNA methylation patterns during development and possibly during adulthood in response to new signals. These patterns have to be renewed once cells undergo division, i.e., duplicate their genome. Of the three DNA methyltransferases identified in mammals, DNMT1 shows preference for hemimethylated DNA *in vitro*, which is consistent with its role as maintenance DNMT, while DNMT3a and DNMT3b can methylate unmethylated DNA supportive of roles as *de novo* methylases. The activity of these enzymes is crucial to the vast array of developmental programs in mammals and is, therefore, tightly regulated. During early embryogenesis, epigenetic silencing of genes from either maternal or paternal origins occurs predominantly through the DNA methylation activity of the "maintenance" methyltransferase DNMT1 while further tissue-specific gene expression and DNA methylation during later postnatal development requires also the activity of the "*de novo*" methyltransferases DNMT3a and DNMT3b (for review see Turek-Plewa and Jagodziński, 2005).

In general, the endpoint of both DNA methylation processes is either long-term silencing or fine-tuning of gene expression potential. Though methylated CpG dinucleotides can directly interfere with transcription factor binding, most effects of repression seem to occur indirectly, via recruitment of methyl-CpG binding domain (MBD) proteins and their associated repressor complexes (for review see Jørgensen and Bird, 2002). The MBD family of proteins, comprising MBD1, MBD2, MBD3, MBD4, and Kaiso in addition to the founding member MeCP2 assemble at methylation marks to provide a platform for the recruitment of corepressor complexes including HDACs that can rewrite histone marks evoking subsequent chromatin compaction and transcriptional suppression. These complexes can additionally recruit DNMTs to promote, maintain and enforce gene repression, compatible with a reciprocal cross talk between DNA methylation and chromatin marks in the regulation of gene transcription.

Although promoter and enhancer regions appear to attract most attention in regard to DNA methylation and gene transcription, it is becoming increasingly clear that methylation at other gene elements play important regulatory roles. For example, increased DNA methylation within the body of genes is typically associated with active transcription (Ball et al., 2009), while DNA methylation at 3′ and intragenic regions may play distinct roles on regulating gene expression (for review see Suzuki and Bird, 2008), possibly controlling activity of intragenic non-coding RNAs. Non-coding RNA are functional RNA molecules that are not translated into a protein and can be involved in a variety of RNA-mediated silencing pathways with increasing evidence indicating that the regulation of these factors could play key roles in neural development and in neuropsychiatric disorders (for review see Qureshi and Mehler, 2010).

As a final point, a new epigenetic mark, 5-hydroxymethylcytosine, has been recently discovered and hailed as the "6th base." This modification of CpG dinucleotides appears to be particularly abundant in human and mouse brains and to increase during aging in mouse hippocampus and cerebellum (e.g., Song et al., 2011). Considering that it can be generated by enzymatic oxidation of methylated cytosine residues, it appears possible that such modifications might regulate gene expression, though any possible role in brain development or function has yet to be explored in detail.

THE EMERGING ROLE OF EPIGENETICS IN MENTAL HEALTH

The billions of neurons in a single brain have the same DNA sequence yet are differentiated for their diverse functions through epigenetic programming during pre- and postnatal development and possibly throughout life. Epigenetic mechanisms are therefore gatekeepers to brain development, differentiation and maturation, and ultimately, associated disease processes.

GENETIC DEFECTS IN THE EPIGENETIC MACHINERY

Deregulation of epigenetic pathways can lead to either silencing or inappropriate expression of specific sets of genes manifesting with diseases. A growing understanding in this field is leading to the identification of an expanding number of epigenetic diseases comprising various cancers, neurodegenerative disease, syndromes characterized by chromosomal instabilities, mental retardation, and imprinting disorders (for review see Haluskov́a, 2010).

In the nervous system epigenetic marks govern basic cellular processes such as synaptic plasticity and complex behaviors like memory and learning. Genetic defects in the epigenetic machinery, triggering faulty marking, can lead to severe defects in brain development, and manifest as devastating diseases such as the Rett syndrome, Rubinstein–Taybi syndrome, Fragile X syndrome, Alzheimer's disease, Huntington's disease, and psychiatric disorders such as autism, schizophrenia, addiction, and depression (for review see Grafodatskaya et al., 2010).

There are a large number of genes encoding epigenetic regulators that, when mutated, can give rise to mental retardation. Though one might assume that different epigenetic factors would orchestrate the expression of a large number of potentially unrelated genes, disruptions in distinct epigenetic regulators seemingly lead to symptomatically similar mental retardation syndromes (Kramer and van Bokhoven, 2009). Ergo, it is conceivable that mental retardation does not take root in changes of specific target gene(s) but by the inability of concerned neurons to respond adequately to environmental signals under conditions of greatly distorted transcriptional homeostasis (Ramocki and Zoghbi, 2008).

One of the most common causes of mental retardation in females is Rett syndrome, a progressive neurodevelopmental disorder resulting from mutations in the methyl-CpG binding protein MeCP2 located on the X chromosome. Interestingly, less disruptive gene mutations or alterations in expression of this gene also appear to underlie some cases of autism (for review see Gonzales and LaSalle, 2010), along with further members of the MBD family in a small number of cases (Cukier et al., 2010). Another severe X-linked form of mental retardation (ATRX; alpha thalassemia/mental retardation syndrome X-linked) results from mutations of a gene coding for a member of the SNF2 subgroup of a superfamily of proteins involved in chromatin remodeling (Picketts et al., 1996). Further defects affecting proteins involved in histone modification leading to mental retardation are mutations of CBP, a protein with HAT function, underlying Rubinstein–Taybi syndrome (Petrij et al., 1995) and alterations in RSK2, involved in histone phosphorylation and interaction with CBP, leading to Coffin–Lowry syndrome, an X-linked mental retardation disorder characterized by psychomotor and growth retardation (Hanauer and Young, 2002). Defects in proteins important for histone methylation are the H3K4-specific histone demethylase JARID1C resulting in X-linked mental retardation (Jensen et al., 2005), the nuclear receptor set domain containing protein 1 (NSD1) gene causing Sotos syndrome and Weaver syndrome (Tatton-Brown and Rahman, 2007), the histone lysine methyltransferase GLP/EHMT1 gene characterized by severe mental retardation (Kleefstra et al., 2006) and finally, MLL1, a H3K4-specific methyltransferase involved in hippocampal synaptic plasticity, that might underlie in the cortical dysfunction of some cases of schizophrenia (for review see Akbarian and Huang, 2009). The development of, often severe, mental retardation in these syndromes supports the importance of functional epigenetic machinery in the regulation of early brain development. Following on, it could be expected that perturbations in the regulation and expression of various epigenetic components might then lead to further mental pathologies.

ALTERATIONS IN EPIGENETIC REGULATION

There are a growing number of studies indicating aberrant epigenetic marks in the development of mental pathologies later in life, though whether changes originate during early development or in later life as a response to an environmental exposure remain important questions. For example, DNA hypomethylation at the promoter of the gene for catechol-O-methyltransferase (COMT), an enzyme regulating the level of dopamine, has been found to associate with schizophrenia and bipolar disorder (Abdolmaleky et al., 2006). At the promoter region of the RELN gene, encoding a protein implicated in long-term memory, a number of studies have evidenced hypermethylation, correlating with reduced expression, in schizophrenia (e.g., Grayson et al., 2005). Within the frontopolar cortex, a further study discovered DNA hypermethylation at the gamma-aminobutyric acid receptor alpha1 subunit (GABA-A) promoter region, in suicide and MDD brains that correlated with altered DNMT mRNA expression (Poulter et al., 2008), while another investigation reported alterations in DNA methylation and mRNA expression of the peptidylprolyl isomerase E-like (PPIEL) gene in monozygotic twins discordant for bipolar disorder (Kuratomi et al., 2008).

Monozygotic twin pairs share a virtually identical genome though may differ to various extents in their pre- and postnatal environments, making them highly informative in understanding how epigenetic variation could affect complex traits (for review see Bell and Spector, 2011). Indeed, twins frequently differ in their prevalence of mental disorders with a number of studies reporting differences in DNA methylation between monozygotic twins discordant for schizophrenia (e.g., Petronis et al., 2003) and a more recent report detecting lower levels of DNA methylation in the temporal cortex of Alzheimer-affected twins (Mastroeni et al., 2009). A further genome-wide screen detected substantial variability in DNA methylation between twins (Kaminsky et al., 2009), which may relate to the earlier findings, in which DNA methylation profiles of young monozygotic twin pairs were shown to be more epigenetically similar than older monozygotic twins (Fraga et al., 2005). This would therefore suggest that epigenetic changes increase with age, following the view that epigenetic mechanisms such as DNA methylation deteriorate with age and may even accelerate the aging process (Murgatroyd et al., 2010b; Rodríguez-Rodero et al., 2010). However, the influence of genetic factors should also be considered as reports have found higher epigenetic variation in dizygotic than in monozygotic twins (Kaminsky et al., 2009) and intra-individual changes in DNA methylation showing degrees of familial clustering (Bjornsson et al., 2008). Finally, the possible influence of random stochastic factors may further complicate such studies with reports that even genetically identical laboratory animals living under the same controlled environmental conditions, nevertheless develop phenotypic and epigenetic differences (e.g., Vogt et al., 2008).

EPIGENETICS AND AGING
The relationship between DNA methylation and aging was originally proposed by Berdyshev, who discovered that genomic global DNA methylation decreases with age in spawning humpbacked salmon (Berdyshev et al., 1967). This was later backed-up by further evidence for the presence of gradual global losses of methylation in various mouse, rat, and human tissues (e.g., Fuke et al., 2004). Much of this global hypomethylation may result from the fact that different types of interspersed repetitive sequences, that make up the major bulk of genomes, appear to be targeted at single time-points to varying degrees by age-associated hypomethylation (Jintaridth and Mutirangura, 2010). In general terms, age-associated hypermethylation is thought to preferentially affect loci at CpG islands, while loci devoid of CpG islands lose methylation with age. Although an increase in promoter methylation with aging is generally accepted, such as from studies in human prostate and colon tissues (e.g., Kwabi-Addo et al., 2007), recent evidence from Bjornsson et al. suggest a more complex picture with both increases and decreases in intra-individual global methylation levels over time (Bjornsson et al., 2008). Certainly, epigenetic dysregulation with age appears to be a highly tissue-dependent phenomenon. Furthermore, there appear to be subsets of genes that are tissue-specifically affected by age-associated DNA methylation changes, such as genes involved in metabolism and metabolic regulation in liver and visceral adipose tissues (Thompson et al., 2010) or CpG sites physically close to genes involved in DNA binding and regulation of transcription in various brain regions (Hernandez et al., 2011). This later study provides a particularly strong argument that specific age-related DNA methylation changes may have quite broad impacts on gene expression in the human brain. We may, however, have to readdress some of our preconceptions regarding age and aging in relation to epigenetic changes concerning a new study of various mouse tissues in which a majority of DNA methylation changes found in adulthood were preceded by similar DNA methylation changes in juveniles, and that the expression levels of genes near progressively methylated and demethylated CpG sites were already significantly up- or down-regulated, respectively, in young mice (Takasugi, 2011). This would imply that the epigenome matures continuously throughout lifespan and that affects of aging emerge gradually over time.

Compatible with this view, a growing number of reports in the literature challenge the conventional view of a locked state for DNA methylation, demonstrating that DNA methylation remains an active process in post-mitotic cells (i.e., neurons). For example, DNMTs are expressed and regulated in the adult brain (e.g., Brown et al., 2008) and evidence continues to mount that epigenetic mechanisms are able to dynamically control changes in gene activity throughout the lifespan as a result of exposure to a variety of environmental factors during aging, as previously described.

Overall, these findings suggest the presence of several mechanisms regulating methylation that are possibly adjusted at different steps during development, maturation and aging by processes that are responsive to numerous environmental and genetic factors.

THE EPIGENOME AND EARLY LIFE ADVERSITY
Aside from controlling constitutive gene expression, epigenetic mechanisms can also serve to fine-tune gene expression potential in response to environmental cues. DNA methylation has been the most studied in regard to understanding early life experiences and the epigenetic programming of their neurobiological sequelae. Indeed, the stable nature of DNA methylation renders it an ideal template for underpinning sustained gene effects controlling brain function and behavior from early development to old age. Thus we and others have proposed that conditions of early life environment can evoke changes in DNA methylation facilitating epigenetic programming of critical genes involved in regulating stress responsivity that may in turn manifest with neuroendocrine and behavioral symptoms in adulthood (e.g., McGowan et al., 2009; Murgatroyd et al., 2010a; **Figure 3**).

MATERNAL CARE AND EPIGENETIC PROGRAMMING OF GR
One well-characterized model established to study the effects of early life environment on stress programming examines variations in the quality of early postnatal maternal care, as measured by levels of licking and grooming. Studies revealed that rat pups receiving

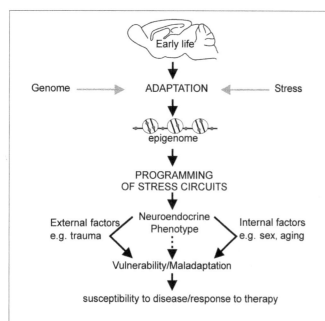

FIGURE 3 | Early life experience can persistently alter expression levels of key genes through epigenetic marking which can underpin changes in behavior, neuroendocrine, and stress responsivity throughout later life. Collectively, this process is referred to as epigenetic programming. The nature of the environment throughout later life, in addition to the impact of biological processes associated with aging and genetic sex, may exacerbate the effects of programming established during early life resulting in increased vulnerability to mood disorders.

high levels of maternal care during early life developed sustained elevations in GR expression within the hippocampus and decreased hippocampal sensitivity to glucocorticoid hormones (Liu et al., 1997). In addition, these rats showed decreased hypothalamic CRH levels and reduced HPA axis responses to stress (Francis et al., 1999) when compared to animals reared by mothers showing low levels of maternal care. Analysis of the molecular mechanisms underlying the long-lasting programming of the GR revealed an important role for epigenetic regulation. The investigators evidenced that the enhanced hippocampal GR expression in animals receiving high levels of maternal care associated with a persistent DNA hypomethylation at specific CpG dinucleotides within the hippocampal GR exon 1_7 promoter and increased histone acetylation. These epigenetic modifications facilitated binding of the transcriptional activator nerve growth factor-inducible protein A (NGF1a) to this region, providing a plausible mechanism for the epigenetic programming of gene function by maternal care during early life (Weaver et al., 2004). Interestingly, a further study using a different paradigm of MS in another species of rat found that corticosterone release and increased NGF1a expression failed to induce changes in DNA methylation levels at the same hippocampal GR promoter (Daniels et al., 2009), supporting again the idea that variations in the genetic make up, and environmental disparities, are critical determinants in organization of the epigenome. In support of this idea, subsequent studies detected altered GR promoter methylation in human postmortum hippocampal tissue of depressed suicide patients who suffered from a history of early life abuse and neglect (McGowan et al., 2009). In contrast, suicide patients who were not exposed to early life adversity, or patients suffering from major depression only, revealed no epigenetic marking of hippocampal GR (Alt et al., 2010).

MATERNAL SEPARATION STRESS AND EPIGENETIC PROGRAMMING OF AVP

Work in our lab evidenced that MS stress in mice, involving separating pups from their mothers for 3 h each day during the first 10 days of life, induced life-long sustained expression of hypothalamic AVP underlying elevated corticosterone secretion, heightened endocrine responsiveness to subsequent stressors, and altered feedback inhibition of the HPA axis. Starting at 10 days of life, directly following the period of MS, and lasting for at least 1 year, elevated AVP expression was specific to the parvocellular subpopulation of PVN neurons while hypothalamic CRH and hippocampal GR expression remained unaltered. Importantly, this altered expression associated with reduced levels of DNA methylation in the PVN at particular CpG dinucleotides within an enhancer region important for AVP gene activity (Murgatroyd et al., 2009). We further showed that hypomethylation at this region reduced the ability of MeCP2 to bind and recruit repressive histone complexes such as HDACs and DNMTs (Murgatroyd, unpublished), supporting previous evidences for a role of MeCP2 as an epigenetic platform upon which histone deacetylation, H3K9 methylation, and DNA methylation are carried out to confer transcriptional repression and gene silencing (e.g., Murgatroyd et al., 2010a).

We then examined the signals controlling MeCP2 occupancy at this early step. Experience-driven synaptic activity causes membrane depolarization and calcium influx into select neurons, which in turn induce a wide variety of cellular responses, connecting neuronal activity to transcriptional regulation (Greer and Greenberg, 2008). Furthermore, neuronal depolarization has previously been shown to trigger Ca^{2+}-dependent phosphorylation of MeCP2, causing dissociation of MeCP2 from the *BDNF* promoter and consequently gene derepression (e.g., Martinowich et al., 2003). Subsequent studies revealed that CaMKII (Ca^{2+}/calmodulin-dependent protein kinase II) was able to mediate this phosphorylation of rat MeCP2 at serine 421 (Zhou et al., 2006), and the homologous serine residue 438 in the mouse (Murgatroyd et al., 2009). Analysis of 10-day-old early life stressed mice revealed increased CaMKII and phospho-MeCP2 immunoreactivity that promoted MeCP2 dissociation at the AVP enhancer and depression. However, though early life stressed mice tested in adulthood (6 week) still showed reduced MeCP2 binding at the AVP enhancer, the levels of MeCP2 phosphorylation and CaMKII activation in the PVN no longer differed to those of control animals. Instead, evolving differences in DNA methylation at this region underlie reduced MeCP2 occupancy in early life stressed mice. Taken together, the initial stimulus of early life stress initiates a loss of MeCP2 occupancy that subsequently leads to the hard-coding of the early life experience at the level of DNA methylation (**Figure 4**). Interestingly, in the control mice an age-associated demethylation also occurred though, critically, the region of the enhancer marked by early life stress was spared, supporting, the importance of this region in AVP regulation (Murgatroyd et al., 2010b).

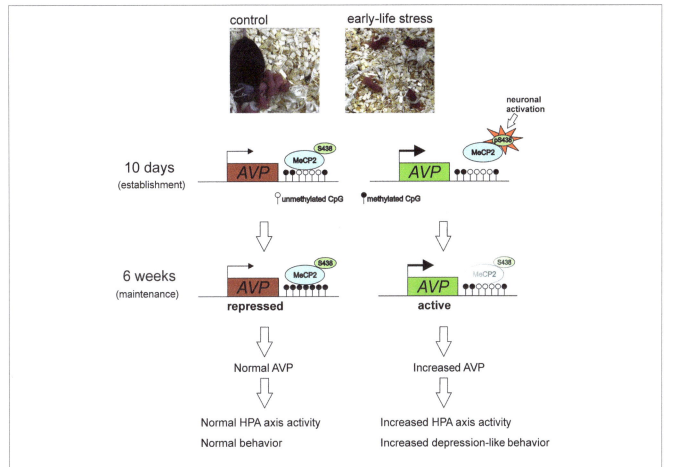

FIGURE 4 | **Experience-dependent activation of neurons in the PVN during early life inhibits MeCP2 binding to and repressing the *AVP* gene in stressed mice.** This further favors DNA hypomethylation underpinning reduced MeCP2 occupancy at the AVP enhancer and maintaining epigenetic control of AVP expression into later life.

ADDITIONAL TARGETS FOR EPIGENETIC PROGRAMMING OF THE HPA AXIS

A growing number of studies support the role of epigenetic modifications in the control of genes regulating the HPA axis. Two recent ones demonstrate epigenetic programming of hypothalamic CRH in response to stress in either the prenatal period or during adulthood. Pregnant mice subjected to chronic variable stressors during early gestation revealed a hypomethylation at the CRH promoter in the hypothalamus of the offspring in adulthood (Mueller and Bale, 2008). Moreover, chronic social stress in adult mice caused a hypomethylation of the CRH promoter in the PVN of a subset of animals displaying subsequent social avoidance (Elliott et al., 2010).

A number of studies describe epigenetic regulation of the *POMC* gene (pro-opiomelanocortin, coding for ACTH), which is a downstream target of AVP and CRH signaling. Hypermethylation of the promoter region leads to silencing of expression that appears to be regulated by cortisol (e.g., Mizoguchi et al., 2007). Recent studies suggest epigenetic programming of POMC by nutritional cues such as overfeeding or anorexia (e.g., Ehrlich et al., 2010), while other research suggested an association with alcohol craving (Muschler et al., 2010). These preliminary findings warrant further studies to address the question of whether epigenetic programming of the HPA axis by early life experiences extends to the pituitary gland (POMC) in addition to hippocampal (GR) and hypothalamic (AVP and CRH) tissues.

EPIGENETIC PROGRAMMING BEYOND THE HPA AXIS

Aside from the HPA axis, additional pathways and epigenetic targets of early life stress seem to exist. For example, rats reared in a hostile postnatal environment exhibited promoter hypermethylation associating with reduced expression of brain-derived neutrotrophic factor (BDNF) in the prefrontal cortex in adulthood (Roth et al., 2009). BDNF is a neurotrophin that regulates neurodevelopment, neuroplasticity, and neuronal functions. It is further involved in the pathogenesis of psychiatric and neurodegenerative disorders and there is a growing body of literature linking epigenetic gene regulation of the *BDNF* gene with brain plasticity and cognitive function (e.g., Lubin et al., 2008).

Neuroendocrine systems associated with female sexual and maternal behavior and the development of the GABA system also appear to be influenced by alterations in the early life environment. Female rat offspring of high-maternal care mothers developed a hypomethylation of the estrogen receptor-alpha (ERα) promoter in the medial preoptic area correlating with increased binding of the transcription factor STAT5 and elevated ERα expression

(Champagne et al., 2006). This study indicates that epigenetic programming can take place in a sex-specific manner which could shed new light on the long standing question of a sex bias in numerous diseases (for review see Menger et al., 2010) Additionally, rat pups receiving high-maternal care showed enhanced hippocampal glutamic acid decarboxylase 1 (GAD1) mRNA expression, decreased cytosine methylation, and increased histone 3-lysine 9 acetylation (H3K9ac) of the GAD1 promoter (Zhang et al., 2010). Furthermore, DNMT1 expression was also significantly lower in the offspring of those rats that received high-maternal care (Zhang et al., 2010). This is interesting, as a number of studies suggest the regulation of components of the epigenetic machinery in response to stressors. For example, recent work has shown that chromatin remodeling in various brain regions, including the hippocampus, is associated with the effects of stress in a variety of models (e.g., Hunter et al., 2009).

Digressing from the literature of early life induced epigenetic changes; one recent study found that traumatic stress during adulthood can also drive epigenetic changes in the brain. Adult rats exposed to severe chronic psychosocial stress showed increased BDNF promoter methylation in the hippocampal regions associating with reduced expression of this gene (Roth et al., 2011). Another neurotrophin known to be important for the regulation of brain plasticity and implicated in depression, is glial cell-derived neurotrophic factor (GDNF). Examining two genetically distinct mouse strains exhibiting different behavioral responses to chronic stress, researches recently discovered GDNF in the nucleus accumbens to be epigenetically silenced following adulthood stress only in the stress-vulnerable mice (Uchida et al., 2011), again supporting the importance of dynamic epigenetic changes in response to environmental cues lasting into adulthood.

CLINICAL STUDIES OF EPIGENETIC PROGRAMMING BY EARLY LIFE ADVERSITY

Evidence is beginning to emerge that the findings of epigenetic programming in animal models may extrapolate to human studies and psychopathologies associated with severe abuse or neglect during childhood. McGowan et al. (2008) found that suicide subjects who had a history of early childhood neglect or abuse exhibited with hypermethylation at the ribosomal RNA (rRNA) promoter. rRNA genes encode ribosomal RNA, important for protein synthesis, leading to the consideration that such reductions in rRNA levels might reflect a reduced capacity for protein synthesis in the hippocampus of suicide victims. Though how this may contribute to the pathology is yet to be determined. Subsequent studies of postmortem tissue by the same researchers further evidenced a hypermethylation of the *GR* gene promoter among suicide victims with a history of abuse in childhood, but not among controls or suicide victims who did not suffer such early life stress (McGowan et al., 2009). This data appear consistent with previous studies demonstrating that the epigenetic status of the homologous *GR* gene promoter is regulated by parental care during early postnatal development in rats (Weaver et al., 2004). Although indirect, this correlation in the human study suggests that epigenetic mechanisms, thought to play a role in vulnerability to stress-related conditions in rodents, might extrapolate to humans. However, it should be noted that further work is necessary to establish a causal link for this epigenetic modification to general depressive behavior in humans. Furthermore, an independent follow-up study failed to identify similar DNA methylation at the GR promoter or alterations in major depression (Alt et al., 2010), again pointing to the importance of inter-individual genetic and environmental variations.

Overall, these studies suggest that epigenetic processes could mediate the effects of the early environment on gene expression and that stable epigenetic marks such as DNA methylation might then persist into adulthood and influence vulnerability for psychopathology through effects on intermediate levels of function such as activity of the HPA axis.

FUTURE RESEARCH

With the advent of new high-throughput sequencing technologies research is now beginning to move on from the single-gene scale to epigenome-wide analyses of all epigenetic marks throughout a genome in a specific tissue. Given that epigenetic modifications are sensitive to changes in the environment, it might be anticipated that these efforts will identify epigenomic signatures for mental disorders and molecular dysregulations resulting from early life stress (Albert, 2010). While such a strategy appears highly attractive in the field of cancer research addressing clonally expanded cell populations, rather than heterogenous tissues, the field of epigenetic association studies in mental illnesses might be more challenging. Epigenetic modifications reported to date in animal models and postmortem brain tissues are seldom "all or none" but gradual, and seem to occur in a highly cell-type-specific manner. In this view, the extraordinary complexity and heterogeneity of neural tissues poses a major hurdle to derive epigenetic biomarkers in psychiatric disease.

EPIGENETIC BIOMARKERS

Ultimately, the identification of "epigenetic biomarkers" in distinct genomic regions may provide important information for the understanding of biological processes underlying mental diseases and thus allow for the development and design of new therapeutics. Though expression and DNA methylation changes in the brain are more obviously relevant to changes in behavior, comparable changes in blood might provide a clinically valuable surrogate, given the easy access to this tissue in patients. Some early studies have shown partial correlations in gene expression between various brain regions and blood (e.g., Brown et al., 2001), which have been supported by following data demonstrating epigenetic differences in lymphocytes associating with the brain in Rett syndrome and Alzheimer's disease (e.g., Wang et al., 2008). Recently it was described that chronic corticosterone exposure in mice stimulated parallel increases in *FKBP5* expression between brain tissues and blood together with some, generally subtle, alterations in DNA methylation at the promoter of this gene (Lee et al., 2010). However, the other candidate HPA axis genes tested in this study – namely, *NR3C1*, *HSP90*, *CRH*, and *CRHR1* – failed to show such effects while further studies in this area of research also describe little correlation (e.g., Yuferov et al., 2011). Consequently, the prospect of diagnostic epigenetic testing for mental diseases using markers in the blood appears so far unresolved, and certainly further research is required.

A MATTER OF TIMING

Many of the studies surveyed in this review highlight the importance of the temporal nature of brain developmental processes in relation to the effects that environmental stressors can have on epigenetic programming of long-term changes in neurodevelopment and behavior. Developing brain regions typically pass through critical "windows" of sensitivity that stretch over different perinatal periods. Therefore, it stands to reason that the impact of stressors at different time-points will confer more pronounced and long-lasting effects within brain regions that are actively developing at that particular time. For example, late prenatal and early postnatal life is the critical period for hippocampal development, possibly explaining why environmental exposures during this time strongly associate with cellular, morphological and epigenetic changes within these structures (for review see McCrory et al., 2010). In contrast, environmental exposures during later life tend to confer their phenotypic effects by altering other areas of the brain. For example, repeated restraint stress in adult rats fails to cause long-term hippocampal-related effects such as those observed following similar stress exposure during prenatal and early postnatal life (Conrad et al., 1999). On the other hand, substantial cortical development and differentiation is known to continue well into adolescence (e.g., Wang and Gao, 2009), possibly explaining why these regions are more susceptible to epigenetic changes in response to later life environmental factors.

In addition to the temporal nature of brain development, we should also consider the temporal and gene-specific manner in which epigenetic marks are established. This will be of crucial importance in understanding how experience-dependent epigenetic marks may undergo the transition from a preliminary labile state to a hard-coded stable print. Indeed, in our studies epigenetic marking of the methylation landmarks in the AVP enhancer persisted under vasopressin receptor blockade in adult (3 month) mice consistent with the concept that the early life stress had already engraved a lasting cellular memory (Murgatroyd et al., 2010a). The question however remains of whether critical "windows" for timely psychotherapeutic and pharmacological interventions following exposure to severe trauma might exist at periods prior to the establishment of stable epigenetic marks. In this view, therapeutic interventions might then re-stimulate or inhibit those same neurons and genes epigenetically programmed earlier in life and reverse these changes. Apparently, timing, quality and duration of such environmental stimulations might be highly specific and context-dependent in regard to the exact nature of the early life stressor.

Nevertheless, studies in rats have demonstrated that environmental enrichment during puberty can alleviate some of the anxiety-related effects of ELS (e.g., Imanaka et al., 2008). This result appears consistent with observations from the clinic. For example, infants who have experienced previous maltreatment, if placed in environments in which positive parenting strategies are being used, show significant improvements in behavior and cortisol regulation (e.g., Fisher et al., 2007). A further study in foster children has revealed that a relational-based intervention focused more on social interactions with caregivers proved to be far more efficient in reducing cortisol levels when compared to an intervention focused more on enhancing cognitive skills (Dozier et al., 2008), bringing us back to the importance of the early life attachment system. Considering these observations, further preclinical studies addressing the effects of such environmental enrichment following early life stress could focus on whether critical time-windows exist for heightened sensitivity to stress, bearing in mind the temporal aspects of brain development and epigenetic mechanisms, and adaptability to ameliorative effects of an enriched environment.

A further option to modify the effects of early life stress could be to target DNMTs and chromatin remodeling enzymes. Though such histone-modifying and DNA methylation-targeting drugs are proving highly attractive to cancer therapeutics, it remains to be seen whether they have any real potential in the realm of psychiatric diseases. Nonetheless, it is notable that the frequently used mood stabilizer valproate (VPA) has been shown to modulate the epigenome by inhibiting HDACs and can additionally promote demethylation in brain cells (e.g., Perisic et al., 2010). However, much caution centers on the fact that most currently available "epigenetic drugs" suffer from a lack of specificity at both the levels of tissue and the genome. This field may yet advance with research targeting specific histone-modifying enzymes, such as G9a, that may be selective enough to ameliorate addiction or mental illness (Maze et al., 2010). Another interesting approach to regulate methylation relies on treatment with the methyl donor L-methionine, or folic acid supplementation during gestation. Intriguingly, there are a number of recent reports linking low folate levels during pregnancy with behavioral symptoms in children (e.g., Schlotz et al., 2010). Although effects in gene expression and behavior have been reported (e.g., Weaver et al., 2005), the mechanisms of how such treatment could be able to target and induce such effects in specific regions of the brain is still yet not properly understood.

In sum, understanding how early life experiences can give rise to lasting epigenetic memories conferring increased risk for mental disorders is emerging at the epicenter of modern psychiatry. Whether suitable social or pharmacological interventions could reverse deleterious epigenetic programming triggered by adverse conditions during early life, should receive highest priority on future research agendas. Progress in this field will further garner public interest, a general understanding and appreciation of the consequences of childhood abuse and neglect for victims in later life.

ACKNOWLEDGMENT

This work was funded by the European Union (CRESCENDO – European Union Contract number LSHM-CT-2005-018652).

REFERENCES

Abdolmaleky, H. M., Cheng, K. H., Faraone, S. V., Wilcox, M., Glatt, S. J., Gao, F., Smith, C. L., Shafa, R., Aeali, B., Carnevale, J., Pan, H., Papageorgis, P., Ponte, J. F., Sivaraman, V., Tsuang, M. T., and Thiagalingam, S. (2006). Hypomethylation of MB-COMT promoter is a major risk factor for schizophrenia and bipolar disorder. Hum. Mol. Genet. 15, 3132–3145.

Aguilera, G., and Rabadan-Diehl, C. (2000). Vasopressinergic regulation of the hypothalamic-pituitary-adrenal axis: implications for stress adaptation. Regul. Pept. 96, 23–29.

Akbarian, S., and Huang, H. S. (2009). Epigenetic regulation in human brain-focus on histone lysine methylation. Biol. Psychiatry 65, 198–203.

Albert, P. R. (2010). Epigenetics in mental illness: hope or hype? J. Psychiatry Neurosci. 35, 366–368.

Alt, S. R., Turner, J. D., Klok, M. D., Meijer, O. C., Lakke, E. A., Derijk, R. H., and Muller, C. P. (2010). Differential expression of glucocorticoid receptor transcripts in major depressive disorder is not epigenetically programmed. *Psychoneuroendocrinology* 35, 544–556.

Ball, M. P., Li, J. B., Gao, Y., Lee, J. H., LeProust, E. M., Park, I. H., Xie, B., Daley, G. Q., and Church, G. M. (2009). Targeted and genome-scale strategies reveal gene-body methylation signatures in human cells. *Nat. Biotechnol.* 27, 361–368.

Bell, J. T., and Spector, T. D. (2011). A twin approach to unraveling epigenetics. *Trends Genet.* 27, 116–125.

Berdyshev, G. D., Korotaev, G. K., Boiarskikh, G. V., and Vaniushin, B. F. (1967). Nucleotide composition of DNA and RNA from somatic tissues of humpback and its changes during spawning. *Biokhimiia* 32, 988–993.

Bilezikjian, L. M., Blount, A. L., and Vale, W. W. (1987). The cellular actions of vasopressin on corticotrophs of the anterior pituitary: resistance to glucocorticoid action. *Mol. Endocrinol.* 1, 451–458.

Bjornsson, H. T., Sigurdsson, M. I., Fallin, M. D., Irizarry, R. A., Aspelund, T., Cui, H., Yu, W., Rongione, M. A., Ekstrom, T. J., Harris, T. B., Launer, L. J., Eiriksdottir, G., Leppert, M. F., Sapienza, C., Gudnason, V., and Feinberg, A. P. (2008). Intra-individual change over time in DNA methylation with familial clustering. *JAMA* 299, 2877–2883.

Bowlby, J. (1982). Attachment and loss: retrospect and prospect. *Am. J. Orthopsychiatry* 52, 664–678.

Bremner, J. D., Licinio, J., Darnell, A., Krystal, J. H., Owens, M. J., Southwick, S. M., Nemeroff, C. B., and Charney, D. S. (1997). Elevated CSF corticotropin-releasing factor concentrations in posttraumatic stress disorder. *Am. J. Psychiatry* 154, 624–629.

Brown, S. E., Weaver, I. C. G., Meaney, M. J., and Szyf, M. (2008). Regional-specific global cytosine methylation and DNA methyltransferase expression in the adult rat hippocampus. *Neurosci. Lett.* 440, 49–53.

Brown, V., Jin, P., Ceman, S., Darnell, J. C., O'Donnell, W. T., Tenenbaum, S. A., Jin, X., Feng, Y., Wilkinson, K. D., Keene, J. D., Darnell, R. B., and Warren, S. T. (2001). Microarray identification of FMRP-associated brain mRNAs and altered mRNA translational profiles in fragile X syndrome. *Cell* 107, 477–487.

Bunck, M., Czibere, L., Horvath, C., Graf, C., Frank, E., Kessler, M. S., Murgatroyd, C., Müller-Myhsok, B., Gonik, M., Weber, P., Pütz, B., Muigg, P., Panhuysen, M., Singewald, N., Bettecken, T., Deussing, J. M., Holsboer, F., Spengler, D., and Landgraf, R. (2009). A hypomorphic vasopressin allele prevents anxiety-related behavior. *PLoS ONE* 4, e5129. doi: 10.1371/journal.pone.0005129

Carpenter, L. L., Shattuck, T. T., Tyrka, A. R., Geracioti, T. D., and Price, L. H. (2010). Effect of childhood physical abuse on cortisol stress response. *Psychopharmacology (Berl.)* 214, 367–375.

Champagne, F., Weaver, I., Diorio, J., Dymov, S., Szyf, M., and Meaney, M. J. (2006). Maternal care associated with methylation of the estrogen receptor-alpha1b promoter and estrogen receptor-alpha expression in the medial preoptic area of female offspring. *Endocrinology* 147, 2909–2915.

Conrad, C. D., LeDoux, J. E., Magariños, A. M., and McEwen, B. S. (1999). Repeated restraint stress facilitates fear conditioning independently of causing hippocampal CA3 dendritic atrophy. *Behav. Neurosci.* 113, 902–913.

Coplan, J. D., Smith, E. L., Altemus, M., Scharf, B. A., Owens, M. J., Nemeroff, C. B., Gorman, J. M., and Rosenblum, L. A. (2001). Variable foraging demand rearing: sustained elevations in cisternal cerebrospinal fluid corticotropin-releasing factor concentrations in adult primates. *Biol. Psychiatry* 50, 200–204.

Cukier, H. N., Rabionet, R., Konidari, I., Rayner-Evans, M. Y., Baltos, M. L., Wright, H. H., Abramson, R. K., Martin, E. R., Cuccaro, M. L., Pericak-Vance, M. A., and Gilbert, J. R. (2010). Novel variants identified in methyl-CpG-binding domain genes in autistic individuals. *Neurogenetics* 11, 291–303.

Daniels, W. M., Fairbairn, L. R., van Tilburg, G., McEvoy, C. R., Zigmond, M. J., Russell, V. A., and Stein, D. J. (2009). Maternal separation alters nerve growth factor and corticosterone levels but not the DNA methylation status of the exon 1(7) glucocorticoid receptor promoter region. *Metab. Brain Dis.* 24, 615–627.

De Bellis, M. D., and Kuchibhatla, M. (2006). Cerebellar volumes in pediatric maltreatment-related posttraumatic stress disorder. *Biol. Psychiatry* 60, 697–703.

De Kloet, E. R., Vreugdenhil, E., Oitzl, M. S., and Joëls, M. (1998). Brain corticosteroid receptor balance in health and disease. *Endocr. Rev.* 19, 269–301.

Dempster, E. L., Burcescu, I., Wigg, K., Kiss, E., Baji, I., Gadoros, J., Tamás, Z., Kapornai, K., Daróczy, G., Kennedy, J. L., Vetró, A., Kovacs, M., Barr, C. L., and International Consortium for Childhood-Onset Mood Disorders. (2009). Further genetic evidence implicates the vasopressin system in childhood-onset mood disorders. *Eur. J. Neurosci.* 30, 1615–1619.

Dozier, M., Peloso, E., Lewis, E., Laurenceau, J. P., and Levine, S. (2008). Effects of an attachment-based intervention on the cortisol production of infants and toddlers in foster care. *Dev. Psychopathol.* 20, 845–859.

Dudley, K. J., Li, X., Kobor, M. S., Kippin, T. E., and Bredy, T. W. (2011). Epigenetic mechanisms mediating vulnerability and resilience to psychiatric disorders. *Neurosci. Biobehav.* doi:10.1016/j.neubiorev.2010.12.016. [Epub ahead of print].

Ehrlich, S., Weiss, D., Burghardt, R., Infante-Duarte, C., Brockhaus, S., Muschler, M. A., Bleich, S., Lehmkuhl, U., and Frieling, H. (2010). Promoter specific DNA methylation and gene expression of POMC in acutely underweight and recovered patients with anorexia nervosa. *J. Psychiatr. Res.* 44, 827–833.

Eiland, L., and McEwen, B. S. (2010). Early life stress followed by subsequent adult chronic stress potentiates anxiety and blunts hippocampal structural remodeling. *Hippocampus.* doi:10.1002/hipo.20862. [Epub ahead of print].

Elliott, E., Ezra-Nevo, G., Regev, L., Neufeld-Cohen, A., and Chen, A. (2010). Resilience to social stress coincides with functional DNA methylation of the Crf gene in adult mice. *Nat. Neurosci.* 13, 1351–1353.

Fernández-Teruel, A., Giménez-Llort, L., Escorihuela, R. M., Gil, L., Aguilar, R., Steimer, T., and Tobeña, A. (2002). Early-life handling stimulation and environmental enrichment: are some of their effects mediated by similar neural mechanisms? *Pharmacol. Biochem. Behav.* 73, 233–245.

Fisher, P. A., Stoolmiller, M., Gunnar, M. R., and Burraston, B. O. (2007). Effects of a therapeutic intervention for foster preschoolers on diurnal cortisol activity. *Psychoneuroendocrinology* 32, 892–905.

Fraga, M. F., Ballestar, E., Paz, M. F., Ropero, S., Setien, F., Ballestar, M. L., Heine-Suñer, D., Cigudosa, J. C., Urioste, M., Benitez, J., Boix-Chornet, M., Sanchez-Aguilera, A., Ling, C., Carlsson, E., Poulsen, P., Vaag, A., Stephan, Z., Spector, T. D., Wu, Y. Z., Plass, C., and Esteller, M. (2005). Epigenetic differences arise during the lifetime of monozygotic twins. *Proc. Natl. Acad. Sci. U.S.A.* 102, 10604–10609.

Francis, D., Diorio, J., Liu, D., and Meaney, M. J. (1999). Nongenomic transmission across generations of maternal behavior and stress responses in the rat. *Science* 286, 1155–1158.

Fries, A. B., and Pollak, S. D. (2004). Emotion understanding in postinstitutionalized Eastern European children. *Dev. Psychopathol.* 16, 355–369.

Fuke, C., Shimabukuro, M., Petronis, A., Sugimoto, J., Oda, T., Miura, K., Miyazaki, T., Ogura, C., Okazaki, Y., and Jinno, Y. (2004). Age related changes in 5-methylcytosine content in human peripheral leukocytes and placentas: an HPLC-based study. *Ann. Hum. Genet.* 68, 196–204.

Gluckman, P. D., Hanson, M. A., Cooper, C., and Thornburg, K. L. (2008). Effect of in utero and early-life conditions on adult health and disease. *N. Engl. J. Med.* 359, 61–73.

Goekoop, J. G., de Winter, R. P., de Rijk, R., Zwinderman, K. H., Frankhuijzen-Sierevogel, A., and Wiegant, V. M. (2006). Depression with above-normal plasma vasopressin: validation by relations with family history of depression and mixed anxiety and retardation. *Psychiatry Res.* 141, 201–211.

Gonzales, M. L., and LaSalle, J. M. (2010). The role of MeCP2 in brain development and neurodevelopmental disorders. *Curr. Psychiatry Rep.* 12, 127–134.

Grafodatskaya, D., Chung, B., Szatmari, P., and Weksberg, R. (2010). Autism spectrum disorders and epigenetics. *J. Am. Acad. Child Adolesc. Psychiatry* 49, 794–809.

Grayson, D. R., Jia, X., Chen, Y., Sharma, R. P., Mitchell, C. P., Guidotti, A., and Costa, E. (2005). Reelin promoter hypermethylation in schizophrenia. *Proc. Natl. Acad. Sci. U.S.A.* 102, 9341–9346.

Greer, P. L., and Greenberg, M. E. (2008). From synapse to nucleus: calcium-dependent gene transcription in the control of synapse development and function. *Neuron* 59, 846–860.

Halusková, J. (2010). Epigenetic studies in human diseases. *Folia Biol. (Praha)* 56, 83–96.

Hanauer, A., and Young, I. D. (2002). Coffin-Lowry syndrome: clinical and molecular features. *J. Med. Genet.* 39, 705–713.

Heim, C., Mletzko, T., Purselle, D., Musselman, D. L., and Nemeroff, C. B. (2008). The dexamethasone/corticotropin-releasing factor test in men with major depression: role of childhood trauma. *Biol. Psychiatry* 63, 398–405.

Heim, C., and Nemeroff, C. B. (2002). Neurobiology of early life stress: clinical studies. *Semin. Clin. Neuropsychiatry* 7, 147–159.

Hernandez, D. G., Nalls, M. A., Gibbs, J. R., Arepalli, S., van der Brug, M., Chong,

S., Moore, M., Longo, D. L., Cookson, M. R., Traynor, B. J., and Singleton, A. B. (2011). Distinct DNA methylation changes highly correlated with chronological age in the human brain. *Hum. Mol. Genet.* 20, 1164–1172.

Heuser, I., Yassouridis, A., and Holsboer, F. (1994). The combined dexamethasone/CRH test: a refined laboratory test for psychiatric disorders. *J. Psychiatr. Res.* 28, 341–356.

Hochberg, Z., Feil, R., Constancia, M., Fraga, M., Junien, C., Carel, J. C., Boileau, P., Le Bouc, Y., Deal, C. L., Lillycrop, K., Scharfmann, R., Sheppard, A., Skinner, M., Szyf, M., Waterland, R. A., Waxman, D. J., Whitelaw, E., Ong, K., and Albertsson-Wikland, K. (2010). Child health, developmental plasticity, and epigenetic programming. *Endocr. Rev.* 32, 159–224.

Holmes, A., le Guisquet, A. M., Vogel, E., Millstein, R. A., Leman, S., and Belzung, C. (2005). Early life genetic, epigenetic and environmental factors shaping emotionality in rodents. *Neurosci. Biobehav. Rev.* 29, 1335–1346.

Holsboer, F. (2000). The corticosteroid receptor hypothesis of depression. *Neuropsychopharma* 23, 477–501.

Hunter, R. G., McCarthy, K. J., Milne, T. A., Pfaff, D. W., and McEwen, B. S. (2009). Regulation of hippocampal H3 histone methylation by acute and chronic stress. *Proc. Natl. Acad. Sci. U.S.A.* 106, 20912–20917.

Huot, R. L., Gonzalez, M. E., Ladd, C. O., Thrivikraman, K. V., and Plotsky, P. M. (2004). Foster litters prevent hypothalamic-pituitary-adrenal axis sensitization mediated by neonatal maternal separation. *Psychoneuroendocrinology* 29, 279–289.

Illingworth, R. S., and Bird, A. P. (2009). CpG islands–"a rough guide" *FEBS Lett.* 583, 1713–1720.

Imanaka, A., Morinobu, S., Toki, S., Yamamoto, S., Matsuki, A., Kozuru, T., and Yamawaki, S. (2008). Neonatal tactile stimulation reverses the effect of neonatal isolation on open-field and anxiety-like behavior, and pain sensitivity in male and female adult Sprague-Dawley rats. *Behav. Brain Res.* 186, 91–97.

Jaenisch, R., and Bird, A. (2003). Epigenetic regulation of gene expression: how the genome integrates intrinsic and environmental signals? *Nat. Genet.* 33, 245–254.

Jensen, L. R., Amende, M., Gurok, U., Moser, B., Gimmel, V., Tzschach, A., Janecke, A. R., Tariverdian, G., Chelly, J., Fryns, J. P., Van Esch, H., Kleefstra, T., Hamel, B., Moraine, C., Gecz, J., Turner, G., Reinhardt, R., Kalscheuer, V. M., Ropers, H. H., and Lenzner, S. (2005). Mutations in the JARID1C gene, which is involved in transcriptional regulation and chromatin remodeling, cause X-linked mental retardation. *Am. J. Hum. Genet.* 76, 227–236.

Jenuwein, T., and Allis, C. D. (2001). Translating the histone code. *Science* 293, 1074–1080.

Jintaridth, P., and Mutirangura, A. (2010). Distinctive patterns of age-dependent hypomethylation in interspersed repetitive sequences. *Physiol. Genomics* PMID: 20145203. 41, 194–200.

Jørgensen, H. F., and Bird, A. (2002). MeCP2 and other methyl-CpG binding proteins. *Ment. Retard. Dev. Disabil. Res. Rev.* 8, 87–93.

Kaminsky, Z. A., Tang, T., Wang, S. C., Ptak, C., Oh, G. H., Wong, A. H., Feldcamp, L. A., Virtanen, C., Halfvarson, J., Tysk, C., McRae, A. F., Visscher, P. M., Montgomery, G. W., Gottesman, I. I., Martin, N. G., and Petronis, A. (2009). DNA methylation profiles in monozygotic and dizygotic twins. *Nat. Genet.* 41, 240–245.

Kessler, M. S., Murgatroyd, C., Bunck, M., Czibere, L., Frank, E., Jacob, W., Horvath, C., Muigg, P., Holsboer, F., Singewald, N., Spengler, D., and Landgraf, R. (2007). Diabetes insipidus and, partially, low anxiety-related behaviour are linked to a SNP-associated vasopressin deficit in LAB mice. *Eur. J. Neurosci.* 26, 2857–2864.

Kleefstra, T., Brunner, H. G., Amiel, J., Oudakker, A. R., Nillesen, W. M., Magee, A., Geneviève, D., Cormier-Daire, V., van Esch, H., Fryns, J. P., Hamel, B. C., Sistermans, E. A., de Vries, B. B., and van Bokhoven, H. (2006). Loss-of-function mutations in euchromatin histone methyl transferase 1 (EHMT1) cause the 9q34 subtelomeric deletion syndrome. *Am. J. Hum. Genet.* 2, 370–377.

Kramer, J. M., and van Bokhoven, H. (2009). Genetic and epigenetic defects in mental retardation. *Int. J. Biochem. Cell Biol.* 41, 96–107.

Kuratomi, G., Iwamoto, K., Bundo, M., Kusumi, I., Kato, N., Iwata, N., Ozaki, N., and Kato, T. (2008). Aberrant DNA methylation associated with bipolar disorder identified from discordant monozygotic twins. *Mol. Psychiatry* 13, 429–441.

Kwabi-Addo, B., Chung, W., Shen, L., Ittmann, M., Wheeler, T., Jelinek, J., and Issa, J. P. (2007). Age-related DNA methylation changes in normal human prostate tissues. *Clin. Cancer Res.* 13, 3796–3802.

Ladd, C. O., Huot, R. L., Thrivikraman, K. V., Nemeroff, C. B., and Plotsky, P. M. (2004). Long-term adaptations in glucocorticoid receptor and mineralocorticoid receptor mRNA and negative feedback on the hypothalamo-pituitary-adrenal axis following neonatal maternal separation. *Biol. Psychiatry* 55, 367–375.

Lee, R. S., Tamashiro, K. L., Yang, X., Purcell, R. H., Harvey, A., Willour, V. L., Huo, Y., Rongione, M., Wand, G. S., and Potash, J. B. (2010). Chronic corticosterone exposure increases expression and decreases deoxyribonucleic acid methylation of Fkbp5 in mice. *Endocrinology* 151, 4332–4343.

Liu, D., Diorio, J., Tannenbaum, B., Caldji, C., Francis, D., Freedman, A., Sharma, S., Pearson, D., Plotsky, P. M., and Meaney, M. J. (1997). Maternal care, hippocampal glucocorticoid receptors, and hypothalamic-pituitary-adrenal responses to stress. *Science* 277, 1659–1662.

Lopez, M. F., Doremus-Fitzwater, T. L., and Becker, H. C. (2010). Chronic social isolation and chronic variable stress during early development induce later elevated ethanol intake in adult C57BL/6J mice. *Alcohol.* doi: 10.1016/j.alcohol.2010.08.017. [Epub ahead of print].

Lubin, F. D., Roth, T. L., and Sweatt, J. D. (2008). Epigenetic regulation of bdnf gene transcription in the consolidation of fear memory. *J. Neurosci.* 28, 10576–10586.

Martinowich, K., Hattori, D., Wu, H., Fouse, S., He, F., Hu, Y., Fan, G., and Sun, Y. E. (2003). DNA methylation-related chromatin remodeling in activity-dependent BDNF gene regulation. *Science* 302, 890–893.

Mastroeni, D., McKee, A., Grover, A., Rogers, J., and Coleman, P. D. (2009). Epigenetic differences in cortical neurons from a pair of monozygotic twins discordant for Alzheimer's disease. *PLoS ONE* 4, e6617. doi: 10.1371/journal.pone.0006617

Maze, I., Covington, H. E. III, Dietz, D. M., LaPlant, Q., Renthal, W., Russo, S. J., Mechanic, M., Mouzon, E., Neve, R. L., Haggarty, S. J., Ren, Y., Sampath, S. C., Hurd, Y. L., Greengard, P., Tarakhovsky, A., Schaefer, A., and Nestler, E. J. (2010). Essential role of the histone methyltransferase G9a in cocaine-induced plasticity. *Science* 327, 213–216.

McCrory, E., De Brito, S. A., and Viding, E. (2010). Research review: the neurobiology and genetics of maltreatment and adversity. *J. Child Psychol. Psychiatry* 51, 1079–1095.

McGowan, P. O., Sasaki, A., D'Alessio, A. C., Dymov, S., Labonte, B., Szyf, M., Turecki, G., and Meaney, M. J. (2009). Epigenetic regulation of the glucocorticoid receptor in human brain associates with childhood abuse. *Nat. Neurosci.* 12, 342–348.

McGowan, P. O., Sasaki, A., Huang, T. C. T., Unterberger, A., Suderman, M., Ernst, C., Meaney, M. J., Turecki, G., and Szyf, M. (2008). Promoter-wide hypermethylation of the ribosomal RNA gene promoter in the suicide brain. *PLoS ONE* 3, e2085. doi: 10.1371/journal.pone.0002085

Meaney, M. J., Diorio, J., Francis, D., Widdowson, J., LaPlante, P., Caldji, C., Sharma, S., Seckl, J. R., and Plotsky, P. M. (1996). Early environmental regulation of forebrain glucocorticoid receptor gene expression: implications for adrenocortical responses to stress. *Dev. Neurosci.* 18, 49–72.

Menger, Y., Bettscheider, M., Murgatroyd, C., and Spengler, D. (2010). Sex differences in brain epigenetics. *Epigenomics* 2, 807–821.

Meynen, G., Unmehopa, U. A., van Heerikhuize, J. J., Hofman, M. A., Swaab, D. F., and Hoogendijk, W. J. (2006). Increased arginine vasopressin mRNA expression in the human hypothalamus in depression: a preliminary report. *Biol. Psychiatry* 60, 892–895.

Mizoguchi, Y., Kajiume, T., Miyagawa, S., Okada, S., Nishi, Y., and Kobayashi, M. (2007). Steroid-dependent ACTH-produced thymic carcinoid: regulation of POMC gene expression by cortisol via methylation of its promoter region. *Horm. Res.* 67, 257–262.

Moles, A., Kieffer, B. L., and D'Amato, F. R. (2004). Deficit in attachment behavior in mice lacking the mu-opioid receptor gene. *Science* 304, 1983–1986.

Mueller, B. R., and Bale, T. L. (2008). Sex-specific programming of offspring emotionality after stress early in pregnancy. *J. Neurosci.* 28, 9055–9065.

Murgatroyd, C., Patchev, A. V., Wu, Y., Micale, V., Bockmühl, Y., Fischer, D., Holsboer, F., Wotjak, C. T., Almeida, O. F., and Spengler, D. (2009). Dynamic DNA methylation programs persistent adverse effects of early-life stress. *Nat. Neurosci.* 12, 1559–1566.

Murgatroyd, C., Wigger, A., Frank, E., Singewald, N., Bunck, M., Holsboer, F., Landgraf, R., and Spengler, D. (2004). Impaired repression at a vasopressin promoter polymorphism underlies overexpression of vasopressin in a rat model of trait anxiety. *J. Neurosci.* 24, 7762–7770.

Murgatroyd, C., Wu, Y., Bockmühl, Y., and Spengler, D. (2010a). Genes learn from stress: How infantile trauma programs us for depression? *Epigenetics* 5, 194–199.

Murgatroyd, C., Wu, Y., Bockmühl, Y., and Spengler, D. (2010b). The Janus face of DNA methylation in aging. *Aging (Albany, NY)* 2, 107–110.

Muschler, M. A., Hillemacher, T., Kraus, C., Kornhuber, J., Bleich, S., and Frieling, H. (2010). DNA methylation of the POMC gene promoter is associated with craving in alcohol dependence. *J. Neural Transm.* 117, 513–519.

Nemeroff, C. B., Owens, M. J., Bissette, G., Andorn, A. C., and Stanley, M. (1988). Reduced corticotropin releasing factor binding sites in the frontal cortex of suicide victims. *Arch. Gen. Psychiatry* 45, 577–579.

O'Connor, T. G., and Rutter, M. (2000). Attachment disorder behavior following early severe deprivation: extension and longitudinal follow-up. English and Romanian adoptees study team. *J. Am. Acad. Child Adolesc. Psychiatry* 39, 703–712.

Perisic, T., Zimmermann, N., Kirmeier, T., Asmus, M., Tuorto, F., Uhr, M., Holsboer, F., Rein, T., and Zschocke, J. (2010). Valproate and amitriptyline exert common and divergent influences on global and gene promoter-specific chromatin modifications in rat primary astrocytes. *Neuropsychopharmacology* 35, 792–805.

Petrij, F., Giles, R. H., Dauwerse, H. G., Saris, J. J., Hennekam, R. C., Masuno, M., Tommerup, N., van Ommen, G. J., Goodman, R. H., and Peters, D. J. (1995). Rubinstein-Taybi syndrome caused by mutations in the transcriptional co-activator CBP. *Nature* 376, 348–351.

Petronis, A., Gottesman, I. I., Kan, P., Kennedy, J. L., Basile, V. S., Paterson, A. D., and Popendikyte, V. (2003). Monozygotic twins exhibit numerous epigenetic differences: clues to twin discordance? *Schizophr. Bull.* 29, 169–178.

Picketts, D. J., Higgs, D. R., Bachoo, S., Blake, D. J., Quarrell, O. W., and Gibbons, R. J. (1996). ATRX encodes a novel member of the SNF2 family of proteins: mutations point to a common mechanism underlying the ATR-X syndrome. *Hum. Mol. Genet.* 5, 1899–1907.

Plotsky, P. M., and Meaney, M. J. (1993). Early, postnatal experience alters hypothalamic corticotropin-releasing factor (CRF) mRNA, median eminence CRF content and stress-induced release in adult rats. *Brain Res. Mol. Brain Res.* 18, 195–200.

Poulter, M. O., Du, L., Weaver, I. C., Palkovits, M., Faludi, G., Merali, Z., Szyf, M., and Anisman, H. (2008). GABAA receptor promoter hypermethylation in suicide brain: implications for the involvement of epigenetic processes. *Biol. Psychiatry* 64, 645–652.

Qureshi, I. A., and Mehler, M. F. (2010). Genetic and epigenetic underpinnings of sex differences in the brain and in neurological and psychiatric disease susceptibility. *Prog. Brain Res.* 186, 77–95.

Raadsheer, F. C., Hoogendijk, W. J., Stam, F. C., Tilders, F. J., and Swaab, D. F. (1994). Increased numbers of corticotropin-releasing hormone expressing neurons in the hypothalamic paraventricular nucleus of depressed patients. *Neuroendocrinology* 60, 436–444.

Ramocki, M. B., and Zoghbi, H. Y. (2008). Failure of neuronal homeostasis results in common neuropsychiatric phenotypes. *Nature* 455, 912–918.

Razin, A., and Cedar, H. (1977). Distriubtion of 5-methylcytosine in chromatin. *Proc. Natl. Acad. Sci. U.S.A.* 74, 2725–2728.

Rodríguez-Rodero, S., Fernández-Morera, J. L., Fernandez, A. F., Menéndez-Torre, E., and Fraga, M. F. (2010). Epigenetic regulation of aging. *Discov. Med.* 10, 225–233.

Roth, T. L., Lubin, F. D., Funk, A. J., and Sweatt, J. D. (2009). Lasting epigenetic influence of early-life adversity on the BDNF gene. *Biol. Psychiatry* 65, 760–769.

Roth, T. L., Zoladz, P. R., Sweatt, J. D., and Diamond, D. M. (2011). Epigenetic modification of hippocampal Bdnf DNA in adult rats in an animal model of post-traumatic stress disorder. *J. Psychiatr. Res.* doi:10.1016/j.psychires.2011.01.013. [Epub ahead of print].

Rupprecht, R., Lesch, K. P., Muller, U., Beck, G., Beckmann, H., and Schulte, H. M. (1989). Blunted adrenocorticotropin but normal beta-endorphin release after human corticotropin-releasing hormone administration in depression. *J. Clin. Endocrinol. Metab.* 69, 600–603.

Rutter, M. (1998). Developmental catch-up, and deficit, following adoption after severe global early privation English and Romanian adoptees (ERA) study team. *J. Child Psychol. Psychiatry* 39, 465–476.

Sanchez, M. M., McCormack, K., Grand, A. P., Fulks, R., Graff, A., and Maestripieri, D. (2010). Effects of sex and early maternal abuse on adrenocorticotropin hormone and cortisol responses to the corticotropin-releasing hormone challenge during the first 3 years of life in group-living rhesus monkeys. *Dev. Psychopathol.* 22, 45–53.

Sartre, J.-P. (1964). Les Mots. *Paris:Gallimard* 254–255.

Schlotz, W., Jones, A., Phillips, D. I., Gale, C. R., Robinson, S. M., and Godfrey, K. M. (2010). Lower maternal folate status in early pregnancy is associated with childhood hyperactivity and peer problems in offspring. *J. Child Psychol. Psychiatry* 51, 594–602.

Schore, A. N. (2000). Attachment and the regulation of the right brain. *Attach. Hum. Dev.* 2, 23–47.

Seckl, J. R., and Meaney, M. J. (2004). Glucocorticoid programming. *Ann. N.Y. Acad. Sci.* 1032, 63–84.

Sedlak, A. J., and Broadhurst, D. D. (1996). *Third National Incidence Study of Child Abuse and Neglect*. Washington, DC: U.S. Department of Health and Human Services, National Center on Child Abuse and Neglect.

Smotherman, W. P., Bell, R. W., Starzec, J., Elias, J., and Zachman, T. A. (1974). Maternal responses to infant volalizations and olfactory cues in rats and mice. *Behav. Biol.* 15, 55–66.

Song, C. X., Szulwach, K. E., Fu, Y., Dai, Q., Yi, C., Li, X., Li, Y., Chen, C. H., Zhang, W., Jian, X., Wang, J., Zhang, L., Looney, T. J., Zhang, B., Godley, L. A., Hicks, L. M., Lahn, B. T., Jin, P., and He, C. (2011). Selective chemical labeling reveals the genome-wide distribution of 5-hydroxymethylcytosine. *Nat. Biotechnol.* 29, 68–72.

Suzuki, M. M., and Bird, A. (2008). DNA methylation landscapes: provocative insights from epigenomics. *Nat. Rev. Genet.* 9, 465–476.

Takasugi, M. (2011). Progressive age-dependent DNA methylation changes start before adulthood in mouse tissues. *Mech. Ageing Dev.* 132, 65–71.

Tarullo, A. R., and Gunnar, M. R. (2006). Child maltreatment and the developing HPA axis. *Horm. Behav.* 50, 632–639.

Tatton-Brown, K., and Rahman, N. (2007). Sotos syndrome. *Eur. J. Hum. Genet.* 3, 264–271.

Thompson, R. F., Atzmon, G., Gheorghe, C., Liang, H. Q., Lowes, C., Greally, J. M., and Barzilai, N. (2010). Tissue-specific dysregulation of DNA methylation in aging. *Aging Cell* 9, 506–518.

Turek-Plewa, J., and Jagodziński, P. P. (2005). The role of mammalian DNA methyltransferases in the regulation of gene expression. *Cell Mol. Biol. Lett.* 10, 631–647.

Tyrka, A. R., Price, L. H., Gelernter, J., Schepker, C., Anderson, G. M., and Carpenter, L. L. (2009). Interaction of childhood maltreatment with the corticotropin-releasing hormone receptor gene: effects on hypothalamic-pituitary-adrenal axis reactivity. *Biol. Psychiatry* 66, 681–685.

Uchida, S., Hara, K., Kobayashi, A., Otsuki, K., Yamagata, H., Hobara, T., Suzuki, T., Miyata, N., and Watanabe, Y. (2011). Epigenetic status of Gdnf in the ventral striatum determines susceptibility and adaptation to daily stressful events. *Neuron* 69, 359–372.

van Oers, H. J., de Kloet, E. R., and Levine, S. (1999). Persistent effects of maternal deprivation on HPA regulation can be reversed by feeding and stroking, but not by dexamethasone. *J. Neuroendocrinol.* 11, 581–588.

Vazquez, D. M., Bailey, C., Dent, G. W., Okimoto, D. K., Steffek, A., López, J. F., and Levine, S. (2006). Brain corticotropin-releasing hormone (CRH) circuits in the developing rat: effect of maternal deprivation. *Brain Res.* 1121, 83–94.

Veenema, A. H., Blume, A., Niederle, D., Buwalda, B., and Neumann, I. D. (2006). Effects of early life stress on adult male aggression and hypothalamic vasopressin and serotonin. *Eur. J. Neurosci.* 24, 1711–1720.

Vogt, G., Huber, M., Thiemann, M., van den Boogaart, G., Schmitz, O. J., and Schubart, C. D. (2008). Production of different phenotypes from the same genotype in the same environment by developmental variation. *J. Exp. Biol.* 211, 510–523.

Wang, H.-X., and Gao, W.-J. (2009). Cell type-specific development of NMDA receptors in the interneurons of rat prefrontal cortex. *Neuropsychopharmacology* 34, 2028–2040.

Wang, S. C., Oelze, B., and Schumacher, A. (2008). Age-specific epigenetic drift in late-onset Alzheimer's disease. *PLoS ONE* 3, e2698. doi: 10.1371/journal.pone.0002698

Weaver, I. C., Cervoni, N., Champagne, F. A., D'Alessio, A. C., Sharma, S., Seckl, J. R., Dymov, S., Szyf, M., and Meaney, M. J. (2004). Epigenetic programming by maternal behaviour. *Nat. Neurosci.* 7, 847–854.

Weaver, I. C., Champagne, F. A., Brown, S. E., Dymov, S., Sharma, S., Meaney, M. J., and Szyf, M. (2005). Reversal of maternal programming of stress responses in adult offspring through methyl supplementation: altering epigenetic marking later in life. *J. Neurosci.* 25, 11045–11054.

Weber, M., Hellmann, I., Stadler, M. B., Ramos, L., Pääbo, S., Rebhan, M., and Schübeler, D. (2007). Distribution, silencing potential and evolutionary impact of promoter DNA methylation in the human genome. *Nat. Genet.* 39, 457–466.

Yuferov, V., Nielsen, D. A., Levran, O., Randesi, M., Hamon, S., Ho, A., Morgello, S., and Kreek, M. J. (2011). Tissue-specific DNA methylation of the human prodynorphin gene in post-mortem brain tissues and PBMCs. *Pharmacogenet. Genomics.* 21, 185–196.

Zhang, T. Y., Hellstrom, I. C., Bagot, R. C., Wen, X., Diorio, J., and Meaney, M. J. (2010). Maternal care and DNA methylation of a glutamic acid decarboxylase 1 promoter in rat hippocampus. *J. Neurosci.* 30, 13130–13137.

Zhou, Z., Hong, E. J., Cohen, S., Zhao, W. N., Ho, H. Y., Schmidt, L., Chen, W. G., Lin, Y., Savner, E., Griffith, E. C., Hu, L., Steen, J. A., Weitz, C. J., and Greenberg, M. E. (2006). Brain-specific phosphorylation of MeCP2 regulates activity-dependent Bdnf transcription, dendritic growth, and spine maturation. *Neuron* 52, 255–269.

The emergence of spanking among a representative sample of children under 2 years of age in North Carolina

Adam J. Zolotor[1]*, T. Walker Robinson[2], Desmond K. Runyan[3], Ronald G. Barr[4] and Robert A. Murphy[5]

[1] Department of Family Medicine and Injury Prevention Research Center, University of North Carolina, Chapel Hill, NC, USA
[2] Department of Pediatrics, Duke University Medical Center, Durham, NC, USA
[3] Robert Wood Johnson Clinical Scholar Program, Departments of Social Medicine and Pediatrics, University of North Carolina, Chapel Hill, NC, USA
[4] Department of Pediatrics and Developmental Neurosciences and Child Health, Child and Family Research Institute, University of British Columbia, Vancouver, BC, Canada
[5] Center for Child & Family Health and Department of Psychiatry & Behavior Sciences, Duke University Medical Center, Durham, NC, USA

*Correspondence:
Adam J. Zolotor, Department of Family Medicine and Injury Prevention Research Center, University of North Carolina, CB #9595, Chapel Hill, NC 27599-7595, USA.
e-mail: ajzolo@med.unc.edu

Spanking is common in the United States but less common in many European countries in which it has been outlawed. Being spanked has been associated with child abuse victimization, poor self-esteem, impaired parent–child relationships, and child and adult mental health, substance abuse, and behavioral consequences. Being spanked as a child has also been shown to increase the likelihood of abusing one's own children or spouse as an adult. Spanking of very young children less than two is almost never recommended even among experts that consider spanking as reasonable in some circumstances. Using a cross-sectional anonymous telephone survey, we describe spanking rates among a representative sample of North Carolina mothers of children less than 2 years old and the association of spanking with demographic characteristics. A substantial proportion of mothers admit to spanking their very young children. The rate of spanking in the last year among all maternal respondents was 30%. Over 5% of the mothers of 3-month olds reported spanking. Over 70% of the mothers of 23-month olds reported spanking. Increased spanking was associated with higher age of the child and lower maternal age. With every month of age, a child had 27% increased odds of being spanked. Early spanking has been shown to be associated with poor cognitive development in early childhood. Further, early trauma has been shown to have significant effects on the early developing brain. It is therefore critical that health and human services professionals address the risk of corporal punishment as a method of discipline early in the life of the child. The spanking of very young children may be an appropriate locus for policy and legislative debates regarding corporal punishment.

Keywords: spanking, corporal punishment, early childhood, survey research

INTRODUCTION

There is mounting evidence that corporal punishment is detrimental to the health and development of children, yet recent studies from the USA have reported that 45–95% of children were spanked in the previous year (Straus and Stewart, 1999; Theodore et al., 2005; Vittrup et al., 2006; Zolotor et al., 2011). Some studies focusing on early childhood have shown similarly high rates for young children with the risk of even more deleterious consequences. Studies over the last decade have described 29–77% of parents reporting spanking children less than age of 2 years of age (Straus and Stewart, 1999; Wissow, 2001; Regalado et al., 2004; Slade and Wissow, 2004; Socolar et al., 2005, 2007). To date, no studies have measured rates by age in months spanking during this early developmental period, although increasing infant age is clearly associated with increased use of spanking (Combs-Orme and Cain, 2008).

Spanking has numerous deleterious consequences on child health and development. A systematic review of the consequences of spanking which included 88 empirical studies reported that spanking was associated with moral internalization, aggression, delinquent and antisocial behavior, poorer quality of the parent–child relationship, poorer mental health, and an increased likelihood of being a victim of physical abuse. Furthermore, spanking during childhood was associated in later adulthood with aggression, criminal and antisocial behavior, poorer mental health, and adult abuse of one's own child or spouse. The only benefit of corporal punishment identified in this systematic review was improved immediate compliance (Gershoff, 2002).

The age of spanking occurrence may have an impact on the developmental and behavioral consequences of spanking. Numerous studies have shown that earlier abuse and neglect has a greater impact on development than later abuse and neglect (Keiley et al., 2001; Kaplow and Widom, 2007; Kotch et al., 2008). Less is known about the consequences of early spanking relative to later spanking regarding differential developmental consequences. One longitudinal study of discipline at age three found that, among girls, physical discipline was associated with a lower IQ (Smith and Brooks-Gunn, 1997). A subsequent study with a much larger sample and more effective control of confounding variables reported that spanking at 1 year of age was associated with aggressive behavior at 2 years of age and lower developmental scores at three compared to children that were not spanked (Berlin et al., 2009). A recent prospective cohort study reported that spanking at three was associated with increased aggressive behavior at five, further reinforcing that the groundwork for adverse developmental and behavioral consequences of spanking may be laid at a young age (Taylor et al., 2010).

Spanking has been associated repeatedly with physical abuse. Child protective service substantiated abuse often results from escalated spanking (Kadushin and Martin, 1981). It is consistently reported that abusive parents are far more likely to spank then non-abusive parents (Gershoff, 2002). A recent study reported that spanking frequency and intensity (use of an object) was associated with increasing probability of self-reported abuse (Zolotor et al., 2008).

Being spanked as a child has been shown to be associated with later abuse of one's own child or spouse in several studies. The study of intergenerational transmission of violence is particularly challenging because of the long time lag between a child's own spanking or other assault and the number and complexity of intervening variables. Seven cross-sectional studies on the effects of spanking report a consistent relationship between being spanked and later abuse of one's own child and spouse (Straus and Gelles, 1990; Gershoff, 2002; Straus and Donnelly, 2005). This association may be the result of other consequences of spanking (such as increased aggression) or due to social learning theory in which children who are spanked themselves "learn" to use violence for resolution of conflict at a young age.

Given the convergent evidence that early abuse and neglect may be more harmful than later abuse and neglect and the similar developmental and behavioral consequences of spanking, we felt that a more detailed understanding of when spanking begins to occur in early childhood would help to better understand these relationships. Further, if it is desirable to curb spanking and/or give parents alternate tools for discipline, it is important to understand when such behaviors begin to occur. We therefore conducted a cross-sectional survey of mothers of children less than approximately 2 years of age in North Carolina (NC) to examine the age-dependent trajectory of rates of spanking. Mothers were asked to report their own disciplinary practices as well as those of spouses or partners involved in raising the child. For the purposes of this study, spanking is defined as being "hit on the buttocks with the hand only." Our primary goal was to describe the pattern of adoption of spanking by mothers as a disciplinary practice in very young children. A secondary goal was to determine whether rates of early spanking were significantly different among mothers with differing demographic backgrounds.

MATERIALS AND METHODS
STUDY DESIGN AND SAMPLING
An anonymous telephone survey on child rearing was administered to a stratified probability sample of North Carolina mothers. The target population consisted of all live births to English or Spanish-speaking mothers born in North Carolina between October 1, 2005 and July 31, 2007. The anticipated sample size was 3450 subjects. Subjects were selected using a random selection procedure from birth certificates. A total of 38,334 live birth certificates were selected. Strata were created based on mother's education, age, and tobacco or alcohol as indicated on the birth certificate. Proportional sampling was done at random from each stratum. Each mother's name and address from a birth certificate was provided to a survey research firm (GENESYS Sampling Systems, Fort Wayne, Pennsylvania) which was back-matched on publicly available telephone numbers for calling.

To be eligible to participate in the study, a selected birth certificate had to be matched with a current telephone number of a North Carolina household. A child born between October 1, 2005 and July 21, 2007 needed to reside in the household. A referent child was selected at random. The mother or female guardian of the referent child had to speak English or Spanish and the interview was conducted in her preferred language. There was no attempt to verify birth certificate matching to minimize the threat of breach of confidentiality. Because of the time lag for birth certificate completion, matching, and entry into the field, we expected to have few subjects with infants less than 3 months of age. Further, we attempted to include mothers of children through 24 months of age in the sample by selection of birth certificates, though considered mothers of children through 30 months to meet eligibility criteria.

The survey was conducted from October 1, 2007 to April 7, 2008 at the Survey Research Unit of the University of North Carolina. Blaise 4.6 (Statistics, Netherlands), a computer-assisted telephone interview software package by Statistics Netherlands, was used when administering the survey. A minimum of 12 call-back attempts were on a rotating schedule. Calls could be scheduled at the preference of the subject. Interviewers were trained according to standard procedures at the Survey Research Unit and the lead author about the contents and purpose of this survey. The survey was translated into Spanish and independently back-translated. All respondents were given phone numbers for parenting resources as part of a routine "debriefing." After initially connecting with a potential respondent and prior to administering the survey, the phone number and identity of the respondent was purged from the computer system. The respondent was therefore not traceable, thus allowing for a truly anonymous survey. It was approved by the University of North Carolina School of Medicine Institutional Review Board.

MEASURES
The survey was designed to describe parenting behaviors, disciplinary practices, and family and community characteristics. The parenting behaviors were assessed using questions selected from the Parent Child Conflict Tactics Scales (PCCTS; Straus et al., 1998). The PCCTS asks parents about a variety of positive and negative discipline techniques, including positive and negative reinforcement, corporal punishment, and potentially abusive behaviors. In addition, supplemental questions for neglect were asked from the PCCTS. Questions from the PCCTS were asked of both the responding mother's behaviors toward the index child and the behavior of her partner toward the index child (two separate questions). Respondents are asked to indicate how many times they have used each practice in the last year, varying from none to more than 20 times. Then, if the answer is "not in the past year," they are asked if they have ever used this practice. Additional questions include family composition, employment, and ethnicity so that the data could be weighted to provide population estimates for the state. The use of anonymous surveys to assess potentially abusive caregiver behaviors utilizes the work of Straus which shows that caregivers are willing to report harsh and socially disapproved of forms of discipline (Straus and Gelles, 1990). The PCCTS has been widely used to assess parenting practices (Tajima, 2000; Theodore et al., 2005; Zolotor et al., 2008 #48)

STATISTICAL ANALYSIS

Sample weights addresses the disproportionality in the sample arising from the sampling process. Variables included in the weighting process included mother's education, mother's age, tobacco or alcohol use during pregnancy (stratification variables), and marital status, race/ethnicity of mother, urbanization of county, and father's education. These weighting procedures allow the survey results to best approximate the true frequencies of behaviors for the target population in North Carolina.

Spanking frequencies were determined for each month-long age category, for a total of 25 categories between 3 and 25 months. These proportions are summarized using a simple histogram. Mothers were dichotomized as spankers or non-spankers of the index child. Among self-reported spankers, we assessed the number of times each mother reported spanking their child in the previous year. Spankers and non-spankers were then compared according to selected maternal, child, and demographic characteristics one at a time. These included maternal age, marital status, educational level, ethnicity, household income, as well as age and sex of the child. Survey-weighted bivariate logistic regression analyses were conducted for each independent variable. Survey-weighted multiple logistic regression was then used to examine the potential associations between spanking and these maternal demographic characteristics in full multivariate models. Models were reduced to maximize statistical power by eliminating demographic variables that were related at a statistical level of significance greater than 0.10. Analysis was conducted using Stata version 10.0 (Stata Corp., College Station, TX, USA).

RESPONSE RATE

A large number of birth certificates (38,334) were back-matched for telephone numbers due to anticipated changes in address, phone number, and unlisted numbers. Forty-nine percent of names and addresses (18,789) were matched to a telephone number. Of these, 12,828 were entered into calling, 2884 subjects completed the interview, and 62 subjects partially completed the interview. This resulted in a total sample of 2946 mothers. There were 1248 respondents determined to be eligible but who did not complete a sufficient part of the interview for inclusion, 3024 numbers of unknown eligibility, and 5610 numbers found to be ineligible.

Response rate was determined using the American Association for Public Opinion Research Standard Definitions (2008). Unknown numbers were adjusted for eligibility status and inclusion in the denominator by determining the proportion which, if contacted, should have been eligible. This is a conservative approach to the determination of response rates known as response rate option 4 (American Association of Public Opinion Research, 2008). This approach yielded a conservative response rate of 53.6%.

RESULTS
SUBJECT CHARACTERISTICS

Table 1 reports both unweighted and weighted maternal and family characteristics for the 2946 maternal respondents, while Table 2 separates the maternal respondents into those who had and had not spanked the index child. The majority of mothers surveyed were married, middle to high income, and of Caucasian ethnicity. Nearly (48%) half of mothers surveyed were college graduates. More than

Table 1 | Description of survey respondents (N = 2946).

Characteristic	Unweighted percent	Weighted percent
AGE OF CHILD, MONTHS		
3–7	20.2	19.0
8–12	25.0	25.8
13–17	21.9	22.0
18–22	21.9	21.0
23–27	11.1	12.2
SEX OF CHILD		
Male	52.0	51.8
Female	48.0	48.3
MATERNAL AGE		
14–20	7.0	12.5
21–35	76.7	75.3
36–49	16.4	12.3
MARITAL STATUS		
Married	81.6	60.6
Single	18.4	39.4
EDUCATION STATUS		
Less than high school	10.9	18.3
HS grad/some college	40.7	46.7
College graduate or higher	48.4	35.0
ETHNICITY/RACE (MUTUALLY EXCLUSIVE CATEGORIES)		
African American/Black	12.3	19.9
Asian/Pacific Islander	2.2	1.5
Hispanic	10.5	15.2
White/Caucasian	74.2	62.4
Native American/Indian	0.7	0.9
Other	0.1	0.6
ANNUAL HOUSEHOLD INCOME		
Less than $40,001	29.0	42.1
40,001–80,000	35.4	31.6
80,001+	35.6	26.3

99% of respondents were the biological mother of the index child. The index children were between 3 and 27 months of age. There were roughly equal numbers of boys and girls.

SPANKING RATE

Of the 2946 mothers surveyed, nearly 1/3 (29.9%) reported spanking their child in the past year. This figure is very similar to the 30.0% prevalence of spanking of children less than 2 years old in a 2002 survey of North Carolina and South Carolina mothers ($n = 115$ of 384 mothers of children less than 2; Theodore et al., 2005). Frequency of spanking among spankers in the past year is graphically represented in **Figure 1**. Notably, 10.8% of those who had spanked their index child at least once responded that they had spanked their child more than 20 times in the past year.

MATERNAL AND FAMILY CHARACTERISTICS PREDICTING SPANKING

The relationships between respondents of differing demographic characteristics and the use of spanking as a disciplinary method were examined using survey-weighted multivariate logistic regression models. Three maternal characteristics predicted reported

Table 2 | Weighted comparison of spankers and non-spankers (N = 2946).

Characteristic	Weighted percent		Number
	Spankers	Non-spankers	All respondents
AGE OF CHILD, MONTHS			
3–7	1.4	98.6	577
8–12	8.6	91.4	715
13–17	32.6	67.4	628
18–22	57.1	42.9	626
23–27	64.0	36.0	317
SEX OF CHILD			
Male	31.9	66.6	1533
Female	27.7	72.3	1413
MATERNAL AGE			
14–20	33.4	66.6	205
21–35	30.6	69.4	2258
36–49	24.7	75.3	483
MARITAL STATUS			
Married	30.1	69.9	2405
Single	29.5	70.5	541
EDUCATION STATUS			
Less than high school	26.7	73.3	322
HS grad/some college	29.3	70.7	1199
College graduate or higher	32.3	67.7	1425
ETHNICITY/RACE			
African American/Black	26.2	73.8	362
Asian/Pacific Islander	28.9	71.1	64
Hispanic	21.8	78.2	308
White/Caucasian	32.8	67.2	2187
Native American/Indian	40.7	59.4	21
Other	29.9	70.1	4
ANNUAL HOUSEHOLD INCOME			
Less than $40,001	27.8	72.2	800
40,001–80,000	33.4	66.6	977
80,001+	29.2	70.8	984

spanking in our final multivariable logistic regression model (see **Table 3**). Spanking was inversely associated with maternal age. Increasing maternal age was associated with a decrease in the odds of spanking. For each year of age, mothers were at 2% lower odds of reporting spanking ($p = 0.001$). There was a significant relationship between spanking occurrence and maternal ethnicity. Mothers of Asian, Native American, and other ethnic groups participated in the survey in low numbers. Estimates of these associations with spanking are imprecise. Hispanic mothers had one-fourth the odds of spanking compared to white mothers (OR = 0.25; $p < 0.001$) and black mothers were also less likely to spank (OR = 0.60, $p = 0.01$). Finally, household income was unrelated to spanking occurrence as was reported maternal education.

As expected, there was a significant relationship between increased child age and maternal spanking practices. Mothers had 1.27 times the odds of spanking their child with each increasing month of the child's life ($p < 0.001$). Mothers of boys were at higher odds of spanking than mothers of girls (OR 1.27, $p = 0.05$). **Figure 2** shows a simple histogram of spanking by child age in months. This figure demonstrates the age at which a majority of mothers report spanking occurs between 18 and 19 months of age.

DISCUSSION

Among mothers in North Carolina, spanking of children under the age of two is quite common. Almost one-third of mothers (30.0%) of young children spanked their child in the past year, some more than 20 times. This rate closely resembles that reported by Slade and Wissow (2004; 38.7% in a nationally representative sample), Socolar et al. (2005; 29% among a NC sample), and a similar 2002 study of North and South Carolina maternal discipline practices in children 0–2 years of age (30.0% among a small sample; Theodore et al., 2005). Unlike these three earlier studies, however, our survey enabled a month-by-month examination of spanking trends in children aged 3–24 months. Multivariate logistic regression showed significant differences in rates of spanking differences among mothers of different ages and ethnicities as well as children of different ages and sex.

While much of the spanking literature has assessed the relationship between parental demographics and spanking across the entire pediatric age spectrum, this study focuses on very young children. Our results support earlier evidence that older mothers are less likely to spank (Smith and Brooks-Gunn, 1997; Day et al., 1998; Eamon, 2001; Wissow, 2001; Regalado et al., 2004). Older mothers may have a better understanding of child development and more experience with children. Contrary to much of the literature associating African American ethnicity with higher spanking prevalence (Smith and Brooks-Gunn, 1997; Day et al., 1998; Socolar et al., 1999; Straus and Stewart, 1999; Pinderhughes et al., 2000; Wissow, 2001; Horn et al., 2004; Regalado et al., 2004; Barkin et al., 2007), we found African American mothers reported spanking less often than white mothers. Black mothers may be less likely to spank very young children, but this relationship may not persist as children age. Hispanic mothers also reported spanking less often than white mothers.

Our analysis of the relationship of household income with spanking yielded no significant association. Previous reports of this relationship have been equivocal. Seven studies have found a direct relationship between decreased income and increased spanking practices (Giles-Sims et al., 1995; Smith and Brooks-Gunn, 1997; Socolar et al., 1999; Straus and Stewart, 1999; Pinderhughes et al., 2000; Wissow, 2001; Regalado et al., 2004), four studies found no relationship between income and spanking prevalence (Buntain-Ricklefs et al., 1994; Day et al., 1998; Horn et al., 2004; Grogan-Kaylor and Otis, 2007), and one study reported equivocal results (Socolar et al., 2005). In our study, mothers at the lowest end of the economic spectrum (<$40,000 per year) were not more likely to spank than mothers in households earning more than $80,000 per year, though households earning in a mid-range income of $40,000–80,000 per year reported spanking at higher rates, but this was not statistically significant. It may be that spanking in the US today is no longer associated with economic status, or that our crude measure of economic status failed to capture these differences.

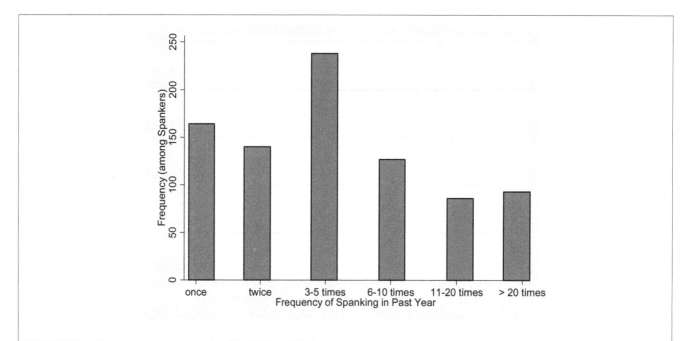

FIGURE 1 | Spanking frequency among spankers (N = 875). Note: This figure does not include the 2027 mothers (70%) who reported not spanking in the past year.

Table 3 | Logistic regression models of spanking behavior on maternal characteristics (N = 2790).

Independent variables	Models					
	Bivariate		Full multivariate[1]		Final multivariate[2]	
	Odds ratio	p-value	Odds ratio	p-value	Odds ratio	p-value
Age of child, months	1.24	<0.001***	1.23	<0.001***	1.27	<0.001***
Sex of child (girl Ref)	1.22	0.04*	1.27	0.06	1.27	0.05*
Maternal age, years	0.98	0.03*	0.96	0.001***	0.95	<0.001***
Marital status (married as reference)	0.97	0.79	0.80	0.23	–	–
EDUCATIONAL STATUS						
Less than HS (Ref)	1.00	–	1.00	–	1.00	–
HS grad/some college	1.14	0.04*	1.33	0.27	1.32	0.28
College graduate	1.31	0.09	1.79	0.05*	1.65	0.06
ETHNICITY						
Black	0.73	0.03*	0.57	0.01**	0.60	0.01**
Asian	0.83	0.59	0.78	0.64	0.75	0.56
Hispanic	0.57	0.02*	0.25	<0.001***	0.25	<0.001***
White (Ref)	1.00	–	1.00	–	1.00	–
Native American	1.40	0.66	1.25	0.65	1.29	0.59
Other	1.99	0.57	1.66	0.56	1.46	0.67
INCOME LEVEL						
<$40,000 (Ref)	1.00	–	1.00	–	–	–
$40–80,000	1.29	0.03*	0.80	0.19	–	–
$80,000+	1.00	0.48	1.09	0.64	–	–

*p < 0.05.
**p < 0.01.
***p < 0.001.
[1]Full model from survey-weighted logistic regression controlling for all other demographic variables in table.
[2]Reduced model maintains all demographic variables with p-value > 0.1 (in the case of categorical variables, all variables maintained in model).

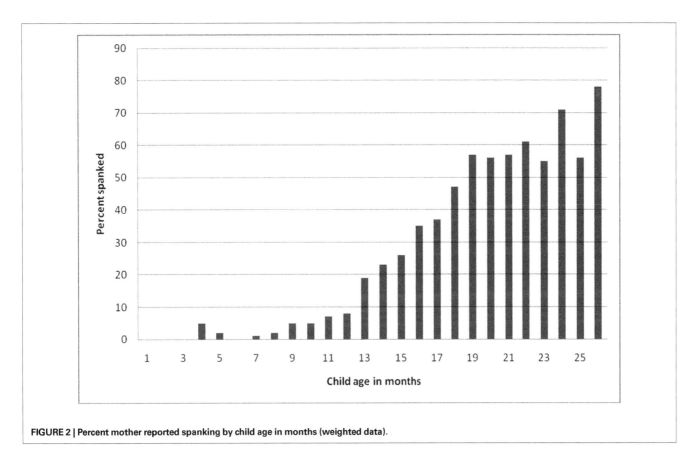

FIGURE 2 | Percent mother reported spanking by child age in months (weighted data).

Despite past studies associating differential spanking prevalence with maternal marital status (Giles-Sims et al., 1995; Smith and Brooks-Gunn, 1997; Regalado et al., 2004) and educational attainment (Smith and Brooks-Gunn, 1997; Day et al., 1998; Socolar et al., 1999; Eamon, 2001; Barkin et al., 2007), neither characteristic significantly predicted spanking in our study. Our study found, as have several others, (Giles-Sims et al., 1995; Smith and Brooks-Gunn, 1997; Day et al., 1998; Pinderhughes et al., 2000; Wissow, 2001), that the sex of the child predicted spanking prevalence with boys being more likely to be spanked. The lack of association between maternal education has been previously reported in another large nationally representative study (Grogan-Kaylor and Otis, 2007). As expected, most prevalence studies have shown an inverse relationship between child age and spanking prevalence throughout the early childhood years (Buntain-Ricklefs et al., 1994; Day et al., 1998; Regalado et al., 2004), a finding also supported by our study.

This study suggests that the 1996 American Academy of Pediatrics (AAP) panel conclusions (Bauman and Friedman, 1998) that children under the age of 2 should not be spanked and the 1998 AAP recommendation (Stein and Perrin, 1998) against spanking as a primary disciplinary practice, particularly in children under 18 months of age, are not being followed consistently. In *Bright Futures,* the AAP's Guidelines for Health Supervision of Infants, Children, and Adolescents (American Academy of Pediatrics. Committee on Psychosocial Aspects of Child and Family Health., 2002), discipline is first mentioned as a component of anticipatory guidance during the 9-month visit, at which point health care providers are advised to discuss parenting expectations, consistency, behavior management, and cultural beliefs about child-rearing. In our study, 8% of mothers of children aged 3–9 months of age already report having spanked their child by this time. As for spanking practices in older children (9- to 24-month olds), child health care providers may not address issues of child discipline in the periodic well-child visits, although it also may be that their advice is not being heeded as other cultural forces regarding spanking may be operating. Our results indicate that pediatric health care professionals should begin discussing discipline strategies with parents as early as the 2- or 4-month visit. Each visit thereafter should seek to assess the success of current discipline strategies, reinforcing practices other than spanking. Several intensive home visiting programs have been shown to reduce spanking or improve positive discipline. Healthy Families America and Healthy Start have shown a reduction in harsh parenting (Duggan et al., 2004; DuMont et al., 2008). The Nurse Family Partnership has shown improved maternal responsivity and use of positive discipline (Olds et al., 2002). Incredible Years has reported less harsh discipline (verbal and physical), less physical punishment, more positive discipline, and improved child behavior (Letarte et al., 2010). A particular therapeutic model, Parent Child Interaction Therapy has been shown to improve positive parental responses to appropriate behavior (Thomas and Zimmer-Gembeck, 2011). Public health interventions such as media coverage and legislative efforts may also reduce the early spanking practices of the public.

Further research continues to be needed in the area of child discipline. Studies of association between early spanking to later outcomes such as aggression or antisocial behavior are methodologically difficult. Efforts to show causal connections between spanking and later negative outcomes need to be undertaken while controlling for other discipline styles and practices. The study of spanking and public discourse about spanking policy and practice tend to be polarizing and based the importance of values such as parents' rights, children's rights, autonomy, and justice. These are important values to consider in the application of spanking research to public discourse. However, with limited exceptions, most parenting experts that advocate for corporal punishment do not recommend the use of this type of discipline for children less than two. More empiric evidence on the consequences of spanking, and especially early spanking, may sway parents, practitioners, and policy makers. By learning alternatives to spanking parents may come to understand that children need not learn through fear, and that the hard and important lessons of childhood can be taught in other ways.

There were a number of limitations to this study. First, this is a survey of mothers in the state of North Carolina and may not, therefore, be representative of mothers across the USA. Earlier national studies noted higher rates of spanking in the southeastern USA (Giles-Sims et al., 1995; Straus and Stewart, 1999); therefore rates may be lower in other regions. However, regional studies that include the deep South versus the Southeast show that North Carolina rates of spanking are similar to those of the southeast and the whole United States and less similar to those of the South which include the deep South (Zolotor et al., 2011). Second, while respondents described their spouse or partner's discipline practices, we did not specifically ask spouses or partners about such practices. Third, our phone survey included very few cell phone users, potentially limiting the generalizability of our conclusions to cell phone only users. Finally, self-reported disciplinary practices may be underestimations of actual prevalence due to the potential social stigma, even in an anonymous survey, against reporting the use of parental corporal punishment to an unknown surveyor.

The AAP states unequivocally that children under two should not be spanked. Notwithstanding this position, almost one-third of mothers in our survey reported spanking their infant on the buttocks by their second birthday. Not all mothers, however, are equally likely to spank their infant. This study suggests that younger maternal age, non-Hispanic ethnicity, and middle household incomes are associated with a higher likelihood of spanking before the age of 2. Pediatric health care professionals, public health and child development workers should assist parents of very young children in developing a discipline skill set including positive and negative reinforcement without physical punishment as well as setting appropriate behavioral expectations for such children. The goal of such interventions is not to ostracize mothers who seem more likely to spank their infants; rather, the goal is to provide support, offer alternatives, and ultimately prevent disciplinary practices that in some cases may escalate to child abuse. Further, the spanking of young children may be an appropriate locus for starting policy and legislative discussions around a parents "right" to spank, given the near universal professional and scientific opinion about the negative effects of spanking on such young children.

ACKNOWLEDGEMENTS

This study was supported by the Centers for Disease Control and Prevention grant number 1 U49 CE001275-01. The authors wish to thank Dr. Terrill Bravender, MD, MPH, of Nationwide Children's Hospital, Columbus, OH, USA; Dr. Margaret Gourlay, MD, MPH, of UNC Department of Family Medicine; Dr. Phyllis Fleming, Ph.D., of UNC Center for Health Promotion and Disease Prevention; Dr. Michael Foster, Ph.D., of UNC School of Public Health; and Dr. Catherine Zimmer, Ph.D, of UNC's Odum Institute for Research in Social Science for assistance with the analysis and preparation of the manuscript.

REFERENCES

American Academy of Pediatrics. Committee on Psychosocial Aspects of Child and Family Health. (2002). *Guidelines for Health Supervision III*, 3rd Edn. Elk Grove Village, IL: American Academy of Pediatrics.

American Association of Public Opinion Research. (2008). *Standard Definitions: Final Dispositions of Case Codes and Outcome Rates for Surveys*. Lenexa, KS: American Association of Public Opinion Research.

Barkin, S., Scheindlin, B., Ip, E. H., Richardson, I., and Finch, S. (2007). Determinants of parental discipline practices: a national sample from primary care practices. *Clin. Pediatr. (Phila.)* 46, 64–69.

Bauman, L. J., and Friedman, S. B. (1998). Corporal punishment. *Pediatr. Clin. North Am.* 45, 403–414.

Berlin, L. J., Ispa, J. M., Fine, M. A., Malone, P. S., Brooks-Gunn, J., Brady-Smith, C., Ayoub, C., and Bai, Y. (2009). Correlates and consequences of spanking and verbal punishment for low-income white, african american, and mexican american toddlers. *Child Dev.* 80, 1403–1420.

Buntain-Ricklefs, J. J., Kemper, K. J., Bell, M., and Babonis, T. (1994). Punishments: what predicts adult approval. *Child Abuse Negl.* 18, 945–955.

Combs-Orme, T., and Cain, D. S. (2008). Predictors of mothers' use of spanking with their infants. *Child Abuse Negl.* 32, 649–657.

Day, R. D., Peterson, Gary W., and McCracken, Coleen. (1998). Predicting Spanking of Younger and Older Children by Mothers and Fathers. *J. Marriage Fam.* 60, 79–94.

Duggan, A., Fuddy, L., Burrell, L. Higman, S. M., McFarlane, E., Windham, A., and Sia, C. (2004). Randomized trial of a statewide home visiting program to prevent child abuse: impact in reducing parental risk factors. *Child Abuse Negl.* 28, 623–643.

DuMont, K., Mitchell-Herzfeld, S., Greene, R., Lee, E. Lowenfels, A. Rodrigues, M., and Dorabawila, V. (2008). Healthy Families New York (HFNY) randomized trial: effects on early child abuse and neglect. *Child Abuse Negl.* 32, 295–315.

Eamon, M. K. (2001). Antecedents and socioemotional consequences of physical punishment on children in two-parent families. *Child Abuse Negl.* 25, 787–802.

Gershoff, E. T. (2002). Corporal punishment by parents and associated child behaviors and experiences: a meta-analytic and theoretical review. *Psychol. Bull.* 128, 539–579.

Giles-Sims, J., Straus, M. A., and Sugarman, D. B. (1995). Child, maternal, and family characteristics associated with spanking. *Fam. Relat.* 44, 170–176.

Grogan-Kaylor, A., and Otis, M. (2007). The predictors of parental use of corporal punishment. *Fam. Relat.* 56, 80–91.

Horn, I. B., Cheng, T. L., and Joseph, J. (2004). Discipline in the African American community: the impact of socioeconomic status on beliefs and practices. *Pediatrics* 113, 1236–1241.

Kadushin, A., and Martin, J. A. (1981). *Child Abuse: An Interactional Event*. New York, NY: Columbia Univeristy Press.

Kaplow, J. B., and Widom, C. S. (2007). Age of onset of child maltreatment predicts long-term mental health outcomes. *J. Abnorm. Psychol.* 116, 176–187.

Keiley, M. K., Howe, T. R., Dodge, K. A., Bates, J. E., and Pettit, G. S. (2001). The timing of child physial maltreatment: a cross-domain gwoth analysis of impact on adolescent externalizing and internalizing symptoms. *Dev. Psychopathol.* 13, 8911–8912.

Kotch, J. B., Lewis, T., Hussey, J. M., English, D., Thompson, R., Litrownik, A. J., Runyan, D. K., Bangdiwala, S. I., Margolis, B., and Dubowitz, H. (2008). Importance of early neglect for childhood aggression. *Pediatrics* 121, 725–731.

Letarte, M. J., Normandeau, S., and Allard, J. (2010). Effectiveness of a parent training program "Incredible Years" in a child protection service. *Child Abuse Negl.* 34, 253–261.

Olds, D. L., Robinson, J., O'Brien, R., Luckey, D. W., Pettitt, L. M., Henderson, C. R., Ng, R. K., Sheff, K. L., Korfmacher, J., Hiatt, S., and Talmi, A. (2002). Home visiting by paraprofessionals and nurses: a randomized, controlled trial. *Pediatrics* 110, 486–496.

Pinderhughes, E. E., Dodge, K. A., Bates, J. E., Pettit, G. S., and Zelli, A. (2000). Discipline responses: influences of parents' socioeconomic status, ethnicity, beliefs about parenting, stress, and cognitive-emotional processes. *J. Fam. Psychol.* 14, 380–400.

Regalado, M., Sareen, H., Inkelas, M., Wissow, L. S., and Halfon, N. (2004). Parents' discipline of young children: results from the National Survey of Early Childhood Health. *Pediatrics* 113(Suppl.), 1952–1958.

Slade, E. P., and Wissow, L. S. (2004). Spanking in early childhood and later behavior problems: a prospective study of infants and young toddlers. *Pediatrics* 113, 1321–1330.

Smith, J. R., and Brooks-Gunn, J. (1997). Correlates and consequences of harsh discipline for young children. *Arch. Pediatr. Adolesc. Med.* 151, 777–786.

Socolar, R. R., Savage, E., and Evans, H. (2007). A longitudinal study of parental discipline of young children. *South. Med. J.* 100, 472–477.

Socolar, R. R., Savage, E., Keyes-Elstein, L., and Evans, H. (2005). Factors that affect parental disciplinary practices of children aged 12 to 19 months. *South. Med. J.* 98, 1181–1191.

Socolar, R. R., Winsor, J., Hunter, W. M., Catellier, D., and Kotch, J. B. (1999). Maternal disciplinary practices in an at-risk population. *Arch. Pediatr. Adolesc. Med.* 153, 927–934.

Stein, M. T., and Perrin, E. L. (1998). Guidance for effective discipline. American Academy of Pediatrics. Committee on Psychosocial Aspects of Child and Family Health. *Pediatrics* 101(Pt 1), 723–728.

Straus, M. A., and Donnelly, D. A. (2005). *Beating the Devil Out of Them: Corporal Punishment in American Families and its Effects on Children*. New Brunswick, NJ: Transaction Publishers.

Straus, M. A., and Gelles, R. J. (1990). *Physical Violence in American Families: Risk Factors and Adaptations to Violence in 8,145 Families*. New Brunswick, NJ: Transaction Publishers.

Straus, M. A., Hamby, S. L., Finkelhor, D., Moore, D. W., and Runyan, D. (1998). Identification of child maltreatment with the Parent-Child Conflict Tactics Scales: development and psychometric data for a national sample of American parents. *Child Abuse Negl.* 22, 249–270.

Straus, M. A., and Stewart, J. H. (1999). Corporal punishment by American parents: national data on prevalence, chronicity, severity, and duration, in relation to child and family characteristics. *Clin. Child Fam. Psychol. Rev.* 2, 55–70.

Tajima, E. A. (2000). The relative importance of wife abuse as a risk factor for violence against children. *Child Abuse Negl.* 24, 1383–1398.

Taylor, C. A., Manganello, J. A., Lee, S. J., and Rice, J. C. (2010). Mothers' spanking of 3-year-old children and subsequent risk of children's aggressive behavior. *Pediatrics* 125(5), e1057-1065.

Theodore, A. D., Chang, J. J., Runyan, D. K., Hunter, W. M., Bangdiwala, S. I., and Agans, R. (2005). Epidemiologic features of the physical and sexual maltreatment of children in the Carolinas. *Pediatrics* 115, e331–e337.

Thomas, R., and Zimmer-Gembeck, M. J. (2011). Accumulating evidence for parent-child interaction therapy in the prevention of child maltreatment. *Child Dev.* 82, 177–192.

Vittrup, B., Holden, G. W., and Buck, J. (2006). Attitudes predict the use of physical punishment: a prospective study of the emergence of disciplinary practices. *Pediatrics* 117, 2055–2064.

Wissow, L. S. (2001). Ethnicity, income, and parenting contexts of physical punishment in a national sample of families with young children. *Child Maltreat.* 6, 118–129.

Zolotor, A. J., Theodore, A. D., Chang, J. J., Berkoff, M. C., and Runyan, D. K. (2008). Speak softly—and forget the stick. Corporal punishment and child physical abuse. *Am. J. Prev. Med.* 35, 364–369.

Zolotor, A. J., Theodore, A. D., Runyan, D. K., Chang, J. J., and Laskey, A. L. (2011). Corporal punishment and physical abuse: population-based trends for three-to-11-year-old children in the United States. *Child Abuse Rev.* 20, 57–66.

Social behavior of offspring following prenatal cocaine exposure in rodents: A comparison with prenatal alcohol

Sonya K. Sobrian[1]* and R. R. Holson[2]

[1] Department of Pharmacology, College of Medicine, Howard University, Washington, DC, USA
[2] Psychology, New Mexico Institute of Mining and Technology, Socorro, NM, USA

*Correspondence:
Sonya K. Sobrian, Department of Pharmacology, College of Medicine, Howard University, 520 West Street, Northwest, Washington, 20059 DC, USA
e-mail: ssobrian@howard.edu

Clinical and experimental reports suggest that prenatal cocaine exposure (PCE) alters the offsprings' social interactions with caregivers and conspecifics. Children exposed to prenatal cocaine show deficits in caregiver attachment and play behavior. In animal models, a developmental pattern of effects that range from deficits in play and social interaction during adolescence, to aggressive reactions during competition in adulthood is seen. This review will focus primarily on the effects of PCE on social behaviors involving conspecifics in animal models. Social relationships are critical to the developing organism; maternally directed interactions are necessary for initial survival. Juvenile rats deprived of play behavior, one of the earliest forms of non-mother directed social behaviors in rodents, show deficits in learning tasks and sexual competence. Social behavior is inherently complex. Because the emergence of appropriate social skills involves the interplay between various conceptual and biological facets of behavior and social information, it may be a particularly sensitive measure of prenatal insult. The social behavior surveyed include social interactions, play behavior/fighting, scent marking, and aggressive behavior in the offspring, as well as aspects of maternal behavior. The goal is to determine if there is a consensus of results in the literature with respect to PCE and social behaviors, and to discuss discrepant findings in terms of exposure models, the paradigms, and dependent variables, as well as housing conditions, and the sex and age of the offspring at testing. As there is increasing evidence that deficits in social behavior may be sequelae of developmental exposure alcohol, we compare changes in social behaviors reported for prenatal alcohol with those reported for prenatal cocaine. Shortcomings in the both literatures are identified and addressed in an effort to improve the translational value of future experimentation.

Keywords: prenatal cocaine, social interactions, play behavior/fighting, aggression, scent marking, maternal behavior, prenatal alcohol

INTRODUCTION

Social behavior is inherently complex. The socialization of human beings begins very early and continues throughout the lifespan. Social relationships are critical to the developing organism. Maternally directed interactions are necessary for initial survival, and attachment behaviors in the infant are part of a social behavior system that operates to ensure that the primary caretaker is nearby to protect and nurture the infant (Bowlby, 1988). Theories concerning social development of the child have focused on the mother–infant dyad (Tronick and Cohn, 1989), where the interaction is both the result of the infant's behaviors and the responses of the mother/caretaker to those behaviors. Interacting with one's own infant is reported to be a rewarding and pleasurable experience. This behavior promotes maternal–infant attachments, which ensures optimal care for the developing infant in the face of competing demands (Strathearn et al., 2008).

Play behavior is one of the earliest forms of non-mother directed social behaviors. Children and most other young mammals devote a significant amount of time and energy playing together. Social play is not just a pleasurable activity. It has been suggested that it is an affiliative form of behavior functioning to facilitate social development. Social play is rewarding and serves as a natural reinforcer that is crucial for the development of behavioral flexibility, the acquisition of social communication and cognitive competence, and may function to establish social organization and maintain cohesion in a group, or facilitate the ability to cope with social conflicts (Thor and Holloway, 1984; Pellis and Pellis, 1998; Auger and Olesen, 2009; Trezza et al., 2010). With respect to the sex differences in social play, theories emphasize either social or motor learning functions. In juvenile male non-human primates, social rank correlates with the number of peer social interactions in the form of play fighting (Meaney, 1989). Females spend more time competing for interaction with infants, whereby they acquire the motor skills necessary for handling infants (Meaney, 1989). In general social play behaviors facilitate different aspects of social development which contribute to the acquisition of adaptive social functioning in adulthood (Thor and Holloway, 1984).

WHILE PLAY DECLINES AS THE CHILD AGES, SOCIAL INTERACTIONS CONTINUE THROUGHOUT THE LIFESPAN

Social behavior in an adult individual is the result of a complex interaction of genetics, brain development, early childhood experiences pertaining to socialization, and learning throughout the lifespan. These factors combine to affect social cognition and motivation (Kelly et al., 2000).

Moreover, abnormalities in socialization or in the social learning processes can impact social interactions and behaviors throughout the lifespan. Because the emergence of normal appropriate social skills involves the proper interplay between various conceptual and biological facets of behavior and social information, social behaviors may be a particularly sensitive measure of prenatal insult (Chae and Covington, 2009). However, human studies of prenatal insults, especially those involving drugs, are limited in experimental designs available. Animal models afford better control of pre- and peri-natal care, the postnatal environment, nutritional factors, dose and timing of cocaine administration and ploy drug exposure in order to examine behavioral outcomes of prenatal manipulations (Gendle et al., 2004; Chae and Covington, 2009). In addition, they can determine if the maternal–infant interaction is altered by drug-induced changes in the behavior of the offspring. The use of experimental cross-fostering, where offspring from 1 litter is given to an unrelated dam from a different (control) treatment group, typically at birth, allows for the successful empirical dissection of maternal versus pup effects (see Wolf et al., 2011 for review). The impact of environmental factors can also be assessed by housing post-weaning offspring in enriched, impoverished or standard caging conditions. These various rearing environments can facilitate the examination of simple social processes and establish more clearly the degree to which the changes in social behavior are the direct result of cocaine-induced changes. Moreover, social behavior in rats has been shown to follow similar principles as in humans, and is also a function of genetics, teratogenic influences, early maternal–infant interactions, and later social learning (Kelly et al., 2000). This review will focus primarily on the effects of prenatal cocaine on social behaviors involving conspecifics in rodent models; the effects of developmental alcohol exposure on these behaviors is included as a control. The social behaviors reviewed include social interaction, play fighting/solicitation, and aggressive behaviors, as well as maternal care, maternal aggression, and mother–infant communication. Sexual behavior was not included as it does not parallel the variables in the clinical articles included in this volume.

PRENATAL COCAINE AND SOCIAL BEHAVIOR

A significant body of literature published during the past 25 years has identified effects of prenatal cocaine exposure (PCE) on growth and development in children. PCE has been shown to influence the ontogeny of motor, cognitive, social skills, and emotional behaviors. Both dose- and gender-specific effects have been identified following PCE, with social behaviors more likely disrupted in boys prenatally exposed to higher levels of cocaine (Delaney-Black et al., 1998; Tronick et al., 2005). Although effects are small, they are first evident in the neonate, remain throughout early childhood, and have been documented in adolescents (Chae and Covington, 2009). The magnitude of the effects may be masked, in part, by confounding factors in study designs. Most children reported in studies in the literature come from low-income backgrounds and consequently have been exposed to multiple medical and social risk factors associated with long-term poverty, that include poor prenatal care, peri-natal complications, and impoverished parenting styles. The fact that exposure to multiple risk factors has compromising effects on children's outcomes may overshadow any specific effects of PCE (Rodning et al., 1989; Tronick and Beeghly, 1999). Moreover, clinical studies involving drugs of abuse often entail exposure to drugs other than the one of interest, and as a result behavioral alterations may reflect insults other than those due to the specific action of cocaine.

Despite the exponential increase in the number of experimental studies published since the 1980s on the effects of PCE, only a small percentage have focused on social behaviors. Rodents are most often used, with rats being the preferred species; mice were used in only two of the studies discussed (Hahn et al., 2000; Estelles et al., 2005). We did not find published studies of PCE and social behavior that used primates or other mammalian species. While the focus of this review is on prenatal exposure, several studies with combined prenatal–postnatal (lactational) exposure, as well as those in which cocaine was administered to pre-weaning rats or females prior to mating have been included (see **Table 1**).

Although the number of studies is limited, there are trends in the data that suggest reliable effects of developmental exposure to cocaine for individual categories of social behavior. **Table 1** summarizes these findings collapsed across both species; exposure period and housing conditions are indicated. When not specified, cocaine was administered prenatally to rat dams and animals were raised in a standard housing environment. Detailed summaries of results are provided in the following text. These will be preceded by a brief review of the relevance of the behavior, and pertinent clinical findings.

PRENATAL COCAINE AND MATERNAL BEHAVIORS

Maternal substance abuse has been associated with deficits in parental functioning. Mothers recovering from cocaine addiction experience difficulties in their maternal roles as care givers, and are described as more passive and disengaged in interactions with their newborns than non-drug-using mothers (see Johnson et al., 2002 for review). It is possible that some of these deficits in maternal care are influenced by the state-traits of PCE infant; these infants are frequently irritable and hyper-aroused by environmental stimuli, responses which might elicit less care and establish a cycle of passivity in which the caretaker becomes more and more passive in attempts at interaction (Chasnoff et al., 1987). Maternal interaction with their young children continue to be problematic, as exemplified by reduced mother–child play interactions and increased hostility toward the child (see Febo and Ferris, 2007 for review).

Although frequently associated with poor parenting outcomes, maternal drug use is not always related to deficits in parenting skills. No differences between cocaine-using and comparison mothers were noted in sensitivity, social–emotional and cognitive growth fostering, and response to infant distress on a

Table 1 | Effects of developmental cocaine exposure on maternal behaviors in dams and first generation offspring compared to controls.

Behavior	Enhanced	No effect	Impaired/reduced
Maternal care (F_0 dams)	**2** Peeke et al. (1994; pre-mating, gestational, and lactational cocaine: PPD 1–20) Nephew and Febo (2010; pre-mating cocaine: PPD 2)	**9** Johns et al. (2005; PPD 5 or 10) Nelson et al. (1998; PPD 3) Sobrian et al. (1990; 1995; PPD 1) Heyser et al. (1992; PPD 2, 5–9) Tonkiss et al. (1995; pre-mating and gestational cocaine: PPD 2–12) McMurray et al. (2008a; PPD 8 and 12) Nephew and Febo (2010; pre-mating cocaine: PPD 9 and 16)	**8** Johns et al. (1994b; 2005; PPD 1) Nelson et al. (1998; PPD 1) Kinsley et al. (1994; PPD 1–2) McMurray et al. (2008a; IC: gestational and lactational: PPD 8)
Acute cocaine (F_0 dams)		Vernotica et al. (1996; single acute cocaine injection PPD 1, testing: 16 h later)	Vernotica et al. (1996; single acute cocaine injection PPD 1. Testing: 4 hrs later) Kinsley et al. (1994; single acute cocaine injection on PPD 5–6)
Intergenerational effects (F_1 offspring)	**1** McMurray et al. (2008a; IC: gestational and lactational: PND 60 mated; tested at PPD 8)	**2** Johns et al. (2005; adult mated; tested at PPD 5 or 10) Johns et al. (2007; tested at PND 28: Pup-induced retrieval-M and F)	**3** Johns et al. (2005; adult mated; tested at PPD 1) Johns et al. (2007; PND 60: M) McMurray et al. (2008a; PND 60 mated; tested at PPD 8)
Maternal aggression (F_0 dams)	**8** Heyser et al. (1992; PPD 10) Johns et al. (1997; PPD 6) Johns et al. (1998a,b; PPD 6, 8, and 10) Lubin et al. (2001; PPD 2, 3, and 5) Johns et al. (2010; PPD 31–35) Nephew and Febo (2010; pre-mating cocaine: PPD 2)	**1** McMurray et al. (2008a; CC: PPD8 and CC and IC: PPD 12)	**1** McMurray et al. (2008a; IC: PPD8)
Intergenerational effects (F_1 dams)	McMurray et al. (2008a; PPD 8)		
Mother–infant communication (ultrasonic vocalizations)	**1** Hahn et al. (2000; M and F; mice: BALB/cJ and DBA/2J: tested at PND 2–4)	**4** Meyer et al. (1992; M and F; tested at PND 11) and Hahn et al. (2000); M and F; mice: SLJ/J: tested at PND 2–4) Barron and Gilbertson (2005) (M and F; neonatal cocaine: PND 4–10. Tested at PND 14) Barron et al. (2000; M and F; Neonatal cocaine: PND 4–10. Tested at PND 14)	**1** Hahn et al. (2000; M and F; mice: BALB/cJ and DBA/2J. Tested at PND 2–4)

Numbers in bold refer to number of findings for each outcome. Unless otherwise stipulated, cocaine exposure is gestational, and subjects are rats. PND: postnatal day at which ultrasonic vocalization was tested; PPD: postpartum day on which maternal behavior was tested; CC: chronic cocaine during gestation; IC: intermittent cocaine during gestation and lactation; F_1: first generation dams. F= females; M= males.

measure of maternal behavior during infant feeding (Neuspiel et al., 1991), or maternal responsivity during free-play (Black et al., 1993). In explaining the impact of prenatal cocaine use on the mother–child parenting outcomes, confounding factors such as maternal psychological functioning and socioeconomic resources must be considered (Jeremy and Bernstein, 1984; Sood et al., 2005). These factors alone or in combination with maternal substance abuse may better explain the impact of prenatal drug use on mother–child relationship outcomes. Moreover, women who use cocaine during pregnancy often continue drug use after delivery, and postnatal maternal substance use is also associated with a number of environmental risk factors that may impact parent–child interactions (Johnson et al., 2002).

Maternal care

Poly drug use and other confounding factors in human cocaine abusers (i.e., the availability of prenatal care, socioeconomic status, and environmental conditions in the home) have promoted the use of animal models in which these variables can be more easily controlled. Maternal care behavior has been well characterized in rat models. Female rats show little interest in infants of their own species until shortly before parturition. Approximately 24 h prior to delivery, they show an intense interest in pups from other litters with nest building, retrieval, grooming, and defense of the young. These behaviors persist through lactation and then abate with weaning (Winslow and Insel, 2002). Moreover, individual variations in key behaviors have been linked to alterations in offspring development (Insel, 2003; Sousa et al., 2006). In general, early care giving experiences can influence the subsequent maternal behavior, stress–susceptibility, and emotionality of the offspring (Sousa et al., 2006; Strathearn and Mayes, 2010).

Environmental insults can give rise to disruptions in mother–pup interactions, and such disruptions of the social milieu can influence behavioral development and brain function of the offspring independent of any direct effect of the drug (Tonkiss et al., 1995). Maternal behavior in rats is a complex interplay of hormonal milieu of the dam and the behavior of both the pup and dam. Disruption of the behavior in the maternal–pup dyad is known to have a critical impact on the long-term outcome of the pup and in particular on the socio-emotional behavior of the pup (Meaney, 2001). As in humans, alterations in early maternal–infant interactions may occur because of drug-induced behavioral abnormalities in either or both the rodent pup and/or the mother, resulting in altered dynamics of the maternal–infant interaction (Kelly et al., 2000).

Exposure of the dams to cocaine, either prior to or during gestation and/or during lactation alters maternal care of infants (**Table 1**). This effect is short lived, and does not require multiple daily cocaine doses. Following daily gestational cocaine exposure, Johns et al. (1994b, 2005) found impaired maternal behavior on postpartum day (PPD) 1 but not PPDs 5 or 10; Nelson et al. (1998) found similar effects on PPD 1 but not 3. However, intermittent cocaine exposure during both gestation and lactation extends the impairment in maternal behavior until PPD 8 (McMurray et al., 2008a). Moreover, Vernotica et al. (1996) reported that a single postnatal cocaine injection on PPD 1 impaired maternal behavior 4 h but not 16 h later. Similarly, Kinsley et al. (1994) saw a short-term decrement in maternal behavior on PPD 5 or 6 following a single cocaine injection.

Enhanced maternal behavior has been reported in two studies, both of which involved pre-mating cocaine exposure. Peeke et al. (1994), who dosed dams with cocaine 21 days prior to mating, as well as throughout gestation and for 2 weeks postpartum, reported that exposed dams spent more time nursing throughout lactation. However, enhanced maternal behavior was seen only on PPD 2 but not PPD 9 or 16 with only a 10-day pre-mating exposure (Nephew and Febo, 2010).

Developmental cocaine exposure failed to affect maternal behavior in nine studies. This lack of effect is seen primarily following gestational cocaine exposure alone (Sobrian et al., 1990, 1995; Heyser et al., 1992; Nelson et al., 1998; Johns et al., 2005; McMurray et al., 2008a), and is evident during both early (Sobrian et al., 1990, 1995; Tonkiss et al., 1995; Vernotica et al., 1996; Nelson et al., 1998), and mid (Heyser et al., 1992; Tonkiss et al., 1995; Johns et al., 2005; McMurray et al., 2008a) lactation.

Intergenerational effects of gestational cocaine exposure on the maternal behavior have been assessed in the female offspring of dams exposed to cocaine during pregnancy (first generation dams: F_1). Gestational exposure to cocaine either impaired (Johns et al., 2005; McMurray et al., 2008a) or had not effect on (Johns et al., 2005) the maternal behavior of F_1 dams. In the Johns et al. (2005) study, the direction of the change was the same for the F_1 dams as those reported for their F_0 mothers. In contrast, with the McMurray et al. (2008a) study, it was the F_1 dams of the chronic gestational cocaine F_0 dams that showed an impairment, an effect not seen in the original dams. In contrast, F_1 dams, whose mothers were exposed to intermittent cocaine during both gestation and lactation, showed enhanced maternal care of their pups.

In a similar study, first generation adolescent and young adult offspring were exposed to pups to induce maternal behavior (Johns et al., 2007). When testing occurred at PND 28, gestational cocaine exposure did not impair male or female juveniles' interactions with 1- to 5-day-old pups (Johns et al., 2007). Subsequently however, 60-day-old male rats did display impaired maternal care of neonates (Johns et al., 2007; females were not tested on PND 60). Taken together, these studies indicate that the effects of developmental cocaine exposure are intergenerational, at least for some aspects of maternal behavior. Clearly, it is an intriguing finding that deserves more study.

Maternal aggression

Interacting with one's own infant is reported to be a rewarding and pleasurable experience, which promotes maternal–infant attachments, and ensures optimal care for the developing infant in the face of competing demands (Strathearn and Mayes, 2010). However, cocaine abuse is highly correlated with maternal neglect and poorer maternal–infant interactions; mothers who are addicted to cocaine appear to be not only less appropriately responsive to their infants, but also find these interactions less rewarding and stress provoking, a situation which may engender child neglect and abuse (Mayes et al., 1997). It has also been reported that in their interactions with young children, drug-using mothers are less likely to use positive reinforcement and more likely to threaten physical discipline than non-drug-using mothers (Johnson et al., 2002). Moreover, there is a higher incidence of foster care placements and allegations of physical abuse, sexual abuse, and neglect among cocaine-exposed 2 year olds compared with non-drug-exposed 2 year olds (Wasserman and Leventhal, 1993).

Maternal aggression has been defined as a subset of maternal behaviors in mammals that is aimed at intruders into the post-parturient female's nest area or at those threatening her young (Blanchard et al., 2003). In rat, both offensive and defensive aggressive behaviors have been well characterized (Sousa et al., 2006). While maternal aggressive behavior is generally considered adaptive, excessive, or mal-adaptive attacks can result in injury to pups (Lubin et al., 2001). Maternal aggression can be elicited 48–24 h prior to birth; it peaks during the first 10 PPD (McMurray et al.,

2008a), and drops off sharply in the hours following pup removal (Blanchard et al., 2003).

Cocaine has been reported to disrupt various aspect of maternal behavior, including maternal aggression. **Table 1** lists the effects of chronic and intermittent cocaine during gestation alone or in combination with postnatal lactational exposure on intruder-induced maternal aggression in dams (F_0) and their first generation (F_1) female offspring. The resident/intruder paradigm was used in all seven studies.

Heyser et al. (1992) reported that cocaine-treated dams raising their own offspring were quicker to initiate the first attack on a female intruder at PPD 10. While a similar increase was seen in controls dams, only cocaine-treated females exhibited an increased number of aggressive attacks against the female intruder throughout the testing period. The lack of sustained aggression reported in cocaine-exposed dams rearing cross-fostered normal pups suggested that characteristics of the PCE-pups may contribute to the treatment-induced increase in maternal aggression (Heyser et al., 1992). However, is should be noted that dams exposed to cocaine during pregnancy did not differ from control dams in pup retrieval latency, nest building behavior, time spent in the nest, or time spent suckling pups (Heyser et al., 1992).

Increased aggression was also reported in cocaine-exposed dams tested early in postpartum period. At PPD 6, these females exhibited an increase in threats and attacks toward an intruder, behavior that did not reflect withdrawal from cocaine; increased aggression was seen in dams whose cocaine treatment ended on gestational day 20, and dams who received cocaine throughout lactation (PPD 1–20; Johns et al., 1997). Similar increases in maternal aggression were reported on PPD 6, 8, and 10 for dams treated chronically with cocaine during gestation (Johns et al., 1998a). This increase was hypothesized to reflect altered sensory or perceptual systems that caused stimuli to be viewed as more threatening than they are (Johns et al., 1998a).

When tested during the initial postpartum period at PPD 2, 3, and 5, gestational cocaine exposure produced a non-dose-dependent increase in the duration of the attacks on the male intruder but not fight attack behavior, in general (Lubin et al., 2001). All dams rearing their natural litters exhibited increased aggressive behavior as evidenced by a decreased latency to pin an intruder. The authors suggest that the aggressive behavior seen in this early postpartum period is not as robust as seen during mid-lactation (Lubin et al., 2001). However, pre-mating exposure of the female to cocaine produces an increased aggressive response to a male intruder at PPD 2 (Nephew and Febo, 2010). Female rats sensitized to cocaine within the 2-week period prior to mating exhibited shorter attack latencies and an increased frequency and duration of attacks on PPD 2, but not on PPD 9, suggesting that in contrast to gestational exposure which produces more aggressive behavior from the dams at mid-lactation, the effects of pre-mating cocaine are more robust almost immediately after birth. This increase in maternal aggression was attributed to a possible cross-sensitization between cocaine and the natural reward of maternal care (Nephew and Febo, 2010). At PPD 8, gestational exposure to chronic cocaine (CC) failed to alter defensive or aggressive behaviors in the dams, while dams exposed to intermittent gestational and lactational cocaine (IC) were less aggressive toward a male intruder (McMurray et al., 2008a). However, rearing conditions altered aggressive behavior in IC dams, who exhibited increased threat to a small male intruder only when rearing their biological litter. No significant differences were found in any group on PND 12.

As with maternal behavior, intergenerational effects have been reported for maternal aggression. However, rearing conditions (F_0 dam treatment) rather than prenatal exposure history have been shown to impact the aggressive responses of first generation (F_1) dams. All F_1 dams raised by either CC or IC F_0 dams displayed increased maternal aggression toward a small male intruder when tested on PPD 8; moreover, IC-reared F_1 dams exhibited increases in more aspects of aggressive behavior and threatened intruders more often (McMurray et al., 2008a). These data suggest that F_0 dam treatment, rather than prenatal exposure condition of the litter appears to be the more salient intergenerational factor influencing maternal aggression.

In summary, clearly prenatal exposure to cocaine increases maternal aggression in the resident/intruder paradigm, irrespective of the sex of the intruder. Factors that influence this effect include not only prenatal treatment, but also the postpartum age at testing, and whether the dam is rearing her biological or foster litter. Increased aggression against an intruder has been reliably reported to occur on PPD 2–6; reports of its occurrence on PPD 8, 9, and 10 are mixed, while it is absent at PPDs 12 and 16. There is some suggestion that the effects of PCE on maternal aggression are more robust during mid-gestation. In contrast the reverse is seen following pre-mating cocaine. There is also evidence of intergenerational effects of developmental cocaine exposure on maternal aggression. F_1 dams appear to exhibit higher levels of aggressive behavior than their F_0 dams; as with F_1 dams, this behavior is influenced by PCE and rearing conditions.

Maternal–infant communication

Crying is a universal vocalization in human infants, as well as in the infants of other mammals. It represents an early evolutionary adaptation for maternal contact and sustenance of an infant, where the need to re-establish mother–infant contact is essential for infant survival when contact is lost (Newman, 2007). Human infants prenatally exposed to cocaine show more passive-withdrawn negative engagement (Tronick et al., 2005), and are reported to produce fewer and shorter cries (Hahn et al., 2000).

In rodents, auditory signals produced by pups play an important role in the regulation of the mother–infant relationship. The ultrasonic vocalizations (USV) emitted by neonatal rats and mice are a critical aspect of pup behavior upon separation from the dam (Kelly et al., 2009a). The frequency of ultrasonic calling is a measure of separation distress, which increases with increasing amounts of separation, and reliably elicits maternal search and retrieval behavior. Moreover, call length and call frequency communicate information about individual identity, as well as the age and gender of the caller (Hahn et al., 2000). As USVs have been shown to promote lactation by increasing prolactin release, and also reduce maternal biting and cannibalism (Barron and Gilbertson, 2005), alterations in USVs can negatively impact pup survival.

Table 1 summarizes the results of four studies that investigated the characteristics of USVs after developmental exposure to cocaine. In F_1 mice of three different genotypes, alterations in the call characteristics of USV reflected an interaction between gestational drug exposure and genotype. Overall, PCE influenced two call characteristic of USV on PNDs 2–4: the rate of calling was reduced in two strains, while there was an increase of the beginning pitch of calls in the same two strains. However, pups of one genotype were unaffected by PCE (Hahn et al., 2000). These cocaine effects, though reliable, were small and differences in USVs were strongly influenced by mouse genotype. In a rat model, PCE failed to alter the frequency of isolation-induced USV in male and female offspring at PND 11, while acute exposure prior to testing markedly suppressed this behavior (Meyer et al., 1992). Postnatal cocaine exposure had an effect similar to that seen with PCE. When tested on PND 14, exposure to cocaine on PNDs 4–10 had no effect on either the frequency of vocalization (Barron et al., 2000) or the sonographic waveform analysis in either male or female offspring (Barron and Gilbertson, 2005). Sex differences were not observed in any of the studies.

In summary, neither chronic pre- nor post-natal exposure to cocaine altered isolation-induced USVs in rat. In mice, the direction of the effect following prenatal cocaine was genotype dependent, with a decreased frequency seen in two of the three strains tested. In addition to species differences, it should be noted that the production of USVs decreases with increasing age (Barron and Gilbertson, 2005) and the lack of an effect in older pups could represent a floor effect. However, the fact that acute cocaine prior to testing markedly suppressed USVs at PND 14 (Meyer et al., 1992) does not support this hypothesis. Despite the small number of studies, it would appear that species differences rather than exposure window, i.e., prenatal or postnatal, has the greater influence on the effects of developmental cocaine exposure on USVs.

SOCIAL INTERACTIONS

The necessity of social interactions for normal development has been outlined above. Infants and young children prenatally exposed to cocaine are somewhat aggressive, show poorer social attachment, and display abnormal play behavior in unstructured environments (Chasnoff et al., 1987; Oro and Dixon, 1987). Social interactions are also an important aspect of a rodent's life. They include all sexual and reproductive activities (although these are not be covered in this review), as well as aggressive behavior.

Social interactions are highly complex functions, requiring recruitment of and interaction between multiple neural circuits, with endocrine hormones and pheromonal cues playing a significant role in their coordination and execution (Sousa et al., 2006). This aspect of social behavior differs from play in that it continues throughout the life of the animal.

We have been able to locate four separate studies of gestational cocaine effects on social investigation, with six findings that are presented in **Table 2**. Estelles et al. (2005) assessed social investigation in adult male mice exposed prenatally to cocaine. Following weaning, subjects were reared either in isolation or in an enriched, multiple-animal environment. Animals were placed for 10 min in an open field with an unfamiliar test male; group-reared males showed enhanced social investigation of strangers, while males raised in isolation investigated strangers less than controls.

The remaining three studies utilized rats. Following PCE, Johns and Noonan (1995) tested male offspring at PND 90, and females at PND 60. Single subjects were placed in an open field with two unfamiliar subjects of the same sex for 10 min. Frequency, duration and latency of eight social behaviors were measured. Hence there were 24 behavioral measures per sex. Cocaine-exposed females showed an increased frequency of rough grooming, with no changes on the other 23 variables; males showed increased latency to reciprocate contact, with no changes on the other 23 variables. To what degree these single differences constitute anything more than statistical noise is not clear.

Neugebauer et al. (2004) tested only female offspring exposed to gestational cocaine. On the assumption that female cycling would confound results, all females were ovariectomized prior to testing. Again, pups were reared in either social (enriched) or isolation conditions. Animals were tested on three daily 10 min tests starting at each of three ages (PND 62, 90, and 122). Test animals were exposed to a single novel stranger. Four behavioral variables [play solicitations (see Play), follows, mutual sniffs, and mutual rears] were measured. Gestational exposure to cocaine increased mutual sniffs and mutual rears in both rearing conditions.

Finally, Overstreet et al. (2000) cross-fostered male and female cocaine-exposed pups to non-treated dams at birth. Pairs of rats of the same sex and treatment condition were tested for 5 min on PNDs 30, 60, and 120 days. Total time spent on social interactions was assessed. Results were the same across sexes: males and females exposed to gestational cocaine interacted less on PNDs 30 and 120, but did not differ from controls on PND 60.

Clearly, these findings do not provide evidence for any strong effect of gestational cocaine exposure on subsequent social investigation in offspring. Half the findings report enhanced social investigation, and half report precisely the opposite outcome. Neither sex, species, nor testing paradigms provide any obvious resolution for these disparate results. However, these studies do indicate that social investigation is sensitive to gestational cocaine.

PLAY

Play behavior is essential for the normal development of social skills. PCE has been associated with deficits in this social behavior. Toddlers exposed to cocaine *in utero* were found to differ from controls on measures of attachment and play behavior, and as young children they were somewhat aggressive, showed poor social attachment and displayed abnormal play behavior in unstructured environments (Oro and Dixon, 1987). These drug-exposed children experienced no distress in response to separation from caregivers, did not seek close physical contact, and appeared to show no strong feelings of pleasure or distress. They were unwilling to combine toys and fantasy play, and exhibited decreased representational play. Elements of their play behavior were characterized by the investigators as a soft neurological sign (Rodning et al., 1989; Howard et al., 1990).

Juvenile rats engage in a distinctive form of interactive social behavior commonly referred to as social play, play fighting, or play chasing that is readily observed in pairs or larger groups, and differs from other forms of social activities. Juvenile social

Table 2 | Effects of developmental cocaine exposure on social behaviors in offspring compared to controls.

Behavior	Enhanced	No effect	Impaired/reduced
Social investigation	**3** Estelles et al. (2005; M; social rearing) Johns and Noonan (1995; F) Neugebauer et al. (2004; F; Ovariectomized)	**0**	**3** Estelles et al. (2005; M; isolation rearing) Johns and Noonan (1995; M) Overstreet et al. (2000; M and F)
Play	**2** Magalhaes et al. (2007; M and F; postnatal cocaine – PND 1–28: enriched Rearing) Neugebauer et al. (2004; F; ovariectomized: isolation rearing)	**3** Magalhaes et al. (2006; M and F; standard rearing) Neugebauer et al. (2004; F; ovariectomized: enriched rearing) Wood et al. (1995; M and F)	**3** Magalhaes et al. (2007; M and F; postnatal cocaine – PND 1–28: standard rearing) Magalhaes et al. (2006; M and F; enriched rearing) Wood et al. (1994; M and F)
Aggression	**4** Estelles et al. (2005; M; mice: isolated and group housed. Cocaine challenge, tested: PND 110) Johns et al. (1994a; M; tested: PND 180) Johns and Noonan (1995; M-tested: PND 180; F-tested: PND 60) Wood and Spear (1998; M; tested: PND 33 and 60–70)	**5** Estelles et al. (2005; M; mice: isolated and group housed, tested: PND 110) Goodwin et al. (1992; M; tested: PND 60–70) Johns et al. (1998b; M; pre-and postnatal intermittent cocaine, tested: PND 180) Johns and Noonan (1995; M; tested: PND 90) Wood and Spear (1998; F; tested: PND 33 and 60–70)	**0**
Scent marking		**1** Vorhees et al. (2000; M and F; pre-weaning exposure)	**1** Raum et al. (1990; M)

Numbers in bold refer to number of findings for each outcome. Unless otherwise stipulated, cocaine exposure is gestational and subjects are rats. M, male; F, female; PND, postnatal day.

play behavior (JSPB) is well characterized in the rat, and consists of a flurry of chasing, pouncing, tumbling, and wrestling movements which often terminates after one juvenile assumes a dominance stance over an inverted juvenile partner (i.e., pinning). JSPB occurs mainly before sexual maturity, peaking at a midpoint of the periadolescent period. Although JSPB is sexually dimorphic, with males exhibiting higher levels of social play than females, due to increased rates of play initiation, there are only minor differences in the sequential organization of play. The early social environment can influence JSPB, in that increased maternal grooming can reduce later juvenile social play and vice versa (Thor and Holloway, 1984; Pellis and Pellis, 1998; Magalhaes et al., 2007; Auger and Olesen, 2009).

Table 2 lists the five studies that involved play behavior; rats were used in all studies and cocaine was administered prenatally in all but one (Magalhaes et al., 2007). In an initial study by Wood et al. (1994), both male and female PCE offspring showed play deficits. Both sexes exhibited less pinning during social play, and were pinned more by their same sex-partner. The submissive behavior exhibited by PCE offspring was thought to reflect changes in the animals' overall ability to respond appropriately in play or social situations. In a second study by these investigators (Wood et al., 1995), adolescent play behaviors (pinning and pouncing) were unaffected by exposure to foot-shock, forced swim or white noise stress, suggesting that stress might have normalized play behavior in PCE offspring. However, alterations in play behavior were manifested by the way in which other animals played with cocaine-exposed animals; play partners were more hesitant to initiate and less likely to continue play with PCE adolescents. This latter finding was interpreted as decreased attractiveness of the PCE offspring to conspecifics.

Environmental conditions have been identified as a confounding variable in clinical studies of PCE (van Gelder et al., 2010). A third study reported that environmental manipulations attenuate the behavioral effects of prenatal cocaine on play behaviors (Neugebauer et al., 2004). While rearing in an impoverished environment increased play solicitations in prenatal PCE offspring at PND 60, 90, and 120, those raised in enriched conditions did not differ from controls. Magalhaes et al. (2006) reported that rearing PCE offspring in a standard environment (SE) had no effect on play fighting, solicitation, or social investigation. In contrast, rearing in an enriched environment (EE) decreased both play behavior and social investigation in offspring prenatally exposed to cocaine. This reduction was attributed to the preference of EE-reared animals to explore a novel environment instead of engaging in social play, and to improved social memory in the PCE rats.

These investigators evaluated the effects of EE in rats exposed to cocaine during the first 28 days of postnatal life (Magalhaes et al., 2007). Again, environmental rearing condition interacted with developmental cocaine exposure. However, in contrast to PCE offspring, animals postnatally exposed to cocaine and reared in a SE showed a decreased frequency of play solicitation, while those reared in the EE displayed more invitation to play and comfort behaviors, as well as a decrease in social investigation. The increase in play solicitation suggested that the rearing in an EE enhances the attractiveness of the play partner. An increased display of comfort behavior (i.e., social groom and pile-up behavior) was interpreted as a stress-reducing strategy in a novel environment, while the decrease in social investigation exhibited by postnatal cocaine rats reared in an EE again suggested improved social memory.

The results of these five studies suggest that PCE either impairs or has no effect on play behaviors; outcome differences are seen despite the similarity in dependent variables across studies.

Enhanced play behavior reflects an interaction of the rearing environment and developmental period of cocaine exposure, and is seen only with postnatal cocaine exposure. In both PCE and postnatally exposed cocaine offspring, rearing in an EE appears to improve social memory.

AGGRESSION

While aggressiveness *per se* is not considered abnormal in humans, abnormal aggression has been linked to psychiatric conditions and is seen as a symptom rather than a disorder of its own (see Haller and Kruk, 2006 for a review). Despite the underlying pathology, aggressive behavior is a social, economic, and medical issue (Blanchard et al., 2003).

Childhood aggression can be a serious problem, as such children are more likely to be involved in future juvenile delinquency. Prenatal exposure to cocaine may contribute a risk factor for aggressive behavior problems. Infants born to mothers who used cocaine during pregnancy are characterized as fussy/difficult, unadaptable, and exhibit signs of increased irritability (Chasnoff et al., 1987). There are also reports of increasing externalization problems (aggression, delinquency) in children who were prenatally exposed to cocaine, some as early as 3 years of age (Griffith et al., 1994; Delaney-Black et al., 2000; Richardson et al., 2009), although there are findings to the contrary (Accornero et al., 2002; Bennett et al., 2002).

The expression of aggressive behavior appears to be modulated not only by child-related variables, such as altered emotional regulation and impulse control (Bendersky and Lewis, 1998a,b), but also by increased environmental and maternal risk factors (Bendersky et al., 2006). Women who use cocaine have higher rates of depression and have been found to be less responsive in interactions with their children (Wood et al., 1995; Mayes et al., 1997). Maternal harsh discipline and greater caregiver psychological distress have also been associated with increased behavioral problems in children (Bennett et al., 2002; Minnes et al., 2010). Moreover the lower economic and educational status of the most likely single head of household can create a chaotic living environment that increases the risk of aggression through poor parenting and variables involved in living in marginalized neighborhoods. However, it should be noted that prenatal cocaine-exposed children in adoptive or foster care are rated as having more behavioral problems than those living with maternal or relative caregivers (Linares et al., 2006).

The contribution of the male gender and age to displays of aggressive behavior following PCE has been consistently reported (see Delaney-Black et al., 2000; Anderson and Bushman, 2002; Bendersky et al., 2006 for reviews), although there are reports that girls between 4 and 10 years of age show increased rates of delinquency (Minnes et al., 2010), and higher aggression scores (Sood et al., 2005). While PCE disposes pre-teens to aggressive behavior (Delaney-Black et al., 1998; Bendersky et al., 2006; Linares et al., 2006), social provocation of adolescent or young adult males exposed to heavy/persistent prenatal cocaine is associated with greater escape behavior, inferring greater submission, social withdrawal, or anxiety as opposed to aggressive behavior (Greenwald et al., 2011).

Aggressive behavior in animals is used to establish social hierarchies and to defend territories. Pre-clinical research has provided a detailed description of aggression and defense patterns in rodents. Although components of aggression are similar, patterns of aggressive behavior are usually distinctive in males and females. The identification of target sites for attack, and the motivational antecedents of attack behavior have allowed for the analyses of offensive and defensive aggression strategies and for the use of these maneuvers in maternal behavior (see Blanchard et al., 2003 for review).

Six experimental studies are summarized in **Table 2**. All except one used rats (Estelles et al., 2005). While all used chronic gestational cocaine exposure, two also used intermittent prenatal exposure alone (Johns et al., 1994a, 1998b), and Johns et al. (1998b) used combined intermittent pre and postnatal cocaine exposure. Several paradigms have been used to study aggressive behavior: resident-intruder (Goodwin et al., 1992; Johns et al., 1994a; Johns and Noonan, 1995; Estelles et al., 2005), shock-elicited aggression (Goodwin et al., 1992), and water competition (Wood and Spear, 1998). Although males are most often used for investigating aggressive behavior, three studies tested both male and female offspring (Johns and Noonan, 1995; Johns et al., 1998b; Wood and Spear, 1998).

In mice (Estelles et al., 2005) PCE had no effect on offensive (i.e., attack latency and number) or defensive (i.e., threat, avoidance/flee) aggressive behaviors in adult (PND 110) offspring reared in groups or in isolation. In contrast, housing conditions impacted aggression scores following cocaine challenge. While isolated PCE animals exhibited an increase in defensive aggression, groups housed PCE males were clearly more aggressive, exhibiting increases in both defensive and offensive aggressive behavior.

Rearing conditions have also been shown to exert modest but detectable influence on aggressive behavior. Using a shock-elicited design, Goodwin et al. (1992) reported that prenatal cocaine *per se* did not influence aggressive behavior in adulthood. Irrespective of prenatal treatment exposure, both fostered and non-fostered young adult male offspring, PND 60–70, raised by cocaine-treated dams were more aggressive, exhibiting shorter attack latencies, with no effect on the number of fighting episodes. Moreover, in contrast to mice, no aggression was observed in any offspring in the resident/intruder model.

A series of studies by Johns et al. (1994a, 1998b), Johns and Noonan (1995) investigated the effects of daily or intermittent PCE alone or in combination with postnatal intermittent exposure on aggressive behaviors in male offspring in a resident/intruder paradigm. In all studies, litters were cross-fostered to untreated surrogate dams. Following daily gestational cocaine exposure, male offspring tested at PND 180 exhibited increased duration of circle threat to a male intruder (Johns et al., 1994a). In a similar study (Johns and Noonan, 1995), at PND 180 chronic PCE male offspring tested for aggression exhibited an increased frequency and duration, and decreased latency to chase a male intruder. At PND 90, PCE did not alter any of the 11 measures of aggression scored. Rough grooming can be considered as social interaction or mild aggression. PCE female offspring at PND 60 showed an increase in this behavior toward non-exposed females. However, while intermittent gestational cocaine did not significantly affect aggressive behavior in either male or female pups at PND 30 and 60, combined intermittent gestational and postnatal cocaine increased the incidence and duration, and decreased the latency of PCE males to chase an intruder (Johns et al., 1998b).

Adolescent and young adult rats were tested for aggression in a water competition task (Wood and Spear, 1998). At PND 33, there was an increased incidence of attacks by PCE males, but not females. As young adults, offspring between PND 60–70, again on PCE males engaged in more incidences of boxing during water competition. In contrast, the incidence of attacks exhibited by PCE female offspring did not differ from control females at either.

In summary, these studies suggest that aggressive behavior in PCE rats may be sensitive to the same factors the influence this behavior in humans: age, gender, and environmental rearing/housing conditions. Consistent increases in aggressive behaviors are seen in PCE male rats with increasing age, and while the studies testing females are very limited, it would appear that mild aggression may be present earlier than in males. In humans, the results of a recent laboratory simulation of an aggressive situation, indicates that teenage males show escape/avoidance behavior rather than aggression when presented with a choice (Greenwald et al., 2011). Although aggressive behavior is more often reported in male children following PCE, it is possible that a more subtle or defensive form of aggression is evidenced by females (see Maternal Aggression).

SCENT MARKING

Urinary scent marks have ethologically important roles in social communication among conspecifics in many rodent species. Scent marking behavior is a communication tool for maintaining social relationships in both sexes; however, males mark two to three times more than females (Raum et al., 1990). When deposited in the environment, scent marks convey information on territory ownership in the absent of the owner, social status, as well as reproductive, health, and nutritional status, and enable recognition of individuals. Among males, scent marking and the counter-marking of the scent marks of other males are important components of dominance advertisement, especially among male mice, and strongly influence their aggressive interactions (see Arakawa et al., 2008 for recent review).

In adulthood, prenatal cocaine-exposed males, but not females, exhibited significantly less marking behavior than controls. Males also exhibited demasculinization in some sexual behaviors (Raum et al., 1990). In contrast, pre-weaning exposure to cocaine failed to alter scent marking behavior in PND 80 rats of either sex. Moreover, typical gender differences were seen, with males marking two to three times more than females (Vorhees et al., 2000). Although cocaine alters scent marking behavior in rats, the effect may be function of the developmental exposure period.

SUMMARY

Prenatal cocaine exposure clearly exerts an immediate, short-term negative effect on maternal care of offspring. This finding has important methodological implications. Given the demonstrated long-term effects of abnormal maternal care seen in first generation male and female offspring, such drug-induced impairments confound direct and indirect effects on exposed pups. Presumably these behavioral changes in dams can be parceled out by cross-fostering pups to drug-naive dams at birth. Such cross-fostering should be a common technique until/unless it can be demonstrated that these drug-induced changes in early postnatal maternal care have no long-term effects on offspring.

A consistent finding is that cocaine exposure enhances maternal aggression toward unfamiliar intruders, for more than a week after the final gestational cocaine exposure. Effects are intergenerational, with first generation dams also exhibiting increased maternal aggression. Whether this enhanced aggression is due to drug-induced increases in anxiety/fearfulness or increased combativeness remains to be elucidated.

Finally, a variety of other behaviors appear to be sensitive to developmental cocaine exposure, in that the majority of studies report changes of some kind. Yet the direction of these changes is currently unclear. Thus reported developmental cocaine effects on infant vocalizations, play, social investigation, and scent marking are more or less evenly divided between reports of no effects, enhanced, or diminished/impaired effects. The commonality of such mixed results clearly provides a major challenge to experimenters. Collectively, the above findings provide evidence for clear species or sex differences; the one exception is offspring aggression.

MECHANISTIC CONSIDERATIONS: OXYTOCIN AND ARGININE-VASOPRESSIN

Oxytocin

Evidence from several decades of animal research indicated that the neuropeptides oxytocin (OT) and arginine-vasopressin (AVP) have substantial roles in regulating complex social behaviors and social cognition. Oxytocin (OT), a nine amino acid peptide, is synthesized primarily in magnocellular neurons of the hypothalamus, and is released directly into the bloodstream from the posterior pituitary. Its function on both peripheral reproductive tissue and in the central nervous system (CNS) is now well characterized. As a neurosecretory hormone on reproductive tissue, OT plays a critical role in the onset of parturition and milk ejection during lactation. In the CNS, it is not only responsible for the induction of maternal nurturing behavior, but also for modulating social cognition, and affiliative behavior in both sexes (see Ross and Young, 2009 for review).

Animal studies indicate a role for OT in mediating maternal behavior in rodents and alloparental care in prairie voles, mother–infant bonding in sheep and pup–mother interactions in rodents, social (pair) bonding adult in adult voles, and social recognition in adult rodents. Pharmacological manipulations with exogenous OT, OT antagonists, and antisera indicate that OT plays a more important role in regulating the onset of maternal behavior than in the maintenance of maternal behavior in rat (Fahrbach et al., 1985; van Leengoed et al., 1987). Genetic experiments using OT and OT receptor (OTR) knock out (KO) mice support pharmacological findings in rat of the role of OT in regulating maternal behavior (Nishimori et al., 1996; Young et al., 1996). OTKO mice were more likely to display infanticidal behavior than wild-type mice housed in a social semi-natural environment (Ragnauth et al., 2005), while OTRKO mice are more deficient in maternal behavior than peptide-KO mice (Tankayanagi et al., 2005). There is also evidence that transgenerational transmission of maternal behavior may be mediated by changes in OTR expression (Francis et al., 1999, 2002).

Prairie vole juveniles and some adult females display nurturing behavior toward pups that are not their own. There is evidence that OT may play an important role in this alloparental behavior (Ross and Young, 2009). OTR density in the nucleus accumbens (NAc) is significantly correlated with the display of alloparental behavior in both juvenile and adult virgin females (Olazabal and Young, 2006), and injections of an OT antagonist into the NAc block the expression of maternal-like behavior toward pups in adult females.

There is some evidence in rodents that OT also modulates the pup's response to the mother. OTKO and OTRKO mouse pups emit fewer USV following separation from their dams than their wild-type counterparts (Winslow et al., 2000; Tankayanagi et al., 2005). OT also influences the attraction of the pup to their dam, as OT antagonist blocks the preference for maternal odors in pups at 15 days of age (Nelson and Panksepp, 1996).

Social recognition, which allows social species to distinguish familiar conspecifics from strangers and to remember individuals previously encountered, is necessary for successful group living and survival. While central injections of OT have been shown to enhance the time that a male rat remembers a conspecific (see Choleris et al., 2009 for review), OTR antagonists do not block memory performance. However, while wild-type mice habituate to familiar mice, OTKO males fail to habituate after repeated exposures to the same mouse (Ferguson et al., 2000).

There is a growing body of literature suggesting that in humans OT modulates social perception, social cognition, and social behavior, all of which promote social approach and affiliation (see Heinrichs et al., 2009; Lee et al., 2009 for reviews). Pharmacological studies have suggested that OT is also able to enhance human social cognition (see Heinrichs et al., 2009), a finding that is consistent with the role of OT in social recognition in rodents. Intranasal OT improved identity recognition for neutral and angry faces (Savaskan et al., 2008) and during game play, stimulated behavior consistent with enhanced interpersonal trust which is a prerequisite of social affiliation and social approach in humans (Kosfeld et al., 2005).

Data involving the role of OT in human interpersonal relationships is scarce and inconclusive. However, active maternal behavior during the first trimester and the first postpartum month has been correlated with high plasma concentration of OT (Feldman et al., 2007; Galbally et al., 2011). OT in humans has been associated with both an enhanced ability to interact socially (Nelson and Panksepp, 1996), and a better central control of stress and anxiety in social situations (Kavaliers et al., 2003).

Arginine-vasopressin

Arginine-vasopressin is similar in structure to OT. It is also synthesized in the hypothalamus and released into the bloodstream via the posterior pituitary gland. Like OT, numerous animal studies have also implicated AVP in mating, pair bonding, and adult–infant attachment (Lim and Young, 2006). Whereas OT is involved in the regulation of social approach behavior, social affiliation, and attachment, AVP has primarily been implicated in male-typical social behaviors, including aggression, pair-bond formation, scent marking, and courtship (see Choleris et al., 2009; Heinrichs et al., 2009 for reviews).

In male rats, social recognition of a juvenile conspecific is enhanced by peripheral administration of AVP immediately after exposure (Sekiguchi et al., 1991; Freeberg et al., 1999), and is reversed by an AVP antagonist (Dantzer et al., 1987). Unlike OT, however, AVP appears to play a more important role in social recognition in males than in females. While AVP improves social recognition in both sexes, AVP antagonists impair social memory only in males (Blunthe and Dantzer, 1990). Two AVP receptors in the CNS, V1aR, and V1bR, have been implicated in species and sex differences in social behavior (Donaldson and Young, 2008). While male V1aR KO mice are completely impaired in social recognition, V1bR KO mice, while impaired with respect to WT mice, can distinguish between familiar and unfamiliar conspecifics (Wersinger et al., 2004). Moreover, AVP V1a receptor antagonist selectively blocks aggressive behavior in hamsters (Ferris et al., 2006), and there appears to be an association between *Avpr-1a* receptor gene and partner preference in the male prairie vole (Young and Wang, 2004).

The few studies conducted on the role of AVP in human social behavior suggest behavioral effects similar to those found in animals. In subjects with personality disorders, the positive correlation found between levels of AVP in cerebrospinal fluid and life histories of general aggression was suggested as reflecting an enhancing effect of central AVP in individuals with impulsive aggressive behavior (Coccaro et al., 1998). As has been reported in animal studies, intranasal AVP influences social communication in a sex-specific manner. In men, AVP stimulated agonistic responses to faces of unfamiliar men, while in women the neuropeptide produced affiliative responses to unfamiliar female faces (Thompson et al., 2006). In addition, the *Avpr-1a* seems to be associated with differences in altruistic or prosocial behavior in men and women, and with pair bonding and marital satisfaction in men (Walum et al., 2008).

Prenatal cocaine, maternal behavior, and oxytocin

In lactating rats, maternal aggression serves to protect the nesting environment from intruders. Administration of oxytocin directly into the central nucleus of the amygdala (CeA) or the bed nucleus of the stria terminalis of the lactating rat has been shown to decrease maternal aggression during the postpartum period (Consiglio et al., 2005). In contrast, the infusion of an OT antagonist into the CeA increases maternal aggression to the point that it is not adaptive (Lubin et al., 2003). The role of OT in maternal behavior following gestational cocaine treatment has focused on aggressive behavior in lactating dams. Research, primarily from Johns et al. (1994b, 1997, 1998a, 2004), indicate that chronic exposure to cocaine throughout gestation (i.e., GD 1–20) results in decreased levels of OT, up-regulation of the oxytocin receptor binding density, and decreased receptor affinity in the amygdala, that coincide with significant increases in maternal aggression on PPD 6 (Johns et al., 1994b, 1997, 1998a, 2004; Elliott et al., 2001). However, during the early postpartum period (i.e., PPD 2), gestational exposure to cocaine resulted in an increase in oxytocin mRNA in the paraventricular nucleus, without an effect on receptor binding (McMurray et al., 2008b). Increased maternal aggression has also been reported at PPD 2 following gestational (Lubin et al., 2001) and pre-mating (Nephew and Febo, 2010) cocaine exposure. Prenatal cocaine-induced disruptions in the onset of maternal behavior have been correlated with decreased levels of OT in the ventral tegmental area (VTA), the medial pre-optic area, and the hippocampus (Johns et al., 1997; Jarrett et al., 2006). The intergenerational effects of PCE that have been reported for maternal aggressive behavior have also been seen for OT. First generation dams also had lower levels of OT in the amygdala (McMurray et al., 2008a), but in contrast to their dams, only a strong trend for increased mRNA was found in the supraoptic nucleus (McMurray et al., 2008b). It would therefore appear that gestational cocaine exposure induces wide-spread alterations in OT system dynamics that may mediate heightened maternal aggression in rat during the postpartum period. We are unaware of published studies involving the effects of PCE on vasopressin.

With respect to the possible mechanism that underlies gestational cocaine's effect on OT and postpartum maternal aggression, there is some suggestion that dynamic changes in serotonergic (5-HT) and/or dopaminergic (DA) system may be involved (Johns et al., 2004). Brain structures involved in maternal behavior or aggression, such as the paraventricular nucleus, hippocampus, amygdala, and the VTA contain both OT neurons fibers and/or receptors, as well as DA and 5-HT projections and receptors. Anatomical evidence indicates that OT neurons are in close contact or have synaptic connections with DA and 5-HT neurons, and that OT system dynamics are altered by cocaine and manipulation of these two transmitter systems. Moreover, the fact that pup retrieval and a nursing posture over pups is blocked in parturient dams by infusion of an OT antagonist into either the VTA or the medial pre-optic area highlights the interaction between DA neurons and OT pathways in maternal behavior (see Johns et al., 2004; McMurray et al., 2008b, and Strathearn and Mayes, 2010 for reviews).

DEVELOPMENTAL ETHANOL EXPOSURE AND SOCIAL BEHAVIOR

Evidence linking gestational alcohol exposure in humans to social defects, including a range of misbehaviors, is subject to high levels of confounding variables. Not surprisingly, women who drink during pregnancy in modern industrialized nations differ on a large variety of factors from those who do not. These confounds necessitate independent validation of a biological linkage between social deficits and developmental alcohol exposure in animal models, which provide satisfactory control of the many confounds plaguing human research. Although animal research is still very limited, this review will show that developmental alcohol exposure does indeed impact a range of rodent social behaviors. These data will be compared to findings reviewed with animal models of developmental cocaine exposure to determine whether the effects on social behaviors produced by cocaine exposure are of the same general nature and magnitude as those reported for alcohol-exposed animals.

DEVELOPMENTAL ETHANOL EXPOSURE IN HUMANS

Gestational exposure to alcohol is doubtlessly as old as human consumption of alcoholic beverages, yet it is only in the past half-century that fetal alcohol syndrome (FAS), which occurs in 0.3–2.2 per 1,000 live births in the US (Ripabelli et al., 2006) and is the consequence of heavy drinking during pregnancy, has been identified and characterized. More recently, concern has shifted to the question of the effects the on brain and behavior of the prevalent use of lower levels of drinking during pregnancy, ethanol intake levels below those required for FAS. It is now recognized that prenatal alcohol exposure may produce a broader spectrum of defects, now recognized as fetal alcohol spectrum disorders (FASD; Jones et al., 2010). Infants affected by FASD show not only intellectual impairment, and difficulties in learning, memory, problem-solving, and attention, but also experience additional problems with mental health and social interactions (Ripabelli et al., 2006). These social disorders are variously characterized as conduct disorder, externalizing disorders, or antisocial personality disorder, and have in common a higher level of misbehavior, delinquency, and even criminal conduct. For simplicity, this variety of misbehaviors will discussed under the term "externalizing disorder," realizing that in actuality there can be subtle differences between these various terms.

Evidence for ethanol-induced externalizing disorders in humans

A number of studies have provided evidence for linkages between externalizing disorders, as defined above, and mild (Sood et al., 2001; Sayal et al., 2007), moderate (Olson et al., 1997), and high (Mattson and Riley, 2000; D'Onofrio et al., 2007; Disney et al., 2008) levels of gestational alcohol intake. Although these studies have attempted to control for a variety of common confounds (Schuckit et al., 2003; Huizink and Mulder, 2006; McGee and Riley, 2007) it is unlikely that they have been able to either identify or control for all sources. Despite these uncertainties, results of some studies have already suggested that it is these confounds and not developmental alcohol exposure *per se* which account for subsequent externalizing behaviors in exposed offspring (e.g., Hill et al., 2000).

DEVELOPMENTAL ETHANOL EXPOSURE IN ANIMALS

We have identified 19 published peer-reviewed studies that have investigated a range of social behaviors following developmental exposure, i.e., gestational, postnatal, or combined exposure to ethanol. Of these 19 studies, 16 used rats (Barron and Riley, 1985; Meyer and Riley, 1986; Royalty, 1990; Blanchard and Hannigan, 1994; Kelly and Dillingham, 1994; Wilson et al., 1996; Lugo et al., 2003, 2006; Lawrence et al., 2008; Kelly et al., 2009b; Hamilton et al., 2010; Mooney and Varlinskaya, 2011) and three used mice (Kršiak et al., 1977; Ewart and Cutler, 1979; Hale et al., 1992). There were no studies of primates or other mammalian species. Further, of these 19 studies, 8 exclusively used gestational exposure (Kršiak et al., 1977; Barron and Riley, 1985; Meyer and Riley, 1986; Ness and Franchina, 1990; Royalty, 1990; Hale et al., 1992; Blanchard and Hannigan, 1994; Hamilton et al., 2010), three used exclusively postnatal exposure (Kelly and Dillingham, 1994; Wilson et al., 1996; Wellmann et al., 2010), and the remaining eight studies combined gestational and postnatal exposure (Ewart and Cutler, 1979; Tattoli et al., 2001; Marino et al., 2002; Lugo et al., 2003, 2006; Lawrence et al., 2008; Kelly et al., 2009b; Mooney and Varlinskaya, 2011). There are too few comparable studies within these various exposure periods to allow meaningful comparisons across developmental exposure periods for individual social behavior categories. Consequently studies were collapsed across both species and exposure periods, to get a first approximation of alcohol exposure effects on social behaviors. These 19 studies looked at six different social behaviors; outcomes were reviewed by behavior and summarized in **Table 3**.

Maternal behavior

Three studies in rats have reported reductions in maternal response to neonates following either gestational (Barron and Riley, 1985; Ness and Franchina, 1990) or postnatal exposure (Wilson et al., 1996). These reductions were seen both at an early age (Barron and Riley, 1985; Ness and Franchina, 1990; Wilson et al., 1996) and in adults (Barron and Riley, 1985), and in young rats of both sexes (Barron and Riley, 1985; Ness and Franchina, 1990). In contrast, Marino et al. (2002) reported no effects of combined pre- and postnatal ethanol exposure on the maternal response to neonates. Four studies with three different ethanol exposure periods do not allow strong conclusions, especially in the presence of one negative report. However, the suggestion is clearly that ethanol exposure over a wide developmental range may impair simple pup retrieval behaviors.

Play

The results for play behavior are contradictory. There are two reports of unchanged behavior (Blanchard and Hannigan, 1994; Mooney and Varlinskaya, 2011), four of enhanced play behavior (Meyer and Riley, 1986; Royalty, 1990; Lawrence et al., 2008; Hamilton et al., 2010) and two of reduced play following developmental exposure (Meyer and Riley, 1986; Mooney and Varlinskaya, 2011). Again, as shown in **Table 3**, these various behavioral outcomes do not segregate by sex; all three possible outcomes are

Table 3 | Social behavior in rodents exposed developmentally to ethanol compared to controls.

Behavior	Enhanced	No effect	Impaired/reduced
Maternal care	0	1 Marino et al. (2002; M and F; pre and postnatal exposure)	3 Barron and Riley (1985; M and F) Wilson et al. (1996; M and F; Postnatal exposure) Ness and Franchina (1990; M and F)
Play	4 Hamilton et al. (2010; M and F) Lawrence et al. (2008; M and F; pre and postnatal exposure) Royalty (1990; M and F) Meyer and Riley (1986; F)	2 Blanchard and Hannigan (1994; M) Mooney and Varlinskaya (2011; F; pre and postnatal exposure)	2 Meyer and Riley (1986; M) Mooney and Varlinskaya (2011; M; pre and postnatal exposure)
Social investigation	2 Kelly and Dillingham (1994; F; postnatal exposure) Lugo et al. (2003; M and F; pre and postnatal exposure)	5 Hamilton et al. (2010; F) Hamilton et al. (2010; M and F) Kelly et al. (2009b; M and F; pre and postnatal exposure) Kršiak et al. (1977; M; mouse) Mooney and Varlinskaya (2011; F)	4 Ewart and Cutler (1979; M and F) Hamilton et al. (2010; M) Kelly and Dillingham (1994; M; postnatal exposure) Mooney and Varlinskaya (2011; M)
Aggression	2 Kršiak et al. (1977; M; mouse) Royalty (1990; M)	1 Ewart and Cutler (1979; M and F; mouse: pre- and postnatal exposure)	1 Lugo et al. (2006; M; pre- and postnatal exposure)
Scent marking	0	1 Hale et al. [1992; mice:C56Bl/6J: (M and F); C3H/He (F)]	1 Hale et al. [1992; mice: C3H/He (M)]
Ultrasonic vocalizations	1 Marino et al. (2002; M and F; pre- and postnatal exposure)	1 Wellmann et al. (2010; M and F; postnatal exposure, PND 8–14)	2 Wellmann et al. (2010; M and F; postnatal exposure, PND 1–7) Tattoli et al. (2001; M; pre- and postnatal exposure)

Numbers in bold refer to number of findings. Unless otherwise stipulated, alcohol exposure is gestational and subjects are rats. F, females; M, males; PND, postnatal day.

seen in both sexes, across studies. The increase in play behavior may reflect an enhanced responsiveness to stimulation related to social experiences as a consequence of developmental alcohol exposure (Hamilton et al., 2010). Moreover, alterations in the normal sexually dimorphic patterns of play behavior (Meyer and Riley, 1986) are suggestive of masculinization of females (increased play) and demasculinization of males (decreased play) as a consequence of developmental alcohol exposure. This finding agrees with hormonal and morphological studies suggesting that gestational alcohol can masculinize females and demasculinize males (McGivern et al., 1984; Barron et al., 1988).

Social investigation
Social investigation is the behavioral variable most often measured. However, the results do not provide strong evidence for effects of developmental alcohol in either direction, or on one sex more than the other. Two studies report increases in social investigation (Kelly and Dillingham, 1994; Lugo et al., 2003). Of these two, Kelly and Dillingham (1994) study again suggested that developmental ethanol exposure demasculinizes males and defeminizes females. In contrast, five studies found no changes in social investigation, in one but not both sexes. Hamilton et al. (2010) reported that males but not females show reduced social investigation; however, after 24 h of social isolation neither sex showed changes in social investigation. Similar results were reported in three other studies (Kršiak et al., 1977; Kelly et al., 2009b; Mooney and Varlinskaya, 2011). Finally, four studies reported reductions in social investigation by one or both sexes (Ewart and Cutler, 1979; Kelly and Dillingham, 1994; Hamilton et al., 2010; Mooney and Varlinskaya, 2011).

Aggression
Given the possible link between gestational alcohol exposure and externalizing disorders in humans, it is surprising that so few studies have investigated aggression in rodents following developmental exposure to alcohol. As with play and social investigation, these studies have variously reported increases, (Kršiak et al., 1977; Royalty, 1990), decreases (Lugo et al., 2006), and no change (Ewart and Cutler, 1979) in aggressive behavior, with both the increased and the decreased aggression reported in males.

Scent marking
A single study of scent marking in mice (Hale et al., 1992) found that gestational effects were strain- and sex-dependent. Gestational ethanol had no effect on the scent marking of either sex in the C56Bl/6J strain, but reduced male but not female scent marking in the C3H/He strain.

Summary
Overall, 11 studies reported no effects of developmental ethanol exposure, 9 found increases and 13 found reductions or impairment of some measure of social behavior (**Table 3**). These results do not appear to differ by sex, age at exposure or species, nor did any one type of social behavior stand out as producing a clear developmental ethanol behavioral effect in a single direction. Additional research, including within-laboratory replication, is required, as this research area has been woefully neglected.

However, a plurality of studies (22 of 33) do show some change in social behavior following developmental alcohol exposure, and at the very least suggest that developmental alcohol exposure has some, as yet uncharacterized, impact upon rodent social behaviors. Further, five of the above studies report some degree of sex difference in developmental alcohol effects upon social behaviors (Meyer and Riley, 1986; Hale et al., 1992; Kelly and Dillingham, 1994; Hamilton et al., 2010; Mooney and Varlinskaya, 2011). Such findings combine with the known sex differences in social behaviors to make imperative the inclusion of both sexes in all future studies.

COMPARISON/CONCLUSION

The clinical literature indicates that in humans, prenatal and/or postnatal exposure to either alcohol or cocaine is associated with what we have referred to as externalizing disorders in the offspring, disorders characterized by abnormalities in social behavior. However, such findings are necessarily entangled in a number of confounding factors, which can be addressed in animal studies. While this review has concentrated on the impact of PCE on rodent social behaviors, it has also surveyed findings of developmental ethanol effects on social behaviors.

In comparing these two sets of literature, it is somewhat surprising that for neither substance of abuse has there been a major effort to determine effects of prenatal exposure on measures of social behavior in rodents or any other species. Our inability to characterize the impacts of these substances on social behaviors reflects in part this relative paucity of studies.

With few exceptions, both literatures are marked by a lack of consistent effects. In many cases, results are divided almost evenly between reports of no effects, increases and decreases on a variety of social behaviors as a consequence of prenatal/developmental exposure to cocaine or ethanol. This lack of unanimity also makes it difficult to reliably characterize the effects of either compound on the range of rodent social behaviors surveyed.

Establishing a phenotype of social behavior following developmental exposure to cocaine or alcohol is imperative. It is therefore necessary that future research concentrates on successful within- and between-laboratory replication of results. With exception of Johns and colleagues, even deliberate within-laboratory replication has not been attempted in either arena. Ultimately, only experimental replication will succeed in unraveling the current confusion of reported results. Here it is important to note that failures to replicate are by no means limited to the fields reviewed herein. True within-laboratory replicate experimental design is simply unheard of in the vast bulk of animal research. Until funding agencies and investigators understand replicate design and analysis, and are forced to utilize such designs, much rodent research will continue to be as fundamentally flawed as the studies reviewed here.

A second conclusion relates to methodological issues. The cocaine literature in this area has been marked by an unusually careful attempt to identify and address the confounds found not only in clinical but also in animal research. Thus, unlike the ethanol literature reviewed here, researchers investigating developmental cocaine effects have begun to identify and control for the effects of this drug that are mediated by the behavioral impact of drug exposure on the maternal–neonatal unit. As we have seen, researchers have clearly established that cocaine directly impairs maternal care of offspring, and increases maternal aggression. In view of these findings, it is imperative that future designs using gestational exposure cross-foster offspring to drug-naive dams. Equally, it is also important to characterize the effects of such impaired maternal care on the pups. Such attempts are currently under way (e.g., Johns and colleagues), and are very much encouraged. Since it is also not unlikely that alcohol exposure will impair maternal care of pups, the ethanol research clearly needs to adopt the same approach.

To summarize, increased research, replication of results, and research which controls for confounding of direct drug effects and effects mediated by abnormalities in the mother–pup unit is necessary. With the implementation of the above suggestions, it will be possible to successfully characterize the impact of these common drugs of abuse on the social behavior of rodents, and by extension perhaps humans as well.

REFERENCES

Accornero, V. H., Morrow, C. E., Bandstra, E. S., Johnson, A. L., and Anthony, J. C. (2002). Behavioral outcome of preschoolers exposed prenatally to cocaine: role of maternal behavioral health. *J. Pediatr. Psychol.* 27, 259–269.

Anderson, C., and Bushman, B. (2002). Human aggression. *Annu. Rev. Psychol.* 53, 27–51.

Arakawa, H., Blanchard, D. C., Arakawa, K., Dunlap, C., and Blanchard, R. J. (2008). Scent marking behavior as an odorant communication in mice. *Neurosci. Biobehav. Rev.* 32, 1236–1248.

Auger, A., and Olesen, K. (2009). Brain sex differences and the organization of juvenile social play behavior. *J. Neuroendocrinol.* 21, 519–525.

Barron, S., and Gilbertson, R. (2005). Neonatal ethanol exposure but not neonatal cocaine selectively reduces specific isolation-induced vocalization waveforms in rats. *Behav. Genet.* 35, 93–102.

Barron, S., and Riley, E. P. (1985). Pup-induced maternal behavior in adult and juvenile rats exposed to alcohol prenatally. *Alcohol. Clin. Exp. Res.* 9, 360–365.

Barron, S., Segar, T. M., Yahr, J. S., Baseheart, B. J., and Willford, J. A. (2000). The effects of neonatal ethanol and/or cocaine exposure on isolation-induced ultrasonic vocalizations. *Pharmacol. Biochem. Behav.* 67, 1–9.

Barron, S., Tiernan, S. B., and Riley, E. P. (1988). Effects of prenatal alcohol exposure on the sexually dimorphic nucleus of the preoptic area of the hypothalamus in male and female rats. *Alcohol. Clin. Exp. Res.* 12, 59–64.

Bendersky, M., Bennett, D., and Lewis, M. (2006). Aggression at age 5 as a function of prenatal exposure to cocaine, gender, and environmental risk. *J. Pediatr. Psychol.* 31, 71–84.

Bendersky, M., and Lewis, M. (1998a). Prenatal cocaine exposure and impulse control at two years. *Ann. N. Y. Acad. Sci.* 84, 365–367.

Bendersky, M., and Lewis, M. (1998b). Arousal modulation in cocaine-exposed infants. *Dev. Psychol.* 34, 555–564.

Bennett, D. S., Bendersky, M., and Lewis, M. (2002). Children's intellectual and emotional-behavioral adjustment at 4 years as a function of cocaine exposure, maternal characteristics, and environmental risk. *Dev. Psychol.* 38, 648–658.

Black, M. M., Schuler, M., and Nair, P. (1993). Prenatal drug exposure: neuro-developmental outcome and parenting environment. *J. Pediatr. Psychol.* 18, 605–620.

Blanchard, B. A., and Hannigan, J. H. (1994). Prenatal ethanol exposure: effects on androgen and nonandrogen dependent behaviors and on gonadal development in male rats. *Neurotoxicol. Teratol.* 16, 31–39.

Blanchard, R. J., Wall, P. M., and Blanchard, D. C. (2003). Problems in the study of rodent aggression. *Horm. Behav.* 44, 161–170.

Blunthe, R. M., and Dantzer, R. (1990). Social recognition does not involve vasopressinergic neurotransmission in female rats. *Brain Res.* 535, 310–304.

Bowlby, J. (1988). Developmental psychiatry comes of age. *Am. J. Psychiatry* 145, 1–10.

Chae, S., and Covington, C. (2009). Biobehavioral outcomes in adolescents and young adults prenatally exposed to cocaine: evidence from animal models. *Biol. Res. Nurs.* 10, 318–330.

Chasnoff, I. J., Burns, K. A., and Burns, W. J. (1987). Cocaine use in pregnancy: perinatal morbidity and mortality. *Neurotoxicol. Teratol.* 9, 291–293.

Choleris, E., Clipperton-Allen, A. E., Phan, A., and Kavaliers, M. (2009). Neuroendocrinology of social information processing in rats and mice. *Front. Neuroendocrinol.* 30, 442–459.

Coccaro, E. F., Kavoussi, R. J., Hauger, R. L., Cooper, T. B., and Ferris, C. F. (1998). Cerebrisounal fluid vasopressin levels: correlates with aggression and serotonin function in personality-disordered subjects. *Arch. Gen. Psychiatry* 55, 708–714.

Consiglio, A. R., Borsoi, A., Pereira, G. A., and Lucion, A. B. (2005). Effects of oxyticun microinjected into the central amygdaloid nucleus and bed nucleus of stria terminalis on maternal aggression behavior in rats. *Physiol. Behav.* 85, 354–362.

Dantzer, R., Blunthe, R. M., Koob, G. F., and Le Moal, M. (1987). Modulation of social memory in male rats by neurohypophyseal peptides. *Psychopharmacology* 91, 363–368.

Delaney-Black, V., Covington, C., Templin, T., Ager, J., Martier, S., and Sokol, R. (1998). Prenatal cocaine exposure and child behavior. *Pediatrics* 102, 945–950.

Delaney-Black, V., Covington, C., Templin, T., Ager, J., Nordstrom-Klee, B., Martier, S., Leddick, L., Czerwinski, R. H., and Sokol, R. J. (2000). Teacher-assessed behavior of children prenatally exposed to cocaine. *Pediatrics* 106, 782–791.

Disney, E. R., Iacono, W., McGue, M., Tully, E., and Legrand, L. (2008). Strengthening the case: prenatal alcohol exposure is associated with increased risk for conduct disorder. *Pediatrics* 122, e1225–e1230.

Donaldson, Z. R., and Young, L. J. (2008). Oxytocin vasopressin and the neurogenetics of sociality. *Science* 322, 900–904.

D'Onofrio, B. M., Van Hulle, C. A., Waldman, I. D., Rodgers, J. L., Rathouz, P. J., Lahey, M., and Benjamin, B. (2007). Causal inferences regarding prenatal alcohol exposure and childhood externalizing problems. *Arch. Gen. Psychiatry* 64, 1296–1304.

Elliott, J. C., Lubin, D. A., Walker, C. H., and Johns, J. M. (2001). Acute cocaine alters oxytocin levels in the medial preoptic area and amygdale in lactating rat dams: implications for cocaine-induced changes in maternal behavior and mater aggression. *Neuropeptides* 35, 127–134.

Estelles, J., Rodriguez-Arias, M., Maldonado, C., Aguilar, M., and Minarro, J. (2005). Prenatal cocaine exposure alters spontaneous and cocaine-induced motor and social behaviors. *Neurotoxicol. Teratol.* 27, 449–457.

Ewart, F. G., and Cutler, M. G. (1979). Effect of ethyl alcohol on development and social behaviour in the offspring of laboratory mice. *Psychopharmacology* 62, 247–251.

Fahrbach, S. E., Morrell, J. I., and Pfaff, D. W. (1985). Possible role of endogenous oxytocin in estrogen-facilitated maternal behavior in rats. *Neuorendocrinology* 40, 526–532.

Febo, M., and Ferris, C. F. (2007). Development of cocaine sensitization before pregnancy affects subsequent maternal retrieval of pups and prefrontal cortical activity during nursing. *Neuroscience* 148, 400–412.

Feldman, R., Weller, A., Zagoory-Sharon, O., and Levine, A. (2007). Evidence for a neuroendocrinological foundation of human affiliation: plasma oxytocin levels across pregnancy and the postpartum period predict mother-infant bonding. *Psychol. Sci.* 18, 965–970.

Ferguson, J. N., Young, L. J., Hearn, E. F., Matzuk, M. M., Insel, T. R., and Winslow, J. T. (2000). Social amnesia in mice lacking the oxytocin gene. *Nat. Genet.* 25, 284–288.

Ferris, C. F., Lu, S. F., Messenger, T., Guillon, C. D., Heindel, N., Miller, M., Koppel, G., Bruns, F. R., and Simon, N. G. (2006). Orally active vasopressin V1a receptor antagonist SRX251 selectively blocks aggressive behavior. *Pharmacol. Biochem. Behav.* 83, 169–174.

Francis, D., Diorio, J., Lui, D., and Meaney, M. J. (1999). Nongenomic transmission across generation of maternal behavior and stress responses in the rat. *Science* 286, 1155–1158.

Francis, D. D., Young, L. J., Meaney, M. J., and Insel, T. R. (2002). Naturally occurring differences in maternal care are associated with the expression of oxytocin and vasopressin (V1a) receptors: gender differences. *J. Neuroendocrinol.* 14, 349–353.

Freeberg, T. M., Duncan, S. D., Kast, T. L., and Enstrom, D. A. (1999). Cultural influences on female mate choices; an experimental test of cowbirds, *Molorthrus ater. Anim. Behav.* 57, 421–426.

Galbally, M., Lewis, A. J., Ijzendoorn, M., and Permezel, M. (2011). The role of oxytocin in mother infant-relations: a systemic review of human studies. *Harv. Rev. Psychiatry* 19, 1–14.

Gendle, M. H., White, T. L., Strawderman, M., Mactutus, C. F., Booze, R. M., Levitsky, D. A., and Strupp, B. J. (2004). Enduring effects of prenatal cocaine exposure on selective attention and reactivity to errors: evidence from an animal model. *Behav. Neurosci.* 118, 290–297.

Goodwin, G. A., Heyser, C. J., Moody, C. A., Rajachandran, L., Molina, V. A., Arnold, H. M., McKinzie, D. L., Spear, N. E., and Spear, L. P. (1992). A fostering study of the effects of prenatal cocaine exposure: II. Offspring behavioral measures. *Neurotoxicol. Teratol.* 14, 423–432.

Greenwald, M., Chiodo, L., Hannigan, J., Sokol, R., Janisse, J., and Delaney-Black, V. (2011). Teens with heavy prenatal cocaine exposure respond to experimental social provocation with escape not aggression. *Neurotoxicol. Teratol.* 33, 198–204.

Griffith, D. R., Azuma, S. D., and Chasnoff, I. J. (1994). Three-year outcome of children exposed prenatally to drugs. *J. Am. Acad. Child Adolesc. Psychiatry* 33, 20–27.

Hahn, M., Benno, R., Schanz, N., and Phadia, E. (2000). The effects of prenatal cocaine exposure and genotype on the ultrasonic calls of infant mice. *Pharmacol. Biochem. Behav.* 67, 729–738.

Hale, R. L., Randall, C. M., Becker, H. C., and Middaugh, L. D. (1992). The effect of prenatal ethanol exposure on scent marking in the C57BL/6J and C3H/He mouse strains. *Alcohol* 9, 287–292.

Haller, J., and Kruk, M. R. (2006). Normal and abnormal aggression: human disorders and novel laboratory models. *Neurosci. Biobehav. Rev.* 30, 292–303.

Hamilton, D. A., Akers, K. G., Rice, J. P., Johnson, T. E., Candelaria-Cook, F. T., Maes, L. I., Rosenberg, M., Valenzuela, C. F., and Savage, D. D. (2010). Prenatal exposure to moderate levels of ethanol alters social behavior in adult rats: relationship to structural plasticity and immediate early gene expression in frontal cortex. *Behav. Brain Res.* 207, 290–304.

Heinrichs, M., van Dawans, B., and Domes, G. (2009). Oxytocin, vasopressin, and human social behavior. *Front. Neuroendocrinol.* 30, 548–557.

Heyser, C. J., Molina, V. A., and Spear, L. P. (1992). A fostering study of the effects of prenatal cocaine exposure: I. Maternal behaviors. *Neurotoxicol. Teratol.* 14, 415–421.

Hill, S. Y., Lowers, L., Locke-Wellman, J., and Shen, S. A. (2000). Maternal smoking and drinking during pregnancy and the risk for child and adolescent psychiatric disorders. *J. Stud. Alcohol* 61, 661–668.

Howard, J., Beckwith, L., and Rodning, C. (1990). Adaptive behavior in recovering female phencyclidine/polysubstance abusers. *NIDA Res. Monogr.* 101, 86–95.

Huizink, A. C., and Mulder, E. J. H. (2006). Maternal smoking, drinking or cannabis use during pregnancy and neurobehavioral and cognitive functioning in human offspring. *Neurosci. Biobehav. Rev.* 30, 24–41.

Insel, T. (2003). Is social attachment an addictive disorder? *Physiol. Behav.* 79, 351–357.

Jarrett, T. M., McMurray, C. H., Walker, C. H., and Johns, J. M. (2006). Cocaine treatment alters oxytocin receptor binding but not mRNA production in postpartum rat dams. *Neuropeptides* 40, 161–167.

Jeremy, R. J., and Bernstein, V. J. (1984). Dyads at risk: methadone-maintained women and their four-month-old infants. *Child Dev.* 55, 1141–1154.

Johns, J. M., Elliott, D. L., Hofler, V. E., Joyner, P. W., McMurray, M. S., Jarrett, T. M., Haslup, A. M., Middleton, C. L., Elliott, J. C., and Walker, C. H. (2005). Cocaine treatment and prenatal environment interact to disrupt intergenerational maternal behavior in rats. *Behav. Neurosci.* 119, 1605–1618.

Johns, J. M., Lubin, D. A., Walker, C. H., Joyner, P., Middleton, C., Hofler, V., and McMurray, M. (2004). Gestational treatment with cocaine and fluoxetine alters oxytocin receptor number and binding affinity in lactating rat dams. *Int. J. Dev. Neurosci.* 22, 321–328.

Johns, J. M., McMurray, M. S., Hofler, V. E., Jarrett, T. M., Middleton, C. L., Elliott, D. L., Mirza, R., Haslup, A., Elliott, J. C., and Walker, C. H. (2007). Cocaine disrupts pup-induced maternal behavior in juvenile and adult rats. *Neurotoxicol. Teratol.* 29, 634–641.

Johns, J. M., McMurray, M. S., Joyner, P. W., Jarrett, T. M., Williams, S. K., Cox, E. T., Black, M. A., Middleton, C. L., and Walker, C. H. (2010). Effects of chronic and intermittent cocaine treatment on dominance, aggression and oxytocin levels in post-lactational rats. *Psychopharmacology (Berl.)* 211, 175–185.

Johns, J. M., Means, M. J., Bass, E. W., Means, L. W., Zimmerman, L. I., and McMillen, B. A. (1994a). Prenatal exposure to cocaine: effects on aggression in Sprague-Dawley rats. *Dev. Psychobiol.* 27, 227–239.

Johns, J. M., Noonan, L. R., Zimmerman, L. I., and Pederson, C. A. (1994b). Effects of chronic and acute cocaine treatment on the onset of maternal behavior and aggression in Sprague-Dawley rats. *Behav. Neurosci.* 108, 107–112.

Johns, J. M., Nelson, C. J., Meter, K. E., Lubin, D. A., Couch, C. D., Ayers, A., and Walker, C. H. (1998a). Dose-dependent effects of multiple acute cocaine injections on maternal behavior and aggression in Sprague-Dawley rats. *Dev. Neurosci.* 20, 525–532.

Johns, J. M., Noonan, L. R., Zimmerman, L. I., McMillen, B., Means, L., Walker, C., Lubin, D., Meter, K., Nelson, C., Pedersen, C., Mason, G., and Lauder, J. (1998b). Chronic cocaine treatment alters social/aggressive behavior in Sprague-Dawley rat dams and in their prenatally exposed offspring. *Ann. N. Y. Acad. Sci.* 846, 399–404.

Johns, J. M., and Noonan, L. R. (1995). Prenatal cocaine exposure affects social behavior in Sprague-Dawley rats. *Neurotoxicol. Teratol.* 17, 569–576.

Johns, J. M., Noonan, L. R., Zimmerman, L. I., Li, L., and Pedersen, C. A. (1997). Effects of short- and long-term withdrawal from gestational cocaine treatment on maternal behavior and aggression in Sprague-Dawley rats. *Dev. Neurosci.* 19, 368–374.

Johnson, A. L., Morrow, C. E., Accornero, V. H., Xue, L., Anthony, J. C., and Bandstra, E. S. (2002). Maternal cocaine use: estimated effects on mother-child play interactions in the preschool period. *J. Dev. Behav. Pediatr.* 23, 191–202.

Jones, K. L., Hoyme, H. E., Robinson, L. K., Del Campo, M., Manning, M. A., Prewitt, L. M., and Chambers, C. D. (2010). Fetal alcohol spectrum disorders: extending the range of structural defects. *Am. J. Med. Genet.* 152A, 2731–2735.

Kavaliers, M., Colwell, D. D., Choleris, E., Agmo, A., Muglia, L. J., Ogawa, S., and Pfaff, D. W. (2003). Impaired discrimination of and aversion to parasitized male odors by female oxytocin knockout mice. *Genes Brain Behav.* 2, 220–230.

Kelly, S., Day, N., and Streissguth, A. (2000). Effects of prenatal alcohol exposure on social behavior in humans and other species. *Neurotoxicol. Teratol.* 22, 143–149.

Kelly, S., Goodlett, C., and Hannigan, J. (2009a). Animal models of fetal alcohol spectrum disorders: impact of the social environment. *Dev. Disabil. Res. Rev.* 15, 200–208.

Kelly, S. J., Leggett, D. C., and Cronise, K. (2009b). Sexually dimorphic effects of alcohol exposure during development on the processing of social cues. *Alcohol Alcohol.* 44, 555–560.

Kelly, S. J., and Dillingham, R. R. (1994). Sexually dimorphic effects of perinatal alcohol exposure on social interactions and amygdala DNA and DOPAC concentrations. *Neurotoxicol. Teratol.* 16, 377–384.

Kinsley, C. H., Turco, D., Bauer, A., Beverly, M., Wellman, J., and Graham, A. L. (1994). Cocaine alters the onset and maintenance of maternal behavior in lactating rats. *Pharmacol. Biochem. Behav.* 47, 857–864.

Kosfeld, M., Heindrich, M., Zak, P. J., Fischbacher, U., and Fehr, E. (2005). Oxytocin increases trust in humans. *Nature* 423, 673–676.

Kršiak, M., Elis, J., Pöschlová, N., and Mašek, K. K. (1977). Increased aggressiveness and lower brain serotonin levels in offspring of mice given alcohol during gestation. *J. Stud. Alcohol* 38, 1696–1704.

Lawrence, R. C., Bonner, H. C., Newsom, R. J., and Kelly, S. J. (2008). Effects of alcohol exposure during development on play behavior and c-Fos expression in response to play behavior. *Behav. Brain Res.* 188, 209–218.

Lee, H.-J., Macbeth, A. H., Pagni, J. H., and Young III, W. S. (2009). Oxytocin: the great facilitator of life. *Prog. Neurobiol.* 88, 127–151.

Lim, M. M., and Young, L. J. (2006). Neuropeptidergic regulation of affiliative behaviour and social bonding in animals. *Horm. Behav.* 50, 506–517.

Linares, T. J., Singer, L. T., Kirchner, H. L., Short, E. J., Min, M. O., Hussey, P., and Minnes, S. (2006). Mental health outcomes of cocaine-exposed children at 6 years of age. *J. Pediatr. Psychol.* 31, 85–97.

Lubin, D. A., Elliott, J. C., Black, M. C., and Johns, J. M. (2003). An oxytocin antagonist infused into the central nucleus of the amygdale increases maternal aggressive behavior. *Behav. Neurosci.* 117, 195–201.

Lubin, D. A., Meter, K. E., Walker, C. H., and Johns, J. M. (2001). Dose-related effects of chronic gestational cocaine treatment on maternal aggression in rats on postpartum days 2, 3, and 5. *Prog. Neuropsychopharmacol. Biol. Psychiatry* 25, 1403–1420.

Lugo, J. N., Marino, M. D., Cronise, K., and Kelly, S. J. (2003). Effects of alcohol exposure during development on social behavior in rats. *Physiol. Behav.* 78, 185–194.

Lugo, J. N., Marino, M. D., Gass, J. T., Wilson, M. A., and Kelly, S. J. (2006). Ethanol exposure during development reduces resident aggression and testosterone in rats. *Physiol. Behav.* 87, 330–337.

Magalhaes, A., Summavielle, T., Melo, P., Rosa, R., Tavares, M., and De Sousa, L. (2006). Prenatal exposure to cocaine and enriched environment. *Ann. N. Y. Acad. Sci.* 1074, 620–631.

Magalhaes, A., Summavielle, T., Tavares, M., and De Sousa, L. (2007). Postnatal exposure to cocaine in rats housed in an enriched environment: effects of social interactions. *Hum. Exp. Toxicol.* 26, 303–309.

Marino, M. D., Cronise, K., Lugo, J. N., and Kelly, S. J. (2002). Ultrasonic vocalizations and maternal-infant interactions in a rat model of fetal alcohol syndrome. *Dev. Psychobiol.* 41, 341–351.

Mattson, S. N., and Riley, E. P. (2000). Parent ratings of behavior in children with heavy prenatal alcohol exposure and IQ-matched controls. *Alcohol. Clin. Exp. Res.* 24, 226–231.

Mayes, L. C., Feldman, R., Granger, R., Haynes, O. M., Bornstein, M., and Schottenfeld, R. (1997). The effects of poly drug use with and without cocaine on mother-infant interactions at 3 and 6 months of age. *Infant Behav. Dev.* 20, 489–502.

McGee, C. L., and Riley, E. P. (2007). Social and behavioral functioning in individuals with prenatal alcohol exposure. *Int. J. Disabil. Hum. Dev.* 6, 369–382.

McGivern, R. F., Clancy, A. N., Hill, M. A., and Noble, E. P. (1984). Prenatal alcohol exposure alters adult expression of sexually dimorphic behavior in the rat. *Science* 224, 896–898.

McMurray, M. S., Joyner, P. W., Middleton, C. W., Jarrett, T. M., Elliott, D. L., Black, M. A., Hofler, V. E., Walker, C. H., and Johns, J. M. (2008a). Intergenerational effects of cocaine on maternal aggressive behavior and brain oxytocin in rat dams. *Stress* 11, 398–410.

McMurray, M. S., Cox, E. T., Jarrett, T. M., Williams, S. K., Walker, C. H., and Johns, J. M. (2008b). Impact of gestational cocaine treatment or prenatal cocaine exposure on early postpartum oxytocin mRNA levels and receptor binding in the rat. *Neuropeptides* 24, 641–652.

Meaney, M. (1989). The sexual differentiation of social play. *Psychiatr. Dev.* 7, 247–261.

Meaney, M. J. (2001). Maternal care, gene expression, and the transmission of individual differences in stress reactivity across generations. *Annu. Rev. Neurosci.* 24, 1161–1192.

Meyer, L. S., and Riley, E. P. (1986). Social play in juvenile rats prenatally exposed to alcohol. *Teratology* 34, 1–7.

Meyer, L. S., Sherlock, J. D., and MacDonald, N. R. (1992). Effects of prenatal cocaine on behavioral responses to a cocaine challenge on postnatal day 11. *Neurotoxicol. Teratol.* 14, 183–189.

Minnes, S., Singer, L. T., Kirchner, H. L., Short, E., Lewis, B., Satayathum, S., and Queh, D. (2010). The effects of prenatal cocaine exposure on problem behavior in children 4-10 years. *Neurotoxicol. Teratol.* 32, 443–451.

Mooney, S. M., and Varlinskaya, E. I. (2011). Acute prenatal exposure to ethanol and social behavior: effects of age, sex, and timing of exposure. *Behav. Brain Res.* 216, 358–364.

Nelson, C. J., Meter, K. E., Walker, C. H., Ayers, A. A., and Johns, J. M. (1998). A dose-response study of chronic cocaine on maternal behavior in rats. *Neurotoxicol. Teratol.* 20, 657–660.

Nelson, E., and Panksepp, J. (1996). Oxytocin mediates acquisition of maternally associated odor preference in preweanling rat pups. *Behav. Neurosci.* 110, 583–592.

Nephew, B. C., and Febo, M. (2010). Effect of cocaine sensitization prior to pregnancy on maternal care and aggression in the rat. *Psychopharmacology* 209, 127–135.

Ness, J. W., and Franchina, J. J. (1990). Effects of prenatal alcohol exposure on rat pups' ability to elicit retrieval behavior from dams. *Dev. Psychobiol.* 23, 85–99.

Neugebauer, N. M., Cunningham, S. T., Zhu, J., Bryant, R. I., Middleton, L. S., and Dwoskin, L. P. (2004). Effects of environmental enrichment on behavior and dopamine transporter function in medial prefrontal cortex in adult rats prenatally treated with cocaine. *Brain Res. Dev. Brain Res.* 153, 213–223.

Neuspiel, D. R., Hamel, S. C., Hochberg, E., Greene, J., and Campbell, D. (1991). Maternal cocaine use and infant behavior. *Neurotoxicol. Teratol.* 13, 229–233.

Newman, J. D. (2007). Neural circuits underlying crying and cry responding in mammals. *Behav. Brain Res.* 182, 155–165.

Nishimori, K., Young, L. J., Guo, Q., Wang, Z., Insel, T. R., and Matzuk, M. M. (1996). Oxytocin is required for nursing but is not essential for parturition or reproductive behavior. *Proc. Natl. Acad. Sci. U.S.A.* 93, 11699–11704.

Olazabal, D. E., and Young, L. J. (2006). Species and individual differences in juvenile female alloparental care are associated with oxytocin receptor density in the striatum and the lateral septum. *Horm. Behav.* 49, 681–687.

Olson, H. C., Streissguth, A. P., Sampson, P. D., Barr, H. M., Bookstein, F. L., and Thiede, K. (1997). Association of prenatal alcohol exposure with behavioral and learning problems in early adolescence. *J. Am. Acad. Child Adolesc. Psychiatry* 36, 1187–1194.

Oro, A. S., and Dixon, S. D. (1987). Perinatal cocaine and methamphetamine exposure: maternal and neonatal correlates. *J. Pediatr.* 111, 571–578.

Overstreet, D. H., Moy, S. S., Lubin, D. A., Gause, L. R., Lieberman, J. A., and Johns, J. M. (2000). Enduring effects of prenatal cocaine administration on emotional behavior in rats. *Physiol. Behav.* 70, 149–156.

Peeke, H., Dark, K., Salamy, A., Salfi, M., and Shah, S. (1994). Cocaine exposure prebreeding to weaning: maternal and offspring effects. *Pharmacol. Biochem. Behav.* 48, 403–410.

Pellis, S., and Pellis, V. (1998). Play flighting of rats in comparative perspective: a schema for neurobehavioral analyses. *Neurosci. Biobehav. Rev.* 23, 87–101.

Ragnauth, A. K., Devidze, N., Moy, V., Finley, K., Goodwillis, A., Kow, L. M., Muglia, L. J., and Pfaff, D. W. (2005). Female oxytocin gene-knockout mice, in a semi-natural environment, display exaggerated aggressive behavior. *Genes Brain Behav.* 4, 229–239.

Raum, W. J., McGivern, R. F., Peterson, M. A., Shryne, J. H., and Gorski, R. A. (1990). Prenatal inhibition of hypothalamic sex steroid uptake by cocaine: effects on neurobehavioral sexual differentiation in male rats. *Brain Res. Dev. Brain Res.* 53, 236.

Richardson, G. A., Goldschmidt, L., and Willford, J. (2009). Continued effects of prenatal cocaine use: preschool development. *Neurotoxicol. Teratol.* 31, 325–333.

Ripabelli, G., Cimmino, L., and Grasso, G. M. (2006). Alcohol consumption, pregnancy and fetal alcohol syndrome: implications in public health and preventive strategies. *Ann. Ig.* 18, 391–406.

Rodning, C., Beckwith, L., and Howard, J. (1989). Prenatal exposure to drugs and its influence on attachment. *Ann. N. Y. Acad. Sci.* 562, 352–364.

Ross, H. E., and Young, L. J. (2009). Oxytocin and the neural mechanisms regulating social cognition and affiliative behavior. *Front. Neuroendocrinol.* 30, 534–547.

Royalty, J. (1990). Effects of prenatal ethanol exposure on juvenile play-fighting and postpubertal aggression in rats. *Psychol. Rep.* 66, 551–560.

Savaskan, E., Ehrhardt, R., Schulz, A., Walter, M., and Schachinger, H. (2008). Post-learning intranasal oxytocin modulates human memory for facial identity. *Psychoneuroendocrinology* 33, 368–374.

Sayal, K., Heron, J., Golding, J., and Emond, A. (2007). Prenatal alcohol exposure and gender differences in childhood mental health problems: a longitudinal population-based study. *Pediatrics* 119, E426–E434.

Schuckit, M. A., Smith, T. L., Barnow, S., Preuss, U., Luczak, S., and Radziminski, S. (2003). Correlates of externalizing symptoms in children from families of alcoholics and controls. *Alcohol Alcohol.* 38, 559–567.

Sekiguchi, R., Wolterink, G., and van Ree, J. M. (1991). Analysis of the influence of vasopressin neuropeptides on social recognition of rats. *Eur. Neuropsychopharmacol.* 1, 123–126.

Sobrian, S., Ali, S., Slikker, S. Jr., and Holson, R. (1995). Interactive effects of prenatal cocaine and nicotine exposure on maternal toxicity, postnatal development, and behavior in the rat. *Mol. Neurobiol.* 11, 121–143.

Sobrian, S. K., Burton, L. E., Robinson, L. E., Ashe, W. K., James, H., Stokes, D. L., and Turner, L. M. (1990). Neurobehavioral and immunological effects of prenatal cocaine exposure in rat. *Pharmacol. Biochem. Behav.* 35, 617–629.

Sood, B., Bailey, B., Covington, C., Sokol, R., Ager, J., Janisse, J., Hannigan, J., and Delaney-Black, V. (2005). Gender and alcohol moderate caregiver reported child behavior after prenatal cocaine. *Neurotoxicol. Teratol.* 27, 191–201.

Sood, B., Delaney-Black, V., Covington, C., Nordstrom-Klee, B., Ager, J., Templin, T., Janisse, J., Martier, S., and Sokol, R. J. (2001). Prenatal alcohol exposure and childhood behavior at age 6 to 7 years: I. Dose-response effect. *Pediatrics* 108, e34.

Sousa, N., Almeida, O. F. X., and Wotjak, C. T. (2006). A hitchhiker's guide to behavioral analysis in laboratory rodents. *Genes Brain Behav.* 5(Suppl. 2), 5–24.

Strathearn, L., Li, J., Fonagy, P., and Montague, P. R. (2008). What's in a smile? Maternal brain responses to infant facial cues. *Pediatrics* 122, 40–51.

Strathearn, L., and Mayes, L. (2010). Cocaine addiction in mothers: potential effects on maternal care and infant development. *Ann. N. Y. Acad. Sci.* 1187, 172–183.

Tankayanagi, Y., Yoshida, M., Bielsky, I. F., Ross, H. E., Kawamata, M., Onaka, T., Yanagisawa, T., Kimura, T., Matzuk, M. M., Young, L. J., and Nishimori, K. (2005). Pervasive social deficits, but normal parturition, in oxytocin receptor-deficient mice. *Proc. Natl. Acad. Sci. U.S.A.* 16096–16101.

Tattoli, M., Cagiano, R., Gaetani, S., Ghiglieri, V., Giustino, A., Mereu, G., Trabace, L., and Cuomo, V. (2001). Neurofunctional effects of developmental alcohol exposure in alcohol-preferring and alcohol-nonpreferring rats. *Neuropsychopharmacology* 691–705.

Thompson, R. R., George, K., Walton, J. C., Orr, S. P., and Benson, J. (2006). Sex-specific influences of vasopressin on human social communications. *Proc. Natl. Acad. Sci. U.S.A.* 103, 7889–7894.

Thor, D., and Holloway, W. (1984). Social play in juvenile rats: a decade of methodological and experimental research. *Neurosci. Biobehav. Rev.* 8, 455–464.

Tonkiss, J., Shumsky, J., Shultz, P., Almeida, S., and Galler, J. (1995). Prenatal cocaine but not prenatal malnutrition affects foster mother-pup interactions in rats. *Neurotoxicol. Teratol.* 17, 601–608.

Trezza, V., Baarendse, P. J., and Vanderschuren, L. J. (2010). The pleasures of play: pharmacological insights into social reward mechanisms. *Trends Pharmacol. Sci.* 31, 463–469.

Tronick, E. Z., and Beeghly, M. (1999). Prenatal cocaine exposure, child development, and the compromising effects of cumulative risk. *Clin. Perinatol.* 26, 151–171.

Tronick, E. Z., and Cohn, J. F. (1989). Infant-mother face-to-face interaction: age and gender differences in coordination and the incidence of miscoordination. *Child Dev.* 60, 85–92.

Tronick, E. Z., Messinger, D. S., Weinberg, M. K., Lester, B. M., Lagasse, L., Seifer, R., Bauer, C. R., Shankaran, S., Bada, H., Wright, L. L., Poole, K., and Liu, J. (2005). Cocaine exposure is associated with subtle compromises of infants' and mothers' social-emotional behavior and dyadic features of their interaction in the face-to-face still-face paradigm. *Dev. Psychol.* 41, 711–722.

van Gelder, M. M., Reefhuis, J., Caton, A. R., Werler, M. M., Druschel, C. M., and Roeleveld, N. (2010). Characteristics of pregnant illicit drug users and associations between cannabis use and perinatal outcome in a population-based study. *Drug Alcohol Depend.* 109, 243–247.

van Leengoed, E., Kerker, E., and Swanson, H. H. (1987). Inhibition of postpartum maternal behavior in the rat by injecting an oxytocin antagonist into the cerebral ventricles. *J. Endocrinol.* 112, 275–282.

Vernotica, E. M., Lisciotto, C. A., Rosenblatt, J. S., and Morrell, J. I. (1996). Cocaine transiently impairs maternal behavior in the rat. *Behav. Neurosci.* 110, 315–323.

Vorhees, C. V., Inman-Wood, S. L., Morford, L. L., Reed, T. M., Moran, M. S., Pu, C., and Cappon, G. D. (2000). Evaluation of neonatal exposure to cocaine on learning, activity, startle, scent marking, immobility, and plasma cocaine concentrations. *Neurotoxicol. Teratol.* 22, 255–265.

Walum, H., Westberg, L., Henningsson, S., Neiderhiser, J. M., Reiss, D., Igl, W., Ganiban, J. M., Spotts, E. L., Pederson, N. L., Eriksson, E., and Lichtenstein, P. (2008). Genetic variation in the vasopressin receptor 1a gene (AVPR1A) associates with pair-bonding behavior in humans. *Proc. Natl. Acad. Sci. U.S.A.* 105, 14153–14156.

Wasserman, D. R., and Leventhal, J. M. (1993). Mistreatment of children born to cocaine-dependent mothers. *Am. J. Dis. Child.* 147, 1324–1328.

Wellmann, K., Lewis, B., and Barron, S. (2010). Agmatine reduces ultrasonic vocalization deficits in female rat pups exposed neonatally to ethanol. *Neurotoxicol. Teratol.* 32, 158–163.

Wersinger, S. R., Kelliher, K. R., Zufall, F., Lolait, S. J., O'Carroll, A. M., and Young, W. S. (2004). Socail motivation is reduced in vasopressin 1b receptor null mice despite normal; performance in an olfactory discrimination task. *Horm. Behav.* 46, 638–645.

Wilson, J. H., Kelly, S. J., and Wilson, M. A. (1996). Early postnatal alcohol exposure in rats: maternal behavior and estradiol levels. *Physiol. Behav.* 59, 287–293.

Winslow, J. T., Hearns, E. F., Ferguson, J., Young, L. J., Matzuk, M. M., and Insel, T. R. (2000). Infant vocalization, adult aggression, and fear behavior of an oxytocin null mutant mouse. *Horm. Behav.* 37, 145–155.

Winslow, J. T., and Insel, T. R. (2002). The social deficits of the oxytocin knockout mouse. *Neuropeptides* 36, 221–229.

Wolf, J. B., Leamy, L. J., Roseman, C. C., and Cheverud, J. M. (2011). Disentangling prenatal and postnatal maternal genetic effects reveals persistent prenatal effects on offspring growth in mice. *Genetics* 189, 1069–1082.

Wood, R. D., Bannoura, M. D., and Johanson, I. B. (1994). Prenatal cocaine exposure: effects on play behavior in the juvenile rat. *Neurotoxicol. Teratol.* 16, 139–144.

Wood, R. D., Molina, V. A., Wagner, J. M., and Spear, L. P. (1995). Play behavior and stress responsivity in periadolescent offspring exposed prenatally to cocaine. *Pharmacol. Biochem. Behav.* 52, 367–374.

Wood, R. D., and Spear, L. P. (1998). Prenatal cocaine alters social competition of infant, adolescent and adult rats. *Behav. Neurosci.* 112, 419–431.

Young, W. S. III, Shepard, E., Amico, J., Hennighausen, L., Wagner, K. U., LaMarca, M. E., McKinney, C., and Ginns, E. I. (1996). Deficiency in mouse oxytocin prevents milk ejection, but not fertility or parturition. *J. Neuroendocrinol.* 8, 847–853.

Young, L. J., and Wang, Z. (2004). The neurobiology of pair-bonding. *Nature Neurosci.* 7, 1048–1054.

The impact of childhood maltreatment: A review of neurobiological and genetic factors

Eamon McCrory[1,2]*, Stephane A. De Brito[1,2] and Essi Viding[1]

[1] *Developmental Risk and Resilience Unit, Division of Psychology and Language Sciences, University College London, London, UK*
[2] *Research Programme, The Anna Freud Centre, London, UK*

*Correspondence:
Eamon McCrory, Developmental Risk and Resilience Unit, Division of Psychology and Language Sciences, University College London, 26 Bedford Way, London WC1H 0AP, UK.
e-mail: e.mccrory@ucl.ac.uk

Childhood maltreatment represents a significant risk factor for psychopathology. Recent research has begun to examine both the functional and structural neurobiological correlates of adverse care-giving experiences, including maltreatment, and how these might impact on a child's psychological and emotional development. The relationship between such experiences and risk for psychopathology has been shown to vary as a function of genetic factors. In this review we begin by providing a brief overview of neuroendocrine findings, which indicate an association between maltreatment and atypical development of the hypothalamic–pituitary–adrenal axis stress response, which may predispose to psychiatric vulnerability in adulthood. We then selectively review the magnetic resonance imaging (MRI) studies that have investigated possible structural and functional brain differences in children and adults who have experienced childhood maltreatment. Differences in the corpus callosum identified by structural MRI have now been reliably reported in children who have experienced abuse, while differences in the hippocampus have been reported in adults with childhood histories of maltreatment. In addition, there is preliminary evidence from functional MRI studies of adults who have experienced childhood maltreatment of amygdala hyperactivity and atypical activation of frontal regions. These functional differences can be partly understood in the context of the information biases observed in event-related potential and behavioral studies of physically abused children. Finally we consider research that has indicated that the effect of environmental adversity may be moderated by genotype, reviewing pertinent studies pointing to gene by environment interactions. We conclude by exploring the extent to which the growing evidence base in relation to neurobiological and genetic research may be relevant to clinical practice and intervention.

Keywords: child abuse, maltreatment, neuroscience, MRI, genetics, HPA, psychopathology, resilience

INTRODUCTION

Early adversity, and in particular childhood maltreatment, has been reliably associated with an increased risk of poor outcome across a range of domains, including, physical and mental health, social and academic functioning, and economic productivity (e.g., Lansford et al., 2002; Shirtcliff et al., 2009; Currie and Widom, 2010). Over the last decade, new techniques have allowed researchers to investigate the possible impact of such adversity on both brain structure and function (e.g., Teicher et al., 2003; Caspi and Moffitt, 2006; Lupien et al., 2009). The aim of this review is to present a concise overview of those studies that have investigated the neurobiological impact of childhood maltreatment. Neuroendocrine, neuroimaging, and genetic factors are considered in turn. Space constraints mean that it is not possible to widen the focus to include many related studies of institutionalization or neglect (see instead Gunnar et al., 2006; Neigh et al., 2009). Rather, the primary focus of this review relates to the experience of childhood maltreatment, defined as an experience of physical, sexual, or emotional abuse. However, we occasionally highlight investigations of institutionalization in contexts where there remains a paucity maltreatment-related research (notably in the field of functional resonance imaging)

We first provide a short overview of the hypothalamic–pituitary–adrenal (HPA) axis stress response before considering evidence that maltreatment may alter the functioning of this system in children and adults. The second and third sections review the evidence for changes at the level of regional brain structure and function, respectively. We then consider the evidence from genetic studies, including investigations of gene by environment (GxE) interactions and epigenetic effects in humans and animals, relating these to possible mechanisms associated with vulnerability and resilience. The final sections of the review seek to consider the limitations of current research and consider the degree to which neurobiological research can help advance our clinical understanding of the impact of maltreatment.

STRESS SYSTEMS AND EARLY ADVERSITY
MALTREATMENT AND THE HPA SYSTEM

The HPA axis represents one of the body's core stress response systems. Exposure to stress triggers release of corticotrophin releasing hormone (CRH) and arginine vasopressin (AVP) release from the paraventricular nucleus of the hypothalamus, which in turn stimulate secretion of adrenocortico-trophic hormone (ACTH) that acts on the adrenal cortex to synthesize cortisol. Feedback loops at several levels ensure that the system is returned to homeostasis since chronically elevated cortisol levels can have deleterious effects on health (Lupien et al., 1998).

CHILDREN WHO HAVE EXPERIENCED MALTREATMENT

Findings from studies investigating HPA axis activity in children and adolescents with a history of maltreatment are mixed (Tarullo and Gunnar, 2006). For example, in one study of HPA axis response to CRH stimulus (Kaufman et al., 1997) reported ACTH hyper-responsiveness, but only among a subsample of maltreated children who were depressed and still exposed to a stressful home environment; no differences were found in cortisol measures. By contrast, Hart et al. (1995) in a study of preschoolers who had experienced maltreatment reported a pattern of cortisol suppression in situations of stress that was associated with social competence.

Most studies have collected basal cortisol level data given the ethical and practical implications of pharmacological challenge tests with children. Several studies have reported elevated basal cortisol levels (De Bellis et al., 1999a; Cicchetti and Rogosch, 2001; Carrion et al., 2002) while others have reported cortical suppression (Hart et al., 1995). One explanation for these apparently contradictory findings is that elevation is associated with the presence of a concurrent affective disorder (Tarullo and Gunnar, 2006). For example, two studies have reported a rise in cortisol levels across the day for maltreated children with depression, but no effects in maltreated children without depression (Kaufman, 1991; Hart et al., 1996). This pattern is also consistent with the elevated ACTH response to CRH in the maltreated-depressed group noted above (Kaufman et al., 1997). Other studies have reported similar elevations in relation to maltreated children with post-traumatic stress disorder (PTSD; Carrion et al., 2002) and dysthymic girls who had been sexually abused (De Bellis et al., 1994). While this pattern of elevated cortisol also characterizes non-maltreated children with affective disorders (e.g., Goodyer et al., 1998) it is not clear if maltreatment contributes an additional effect (Cicchetti and Rogosch, 2001; Cicchetti et al., 2001). It should also be noted that several studies of children with antisocial behavior have reported reduced basal cortisol concentrations and lower cortisol levels when exposed to stress (see van Goozen and Fairchild, 2008, for a comprehensive review). It is possible that that exposure to early adversity in these children leads to a pattern of stress habituation over time, a pattern that increases the risk of difficulties in emotional and behavioral regulation; equally, reduced stress responsivity may emerge as a result of genetic factors, or GxE interactions (van Goozen and Fairchild, 2008).

ADULTS WHO HAVE EXPERIENCED MALTREATMENT AS CHILDREN

Heim and colleagues propose that childhood maltreatment increases the risk of developing depression due to a sensitization of the neurobiological systems implicated in stress adaptation and response (Heim et al., 2008). In an early study using the standardized Treir Social Stress Test (requiring public speaking and mental arithmetic) they reported that women with a history of maltreatment with and without depression exhibited an increased ACTH response compared with controls (Heim et al., 2002). A history of childhood abuse was found to be the strongest predictor of ACTH responsiveness; this was amplified by the experience of further trauma in adulthood (Heim et al., 2002). More recently, Heim et al. (2008) used the combined pharmacological test of HPA functioning (the dexamethasone/CRF challenge) with a sample of men with and without childhood maltreatment and current depression. A pattern of increased cortisol response was reported in the context of a failure of the glucocorticoid-mediated negative feedback loop to adequately control HPA activation (Heim et al., 2008). These studies suggest that major depression subsequent to childhood maltreatment is associated with inadequate inhibitory feedback regulation of the HPA axis. We know from animal models that low levels of maternal care are associated with reduced concentration of glucocorticoid receptors in the hippocampus (Liu et al., 1997); it is thus possible that a similar mechanism may account, at least in part, for the observed changes in HPA regulation in humans following maltreatment.

A parallel set of research studies has investigated PTSD in a wide range of populations including those with a prior history of maltreatment. Findings from this literature have been mixed at best (Shea et al., 2004); however a recent systematic review and meta-analysis supports the view that PTSD is associated with a general pattern of hypocortisolism, with reduced cortisol levels, at least in the afternoon (Meewisse et al., 2007). Furthermore, Meewisse et al. (2007) highlight the relationship between lower cortisol levels and PTSD in the context of physical and sexual forms of abuse. These findings therefore indicate a possible distinct patterns of adaptation across the two disorders, with HPA hypoactivity characterizing those with maltreatment-related PTSD (Meewisse et al., 2007) and hyperactivity of the HPA system characterizing maltreated individuals presenting with depression (e.g., Heim et al., 2002). These differing patterns may in part reflect adaptations of the HPA axis to different forms of maltreatment, different periods of onset and chronicity, and differential genetic susceptibility. Equally, methodological confounds may account for some of the reported differences, including the frequently observed comorbidity of depression and PTSD (Newport et al., 2004).

SUMMARY: STRESS SYSTEMS AND EARLY ADVERSITY

Early trauma, including physical, sexual, and emotional abuse is associated with increased risk of psychopathology in childhood and adulthood, as well as social and health problems (Gilbert et al., 2009). There is persuasive evidence from human (and animal) studies of a link between early stress and atypical HPA functioning. Specifically, it appears that childhood maltreatment may lead to atypical responsiveness of the HPA axis to stress, which in turn predisposes to psychiatric vulnerability in later life (van Goozen and Fairchild, 2008). While there is general agreement around this broad principle, the putative mechanisms of how dysregulation of the HPA axis might mediate the link between stress and psychopathology and the precise nature of any interaction remain less clear (see Miller et al., 2007). It is possible that diminished cortisol responsiveness (for example) may emerge if early chronic stress leads to an initial hyper-activation of the HPA system which then progresses over time to a state of hyporeactivity, as a form of adaptation following sustained exposure to ACTH (e.g., Fries et al., 2005).

STRUCTURAL BRAIN DIFFERENCES ASSOCIATED WITH MALTREATMENT

A growing body of research has investigated how stress, and specifically different forms of childhood maltreatment, can influence neural structure and function. These studies have employed both children who have experienced maltreatment and adults reporting childhood histories of early adversity. In the following section we first consider those studies that have investigated differences in brain structure, before considering the evidence from the smaller number of studies that have investigated the impact on brain function.

HIPPOCAMPUS
Children who have experienced maltreatment
A substantial body of animal research has shown that the hippocampus plays a central role in learning and various aspects of memory (Mizomuri et al., 2007) and that memory function is impaired in animals that have been exposed to chronic stress (McEwen, 1999). De Bellis et al. (1999b) were the first to report that maltreated children with PTSD presented with smaller intracranial and cerebral volumes, smaller corpus callosum (CC) and larger lateral ventricular volume compared to healthy, non-maltreated children. It was notable that the expected decrease in hippocampal volume, based on previous studies of adults with PTSD was not observed. Since that time, over 10 structural MRI (sMRI) studies of children and adolescents with PTSD following maltreatment have consistently failed to detect the adult pattern of lower hippocampal volume (e.g., Carrion et al., 2001; Woon and Hedges, 2008; Jackowski et al., 2009; Mehta et al., 2009).

Adults who have experienced maltreatment as children
By contrast, with the exception of one study (Pederson et al., 2004), reduced volume of the hippocampus has generally been reported for adults who have experienced maltreatment as children (Vythilingam et al., 2002; Vermetten et al., 2006; Woon and Hedges, 2008). Two explanations have been proposed to account for the discrepancy of child and adult findings (see Lupien et al., 2009). The *neurotoxicity hypothesis*, based on data from both animal and human studies, postulates that stress-induced prolonged exposure to glucocorticoids can lead to a reduction in hippocampal cell complexity and even lead to cell death (e.g., Sapolsky et al., 1990). Thus, it is possible that in humans, hippocampal volume reduction may result from years or decades of PTSD or chronic stress. In support of this hypothesis, (Carrion et al., 2007) in a longitudinal study reported that cortisol levels and PTSD symptoms at baseline predicted the degree of hippocampal volume reduction over an ensuing 12- to 18-month interval in 15 maltreated children with PTSD. Alternatively, the *vulnerability hypothesis* posits that a smaller hippocampal volume in individuals with PTSD is not a consequence of stress, but rather a predisposing risk factor for the disorder present in some individuals prior to any traumatic experience (e.g., Gilbertson et al., 2002). Further longitudinal studies and studies taking advantage of identical twins discordant for maltreatment exposure are required to distinguish between these competing accounts.

AMYGDALA
Children who have experienced maltreatment
The amygdala plays a key role in evaluating potentially threatening information, fear conditioning, emotional processing, and memory for emotional events (Phelps and LeDoux, 2005). In animal studies chronic stress has been shown to increase dendritic arborization in the amygdala (e.g., Vyas et al., 2003). It would therefore seem reasonable to predict that differences in amygdala structure would be associated with childhood maltreatment (Lupien et al., 2009). Until recently there was a consensus that children with maltreatment-related PTSD did not differ in terms of amygdala volume compared to non-maltreated children (Woon and Hedges, 2008). However, two recent studies have reported increased amygdala volumes in children and adolescents who had experienced early institutionalization and subsequent adoption. Mehta et al. (2009) reported greater amygdala volume in 14 adoptee adolescents who had experienced severe early institutional deprivation in Romania compared to a group of non-deprived, non-adopted UK controls. Similarly (Tottenham et al., 2010) reported greater amygdala volume in 17 mainly preadolescent children who had been adopted out of an orphanage when older that 15 months compared to non-adopted controls or early adopted children. A significant correlation is also reported between amygdala volume and age of adoption, suggesting that early and extended exposure to institutionalized care may lead to atypical development of limbic circuitry. It is noteworthy that the effects of early adversity on the amygdala in these two studies were observed even many years after the adversity had ceased, which is in line with evidence from animal research (Lupien et al., 2009).

Adults who have experienced maltreatment as children
To date only three studies have examined amygdala volume in adults with a history of childhood maltreatment; one found reduced volume in female patients with dissociative identity disorder as compared to healthy females (Vermetten et al., 2006) while the other two reported no measurable differences (Bremner et al., 1997; Andersen et al., 2008). While it is too early to draw definitive conclusions regarding impact of maltreatment on amygdala development, these preliminary findings suggest that the amygdala is vulnerable to early and severe stress in the context of parental loss and institutionalization. However, it appears that less severe, time-limited, and developmentally later exposure has a weaker impact on amygdala volume.

CORPUS CALLOSUM AND OTHER WHITE MATTER TRACTS
Children who have experienced maltreatment
The CC is the largest white matter structure in the brain and controls inter-hemispheric communication of a host of processes, including, but not limited to, arousal, emotion, and higher cognitive abilities (Kitterle, 1995; Giedd et al., 1996). Crucially, in terms of development, nerve fiber connections passing though this region are fully formed before birth with myelination continuing throughout childhood and adulthood (Giedd et al., 1996; Teicher et al., 2004). Teicher et al. (2004) have speculated that different regions of the CC might have different windows of vulnerability to early experience. With the exception of one study (Mehta et al., 2009), decreases in CC volume (particularly middle and posterior

regions) have consistently been reported in maltreated children and adolescents compared to non-maltreated peers (De Bellis et al., 1999b, 2002; De Bellis and Keshavan, 2003; Teicher et al., 2004; Jackowski et al., 2008). Furthermore, preliminary evidence suggests that these effects are characterized by sex-dependent differences (De Bellis and Keshavan, 2003; Teicher et al., 2004). It may be speculated that these structural abnormalities within the CC may be associated with some of the emotional and cognitive impairments that have been reported in maltreated individuals (e.g., Pears et al., 2008).

A recent study that employed diffusion tensor imaging (DTI) found decreased fractional anisotropy values (indicative of decreased white matter fiber tracts coherence or lower density of white matter fiber tracts) in maltreated children in frontal and temporal white matter regions, as compared to non-maltreated children (Govindan et al., 2010). Similar to an earlier DTI study in maltreated children (Eluvathingal et al., 2006), group differences were also observed in the uncinate fasciculus, which connects the orbitofrontal cortex (OFC) to the anterior temporal lobe, including the amygdala (Govindan et al., 2010). Interestingly, the reduction in fractional anisotropy observed by Govindan and colleagues was associated with longer periods within an orphanage and may partly underpin some of the cognitive and socioemotional impairments associated with early severe deprivation.

Adults who have experienced maltreatment as children
A study of adult females with maltreatment-related PTSD has also reported smaller area of the posterior midbody of the CC as compared to healthy controls (Kitayama et al., 2007). More recently, a recent DTI study in a non-clinical sample examined the effects of severe parental verbal abuse (e.g., ridicule, humiliation, and disdain) on brain connectivity; three white matter tracts were reported to show reduced fractional anisotropy (Choi et al., 2009). Again, the researchers hypothesized that these abnormalities may underlie some of the language and emotional regulation difficulties seen in victims of childhood maltreatment.

PREFRONTAL CORTEX
Children who have experienced maltreatment
The prefrontal cortex (PFC) is extensively interconnected with other cortical and subcortical regions consistent with its major role in the control of many aspects of behavior, cognition, and emotion regulation (Fuster, 1997; Davidson et al., 2000; Miller and Cohen, 2001). There are mixed findings from studies comparing PFC volume of children with maltreatment-related PTSD and non-maltreated children. One study reported no group difference (De Bellis et al., 1999b), but another found smaller prefrontal volume and prefrontal white matter (De Bellis et al., 2002) in the maltreated group, while the two most recent studies – one using voxel-based morphometry (VBM; provides a measure of regional volume differences by analyzing spatially normalized brain segments on a voxel-wise basis) investigating PTSD – observed larger gray matter volume of the middle-inferior and ventral regions of the PFC in the clinical groups (Richert et al., 2006; Carrion et al., 2009).

Tensor-based morphometry (TBM) provides a measure of regional volume by examining regional shape differences via analyses of the deformation fields. A recent study used TBM to compare 31 children with documented histories of physical abuse without PTSD to 41 non-abused children matched for age, pubertal stage, and gender (Hanson et al., 2010). One of the largest reported differences was observed in the right OFC. The abused group were found to have significantly smaller brain volumes in this region, differences which in turn correlated with poorer social functioning. Given that the OFC is known to play a key role in emotion and social regulation, the authors suggest that these alterations in OFC structure may partly represent the biological mechanism linking early social learning to later behavioral outcomes. However, we know that cortical thickness of the OFC is susceptible to thinning following prenatal exposure to maternal cigaret smoking and to drug taking, risk factors likely to characterize a proportion of those in a maltreated sample (Lotfipour et al., 2009). Further research will be necessary to tease apart possible risk factors that may influence structural development of this region.

A lack of consistency regarding observed structural differences in the PFC may relate to methodological differences, sample differences in age range of participants, variation in maltreatment type and chronicity, and a focus on different regions within the PFC. In addition, while it is likely that there are specific windows of vulnerability in brain development, we know little about how maltreatment at different points in development impacts different brain regions. In a unique cross-sectional study, Andersen et al. (2008) found that gray matter volume of the frontal cortex was maximally affected by abuse at ages 14–16 years, while the hippocampus and CC were maximally affected at ages 3–5 and 9–10 years respectively, indicating that the frontal cortex in this sample was particularly susceptible to structural change following abuse during the adolescent period. Further work exploring how regional brain differences may emerge depending on the timing of maltreatment is essential if we are to formulate a developmentally informed picture of the impact of such adversity on neurobiological development.

Adults who have experienced maltreatment as children
In contrast to the studies on maltreated children, decreased PFC volume in adults with a history of childhood maltreatment has been a consistent finding. For example, in a non-clinical sample, Tomoda et al. (2009) found that harsh childhood corporal punishment was associated with reduced gray matter volume in the left dorsolateral PFC and the right medial PFC, two brain regions central to higher cognitive processing, such as working memory and to aspects of social cognition, respectively (Miller and Cohen, 2001; Amodio and Frith, 2006). In another study, in comparison to healthy individuals, patients with major depressive disorder who reported a history of childhood maltreatment exhibited reduced volume of the rostral anterior cingulate cortex (ACC), which was negatively correlated with both cortisol levels and maltreatment severity (Treadway et al., 2009). Despite important limitations (such as the lack of information on the age of onset and duration of maltreatment) this study suggests that the rostral ACC, like the hippocampus, might be vulnerable to prolonged glucocorticoid exposure resulting from chronic stress, which in turn may decrease its ability to exert negative feedback control over HPA regulation (Treadway et al., 2009). Finally, a recent study compared healthy

controls and patients with depression and/or anxiety disorders reporting childhood emotional maltreatment before age 16 to a group composed of healthy controls and patients who reported no childhood abuse (van Harmelen et al., 2010). The authors reported that emotional abuse was associated with a reduction in left dorsal medial PFC, even in the absence of physical or sexual abuse in childhood. Crucially, this group difference was independent of gender and could not be attributed to current psychopathology, which support the idea that the observed brain differences might be associated with the experience of maltreatment.

SUMMARY: STRUCTURAL BRAIN DIFFERENCES ASSOCIATED WITH MALTREATMENT

The findings from the structural studies reviewed above are summarized in **Table 1**. It is clear that there is relatively consistent evidence for reduced CC volume in children and adults who have experienced adversity, some evidence of greater amygdala volume in late-adopted previously institutionalized children, and a relatively clear pattern of normal hippocampal volume during childhood, which contrasts with the consistent finding of reduced hippocampal volume seen in adults with histories of abuse. It has recently been suggested that variations in developmental timing and age of measurement may partly account for the observed variability in the findings for structural differences in the amygdala and hippocampus (Tottenham and Sheridan, 2010). The structural findings are more mixed for the PFC in maltreated children, but there is a consistent pattern of decreased PFC volume among adults with childhood histories of maltreatment. However, a recent finding highlights that structural differences in the OFC may be linked to degree of social difficulty in physically abused children even in the absence of PTSD (Hanson et al., 2010).

FUNCTIONAL BRAIN DIFFERENCES ASSOCIATED WITH MALTREATMENT

CHILDREN WHO HAVE EXPERIENCED MALTREATMENT

In contrast to the research examining structural brain differences associated with maltreatment, there are as yet relatively few that have used functional MRI (fMRI). To date, only five fMRI studies have investigated children exposed to early adversity, and only two from the same research group have recruited children who have experienced maltreatment. These studies by Carrion and colleagues investigated cognitively oriented processes. The first, which compared youths with post-traumatic stress symptoms (PTSS) secondary to maltreatment (i.e., trauma related to physical and sexual abuse and exposure to violence) with healthy controls, investigated response inhibition (Carrion et al., 2008). Increased activation in the ACC was reported in maltreated participants as compared to controls. This result is consistent with a model in which impaired cognitive control arises in the context of heightened subcortical reactivity to negative affect, potentially conferring an increased risk for psychopathology (Mueller et al., 2010). The second study used a verbal declarative memory task and compared youths with PTSS secondary to maltreatment with healthy controls (Carrion et al., 2010). During the retrieval component of the task, the youths with PTSS exhibited reduced right hippocampal activity, which was associated with greater severity of avoidance and numbing symptoms.

Three other fMRI studies have investigated the impact of early institutionalization. Using an emotional face processing paradigm, children exposed to such adversity were found to exhibit increased amygdala response to threatening facial cues (Maheu et al., 2010; Tottenham et al., 2011). It is not yet clear if these findings of atypical emotional processing generalize to children who have experienced maltreatment, such as physical, sexual, and emotional abuse. Another study assessed response inhibition and observed increased activation in the ACC in previously institutionalized children as compared to controls (Mueller et al., 2010).

While the main strength of fMRI is its good spatial resolution in relation to brain activity, event-related potentials (ERP) record the brain's electrical activity and yield detailed information about the temporal sequence (resolution in milliseconds) of cognitive operations throughout the brain (i.e., mental chronometry). Much of the existing ERP research has compared the pattern of brain response of maltreated children and healthy children when processing facial expressions, an ability that is usually mastered by the preschool years (Izard and Harris, 1995). When compared with never institutionalized children, institutionalized children who have experienced severe social deprivation show a pattern of cortical hypoactivation when viewing emotional facial expressions (Parker and Nelson, 2005), and familiar and unfamiliar faces (Parker et al., 2005). A second set of important studies by Pollak and colleagues has demonstrated that school-aged children who had been exposed to physical abuse allocate more attention to angry faces (Pollak et al., 1997, 2001) and require more attentional resources to disengage from such stimuli (Pollak and Tolley-Schell, 2003) leading to problems with emotional regulation that may predispose to anxiety (Shackman et al., 2007). Findings consistent with this pattern have also been obtained with toddlers who experienced maltreatment in their first year of life (Cicchetti and Curtis, 2005). It appears therefore that some maltreated children allocate more resources and remain hyper-vigilant to social threat cues in their environment, potentially at the cost of other developmental processes.

ADULTS WHO HAVE EXPERIENCED MALTREATMENT AS CHILDREN

Three fMRI studies using a range of paradigms have compared adults with a history of childhood maltreatment to adults without such a history. Using a flanker task with face stimuli, Grant et al. (2011) observed a robust positive correlation between physical abuse and right amygdala response to sad faces in sample including 20 patients with depression and 16 healthy controls. Importantly, group differences indicated that heightened amygdala response to sad faces was not a characteristic of individuals with depression, but rather of those with a significant history of maltreatment. This pattern of amygdala response to negative faces is consistent with that observed in maltreated children in the studies reviewed above. Dillon et al. (2009) recently investigated reward processing using a monetary incentive delay task and found that adults with a history of childhood maltreatment, relative to peers with no history of adversity, reported higher depressive symptoms, rated reward-predicting cues as less positive, and exhibited a blunted brain response to reward cues in the left pallidus. According to the authors, this result suggests a possible link between childhood adversity and later depressive psychopathology. Given the overlap

Table 1 | Structural magnetic resonance brain imaging studies comparing maltreated to non-maltreated individuals.

Brain regions	Studies[#]	ED	Mean age years	Sample	Summary of results
HIPP	De Bellis et al. (1999b)	No	12.1	44 MP vs. 61 NM	n.s.
	Carrion et al. (2001)	No	11.0	24 MP vs. 24 NM	n.s.
	Mehta et al. (2009)	Yes	16.1	14 M vs. 11 NM	n.s.
	Carrion et al. (2007)	No	10.4	15 MP	Cortisol levels and PTSD symptoms predicted the degree of hippocampal volume reduction
	Pederson et al. (2004)	No	25.1	17 MP vs. 17 M vs. 17 NM	n.s.
	Vythilingam et al. (2002)	No	31.3	21 MD vs. 11 DEP vs. 14 NM	MD < DEP = NM, left hippocampus, right hippocampus: n.s.
	Vermetten et al. (2006)	No	38.7	15 MDI vs. 23 NM	M < NM, left and right hippocampus
AMY	Mehta et al. (2009)	Yes	16.1	14 M vs. 11 NM	M > NM, right amygdala, left amygdala: trend
	Tottenham et al. (2010)	Yes	9.0	34 M vs. 26 NM	M > NM, but only for those adopted after 15 months of age ($n = 17$)
	Vermetten et al. (2006)	No	38.7	15 MDI vs. 23 NM	M < NM, left and right amygdala
	Bremner et al. (1997)	No	41.3	17 MP vs. 17 NM	n.s.
	Andersen et al. (2008)	No	19.7	26 M vs. 17 NM	n.s.
CC/WM	Mehta et al. (2009)	Yes	16.1	14 M vs. 11 NM	n.s.
	De Bellis et al. (1999b)	No	12.1	44 MP vs. 61 NM	M < NM
	De Bellis et al. (2002)	No	11.5	28 MP vs. 66 NM	M < NM
	De Bellis and Keshavan (2003)	No		67 MP vs. 122 NM	M < NM
	Teicher et al. (2004)	No	12.4	51 M vs. 115 NM	M < NM
	Jackowski et al. (2008)	No	10.6	17 MP vs. 15 NM	M < NM
	Govindan et al. (2010)	Yes	11.3	17 M vs. 15 NM	M < NM, FA values in left/right UF, left/right SLF, left/right AF
	Eluvathingal et al. (2006)	Yes	10.2	7 M vs. 7 NM	M < NM, FA values in left uncinate fasciculus
	Kitayama et al. (2007)	No	37.3	9 MP vs. 9 NM	M < NM, area of the posterior midbody of the corpus callosum
	Choi et al. (2009)	No	21.5	16 M vs. 16 NM	M < NM, FA values in left arcuate fasciculus, left cingulum bundle, left body of the fornix
PFC	De Bellis et al. (1999b)	No	12.1	44 MP vs. 61 NM	n.s.
	De Bellis et al. (2002)	No	11.5	28 MP vs. 66 NM	M < NM, PFC volume and PFC white matter
	Richert et al. (2006)	No	11.0	23 MP vs. 23 NM	M > NM, GMV in the middle-inferior and ventral regions of the PFC
	Carrion et al. (2009)*	No	11.0	24 MP vs. 24 NM	Manual tracing: M > NM, GMV in left/right/superior/inferior regions of the PFC; VBM: M > NM, volume of ventral PFC
	Hanson et al. (2010)**	No	11.9	31 M vs. 41 NM	M < NM, orbitofrontal cortex GMV, which correlated negatively with social functioning difficulties
	Tomoda et al. (2009)*	No	21.7	23 M vs. 22 NM	M < NM, gray matter volume in the left dorsolateral PFC and the right medial PFC
	Treadway et al. (2009)*	No	32.8	19 MD vs. 19 NM	M < NM, reduced volume of the rostral ACC
	van Harmelen et al. (2010)*	No	37.6	84 M vs. 97 NM	M < NM, left dorsal medial PFC

ACC, anterior cingulate cortex; AF, arcuate fasciculus; AMY, Amygdala; CC, corpus callosum; DEP, depression; ED, early deprivation; GMV, gray matter volume; HIPP, hippocampus; M, maltreated; MD, maltreated with depression; MDI, maltreated with dissociation; MP, maltreated with PTSD/PTSD symptomatology; NM, non-maltreated; n.s., not statistically significant; PFC, prefrontal cortex; PTSD, post-traumatic stress disorder; SLF, superior longitudinal fasciculus; UF, uncinate fasciculus; VBM, voxel-based morphometry; WM, white matter.
[#]All the studies used manual tracing to define their region of interest except: * Voxel-based morphometry; ** Tensor-based morphometry.

between the brain regions previously identified in sMRI studies in maltreated populations and the projection area of the olfactory system, such as the amygdala, OFC, and hippocampus, Croy et al. (2010) compared neural response to neutral and pleasant olfactory stimulation between female patients from a psychosomatic clinic with ($n = 12$) and without ($n = 10$) a history of childhood abuse. Results indicated that, despite similar group ratings for hedonic and intensity values of the stimuli and normal neural activation in olfactory projection areas, patients with a history of childhood maltreatment displayed increased activation in the posterior cingulate cortex and decreased activation in the subgenual ACC, possibly indicative of altered processing of non-traumatic stimuli.

SUMMARY: FUNCTIONAL BRAIN DIFFERENCES ASSOCIATED WITH MALTREATMENT

Studies of adults using fMRI suggest that the experience of maltreatment may be associated with hyperactivity of the amygdala in response to negative facial affect; such an effect has also been reported in children who have experienced early institutionalization. Studies of maltreated children that have examined response inhibition have observed increased activity in the ACC. The findings from these fMRI studies of children and adults are summarized in **Table 2**. ERP studies have found increased responses to angry faces in prefrontal regions consistent with increased attentional monitoring for social threat.

THE GENETICS OF RESILIENCE AND VULNERABILITY
DO GENETIC DIFFERENCES ACCOUNT FOR INDIVIDUAL DIFFERENCES IN RESILIENCE AND VULNERABILITY?

Many recent studies have measured the biological impact of environmental adversity by taking into account genetic differences that may constrain the stress response and increase the likelihood of resilience vs. vulnerability following maltreatment (Moffitt et al., 2005). Twin and adoption studies have demonstrated that many of the psychiatric outcomes that are associated with maltreatment, such as PTSD, depression, and antisocial behavior, are partly heritable (e.g., Sullivan et al., 2000; Rhee and Waldman, 2002; Koenen et al., 2008). In other words, individual differences in susceptibility to these disorders are partly driven by genetic influences. Despite demonstrable heritable influences, it is not the case that there are genes for PTSD, depression, or antisocial behavior. Rather, there are genetic variants each adding a small increment to the probability that someone may develop or be protected from developing a psychiatric disorder (Plomin et al., 1994). It is believed that these genetic variants act across the lifespan by biasing the functioning of several brain and hormonal circuits, which mediate the body's response to stress (Viding et al., 2006).

For example, linkage and association studies have implicated variants within several genes, such as monoamine oxidase-A (MAOA), Brain-Derived Neurotrophic Factor (BDNF), serotonin transporter (5-HTT), and catechol-O-methyl transferase (COMT) in the etiology of PTSD, depression, and antisocial behavior (e.g., Craig, 2007; Feder et al., 2009). Several issues should be borne in mind when considering these genetic findings. Firstly, for every study reporting a positive association between a gene and a disorder there seem to be an equal or larger number of negative findings. This is not surprising. Given the assumed small main effect of any single gene on behavioral outcome, the reliable detection of a main effect will require a degree of statistical power that is beyond most existing studies. Secondly, although the genes influencing stress reactivity are likely to act in an additive manner, gene–gene interactions have also been reported to drive individual differences in stress reactivity; for example, carrying two risk-associated gene variants may confer a greater level of vulnerability to stress reactivity compared to the combined risk conferred by each separately (e.g., Kaufman et al., 2006). Thirdly, several GxE interaction studies have demonstrated that in addition to conferring vulnerability to environmental adversity, genetic make-up can

Table 2 | Functional magnetic resonance brain imaging studies comparing maltreated to non-maltreated individuals.

Studies	ED	Mean age years	Sample	Task	Summary of results
Maheu et al. (2010)	Yes	13.6	11 M vs. 19 NM	FP	M > NM, left amygdala in response to fearful and angry faces, right amygdala: n.s.
Tottenham et al. (2011)	Yes	10.1	22 M vs. 22 NM	FP	M > NM, in left and right amygdala in response to fearful faces
Carrion et al. (2008)	No	13.5	16 MP vs. 16 NM	GNG	M > NM, in left and right ACC when in contrast no-go minus go trials
Mueller et al. (2010)	Yes	13.0	12 M vs. 21 NM	STOP	M > NM, in left and right ACC when contrast correct change minus correct go
Carrion et al. (2010)	No	13.9	16 MP vs. 11 NM	VDM	M < NM, right HIPP activity negatively correlated with symptoms severity, left HIPP: n.s.
Grant et al. (2011)	No	32.8	10 MD vs. 10 M vs. 16 NM	FTF	M > MD = NM, in right amygdala response to sad faces, left amygdala: n.s.
Dillon et al. (2009)	No	30.8	13 M vs. 21 NM	R/L-P	M < NM, blunted brain response to reward cues in the left pallidus
Croy et al. (2010)	No	39.9	12 M vs. 10 NM	OS	M > NM, increased activation in posterior cingulate cortex and decreased activation in subgenual ACC

ACC, anterior cingulate cortex; ED, early deprivation; FP, face processing; FTF, Flanker task with face stimuli; GNG = Go/No-go; M, maltreated; MD, maltreated with depression; MP, maltreated with PTSD/PTSD symptomatology; NM, non-maltreated; R/L-P, reward/loss processing; STOP, stop task; VDM, verbal declarative memory.

also denote resilience. Finally, the vulnerability effects exerted by the genes do not appear to be disorder specific. In other words, the same risk genes are often implicated in the etiology of several disorders associated with maltreatment/adversity. For example, 5-HTT has been associated with PTSD, depression, and antisocial behavior (e.g., Cicchetti et al., 2007; Feder et al., 2009).

THE INTERACTION OF GENES AND ENVIRONMENT IN CONFERRING RISK OR RESILIENCE

There is intuitive appeal of a biologically driven predisposition (genes) interacting with environmental factors to produce an individual's phenotype (i.e., the classic notion put forward by the stress-diathesis model). GxE research has taken off in recent years following the first seminal reports of gene–environment interaction by Caspi et al. (2002). Much of this work has focused on outcomes of early stress and maltreatment as a function of genotype. Caspi et al. (2002) were the first to report on an interaction of a measured genotype (MAOA) and environment (maltreatment) for a psychiatric outcome and demonstrated that individuals who are carriers of the low activity allele (MAOA-l), but not of the high activity allele (MAOA-H), are at an increased risk for antisocial behavior disorders following maltreatment.

This finding has since been replicated by several other research groups (see Taylor and Kim-Cohen, 2007; Weder et al., 2009) and imaging genetic studies have found that the risk, MAOA-l, genotype is related to hyper-responsivity of the brain's threat detection system and reduced activation in emotion regulation circuits, as well as to structural differences (in males) in key regulatory regions, such as OFC (Meyer-Lindenberg et al., 2006). This work suggests that a mechanism by which MAOA genotype engenders vulnerability to (reactive) aggression following maltreatment may include increased and poorly regulated neural reactivity to threat cues in the environment (Viding and Frith, 2006).

These studies suggest that genotypes potentially serve as predictors of both risk and resilience for adult psychiatric outcomes for people who have survived childhood maltreatment and abuse. GxE research has also suggested that positive environmental influences, such as social support, can buffer genetic and environmental risk for psychopathology and promote resiliency. Kaufman et al. (2006) demonstrated that children with genetic vulnerability (BDNF met allele and two 5-HTT short alleles) and environmental risk (maltreatment) were less likely to develop depression if they had social support. This finding illustrates the importance of considering positive environmental influences (such as contact with a supportive attachment figure) and how these may be protective even in the context of genetic vulnerability.

EPIGENETICS AND THE IMPACT OF EARLY REARING ENVIRONMENT

The risk effects of a gene may never manifest if that gene is not actually expressed. The regulation of gene expression has been proposed as a potential molecular mechanism that can mediate maladaptations (vulnerability) as well as adaptations (resilience) in the brain (Tsankova et al., 2007). These "epigenetic" mechanisms refer to complex processes by which environmental influences can serve to regulate gene activity without altering the underlying DNA sequence. We now know that epigenetic regulation is a candidate mechanism through which care-giving behaviors, at least in animals, may produce long-lasting effects on HPA activity and neuronal function (e.g., Weaver et al., 2004). In other words, epigenetic modification of gene expression may help explain the link between a set of maternal behaviors (high licking and grooming of rat pups early in life) and more modest HPA responses to stress (Weaver et al., 2004). One striking finding from this work is that cross-fostering can reverse the epigenetic methylation changes associated with less attentive maternal care highlighting the ongoing importance of environmental influences (both positive and negative) in shaping the stress response at the biological level. Such reversibility has important implications for intervention.

A recent animal study investigating epigenetic effects of maltreatment employed a rodent model in which infant rats were exposed to stressed caretakers that showed abusive behaviors (Roth et al., 2009). It was reported that early maltreatment produced persisting changes in methylation of BDNF DNA. Critically, the methylation changes altered BDNF gene expression in the adult PFC and hippocampus. This finding is of particular interest as it documents "epigenetic" effects of maltreatment in brain areas that are known to be both structurally and functionally altered in adults following maltreatment. Roth et al. (2009) also observed altered BDNF DNA methylation in the *offspring* of these females that had previously been exposed to maltreatment as pups. This suggests the possibility of a trans-generational transmission of changes in gene expression and behavior associated with early maltreatment, even in a new generation of animals who had not been exposed to such environmental stressors.

We know of only few human epigenetic studies that have assessed the effects of maltreatment on gene expression. McGowan et al. (2009) observed differences in epigenetic regulation of hippocampal glucocorticoid receptor expression (including increased cytosine methylation of an NR3C1 promoter) in suicide victims with a history of childhood abuse, as compared with either suicide victims with no childhood abuse or controls. Interestingly, the epigenetic effects observed in the childhood abuse victims of this human study were comparable to the effects observed for the rats with low licking and grooming and reduced arched back nursing mothers (Weaver et al., 2004). Another recent study suggested that long-lasting changes in methylation of the 5-HTT promoter region could explain some of the association between childhood sexual abuse and symptoms of antisocial personality disorder in women (Beach et al., 2011). To our knowledge, no studies have looked at how baseline genotype differences may limit the extent and nature of epigenetic changes following maltreatment to provide a more mechanistic understanding of maltreatment GxE interactions. Finally, it should be noted that epigenetic processes, such as DNA methylation, regulate tissue specific gene expression. One consequence for human research is that this limits our ability to directly characterize epigenetic modification of neural structures or central tissues implicated in stress regulation. This is in contrast to rodent models where it is possible to assay tissue from cortical structures (e.g., Roth et al., 2009). While researchers have attempted to circumvent this limitation by using post-mortem tissue, this severely constrains the potential of further research in humans. It should be possible, however, to establish the association between patterns of epigenetic modification of accessible tissues, such as T cells in the blood or cells from buccal cheek swabs and specific developmental experiences, such as maltreatment. There is increasing evidence that measuring epigenetic changes longitudinally using such cells can provide meaningful information with regard to pathophysiology (e.g., Mill, 2011).

SUMMARY: GENETICS OF RESILIENCE AND VULNERABILITY

There are genetic influences on individual differences in the psychiatric outcomes associated with maltreatment. Recent GxE interaction studies suggest that certain polymorphisms may confer vulnerability or resilience to maltreatment, for example in terms of later levels of PTSD, depression, or antisocial behavior. Epigenetics is providing an exciting new avenue of research that aims to understand the mechanisms by which gene expression is influenced by exposure to environmental stressors and protective factors.

LIMITATIONS OF CURRENT RESEARCH

It is important to highlight several limitations that characterize many of the research studies investigating maltreatment. Firstly, all, but one (Carrion et al., 2007) of the brain imaging studies included in this review are cross-sectional, therefore no conclusions can be made on the causal effect of maltreatment on the brain; indeed it is possible (albeit unlikely) that the reported brain differences might represent a risk factor for exposure to maltreatment that in turn increases the risk of developing psychopathology. Secondly, the studies on adult samples have all relied on subjective retrospective reporting of maltreatment, which is liable to errors in recall that may reduce the reliability and validity of the data collected. Thirdly, researchers in the field have struggled to recruit and assess samples of children and adults that are readily comparable. Samples labeled "maltreated" have often been highly heterogeneous, drawn from different contexts (e.g., residential settings vs. home environments) and have been characterized by very different maltreatment histories. There is an increasing recognition of the need to improve the construct validity of measures that assess maltreatment type (Herrenkohl and Herrenkohl, 2009) as well as improve our accuracy in gaging maltreatment severity (Litrownik et al., 2005). If findings across studies are to be meaningfully compared, future studies need to meet the challenge of becoming more systematic in delineating maltreatment type, chronicity, frequency, and even perpetrator identity in their samples. There are some notable exceptions where researchers are already working to address these challenges (e.g., Andersen et al., 2008; Cicchetti and Rogosch, 2001). Fourthly, as noted earlier, many studies of adults and children have tended to recruit individuals with PTSD, particularly studies assessing structural brain differences. This approach makes it difficult to tease apart effects unique to maltreatment experience and current psychopathology. However, there now are a number of new studies that have recruited children who have experienced maltreatment but who do not present with PTSD (e.g., Hanson et al., 2010). Finally, it is worth noting the relatively small sample sizes that have characterized some of the studies reviewed here, particularly in several neuroimaging studies. There are undoubtedly real practical barriers that make recruiting such samples of children difficult, but larger samples would certainly improve statistical power, and allow us to better understand individual differences. These limitations should act to caution any strong conclusions regarding the neurobiological developmental trajectories of children experiencing maltreatment.

CLINICAL IMPLICATIONS

There is good evidence that early adversity in the form of childhood maltreatment is associated with poor outcome across a range of domains; in our view the evidence reviewed here suggests that this association is likely to be reflected, at least in part, at the neurobiological level. Specifically it appears that an early hostile environment contributes to stress-induced changes in the child's neurobiological systems that may be adaptive in the short-term but which reap long-term costs. These costs can be conceptualized at both the biological and psychological level. At the biological level we know from animal and human studies that chronic exposure to early stress is associated with atypical levels of stress hormones that may have an effect on the structure and function of the neurobiological systems that underpin social and psychological functioning (e.g., Arborelius et al., 1999; McEwen and Gianaros, 2010). At the psychological level it is possible that attentional and emotional systems adapt, such that they may become more effective in detecting and processing social threat but less able to successfully negotiate other aspects of social interaction (Pollak, 2008). One might speculate that these psychological changes ultimately become manifest as clinical symptoms in some children, for example as attentional difficulties or in the form of reactive aggression.

While neurobiological and genetic research has genuine long-term potential to inform clinical practice (Cicchetti and Gunnar, 2008; McCrory et al., 2010), it has already contributed to a broadening of our developmental narrative when thinking about how disruption to early caregiving can impact on a child's psychological and emotional development. Research at the neuroendocrine level – that has documented changes in the functioning of the HPA axis in children and adults who have experienced maltreatment – is probably the most advanced in this regard. Maternal behavior, for example, has been shown to be predictive of how well very young infants respond to everyday stressors: infants with mothers demonstrating higher quality maternal behavior, including greater sensitivity, show lower cortisol responses (Albers et al., 2008). Similarly, attachment security has been found to be associated with a child's pattern of stress reactivity to novel and stressful environments, such as entering child care for the first time (Ahnert et al., 2004). In securely attached infants the presence of their mother serves a stress protective function, indicated by lower levels of cortisol production when adapting to a novel environment; this contrasts with higher levels of cortisol production in insecurely attached infants (Ahnert et al., 2004). Such variation in normative samples illustrates how sensitively the neurobiological system is calibrated by the behavior of the caregiver who is tasked both with creating a safe micro-environment for the child and with helping the child regulate their own emotional states. In other words, patterns of sensitive, responsive, and attentive caregiving provides an external mechanism that can help regulate glucocorticoid and other stress responses (Nachmias et al., 1996; Gunnar and Donzella, 2002). This review has highlighted the consequences of maltreatment where such scaffolding is markedly absent and a child is forced to regulate their own levels of stress and/or manage heightened levels of negative affect in the environment. Sadly, in some cases it is the caregiver themselves who may be the source of stress for the child. As we have seen, this may lead to developmental adaptation of the HPA axis with psychological and biological consequences that increase long-term vulnerability for psychopathology (Gunnar and Cheatham, 2003).

A greater understanding of how the quality of caregiving can alter a child's stress reactivity has prompted several studies where the effectiveness of an intervention has been partly evaluated by assessing a child's cortisol reactivity under mild stress. Dozier et al. (2006a,b), for example, have investigated patterns of cortisol reactivity in children following an attachment-based intervention for foster parents. Children whose foster parents received this intervention essentially showed a normalization of cortisol responses to a social stressor (Dozier et al., 2008), demonstrating that clinical interventions may have the capacity to help recalibrate a child's stress reactivity.

While these studies investigating the relationship between indices of a child's HPA axis functioning and parenting have clear clinical relevance, the field of brain imaging lags somewhat behind in this regard. As yet, there is limited scope for explicit implications to be drawn from existing brain imaging research. Arguably there are several reasons what this is the case. Firstly, structural brain imaging studies have generally not aimed to explore the functional significance of observed brain differences in maltreated and non-maltreated children. Rather the interpretation of an observed difference is generally made in the context of our existing neurocognitive framework regarding the function of a given region. For many brain regions such a framework remains sparsely delineated, particularly within child samples. There have been a number of notable exceptions to this rule. In a recent study, Hanson et al. (2010) investigated not only structural differences in a region implicated in social functioning (the OFC) but investigated whether such differences were associated with impairments in actual social functioning of the children who participated in the study. Establishing brain–behavior correlations in this way is an important advance in building a more clinically relevant framework within which structural brain imaging findings can be meaningfully interpreted. Ultimately these correlational studies need to be complemented by longitudinal as well as by intervention studies that will allow changes in the child's environment and behavior to be measured alongside changes in brain structure and function. Such an approach is necessary if we are to begin to make even tentative inferences regarding causality.

Secondly our ability to draw clinical implications is constrained by our limited understanding of how neurobiological sensitivity to stress varies across development. This issue is not straightforward for the simple fact that brain areas are characterized by regional variation in rates of maturation; in other words, different brain regions develop at different rates (Gogtay et al., 2004). Therefore a given brain region may be more or less susceptible to the impact of maltreatment at a given stage in development. The consequence of this for researchers is that the same experience may lead to different patterns of brain abnormality depending on when a child is exposed to a given traumatogenic event. Andersen et al. (2008), who employed an innovative cross-sectional design, have reported preliminary evidence for this phenomenon. They aimed to investigate whether the experience of sexual abuse at different ages had specific effects in terms of regional brain volume. Twenty-six young women aged between 18 and 24 who had experienced repeated episodes of childhood sexual abuse were compared with non-abused controls. The authors reported that hippocampal volume was reduced in association with childhood sexual abuse at ages 3–5 years and ages 11–13 years; CC volume was reduced with childhood sexual abuse at ages 9–10 years, and frontal cortex volume was reduced in subjects with childhood sexual abuse at ages 14–16 years. The authors concluded that different brain regions are likely to have unique windows of vulnerability to the effects of traumatic stress. This study highlights the possibility that the same maltreatment experience (in this case, sexual abuse) may have very different effects on brain structure depending on the age at which the abuse was experienced. It might be conjectured that these windows of vulnerability would be differentially susceptible to different forms of traumatic stress or maltreatment; however, further research is required to support such a hypothesis.

For most clinicians, a third limitation of the existing brain imaging literature pertains to the populations of children investigated. As noted earlier, many of the structural studies have focused on children presenting with clinically diagnosed PTSD, making it difficult to identify the specific correlates that are uniquely associated with maltreatment as opposed to those that might reflect predisposition to PTSD. To date the two fMRI studies of emotional processing have recruited children who have experienced early institutionalization and subsequent adoption. These children, who have experienced a diverse range of early stressors – most of which are undocumented – are very unlikely to be representative of the community samples typically referred to social services. Community based familial maltreatment, including physical, sexual, and emotional abuse as well as neglect and domestic violence characterize the majority who present to mental health clinics. These are not rare experiences, with 896,000 cases of substantiated maltreatment in the USA alone during 2005 (U.S. Department of Health and Human Services, Administration on Children, Youth, and Families, 2007). Despite this, we know almost nothing about the functional neural correlates of such experiences in these children, which limits our ability to make clinically informed inferences.

Recent years have increased our understanding of gene–environment interactions that may increase the likelihood of psychopathology in children exposed to maltreatment. From a clinical perspective this helps provide a rationale as to the potential for individual variability in outcome for children exposed to similar traumatic experiences. In the field of GxE research it is recognized that advances will be contingent on improvements in how environmental influences are quantified, and precision in identifying the timing of their occurrence (Lenroot and Giedd, 2011). However, there is preliminary evidence that genetic polymorphisms may also help account for the potential variability in clinical outcome. In a study of 1- to 3-year-old children with externalizing problems Bakermans-Kranenburg et al. (2008) found a moderating role for the dopamine D4 receptor (DRD4) in a video-feedback intervention study designed to improve maternal sensitivity and discipline. The intervention was effective primarily in those children with the DRD4 7-repeat polymorphism. This is the first study to provide preliminary evidence that gene by environment interactions may play an important role in explaining the differential effectiveness of a given intervention. We remain a long way, however, from being able to tailor interventions to specific groups of children on the basis of genetic information. Nonetheless, improving our conceptual understanding of the factors underpinning outcome variability will represent an important advance in our efforts to treat more effectively the wide range of problems that are known to be associated with maltreatment.

CONCLUSION

While there is now accumulating evidence indicating an association between neurobiological change and childhood maltreatment there remains a need for caution in how such evidence is interpreted. Much of the research to date has been based on very mixed samples of children or adults with diverse experiences of early adversity. This partly derives from the complexities inherent in the defining and assessing maltreatment type, given that abusive experiences seldom occur in isolation. Nonetheless greater precision and homogeneity in how groups are characterized in relation to maltreatment experience, age range, socio-economic status, and intellectual ability are required, as too is the need for longitudinal and intervention studies. This will assist in making more meaningful inferences about the significance of any observed neurobiological differences.

Nonetheless, the studies reviewed here support a growing consensus that maltreatment contributes to stress-induced changes in a child's neurobiological systems. While these changes may be adaptive in the short-term it is hypothesized that they contribute to heightened risk for psychopathology over the longer term. There is a need to specify with more precision the psychological factors that may mediate the association with poor behavioral outcome, both in terms of adaptations to psychological processes (e.g., attentional hypervigilance to threat) and in terms of internal representations of self and others (e.g., schemas or internal working models). The longer-term goal is to establish a clearer picture of the links between environmental stress, neurobiological, and neuroendocrine change and the ways in which these may potentiate and shape social, affective, and cognitive development.

ACKNOWLEDGMENTS

Eamon McCrory and Stephane A. De Brito are supported by RES-061-25-0189 from the ESRC, and Eamon McCrory and Essi Viding are also supported by RES-062-23-2202 from ESRC and BARDA-53229 from the British Academy.

REFERENCES

Ahnert, L., Gunnar, M. R., Lamb, M. E., and Barthel, M. (2004). Transition to child care: associations with infant-mother attachment, infant negative emotion, and cortisol elevations. *Child Dev.* 75, 639–650.

Albers, E. M., Marianne Riksen-Walraven, J., Sweep, F. C. G. J., and Weerth, C. D. (2008). Maternal behavior predicts infant cortisol recovery from a mild everyday stressor. *J. Child. Psychol. Psychiatry* 49, 97–103.

Amodio, D. M., and Frith, C. D. (2006). Meeting of minds: the medial frontal cortex and social cognition. *Nat. Rev. Neurosci.* 7, 268–277.

Andersen, S. L., Tomada, A., Vincow, E. S., Valente, E., Polcari, A., and Teicher, M. H. (2008). Preliminary evidence for sensitive periods in the effect of childhood sexual abuse on regional brain development. *J. Neuropsychiatry Clin. Neurosci.* 20, 292–301.

Arborelius, L., Owens, M. J., Plotsky, P. M., and Nemeroff, C. B. (1999). The role of corticotropin-releasing factor in depression and anxiety disorders. *J. Endocrinol.* 160, 1–12.

Bakermans-Kranenburg, M. J., Van Ijzendoorn, M. H., Pijlman, F. T. A., Mesman, J., and Juffer, F. (2008). Experimental evidence for differential susceptibility: dopamine D4 receptor polymorphism (DRD4 VNTR) moderates intervention effects on toddlers' externalizing behavior in a randomized controlled trial. *Dev. Psychol.* 44, 293–300.

Beach, S. R., Brody, G. H., Todorov, A. A., Gunter, T. D., and Philibert, R. A. (2011). Methylation at 5HTT mediates the impact of child sex abuse on women's antisocial behavior: an examination of the Iowa adoptee sample. *Psychosom. Med.* 73, 83–87.

Bremner, J. D., Randall, P., Vermetten, E., Staib, L., Bronen, R. A., Mazure, C., Capelli, S., Mccarthy, G., Innis, R. B., and Charney, D. S. (1997). Magnetic resonance imaging-based measurement of hippocampal volume in posttraumatic stress disorder related to childhood physical and sexual abuse – a preliminary report. *Biol. Psychiatry* 41, 23–32.

Carrion, V. G., Garrett, A., Menon, V., Weems, C. F., and Reiss, A. L. (2008). Posttraumatic stress symptoms and brain function during a response-inhibition task: an fMRI study in youth. *Depress. Anxiety* 25, 514–526.

Carrion, V. G., Haas, B. W., Garrett, A., Song, S., and Reiss, A. L. (2010). Reduced hippocampal activity in youth with posttraumatic stress symptoms: an fMRI study. *J. Pediatr. Psychol.* 35, 559–569.

Carrion, V. G., Weems, C. F., Eliez, S., Patwardhan, A., Brown, W., Ray, R. D., and Reiss, A. L. (2001). Attenuation of frontal asymmetry in pediatric posttraumatic stress disorder. *Biol. Psychiatry* 50, 943–951.

Carrion, V. G., Weems, C. F., Ray, R. D., Glaser, B., Hessl, D., and Reiss, A. L. (2002). Diurnal salivary cortisol in pediatric posttraumatic stress disorder. *Biol. Psychiatry* 51, 575–582.

Carrion, V. G., Weems, C. F., and Reiss, A. L. (2007). Stress predicts brain changes in children: a pilot longitudinal study on youth stress, posttraumatic stress disorder, and the hippocampus. *Pediatrics* 119, 509–516.

Carrion, V. G., Weems, C. F., Watson, C., Eliez, S., Menon, V., and Reiss, A. L. (2009). Converging evidence for abnormalities of the prefrontal cortex and evaluation of midsagittal structures in pediatric posttraumatic stress disorder: an MRI study. *Psychiatry Res.* 172, 226–234.

Caspi, A., Mcclay, J., Moffitt, T., Mill, J., Martin, J., Craig, I. W., Taylor, A., and Poulton, R. (2002). Role of genotype in the cycle of violence in maltreated children. *Science* 297, 851–854.

Caspi, A., and Moffitt, T. E. (2006). Gene-environment interactions in psychiatry: joining forces with neuroscience. *Nat. Rev. Neurosci.* 7, 583–590.

Choi, J., Jeong, B., Rohan, M. L., Polcari, A. M., and Teicher, M. H. (2009). Preliminary evidence for white matter tract abnormalities in young adults exposed to parental verbal abuse. *Biol. Psychiatry* 65, 227–234.

Cicchetti, D., and Curtis, W. J. (2005). An event-related potential study of the processing of affective facial expressions in young children who experienced maltreatment during the first year of life. *Dev. Psychopathol.* 17, 641–677.

Cicchetti, D., and Gunnar, M. R. (2008). Integrating biological measures into the design and evaluation of preventive interventions. *Dev. Psychopathol.* 20, 737–743.

Cicchetti, D., and Rogosch, F. A. (2001). The impact of child maltreatment and psychopathology on neuroendocrine functioning. *Dev. Psychopathol.* 13, 783–804.

Cicchetti, D., Rogosch, F. A., and Cox Kearns, S. (2001). Diverse patterns of neuroendocrine activity in maltreated children. *Dev. Psychopathol.* 13, 677–693.

Cicchetti, D., Rogosch, F. A., and Sturge-Apple, M. L. (2007). Interactions of child maltreatment and serotonin transporter and monoamine oxidase A polymorphisms: depressive symptomatology among adolescents from low socioeconomic status backgrounds. *Dev. Psychopathol.* 19, 1161–1180.

Craig, I. W. (2007). The importance of stress and genetic variation in human aggression. *Bioessays* 29, 227–236.

Croy, I., Schellong, J., Gerber, J., Joraschky, P., Iannilli, E., and Hummel, T. (2010). Women with a history of childhood maltreatment exhibit more activation in association areas following non-traumatic olfactory stimuli: a fMRI study. *PLoS ONE* 5, e9362. doi: 10.1371/journal.pone.0009362

Currie, J., and Widom, C. S. (2010). Long-term consequences of child abuse and neglect on adult economic well-being. *Child Maltreat.* 15, 111–120.

Davidson, R. J., Putnam, K. M., and Larson, C. L. (2000). Dysfunction in the neural circuitry of emotion regulation – a possible prelude to violence. *Science* 289, 591–594.

De Bellis, M. D., Baum, A. S., Birmaher, B., Keshavan, M. S., Eccard, C. H., Boring, A. M., Jenkins, F. J., and Ryan, N. D. (1999a). Developmental traumatology part I: biological stress systems. *Biol. Psychiatry* 45, 1259–1270.

De Bellis, M. D., Keshavan, M. S., Clark, D. B., Casey, B. J., Giedd, J. N., Boring, A. M., Frustaci, K., and Ryan, N. D. (1999b). Developmental traumatology part II: brain development. *Biol. Psychiatry* 45, 1271–1284.

De Bellis, M. D., Chrousos, G. P., Dorn, L. D., Burke, L., Helmers, K., Kling, M. A., Trickett, P. K., and Putnam, F. W. (1994). Hypothalamic-pituitary-adrenal axis dysregulation in sexually abused girls. *J. Clin. Endocrinol. Metab.* 78, 249–255.

De Bellis, M. D., and Keshavan, M. S. (2003). Sex differences in brain maturation in maltreatment-related pediatric posttraumatic stress disorder. *Neurosci. Biobehav. Rev.* 27, 103–117.

De Bellis, M. D., Keshavan, M. S., Shifflett, H., Iyengar, S., Beers, S. R., Hall, J., and Moritz, G. (2002). Brain structures in pediatric maltreatment-related posttraumatic stress disorder: a sociodemographically matched study. *Biol. Psychiatry* 52, 1066–1078.

Dillon, D. G., Holmes, A. J., Birk, J. L., Brooks, N., Lyons-Ruth, K., and Pizzagalli, D. A. (2009). Childhood adversity is associated with left basal ganglia dysfunction during reward anticipation in adulthood. *Biol. Psychiatry* 66, 206–213.

Dozier, M., Manni, M., Gordon, M. K., Peloso, E., Gunnar, M. R., Stovall-Mcclough, K. C., Eldreth, D., and Levine, S. (2006a). Foster children's diurnal production of cortisol: an exploratory study. *Child Maltreat.* 11, 189–197.

Dozier, M., Peloso, E., Lindhiem, O., Gordon, M. K., Manni, M., Sepulveda, S., Ackerman, J., Bernier, A., and Levine, S. (2006b). Developing evidence-based interventions for foster children: an example of a randomized clinical trial with infants and toddlers. *J. Soc. Issues* 62, 767–785.

Dozier, M., Peloso, E., Lewis, E., Laurenceau, J. P., and Levine, S. (2008). Effects of an attachment-based intervention on the cortisol production of infants and toddlers in foster care. *Dev. Psychopathol.* 20, 845–869.

Eluvathingal, T. J., Chugani, H. T., Behen, M. E., Juhász, C., Muzik, O., Maqbool, M., Chugani, D. C., and Makki, M. (2006). Abnormal brain connectivity in children after early severe socioemotional deprivation: a diffusion tensor imaging study. *Pediatrics* 117, 2093–2100.

Feder, A., Nestler, E. J., and Charney, D. S. (2009). Psychobiology and molecular genetics of resilience. *Nat. Rev. Neurosci.* 10, 446–457.

Fries, E., Hesse, J., Hellhammer, J., and Hellhammer, D. H. (2005). A new view on hypocortisolism. *Psychoneuroendocrinology* 30, 1010–1016.

Fuster, J. M. (1997). *The Prefrontal Cortex: Anatomy, Physiology, and Neurophysiology of the Frontal Lobe.* Philadelphia: Lippincott-Raven.

Giedd, J. N., Rumsey, J. M., Castellanos, F. X., Rajapakse, J. C., Kaysen, D., Vaituzis, A. C., Vauss, Y. C., Hamburger, S. D., and Rapoport, J. L. (1996). A quantitative MRI study of the corpus callosum in children and adolescents. *Brain Res. Dev. Brain Res.* 91, 274–280.

Gilbert, R., Kemp, A., Thoburn, J., Sidebotham, P., Radford, L., Glaser, D., and Macmillan, H. L. (2009). Recognising and responding to child maltreatment. *Lancet* 373, 167–180.

Gilbertson, M. W., Shenton, M. E., Ciszewski, A., Kasai, K., Lasko, N. B., Orr, S. P., and Pitman, R. K. (2002). Smaller hippocampal volume predicts pathologic vulnerability to psychological trauma. *Nat. Neurosci.* 5, 1242–1247.

Gogtay, N., Giedd, J. N., Lusk, L., Hayashi, K. M., Greenstein, D., Vaituzis, A. C., Nugent III, T. F., Herman, D. H., Clasen, L. S., Toga, A. W., Rapoport, J. L., and Thompson, P. M. (2004). Dynamic mapping of human cortical development during childhood through early adulthood. *Proc. Natl. Acad. Sci. U.S.A* 101, 8174–8179.

Goodyer, I. M., Herbert, J., and Altham, P. M. E. (1998). Adrenal steroid secretion and major depression in 8- to 16-year-olds, III. Influence of cortisol/DHEA ratio at presentation on subsequent rates of disappointing life events and persistent major depression. *Psychol. Med.* 28, 265–273.

Govindan, R. M., Behen, M. E., Helder, E., Makki, M. I., and Chugani, H. T. (2010). Altered water diffusivity in cortical association tracts in children with early deprivation identified with tract-based spatial statistics (TBSS). *Cereb. Cortex* 20, 561–569.

Grant, M. M., Cannistraci, C., Hollon, S. D., Gore, J., and Shelton, R. (2011). Childhood trauma history differentiates amygdala response to sad faces within MDD. *J. Psychiatr. Res.* 45, 886–895.

Gunnar, M. R., and Cheatham, C. L. (2003). Brain and behavior interface: stress and the developing brain. *Infant Ment. Health J.* 24, 195–211.

Gunnar, M. R., and Donzella, B. (2002). Social regulation of the cortisol levels in early human development. *Psychoneuroendocrinology* 27, 199–220.

Gunnar, M. R., Fisher, P. A., Dozier, M., Fox, N., Levine, S., Neal, C., Pollak, S., Plotsky, P., Sanchez, M., and Vazquez, D. (2006). Bringing basic research on early experience and stress neurobiology to bear on preventive interventions for neglected and maltreated children. *Dev. Psychopathol.* 18, 651–677.

Hanson, J. L., Chung, M. K., Avants, B. B., Shirtcliff, E. A., Gee, J. C., Davidson, R. J., and Pollak, S. D. (2010). Early stress is associated with alterations in the orbitofrontal cortex: a tensor-based morphometry investigation of brain structure and behavioral risk. *J. Neurosci* 30, 7466–7472.

Hart, J., Gunnar, M., and Cicchetti, D. (1995). Salivary cortisol in maltreated children: evidence of relations between neuroendocrine activity and social competence. *Dev. Psychopathol.* 7, 11–26.

Hart, J., Gunnar, M., and Cicchetti, D. (1996). Altered neuroendocrine activity in maltreated children related to symptoms of depression. *Dev. Psychopathol.* 8, 201–214.

Heim, C., Mletzko, T., Purselle, D., Musselman, D. L., and Nemeroff, C. B. (2008). The dexamethasone/corticotropin-releasing factor test in men with major depression: role of childhood trauma. *Biol. Psychiatry* 63, 398–405.

Heim, C., Newport, D. J., Wagner, D., Wilcox, M. M., Miller, A. H., and Nemeroff, C. B. (2002). The role of early adverse experience and adulthood stress in the prediction of neuroendocrine stress reactivity in women: a multiple regression analysis. *Depress. Anxiety* 15, 117–125.

Herrenkohl, R. C., and Herrenkohl, T. I. (2009). Assessing a child's experience of multiple maltreatment types: some unfinished business. *J. Fam. Violence* 24, 485–496.

Izard, C. E., and Harris, P. (1995). "Emotional development and developmental psychopathology," in *Developmental Psychopathology: Vol. I: Theories and Methods*, eds D. Cicchetti and J. Cohen (New York: John Wiley), 467–503.

Jackowski, A. P., De Araújo, C. M., De Lacerda, A. L. T., De Jesus Mari, J., and Kaufman, J. (2009). Neurostructural imaging findings in children with post-traumatic stress disorder: brief review. *Psychiatry Clin. Neurosci.* 63, 1–8.

Jackowski, A. P., Douglas-Palumberi, H., Jackowski, M., Win, L., Schultz, R. T., Staib, L. W., Krystal, J. H., and Kaufman, J. (2008). Corpus callosum in maltreated children with posttraumatic stress disorder: a diffusion tensor imaging study. *Psychiatry Res.* 162, 256–261.

Kaufman, J. (1991). Depressive disorders in maltreated children. *J. Am. Acad. Child Adolesc. Psychiatry* 30, 257–265.

Kaufman, J., Birmaher, B., Perel, J., Dahl, R. E., Moreci, P., Nelson, B., Wells, W., and Ryan, N. D. (1997). The corticotropin-releasing hormone challenge in depressed abused, depressed nonabused, and normal control children. *Biol. Psychiatry* 42, 669–679.

Kaufman, J., Yang, B. Z., Douglas-Palumberi, H., Grasso, D., Lipschitz, D., Houshyar, S., Krystal, J. H., and Gelernter, J. (2006). Brain-derived neurotrophic factor-5-HTTLPR gene interactions and environmental modifiers of depression in children. *Biol. Psychiatry* 59, 673–680.

Kitayama, N., Brummer, M., Hertz, L., Quinn, S., Kim, Y., and Bremner, J. D. (2007). Morphologic alterations in the corpus callosum in abuse-related posttraumatic stress disorder: a preliminary study. *J. Nerv. Ment. Dis.* 195, 1027–1029.

Kitterle, F. (1995). *Hemispheric Communication: Mechanisms and Models.* Hillsdale, NJ: Laurence Erlbaum Associates, Inc.

Koenen, K. C., Nugent, N. R., and Amstadter, A. B. (2008). Gene-environment interaction in post-traumatic stress disorder: review, strategy and new directions for future research. *Eur. Arch. Psychiatry Clin. Neurosci.* 258, 82–96.

Lansford, J. E., Dodge, K. A., Pettit, G. S., Bates, J. E., Crozier, J., and Kaplow, J. (2002). A 12-year prospective study of the long-term effects of early child physical maltreatment on psychological, behavioral, and academic problems in adolescence. *Arch. Pediatr. Adolesc. Med.* 156, 824–830.

Lenroot, R. K., and Giedd, J. N. (2011). Annual research review: developmental considerations of gene by environment interactions. *J. Child Psychol. Psychiatry* 52, 429–441.

Litrownik, A. J., Lau, A., English, D. J., Briggs, E., Newton, R. R., Romney, S., and Dubowitz, H. (2005). Measuring the severity of child maltreatment. *Child Abuse Negl.* 29, 553–573.

Liu, D., Diorio, J., Tannenbaum, B., Caldji, C., Francis, D., Freedman, A., Sharma, S., Pearson, D., Plotsky, P. M., and Meaney, M. J. (1997). Maternal care, hippocampal glucocorticoid receptors, and hypothalamic-pituitary-adrenal responses to stress. *Science* 277, 1659–1662.

Lotfipour, S., Ferguson, E., Leonard, G., Perron, M., Pike, B., Richer, L., Seguin, J. R., Toro, R., Veillette, S., Pausova, Z., and Paus, T. (2009). Orbitofrontal cortex and drug use during adolescence: role of prenatal exposure to maternal smoking and BDNF genotype. *Arch. Gen. Psychiatry* 66, 1244–1252.

Lupien, S. J., De Leon, M., De Santi, S., Convit, A., Tarshish, C., Nair, N. P. V., Thakur, M., Mcewen, B. S., Hauger, R. L., and Meaney, M. J. (1998). Cortisol levels during human aging predict hippocampal atrophy and memory deficits. *Nat. Neurosci.* 1, 69–73.

Lupien, S. J., Mcewen, B. S., Gunnar, M. R., and Heim, C. (2009). Effects of stress throughout the lifespan on the brain, behaviour and cognition. *Nat. Rev. Neurosci.* 10, 434–445.

Maheu, F. S., Dozier, M., Guyer, A. E., Mandell, D., Peloso, E., Poeth, K., Jenness, J., Lau, J. Y., Ackerman, J. P., Pine, D. S., and Ernst, M. (2010). A preliminary study of medial temporal lobe function in youths with a history of caregiver deprivation and emotional neglect. *Cogn. Affect. Behav. Neurosci.* 10, 34–49.

McCrory, E., De Brito, S. A., and Viding, E. (2010). Research review: the neurobiology and genetics of maltreatment and adversity. *J. Child. Psychol. Psychiatry* 51, 1079–1095.

McEwen, B. S. (1999). Stress and hippocampal plasticity. *Annu. Rev. Neurosci.* 22, 105–122.

McEwen, B. S., and Gianaros, P. J. (2010). Central role of the brain in stress and adaptation: links to socioeconomic status, health, and disease. *Ann. N. Y. Acad. Sci.* 1186, 190–222.

McGowan, P. O., Sasaki, A., D'alessio, A. C., Dymov, S., Labonté, B., Szyf, M., Turecki, G., and Meaney, M. J. (2009). Epigenetic regulation of the glucocorticoid receptor in human brain associates with childhood abuse. *Nat. Neurosci.* 12, 342–348.

Meewisse, M. L., Reitsma, J. B., De Vries, G. J., Gersons, B. P. R., and Olff, M. (2007). Cortisol and post-traumatic stress disorder in adults: systematic review and meta-analysis. *Br. J. Psychiatry* 191, 387–392.

Mehta, M. A., Golembo, N. I., Nosarti, C., Colvert, E., Mota, A., Williams, S. C. R., Rutter, M., and Sonuga-Barke, E. J. S. (2009). Amygdala, hippocampal and corpus callosum size following severe early institutional deprivation: the English and Romanian Adoptees Study Pilot. *J. Child. Psychol. Psychiatry* 50, 943–951.

Meyer-Lindenberg, A., Buckholtz, J. W., Kolachana, B., Hariri, A. R., Pezawas, L., Blasi, G., Wabnitz, A., Honea, R., Verchinski, B., Callicott, J. H., Egan, M., Mattay, V., and Weinberger, D. R. (2006). Neural mechanisms of genetic risk for impulsivity and violence in humans. *Proc. Natl. Acad. Sci. U.S.A.* 103, 6269–6274.

Mill, J. (2011). Toward an integrated genetic and epigenetic approach to Alzheimer's disease. *Neurobiol. Aging* 32, 1188–1191.

Miller, E. K., and Cohen, J. D. (2001). An integrative theory of prefrontal cortex function. *Annu. Rev. Neurosci.* 24, 167–202.

Miller, G. E., Chen, E., and Zhou, E. S. (2007). If it goes up, must it come down? Chronic stress and the hypothalamic-pituitary-adrenocortical axis in humans. *Psychol. Bull.* 133, 25–45.

Mizomuri, S. J. Y., Smith, D. M., and Puryear, C. B. (2007). "Mnemonic contributions of hippocampal place cells," in *Neurobiology of Learning and Memory*, eds J. Martinez and R. Kesner (Burlington, MA: Elsevier), 155–190.

Moffitt, T. E., Caspi, A., and Rutter, M. (2005). Strategy for investigating interactions between measured genes and measured environments. *Arch. Gen. Psychiatry* 62, 473–481.

Mueller, S. C., Maheu, F. S., Dozier, M., Peloso, E., Mandell, D., Leibenluft, E., Pine, D. S., and Ernst, M. (2010). Early-life stress is associated with impairment in cognitive control in adolescence: an fMRI study. *Neuropsychologia* 48, 3037–3044.

Nachmias, M., Gunnar, M., Mangelsdorf, S., Parritz, R. H., and Buss, K. (1996). Behavioral inhibition and stress reactivity: the moderating role of attachment security. *Child Dev.* 67, 508–522.

Neigh, G. N., Gillespie, C. F., and Nemeroff, C. B. (2009). The neurobiological toll of child abuse and neglect. *Trauma Violence Abuse* 10, 389–410.

Newport, D. J., Heim, C., Bonsall, R., Miller, A. H., and Nemeroff, C. B. (2004). Pituitary-adrenal responses to standard and low-dose dexamethasone suppression tests in adult survivors of child abuse. *Biol. Psychiatry* 55, 10–20.

Parker, S. W., and Nelson, C. A. (2005). The impact of early institutional rearing on the ability to discriminate facial expressions of emotion: an event-related potential study. *Child Dev.* 76, 54–72.

Parker, S. W., Nelson, C. A., Zeanah, C. H., Smyke, A. T., Koga, S. F., Fox, N. A., Marshall, P. J., and Woodward, H. R. (2005). An event-related potential study of the impact of institutional rearing on face recognition. *Dev. Psychopathol.* 17, 621–639.

Pears, K. C., Kim, H. K., and Fisher, P. A. (2008). Psychosocial and cognitive functioning of children with specific profiles of maltreatment. *Child Abuse Negl.* 32, 958–971.

Pederson, C. L., Maurer, S. H., Kaminski, P. L., Zander, K. A., Peters, C. M., Stokes-Crowe, L. A., and Osborn, R. E. (2004). Hippocampal volume and memory performance in a community-based sample of women with posttraumatic stress disorder secondary to child abuse. *J. Trauma Stress* 17, 37–40.

Phelps, E. A., and LeDoux, J. E. (2005). Contributions of the amygdala to emotion processing: from animal models to human behavior. *Neuron* 48, 175–187.

Plomin, R., Owen, M. J., and Mcguffin, P. (1994). The genetic basis of complex human behaviors. *Science* 264, 1733–1739.

Pollak, S. D. (2008). Mechanisms linking early experience and the emergence of emotions: illustrations from the study of maltreated children. *Curr. Dir. Psychol. Sci.* 17, 370–375.

Pollak, S. D., Cicchetti, D., Klorman, R., and Brumaghim, J. T. (1997). Cognitive brain event-related potentials and emotion processing in maltreated children. *Child Dev.* 68, 773–787.

Pollak, S. D., Klorman, R., Thatcher, J. E., and Cicchetti, D. (2001). P3b reflects maltreated children's reactions to facial displays of emotion. *Psychophysiology* 38, 267–274.

Pollak, S. D., and Tolley-Schell, S. A. (2003). Selective attention to facial emotion in physically abused children. *J. Abnorm. Psychol.* 112, 323–338.

Rhee, S. H., and Waldman, I. D. (2002). Genetic and environmental influences on antisocial behavior: a meta-analysis of twin and adoption studies. *Psychol. Bull.* 128, 490–529.

Richert, K. A., Carrion, V. G., Karchemskiy, A., and Reiss, A. L. (2006). Regional differences of the prefrontal cortex in pediatric PTSD: an MRI study. *Depress. Anxiety* 23, 17–25.

Roth, T. L., Lubin, F. D., Funk, A. J., and Sweatt, J. D. (2009). Lasting epigenetic influence of early-life adversity on the BDNF gene. *Biol. Psychiatry* 65, 760–769.

Sapolsky, R. M., Uno, H., Rebert, C. S., and Finch, C. E. (1990). Hippocampal damage associated with prolonged glucocorticoid exposure in primates. *J. Neurosci.* 10, 2897–2902.

Shackman, J. E., Shackman, A. J., and Pollak, S. D. (2007). Physical abuse amplifies attention to threat and increases anxiety in children. *Emotion* 7, 838–852.

Shea, M. T., Yen, S., Pagano, M. E., Morey, L. C., Mcglashan, T. H., Grilo, C. M., Sanislow, C. A., Stout, R. L., Skodol, A. E., Gunderson, J. G., Bender, D. S., and Zanarini, M. C. (2004). Associations in the course of personality disorders and axis i disorders over time. *J. Abnorm. Psychol.* 113, 499–508.

Shirtcliff, E. A., Coe, C. L., and Pollak, S. D. (2009). Early childhood stress is associated with elevated antibody levels to herpes simplex virus type 1. *Proc. Natl. Acad. Sci. U.S.A.* 106, 2963–2967.

Sullivan, P. F., Neale, M. C., and Kendler, K. S. (2000). Genetic epidemiology of major depression: review and meta-analysis. *Am. J. Psychiatry* 157, 1552–1562.

Tarullo, A. R., and Gunnar, M. R. (2006). Child maltreatment and the developing HPA axis. *Horm. Behav.* 50, 632–639.

Taylor, A., and Kim-Cohen, J. (2007). Meta-analysis of gene-environment interactions in developmental psychopathology. *Dev. Psychopathol.* 19, 1029–1037.

Teicher, M. H., Andersen, S. L., Polcari, A., Anderson, C. M., Navalta, C. P., and Kim, D. M. (2003). The neurobiological consequences of early stress and childhood maltreatment. *Neurosci. Biobehav. Rev.* 27, 33–44.

Teicher, M. H., Dumont, N. L., Ito, Y., Vaituzis, C., Giedd, J. N., and Andersen, S. L. (2004). Childhood neglect is associated with reduced corpus callosum area. *Biol. Psychiatry* 56, 80–85.

Tomoda, A., Suzuki, H., Rabi, K., Sheu, Y.-S., Polcari, A., and Teicher, M. H. (2009). Reduced prefrontal cortical gray matter volume in young adults exposed to harsh corporal punishment. *Neuroimage* 47, T66–T71.

Tottenham, N., Hare, T. A., Millner, A., Gilhooly, T., Zevin, J. D., and Casey, B. J. (2011). Elevated amygdala response to faces following early deprivation. *Dev. Sci.* 14, 190–204.

Tottenham, N., Hare, T. A., Quinn, B. T., Mccarry, T. W., Nurse, M., Gilhooly, T., Millner, A., Galvan, A., Davidson, M. C., Eigsti, I. M., Thomas, K. M., Freed, P. J., Booma, E. S., Gunnar, M. R., Altemus, M., Aronson, J., and Casey, B. J. (2010). Prolonged institutional rearing is associated with atypically large amygdala volume and difficulties in emotion regulation. *Dev. Sci.* 13, 46–61.

Tottenham, N., and Sheridan, M. A. (2010). A review of adversity, the amygdala and the hippocampus: a consideration of developmental timing. *Front. Hum. Neurosci.* 3:68. doi: 10.3389/neuro.09.068.2009

Treadway, M. T., Grant, M. M., Ding, Z., Hollon, S. D., Gore, J. C., and Shelton, R. C. (2009). Early adverse events, HPA activity and rostral anterior cingulate volume in MDD. *PLoS ONE* 4, e4887. doi: 10.1371/journal.pone.0004887

Tsankova, N., Renthal, W., Kumar, A., and Nestler, E. J. (2007). Epigenetic regulation in psychiatric disorders. *Nat. Rev. Neurosci.* 8, 355–367.

U.S. Department of Health and Human Services, Administration on Children, Youth, and Families. (2007). *Child Maltreatment 2005.* Washington, DC: U.S. Government Printing Office.

van Goozen, S. H. M., and Fairchild, G. (2008). How can the study of biological processes help design new interventions for children with severe antisocial behavior? *Dev. Psychopathol.* 20, 941–973.

van Harmelen, A.-L., Van Tol, M.-J., Van Der Wee, N. J. A., Veltman, D. J., Aleman, A., Spinhoven, P., Van Buchem, M. A., Zitman, F. G., Penninx, B. W. J. H., and Elzinga, B. M. (2010). Reduced medial prefrontal cortex volume in adults reporting childhood emotional maltreatment. *Biol. Psychiatry* 68, 832–838.

Vermetten, E., Schmahl, C., Lindner, S., Loewenstein, R. J., and Bremner, J. D. (2006). Hippocampal and amygdalar volumes in dissociative identity disorder. *Am. J. Psychiatry* 163, 630–636.

Viding, E., and Frith, U. (2006). Genes for susceptibility to violence lurk in the brain. *Proc. Natl. Acad. Sci. U.S.A.* 103, 6085–6086.

Viding, E., Williamson, D. E., and Hariri, A. R. (2006). Developmental imaging genetics: challenges and promises for translational research. *Dev. Psychopathol.* 18, 877–892.

Vyas, A., Bernal, S., and Chattarji, S. (2003). Effects of chronic stress on dendritic arborization in the central and extended amygdala. *Brain Res.* 965, 290–294.

Vythilingam, M., Heim, C., Newport, J., Miller, A. H., Anderson, E., Bronen, R., Brummer, M., Staib, L., Vermetten, E., Charney, D. S., Nemeroff, C. B., and Douglas Bremner, J. (2002). Childhood trauma associated with smaller hippocampal volume in women with major depression. *Am. J. Psychiatry* 159, 2072–2080.

Weaver, I. C. G., Cervoni, N., Champagne, F. A., D'alessio, A. C., Sharma, S., Seckl, J. R., Dymov, S., Szyf, M., and Meaney, M. J. (2004). Epigenetic programming by maternal behavior. *Nat. Neurosci.* 7, 847–854.

Weder, N., Yang, B. Z., Douglas-Palumberi, H., Massey, J., Krystal, J. H., Gelernter, J., and Kaufman, J. (2009). MAOA genotype, maltreatment, and aggressive behavior: the changing impact of genotype at varying levels of trauma. *Biol. Psychiatry* 65, 417–424.

Woon, F. L., and Hedges, D. W. (2008). Hippocampal and amygdala volumes in children and adults with childhood maltreatment-related posttraumatic stress disorder: a meta-analysis. *Hippocampus* 18, 729–736.

Permissions

All chapters in this book were first published by Frontiers; hereby published with permission under the Creative Commons Attribution License or equivalent. Every chapter published in this book has been scrutinized by our experts. Their significance has been extensively debated. The topics covered herein carry significant findings which will fuel the growth of the discipline. They may even be implemented as practical applications or may be referred to as a beginning point for another development.

The contributors of this book come from diverse backgrounds, making this book a truly international effort. This book will bring forth new frontiers with its revolutionizing research information and detailed analysis of the nascent developments around the world.

We would like to thank all the contributing authors for lending their expertise to make the book truly unique. They have played a crucial role in the development of this book. Without their invaluable contributions this book wouldn't have been possible. They have made vital efforts to compile up to date information on the varied aspects of this subject to make this book a valuable addition to the collection of many professionals and students.

This book was conceptualized with the vision of imparting up-to-date information and advanced data in this field. To ensure the same, a matchless editorial board was set up. Every individual on the board went through rigorous rounds of assessment to prove their worth. After which they invested a large part of their time researching and compiling the most relevant data for our readers.

The editorial board has been involved in producing this book since its inception. They have spent rigorous hours researching and exploring the diverse topics which have resulted in the successful publishing of this book. They have passed on their knowledge of decades through this book. To expedite this challenging task, the publisher supported the team at every step. A small team of assistant editors was also appointed to further simplify the editing procedure and attain best results for the readers.

Apart from the editorial board, the designing team has also invested a significant amount of their time in understanding the subject and creating the most relevant covers. They scrutinized every image to scout for the most suitable representation of the subject and create an appropriate cover for the book.

The publishing team has been an ardent support to the editorial, designing and production team. Their endless efforts to recruit the best for this project, has resulted in the accomplishment of this book. They are a veteran in the field of academics and their pool of knowledge is as vast as their experience in printing. Their expertise and guidance has proved useful at every step. Their uncompromising quality standards have made this book an exceptional effort. Their encouragement from time to time has been an inspiration for everyone.

The publisher and the editorial board hope that this book will prove to be a valuable piece of knowledge for researchers, students, practitioners and scholars across the globe.

List of Contributors

Thomas F. Tropea
Division of Pediatric Neurology, Department of Pediatrics, Weill Cornell Medical College, New York, NY, USA
College of Osteopathic Medicine, University of New England, Biddeford, ME, USA

Zeeba D. Kabir, Anjali M. Rajadhyaksha and Barry E. Kosofsky
Division of Pediatric Neurology, Department of Pediatrics, Weill Cornell Medical College, New York, NY, USA
Graduate Program in Neurosciences, Weill Cornell Medical College, New York, NY, USA

Gagandeep Kaur
School of Environmental and Biological Sciences, Rutgers, The State University of New Jersey, New Brunswick, NJ, USA

Charles F. Mactutus, Steven B. Harrod, Lauren L. Hord, Landhing M. Moran and Rosemarie M. Booze
Behavioral Neuroscience Program, Department of Psychology, University of South Carolina, Columbia, SC, USA

Yanli Hao, Wen Huang, David A. Nielsen and Therese A. Kosten
Menninger Department of Psychiatry and Behavioral Sciences, Baylor College of Medicine, Houston, TX, USA
Michael E Debakey Veterans Administration Medical Center, Houston, TX, USA

Karen L. Bales
Department of Psychology, University of California, Davis, CA, USA

Ericka Boone, Pamela Epperson and C. Sue Carter
Brain-Body Center, Department of Psychiatry, University of Illinois, Chicago, IL, USA

Gloria Hoffman
Department of Biology, Morgan State University, Baltimore, MD, USA

Marcelo Febo
Department of Psychiatry, The McKnight Brain Institute, University of Florida College of Medicine, Gainesville, FL, USA
Department of Neuroscience, The McKnight Brain Institute, University of Florida College of Medicine, Gainesville, FL, USA

Lisa M. Tarantino and Samantha Meltzer-Brody
Department of Psychiatry, University of North Carolina, Chapel Hill, NC, USA

Patrick F. Sullivan
Department of Psychiatry, University of North Carolina, Chapel Hill, NC, USA
Department of Genetics, University of North Carolina, Chapel Hill, NC, USA

Franc C. L. Donkers, Shane R. Schwikert, Anna M. Evans, Katherine M. Cleary, Diana O. Perkins and Aysenil Belger
Department of Psychiatry, University of North Carolina at Chapel Hill, Chapel Hill, NC, USA

Nicole L. Johnson, Lindsay Carini, Marian E. Schenk, Michelle Stewart and Elizabeth M. Byrnes
Department of Biomedical Science, Cummings School of Veterinary Medicine, Tufts University, North Grafton, MA, USA

Donita L. Robinson
Bowles Center for Alcohol Studies, University of North Carolina, Chapel Hill, NC, USA
Department of Psychiatry, University of North Carolina, Chapel Hill, NC, USA
Curriculum in Neurobiology, University of North Carolina, Chapel Hill, NC, USA

Dawnya L. Zitzman
Bowles Center for Alcohol Studies, University of North Carolina, Chapel Hill, NC, USA

Sarah K. Williams
Department of Psychiatry, University of North Carolina, Chapel Hill, NC, USA
Curriculum in Neurobiology, University of North Carolina, Chapel Hill, NC, USA

Guido Gerig and Sylvain Gouttard
Scientific Computing and Imaging Institute, University of Utah, Salt Lake City, UT, USA

Karen Grewen and Josephine Johns
Department of Psychiatry, University of North Carolina, Chapel Hill, NC, USA

Martin Andreas Styner
Department of Psychiatry, University of North Carolina, Chapel Hill, NC, USA
Department of Computer Science, University of North Carolina, Chapel Hill, NC, USA

List of Contributors

Joohwi Lee
Department of Computer Science, University of North Carolina, Chapel Hill, NC, USA

Matthew McMurray
Department of Psychology, University of North Carolina, Chapel Hill, NC, USA

Fulton T. Crews and Ryan Peter Vetreno
Department of Pharmacology, Bowles Center for Alcohol Studies, The University of North Carolina at Chapel Hill, Chapel Hill, NC, USA
Department of Psychiatry, Bowles Center for Alcohol Studies, The University of North Carolina at Chapel Hill, Chapel Hill, NC, USA

Yu Cai, Hong Yuan, Weili Lin and Hongyu An
Department of Radiology, University of North Carolina at Chapel Hill, Chapel Hill, NC, USA
Biomedical Research Imaging Center, University of North Carolina at Chapel Hill, Chapel Hill, NC, USA

Matthew S. McMurray
Department of Psychology, University of North Carolina at Chapel Hill, Chapel Hill, NC, USA

Ipek Oguz, Martin A. Styner and Josephine M. Johns
Department of Psychology, University of North Carolina at Chapel Hill, Chapel Hill, NC, USA
Department of Psychiatry, University of North Carolina at Chapel Hill, Chapel Hill, NC, USA

Nicole Landi
Yale Child Study Center, Yale University School of Medicine, New Haven, CT, USA
Haskins Laboratories, New Haven, CT, USA

Jessica Montoya, Hedy Kober and Patrick D. Worhunsky
Department of Psychiatry, Yale University School of Medicine, New Haven, CT, USA

Helena J.V. Rutherford and Linda C. Mayes
Yale Child Study Center, Yale University School of Medicine, New Haven, CT, USA

W. Einar Mencl
Haskins Laboratories, New Haven, CT, USA

Marc N. Potenza
Yale Child Study Center, Yale University School of Medicine, New Haven, CT, USA
Department of Psychiatry, Yale University School of Medicine, New Haven, CT, USA
Department of Neurobiology, Yale University School of Medicine, New Haven, CT, USA

Cheryl A. Frye
Department of Psychology, University at Albany-State University of New York, Albany, NY, USA
Department of Biological Sciences, University at Albany-State University of New York, Albany, NY, USA
The Centers for Life Sciences, University at Albany-State University of New York, Albany, NY, USA
Neuroscience Research, University at Albany-State University of New York, Albany, NY, USA

Jason J. Paris and Danielle M. Osborne
Department of Psychology, University at Albany-State University of New York, Albany, NY, USA

Joannalee C. Campbell and Tod E. Kippin
Department of Psychology, University of California, Santa Barbara, CA, USA

Georgia Gleason, Bojana Zupan and Miklos Toth
Department of Pharmacology, Weill Medical College of Cornell University, New York, NY, USA

Chris Murgatroyd and Dietmar Spengler
Max Planck Institute of Psychiatry, Munich, Germany

Adam J. Zolotor
Department of Family Medicine and Injury Prevention Research Center, University of North Carolina, Chapel Hill, NC, USA

T. Walker Robinson
Department of Pediatrics, Duke University Medical Center, Durham, NC, USA

Desmond K. Runyan
Robert Wood Johnson Clinical Scholar Program, Departments of Social Medicine and Pediatrics, University of North Carolina, Chapel Hill, NC, USA

Ronald G. Barr
Department of Pediatrics and Developmental Neurosciences and Child Health, Child and Family Research Institute, University of British Columbia, Vancouver, BC, Canada

Robert A. Murphy
Center for Child & Family Health and Department of Psychiatry & Behavior Sciences, Duke University Medical Center, Durham, NC, USA

Sonya K. Sobrian
Department of Pharmacology, College of Medicine, Howard University, Washington, DC, USA

R. R. Holson
Psychology, New Mexico Institute of Mining and Technology, Socorro, NM, USA

Eamon McCrory and Stephane A. De Brito
Developmental Risk and Resilience Unit, Division of Psychology and Language Sciences, University College London, London, UK
Research Programme, The Anna Freud Centre, London, UK

Essi Viding
Developmental Risk and Resilience Unit, Division of Psychology and Language Sciences, University College London, London, UK

Index

A
Addictive Disorder, 220
Anogenital Region, 27-29, 31-32
Apoptosis, 22, 24
Arginine Vasopressin, 39, 42-43, 59, 184, 223
Auditory Brainstem Response, 25-26
Auditory Stimuli, 13, 15, 20, 148, 179

C
Cerebral Blood Flow, 9, 51, 65-67
Cognitive Development, 1, 102, 198, 233
Corporal Punishment, 198-199, 204-205
Corpus Callosum, 118, 123, 138, 140, 142, 144, 223, 225, 228, 234-235
Corticosterone Secretion, 172, 190
Cortisol Reactivity, 232
Cytosine Methylation, 29, 192, 194, 230

D
Dinucleotide, 128, 186
Dopamine, 1-3, 8-11, 22-26, 37, 47, 61, 63-65, 102, 104-116, 133, 135, 147, 158-161, 167-172, 176-177, 179-181, 188, 221, 232-233
Dopamine Transient, 110-111

E
Electrical Stimulation, 56, 105, 107-108
Electrophysiology, 106
Environmental Stimuli, 106-107, 207
Enzyme Immunoassay, 41, 49
Epigenetic Modification, 230-231
Epigenetic Regulation, 183, 186, 188, 190-191, 193, 195, 230, 235

G
Genotype Effect, 174-177
Gestational Stress, 164, 167, 172-173
Glucocorticoid, 28, 50, 71-72, 113, 129, 161-162, 165-166, 170-171, 178, 181, 184-186, 190, 193-196, 224, 226, 230-231, 235
Glucose Metabolism, 59-60

H
Hippocampus, 11, 27-29, 31-34, 36-37, 54, 63, 73, 114, 120-121, 126-127, 130-132, 135-136, 151, 159-160, 164-166, 168-174, 176, 181, 185-186, 188, 190, 192, 194, 197, 216, 223-230, 236
Histology, 117, 124, 144
Histone Acetylation, 127, 186-187, 190

Homeostasis, 36, 135, 188, 196
Human Psychiatric Syndrome, 70
Hyperexcitability, 131-133
Hypothalamic-pituitary-adrenal, 27, 37, 45, 49, 58, 99, 128, 133, 167, 169, 171-172, 178, 193, 223

I
Immunoblot, 7
Inferior Occipital Gyrus, 153

J
Juvenile Play Behavior, 94

L
Litter Gender Composition, 27-28, 36

M
Macroorchidism, 176
Magnetic Resonance Imaging, 51, 62, 65-66, 117-118, 125-126, 137, 145-146, 223, 233
Maternal Psychiatric Illness, 68
Medial Preoptic Area, 37, 75, 104, 109, 114, 191, 194, 219
Mesolimbic Pathway, 104
Microdialysis, 104, 106, 113-116, 159, 167, 171, 181
Mortality Rate, 140

N
Neuroendocrine, 36-37, 39, 41, 45, 48, 50, 68, 73-74, 102, 158, 160-162, 166-167, 169, 179, 184-186, 189-191, 223, 231, 233-234
Neuroimaging Studies, 51, 59, 118, 231
Neuropeptide, 47-48, 102, 109, 167, 215
Neuroplasticity, 135, 191
Neurotransmitter Activity, 159
Neurotrophic Factor, 1-2, 7, 59, 229
Norepinephrine, 2, 12, 22-23, 102, 134, 159-161, 172
Nuclear Factor Kappa, 126, 128
Nucleotide Polymorphism, 37
Nucleotide Sequence, 29

O
Oncogene, 135
Opioid Receptors, 27-28, 103, 129
Orbitofrontal Cortices, 127, 132

P
Parahippocampal Gyrus, 150-155
Phosphorylation, 1-8, 190, 197

Polymorphism, 28, 35-37, 173, 181, 195, 232-233
Post-traumatic Stress Disorder, 39, 165, 228, 234
Posterior Cingulate, 45, 150, 153, 155, 229
Postpartum Depression, 68-69, 74-76, 174, 181
Prefrontal Cortex, 3, 7, 24, 59-60, 71, 78, 88, 104, 114, 119, 127, 133-135, 147-148, 151, 153, 167, 169-170, 179, 191, 196, 221, 226, 228, 236
Prenatal Cocaine Treatment, 2-5, 8, 12, 17-18, 21
Protein Phosphorylation, 3-6
Psychiatric Disorder, 80, 117, 229
Psychopathology, 39, 50, 88, 126, 133, 169, 173, 179, 183, 186, 223-224, 227, 230-234
Psychostimulant, 1-2, 10, 59, 180

S
Schizophrenia, 78-82, 87-89, 124, 165, 167-168, 177-181, 188-189, 193-194

Signal Transduction, 2, 136
Single Nucleotide, 37, 70
Symptomatology, 180, 228-229, 233

T
Teratogenic Substance, 148
Thalamus, 136, 147, 151-152, 154-155

V
Ventral Striatum, 10, 104, 106-107, 114, 134, 176, 237-238, 243-244
Ventral Tegmental Area, 7, 22, 59, 64, 104, 114-115, 129-130, 160, 168, 180, 216